HIP AND KNEE
PAIN DISORDERS

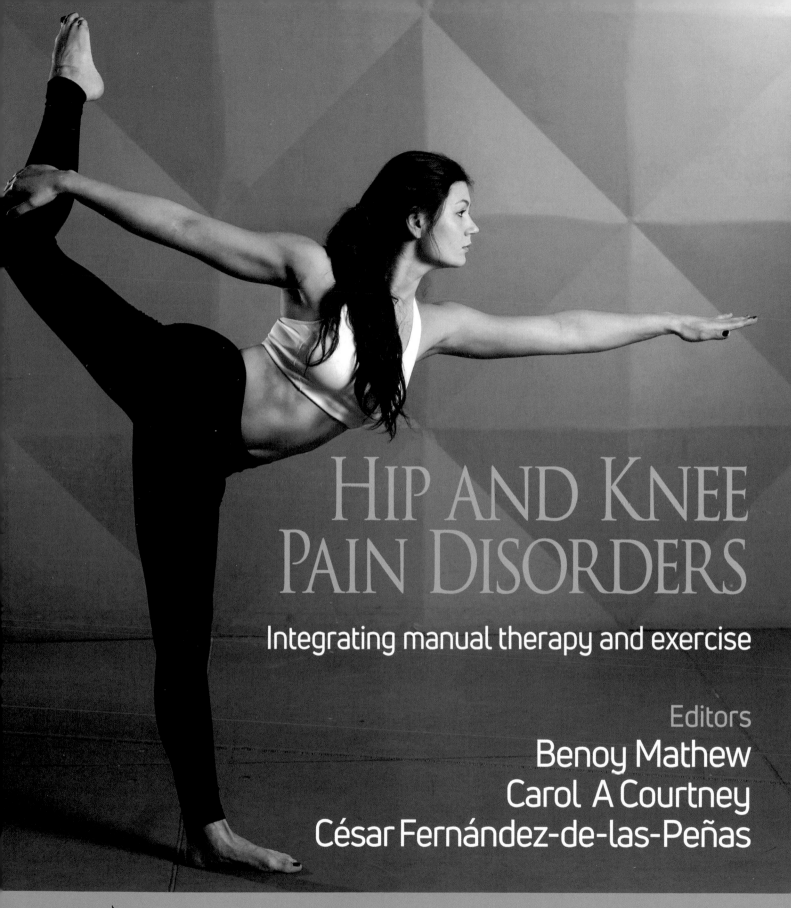

Hip and Knee Pain Disorders

Integrating manual therapy and exercise

Editors

Benoy Mathew
Carol A Courtney
César Fernández-de-las-Peñas

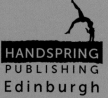

HANDSPRING PUBLISHING Edinburgh

Forewords Alison Grimaldi Cara L. Lewis Vikas Khanduja

HANDSPRING PUBLISHING LIMITED
The Old Manse, Fountainhall,
Edinburgh, East Lothian
EH34 5EY, Scotland
Tel: +44 1875 341 859
Website: www.handspringpublishing.com

First published 2022 in the United Kingdom by Handspring Publishing Limited

ISBN 978-1-913426-13-2
ISBN (Kindle eBook) 978-1-913426-14-9

British Library Cataloguing in Publication Data
A catalogue record for this book is available from the British Library

Library of Congress Cataloging in Publication Data
A catalog record for this book is available from the Library of Congress

Notice
Neither the Publisher nor the Authors assume any responsibility for any loss or injury and/or damage to persons or property arising out of or relating to any use of the material contained in this book. It is the responsibility of the treating practitioner, relying on independent expertise and knowledge of the patient, to determine the best treatment and method of application for the patient.

All reasonable efforts have been made to obtain copyright clearance for illustrations in the book for which the authors or publishers do not own the rights. If you believe that one of your illustrations has been used without such clearance, please contact the publishers and we will ensure that appropriate credit is given in the next reprint.

This book is a guide for personal exploration and is in no way meant to substitute for any type of medical advice – allopathic, Western, Eastern, Indian. It can complement a healing protocol. Ultimately all movement ideas are to be visited with gentleness allowing your body responses and related sensations to guide you.

Commissioning Editor Mary Law
Project Manager Morven Dean
Copy editor Glenys Norquay
Cover, Design Direction Bruce Hogarth
Indexer Aptara
Typesetter Amnet, India
Printer Melita, Malta

The
Publisher's
policy is to use
paper manufactured
from sustainable forests

Contents

Contents *continued*

About the editors

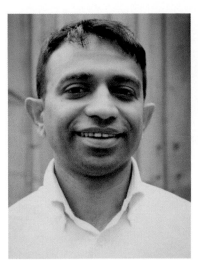

Benoy Mathew PT, MSc, MCSP, PG Cert (MSK US) is a specialist lower limb physiotherapist, an Advanced Practice Physiotherapist, an MSK Sonographer and Shockwave UK Education Lead. He works for the UK National Health Service in London, UK, as well as in private practice.

Benoy has a special interest in chronic hip and groin pathologies and the management of running injuries. He is the clinical lead for shockwave education in the UK. As a trained musculoskeletal sonographer he employs diagnostic ultrasound in his clinical practice. He is passionate about the application of research in clinical practice and has had a number of his own research papers published in internationally peer-reviewed journals.

Benoy teaches regularly on numerous courses, both in the UK and overseas. More than 2500 participants have attended his courses in the last 8 years.

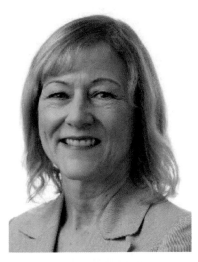

Carol A. Courtney PT, MApplSc, PhD, ATC is Professor of Physical Therapy and Human Movement Sciences at Northwestern University, Chicago, USA. She is a licensed physical therapist and athletic trainer and has been recognized as a Fellow of the American Academy of Orthopaedic Manual Physical Therapists. In 1991 and 1992, she was chosen to serve on the US medical staffs for the Pan American Games in Havana, Cuba, and the Olympic Games in Barcelona, Spain. Dr Courtney has clinical expertise in the management of chronic musculoskeletal pain and sports injury. Her academic focus is on advanced clinical reasoning in orthopedic physical therapy and her research investigates the effects of knee joint injury and osteoarthritis on pain processing and joint function; her work also focuses on the modulation of pain mechanisms through non-pharmacologic interventions, including manual therapy and exercise. She has over 100 peer-reviewed publications, book chapters and conference presentations and has lectured both nationally and internationally on this research.

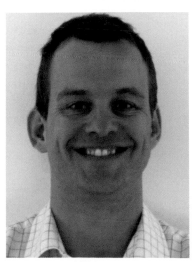

César Fernández-de-las-Peñas PT, PhD, Dr MedSci is full professor at Universidad Rey Juan Carlos (URJC), Madrid, Spain, where he is also leader of the Clinical Pain Research Group on Manual Therapy and Exercise. He combines his research activity with clinical practice as Head, Division of Physical Therapy Department, at the University Physical Therapy Clinic. He has received several awards for his research and clinical practice.

César has published around 550 peer-reviewed publications and is the first-named author of approximately 250. His research activities are concentrated on the neuroscience of pain. In his clinical practice César treats patients with chronic pain disorders. His premise is: "integrating clinical practice with research is the key for our patients."

César is often invited to present keynote lectures at international conferences and he has taught workshops in over 20 countries. He is the main editor of 10 textbooks on manual therapy for chronic musculoskeletal pain including *Temporomandibular Disorders*, also published by Handspring Publishing.

About the contributors

Kyle Adams PhD, PT
Clinical Assistant Professor
Baylor University Doctoral Physical Therapy Program
Baylor University
Waco, TX, USA

Alexandra Anderson PT, DPT, OMT, FAAOMPT
Physical Therapist
University of Illinois Health
Owner
The Physical Therapy Academy
IL, USA

Lars Arendt-Nielsen DM, PhD
Professor
Center for Pain and Neuroplasticity
Aalborg University
Aalborg, Denmark

Alison H. Chang PT, DPT, MS
Associate Professor
Department of Physical Therapy & Human Movement
Sciences
Feinberg School of Medicine
Northwestern University
Chicago, IL, USA

Joshua Cleland PT, PhD, FAPTA
Professor, Director of Research & Faculty
Development, Doctor of Physical Therapy Program
Department of Public Health & Community Medicine
Tufts University
Boston, MA, USA

Chad E. Cook PT, PhD, FAPTA
Professor in Orthopaedic Surgery
Division of Physical Therapy
Duke University
Durham, NC, USA

Jill Cook PhD, BAppSci(Phty)
Professor
La Trobe Sport & Exercise Medicine Research Centre
La Trobe University
Melbourne, Vic, Australia

Megan Donaldson PT, PhD, FAAOMPT
Program Director and Associate Professor
Physical Therapy Program
Department of Public Health & Community Medicine
Tufts University
Boston, MA, USA

Joseph M. Donnelly PT, OCS, FAPTA, FAAOMPT
Professor Physical Therapy
Health Sciences
University of St Augustine
Miami, FL, USA

Alicia J. Emerson DPT, MS, OCS, FAAOMPT
Assistant Professor
Department of Physical Therapy
High Point University
High Point, NC, USA

Katia Ferrar PhD, B HlthSc (Hons), B AppSc (Physio)
Research Fellow
La Trobe Sport & Exercise Medicine
Research Centre
La Trobe University and The Australian Ballet
Adjunct Senior Lecturer
University of South Australia
Bundoora, Vic, Australia

Michelle Finnegan PT, DPT, OCS, MTC, CMTPT, CCTT,
FAAOMPT
Adjunct Assistant Professor
The George Washington University
Washington, DC, USA;
Adjunct Faculty
South College
Knoxville, TN, USA;
Senior Faculty
Myopain Seminars
Bethesda, MD, USA;
Owner
ProMove PT Pain Specialists
Bethesda, MD, USA

Timothy W. Flynn PT, PhD, OCS, FAAOMPT, FAPTA
Professor
School of Physical Therapy

South College
Knoxville, TN, USA

Michael Freeman MSportsPhysio, BHScMPP, APA
Titled Sports and Exercise Physiotherapist
Physiotherapist
The Australian Ballet
Australia;
North Melbourne Football Club
North Melbourne, Australia;
Physio Plus Group
Footscray, Vic, Australia

Alessandra Narciso Garcia PT, PhD
Physiotherapist
Division of Physical Therapy
Department of Orthopaedic Surgery
Duke University
Durham, NC, USA

Benjamin J. Geletka PT, DPT, AAOMPT
Clinical Specialist
University Hospitals
Cleveland, OH, USA

Paul Glynn PT, DPT, OCS, FAAOMPT
Owner
Glynn Physical Therapy LLC
Lexington, MA, USA;
Faculty Partner
Evidence in Motion
San Antonio, TX, USA

Brenton J. Grant BHSc, Master of Physiotherapy
Practice
Physical Therapist
Dignity Health, St Rose Dominican Hospital
Las Vegas, NV, USA

Georgina E. Grant MD, BSC Biological Sciences
Kirk Kerkorian School of Medicine
Las Vegas, NV, USA
Emergency Physician,
University of Nevada Las Vegas School of Medicine
Las Vegas, NV, USA

Dr Derek Griffin PT, PhD, BSc (Hons)
Specialist Musculoskeletal Physiotherapist
Bon Secours Hospital Tralee
Tralee, Ireland

David W. Griswold PhD, DPT
Associate Professor of Physical Therapy
Department of Graduate Studies in Health and
Rehabilitation Sciences
Youngstown State University
Youngstown, OH, USA

Dhinu J. Jayaseelan DPT, OCS, FAAOMPT
Assistant Professor
The George Washington University Program in
Physical Therapy
The George Washington University
Washington, DC, USA

Dr Joanne Kemp PhD, MSportsPhysio, BAppSci(Phys)
APA Sport & Exercise Physiotherapist
Senior Research Fellow
La Trobe Sports & Exercise Medicine Research Centre
La Trobe University
Melbourne, Vic, Australia

Shane Koppenhaver PT, PhD
Clinical Professor
Baylor University Doctoral Physical Therapy Program
Baylor University
Waco, TX, USA

Ken Learman PhD, PT, OCS, FAAOMPT
Professor of Physical Therapy & Director of PhD in
Health Sciences
Youngstown State University
Youngstown, OH, USA

Gregory J. Lehman DC, MScPT
Clinical Educator, Physiotherapist & Chiropractor,
Strength & Conditioning Specialist
Greg Lehman Physiotherapy
Toronto, Canada

Thomas A. Longbottom PT, DPT, NCS
Clinical Associate Professor
Baylor University Doctor of Physical Therapy Program
Baylor University
Waco, TX, USA

Fraser McKinney BSc Hons (Physio), MSc (Sports Physio), BSc Hons (Sports & Exercise Science)
Lead of Rehabilitation
Southampton Football Club Science and Medicine Department
Southampton Football Club
(English Premier League)
Southampton, UK

Alfred Zeev Markovits BPT, PGDip
Musculoskeletal Physiotherapist
Outpatient Physiotherapy
Homerton University Hospital NHS Foundation Trust
London, UK

Elizabeth Marlow BSc (Hons), MSc
Specialist Musculoskeletal Physiotherapist
Ealing Community MSK Service
Clayponds Rehabilitation Hospital
London, UK

Susan Mayes PhD, BAppSci
Director of Artistic Health
The Australian Ballet
Southbank, Vic, Australia
Adjunct Research Fellow
La Trobe University
Melbourne, Vic, Australia

John J. Mischke DPT, OCS, FAAOMPT
Clinical Faculty & Orthopedic Residency Director
School of Physical Therapy & Rehabilitation Science
University of Montana
Missoula, MT, USA

Thomas G.C. Mitchell MSc, BSc (Hons), MCTA
Clinical Lead Physiotherapist
Remedy Physio
Sheffield, UK;
Advanced Physiotherapy Practitioner

Primary Care Sheffield NHS Trust
Sheffield, UK

Scot Morrison PT, OCS, CSCS
Owner & Operator
Physio Praxis
Vancouver, WA, USA

Dr Andrea Mosler BAppSc, MAppSc, PhD
Specialist Sports & Exercise Physiotherapist (FACP)
Fellow of the Australian Sports Medicine Federation (FASMF)
Research Fellow
Sports & Exercise Medicine Research Centre
La Trobe University
Melbourne, Vic, Australia

Sergio Muela-Fernández PT
Fisioterapia Sergio Muela Fernández
Leon, Spain

Bradley J. Myers PT, DPT, DSC
Assistant Professor
Physical Therapy Program
College of Pharmacy and Health Sciences
Campbell University
Buies Creek, NC, USA

Jo Nijs PhD, PT, MT
Professor
Brussels Health Campus Department KIMA
Vrije Universiteit Brussel
Brussels, Belgium
Guest Professor
University of Gothenburg
Gothenburg, Sweden

Michael O'Brien BHSc
Physiotherapist
The Hip & Groin Clinic
Windsor, Vic, Australia;
PhD Candidate
La Trobe Sport & Exercise Medicine
Research Centre
La Trobe University
Melbourne, Vic, Australia

Kristian Kjær Petersen MSc, PhD
Associate Professor
Center for Neuroplasticity & Pain
Department of Health Science & Technology
Aalborg University
Aalborg, Denmark

Gustavo Plaza-Manzano PT, PhD
Professor
Department of Radiology, Rehabilitation &
Physiotherapy
Universidad Complutense de Madrid
Madrid, Spain

Emilio Puentedura PT, DPT, PhD, OCS, FAAOMPT
Professor
Doctor of Physical Therapy Program
Baylor University
Waco, TX, USA

Craig R. Purdam DSc, MSportsPhysio
Professor
School of Allied Health
La Trobe University
Bundoora, Vic, Australia;
Professor
Faculty of Health
University of Canberra
Bruce, SA, Australia

Madhan Kumar Ramanathan PGDipPhty
Chartered Sports Physiotherapist; Specialist Sports
and MSK Physiotherapist
Northamptonshire County Cricket
Northampton, UK

Dr Ebonie Kendra Rio PhD, MSportsPhysio, BAPhysio
(Hons), BAAppSci
Post-Doctoral Research Fellow
La Trobe Sport & Exercise Medicine Research Centre
La Trobe University
Bundoora, Vic, Australia

Rachel Koldenhoven Rolfe PhD, ATC
Assistant Professor,
Department of Health and Human Performance

Texas State University
San Marcos, TX, USA

Nils Runge BSc, MSc
Advanced Physiotherapy Practitioner in Pain
Management
Connect Health
Newcastle upon Tyne, UK;
Advanced Physiotherapy Practitioner
Primary Care Sheffield
Sheffield, UK

Josiah D. Sault DPT, OCS, FAAOMPT
Coordinator of Outpatient Physical Therapy
Department of Occupational & Physical Therapy
University of Illinois Chicago
Chicago, IL, USA

Holly Soper-Doyle BSc (Hons), PGdipVetPhysio
Clinical specialist MSK Physiotherapist
Royal National Orthopaedic Hospital, London;
Honorary Clinical Lecturer University College London,
London;
Physiotherapist and Owner
Integrum Physiotherapy,
London, UK

Suresh Sudula BPT, PGDip, MCSP
Consultant Physiotherapist in MSK Ultrasound
Medway Maritime NHS Foundation Trust
Kent Musculoskeletal Clinic
The Regenerative Clinic
Kent, UK

Martin Thomas MSc, MCSP
First Contact Physiotherapy Practitioner
Harrogate NHS Foundation Trust & Airedale NHS
Foundation Trust
Harrogate, UK

Allison R. Toole PT, FAAOMPT, OPT
Physical Therapist
Outpatient Rehabilitation
Southeast Health
Cape Girardeau, MO, USA

Henrik Bjarke Vægter PT, MSc (Pain Management), PhD
Physical Therapist
Pain Research Group
Pain Center
University Hospital Odense;
Department of Clinical Research
University of Southern Denmark
Odense, Denmark

Richard W. Willy MPT, PhD
Assistant Professor
School of Physical Therapy & Rehabilitation Science
University of Montana
Missoula, MT, USA

Foreword by Alison Grimaldi

For busy clinicians and students alike, sourcing relevant information on musculoskeletal conditions is becoming increasingly more difficult, due to the exponential growth of publications in the rehabilitation field. Paywall restrictions limit access to the full breadth of information, the quality of research studies is highly variable, and clinical implications of many scientific papers are unclear to the reader. The other major challenge is that, despite the plethora of papers emerging on a daily basis, we still have many unanswered questions, and systematic reviews repeatedly confirm that there is inadequate evidence to make firm conclusions on most topics. If we adhered to true "evidence-based" practice, our treatment tool-bag would be rather limited.

This textbook on *Hip and Knee Pain Disorders* sets out to provide a state-of-the-art account of evidence-informed examination and conservative management of hip and knee pain conditions. Evidence-informed practice brings together the evidence base, pathophysiological rationale from basic science, and information from clinical experts to guide decision-making within a clinical reasoning framework. The editors of this text, Benoy Mathew, Carol Courtney, and César Fernández-de-las-Peñas have done all the "leg-work" for their readers. Not only do they share their own extensive expertise in clinical practice and research, but they have brought together more than 50 other specialists in this field, a mix of clinicians and clinician-researchers.

Prior to hearing from these experts, the editors showcase the stories of three patients, two with hip pain and one with knee pain. This is a potent reflection on why we do what we do, namely address the problems experienced by our patients and assist them with the frustrations and barriers they face. The representative voices of these three people and their journeys set the scene for the clinical chapters that follow.

Part I of *Hip and Knee Pain Disorders* provides the evidence base for the subsequent clinical examination and management sections. Experts in their fields provide a clinically interpreted update on epidemiology, and specific conditions in the region including hip and knee tendinopathies and muscle injuries, patellofemoral pain syndrome, osteoarthritis, FAI syndrome, hip dysplasia and instability, and ligament and meniscal injuries of the knee. With this knowledge in hand, Part II provides an evidence-informed, practical guide for clinical examination of hip and knee pain disorders. This section first explores the importance of clinical history and the validity of hip and knee outcome measures in a clinical setting. Detailed examination strategies are then provided, not only for the hip and knee, but for the whole lower quadrant. Chapters on the lumbar spine and sacroiliac joint proximally and the foot and ankle distally, reflect the comprehensive approach taken to examination of both local and remote mechanisms at play in hip and knee conditions. This section also includes a novel chapter on sono-anatomy and ultrasound scanning techniques for the hip and knee, a useful guide for a tool whose value is increasingly being recognized in clinical practice.

Part III covers multidisciplinary management of hip and knee pain disorders in seven comprehensive chapters. After an interrogation of the effectiveness of manual therapy, joint-biased interventions, muscular biased interventions, and clinical neurodynamics are detailed. Information from focus chapters on therapeutic exercise and therapeutic neuroscience is then brought together in a final chapter on multimodal management and how the clinician can integrate hands-on and hands-off interventions for chronic pain in the lower extremity.

Providing over 200,000 words of clinically relevant wisdom and over 300 full-colour photographs, *Hip and Knee Pain Disorders* will no doubt become a desktop staple for clinicians and students involved in musculoskeletal rehabilitation of the lower extremity.

Alison Grimaldi BPhty, MPhty(Sports), PhD

Principal Physiotherapist at Physiotec

Adjunct Research Fellow, University of Queensland

Brisbane, Queensland, Australia.

January 2022

Foreword by Cara L. Lewis

As clinicians and researchers, we are motivated by the stories we hear from the clients, patients, and research participants we meet along the way. This book begins there – with the poignant perspective of three individuals who have experienced hip or knee pain. With these stories as the backdrop, the textbook goes on to expertly integrate the current evidence and clinical knowledge informing best rehabilitative treatment practices for individuals with hip or knee pain disorders.

Each of the three editors, Benoy Mathew, Carol Courtney, and César Fernández-de-las-Peñas, is a skilled clinical scholar. Together, they have selected a talented team of coauthors who are international experts in the field – in terms of both generating and applying the evidence. Each author has advanced knowledge and clinical practice through countless publications and presentations. Here, they have compiled and synthesized the current knowledge of hip and knee pain problems into 21 digestible chapters.

This textbook runs the gamut from epidemiology and examination of hip and knee pain disorders to multidisciplinary management solutions. While discussions of hip and knee disorders often revolve around the newest surgical approach, this textbook highlights effective manual therapy and exercise interventions for this patient population. Part I provides the background knowledge and clinical rationale. Part II walks the reader through the evaluation of individuals with hip and knee pain disorders, beginning with the importance of a clinical history and appropriate outcome measures.

My personal favorite is that, while the authors discuss assessment of the hip and knee, they don't stop there; they continue down the limb, recognizing the contribution of the foot and ankle to any lower extremity pathology. Part III nicely concludes the book by presenting manual therapy and exercise interventions while recognizing the important role of the brain in musculoskeletal pain.

Through 21 chapters and over 300 photos, the authors have created a thorough and accessible textbook, knowledgeably summarizing the critical areas of musculoskeletal pain that affect so many people. *Hip and Knee Pain Disorders* is a valuable resource for any individual (clinician and consumer alike) who wants to better understand hip and knee pain problems and their solutions.

Cara L. Lewis PT, PhD

Associate Professor of Physical Therapy Rehabilitation Sciences (PhD) and Medicine

College of Health & Rehabilitation Sciences Sargent College

Boston University

Boston, MA, USA.

January 2022

Foreword by Vikas Khanduja

It gives me immense pleasure to be writing a foreword for *Hip and Knee Pain Disorders*.

As hip and knee pathologies continue to become more prevalent, so does the demand for a rapid and effective return to function. Aimed at clinicians involved in managing musculoskeletal pathology, this book explores the latest scientific evidence and applies it to appropriate exercise selection and manual therapy techniques in the pre- and post-operative management of hip and knee disorders.

I congratulate the Editors, Benoy Mathew, Carol Courtney, and César Fernández-de-las-Peñas, for putting together this comprehensive text, which provides a state-of-the-art review of evidence-informed examination and management of hip and knee disorders. With the explosion of information on hip and knee pathology in the literature, particularly in the management of the young adult, this book is very timely and offers a comprehensive treatise in this arena.

This book is unique in the fact that the Editors have worked hard in bringing together multimodal approaches (education, exercise programmes, manual therapy, strength and conditioning) for the management of hip and knee pathology, based on clinical experience of the authors as well as evidence in the literature. The book is very user friendly and designed in a way that the reader can pick and choose what interests them the most or relates to a specific clinical scenario that they may be encountering.

The book commences with a remarkable collection of personal case studies that emphasize the psychological and emotional dimensions of care received by patients with hip and knee pathology. As clinicians, we can all learn immensely from the personal journeys of our patients and the importance of understanding the psycho-social impact of their pathologies.

Part 1 then reviews common pathologies including osteoarthritis, tendinopathies around the hip and knee, patello-femoral pathology, meniscal and knee ligament injuries, and pathology in the young adult hip. Chapter 5 covers the contemporary management of Femoro-acetabular Impingement Syndrome (FAIS) and hip dysplasia, a topic very close to my heart. The understanding of the dynamic nature of young adult hip pathology and strategies of management is one of the most rapidly evolving arenas in orthopedics today.

Part 2 explores the clinical examination of the hip and knee. Chapter 10 deals with sonographic anatomy and scanning techniques for the hip and knee, which again is gaining a lot of popularity amongst many musculoskeletal clinicians.

Part 3 discusses the multi-disciplinary management of hip and knee pathology in seven comprehensive chapters.

As anyone who has written a book of this magnitude would appreciate, selecting and coordinating international authors for different chapters, getting relevant permissions, editing and ensuring that the central message is not lost, and liaising with the publishers, it is a mammoth task. I believe the editors have managed this task extremely well, drawing in from the experience of more than 40 authors who are leading experts in this field, contributing a total of 21 chapters with over 400 colour drawings and photographs.

I believe that this textbook provides comprehensive information in an efficient manner resulting in an invaluable aide-memoire in clinic and a reference text at home. I sincerely hope that you enjoy reading the book as much as the team has enjoyed putting it together and this enables you to deliver excellent care for patients with hip and knee pathology globally.

Vikas Khanduja MA (Cantab) MB BS MSc,
FRCS (Orth) PhD

Consultant Orthopaedic Surgeon & Research
Lead (Elective)

Addenbrooke's – Cambridge University Hospital

Chair | ISAKOS & ESSKA Hip Arthroscopy Committee
President Elect | British Hip Society
2021 Royal College of Surgeons Hunterian Professor.
Cambridge, *January 2022*

Preface

The last 20 years have seen a revolution in our understanding of the pathophysiology of hip and knee disorders. Conservative and surgical management of common hip and knee pathologies have developed tremendously. Further, our ability to diagnose, intervene, and rehabilitate has also evolved with new insights. These discoveries have created the need for a comprehensive evidence-based text about the management of hip and knee pain.

As hip and knee pathologies affect many individuals, our goal with *Hip and Knee Pain Disorders: Integrating manual therapy and exercise* was to provide a definitive reference for musculoskeletal clinicians who are involved in the management of patients with hip and knee pain. While many sources provide commentary on treatment techniques or emphasize the research component, they often lack the clinical framework in the management of a patient with hip/knee pain, in the absence of a comprehensive scientific rationale.

The purpose of the book is twofold: first, to serve as a textbook for the musculoskeletal evaluation and differential diagnosis of hip and knee pain and second, to provide a user-friendly guide and reference for clinicians who wish to locate the current evidence and treatment strategies for frequently encountered hip and knee pathologies. Each chapter blends the current evidence with clinical expertise, which provides a unique perspective for the reader. With input and contribution from numerous experts in the field, this book was developed to meet the demands of the clinician and researcher desiring such information. The overall result is 21 chapters dedicated to hip and knee disorders from multiple authors who are the current and future leaders in this field.

Whether you are a beginning or an advanced clinician, we trust that the content of this book will be a valuable tool in your reference armamentarium and clinical practice in the management of hip and knee pain. This book is unique in bringing together multimodal approaches to the management of hip and knee pain by integrating the different therapeutic strategies available from a clinical and evidence-based point of view. Further, the book is packed with photographs and illustrations to help explain the concepts discussed in the text.

The book is divided into three parts. Becoming an effective musculoskeletal practitioner requires the development of a professional skillset and a thorough understanding of the scientific basis of best practice. The first chapter sets the stage by providing an overview of the prevalence, disease burden, and risk factors of common hip and knee/hip pathologies and relevant classification systems. The remainder of Part 1, consists of chapters devoted to commonly encountered pathologies including hip and knee osteoarthritis, patellofemoral pain, FAI syndrome, hip dysplasia, muscle and tendon injuries of the hip/knee, and ligament/meniscus injuries of the knee.

Part 2 includes chapters devoted to detailed examination strategies of not only the hip and knee joint, but also of the lower quadrant. Chapter 10 is a novel chapter which briefly reviews the relevant anatomy and scanning technique of the hip and knee region as part of musculoskeletal clinical evaluation. Patients presenting with hip and knee pain require a methodical history and physical examination with specific diagnostic tests to assess all structures around the hip and the knee. These are explored in detail in Chapter 12. The focus of Chapters 11 and 13 is the relationship between pathology stemming from the sacroiliac joint and lumbar spine, and their contribution to pain syndromes of the hip and knee. Chapter 14 explores the potential impact on the functioning of the hip and knee joint, secondary to foot and ankle impairments.

Part 3 covers multimodal management of hip and knee pain, incorporating manual therapy, muscular-biased intervention, exercise programs, and clinical neurodynamics. Chapter 16 describes several joint-biased interventions for hip and knee pain problems. The clinician should choose the appropriate technique based on proper clinical reasoning and the best evidence available as outlined in Chapter 15. Further, therapy interventions should be individualized to each particular patient based on treatment aims, but also on patient expectations as well as their preferences. Moving beyond local treatment, Chapter 20 explores observed changes within the brain and spinal cord related to hip/knee pain and then discusses treatment options to restore these changes. In the concluding chapter, an integrated clinical approach is recommended using the application of manual (hands-on) intervention with pain neuroscience education (hands-off), within a broader biopsychosocial context.

All of us practicing clinicians should be deliberate in our efforts to provide comprehensive care for our patients. We believe that *Hip and Knee Pain Disorders* presents up-to-date information in a user-friendly and efficient manner providing a valuable clinical resource and reference for use in the management of patients with hip and knee pain. We are delighted that the book is also available in eBook format, which in addition allows readers to access the content online.

Acknowledgments

The Editors would like to acknowledge all the contributing authors of this textbook for the masterful work they have done. This book would not have been possible without their dedication, tireless effort, and passion for this project. We feel privileged to have had the opportunity to work together with these expert clinicians and researchers who bring to you their vast experience and clinical acumen, as well as latest thinking in this field.

We also want to thank the Handspring team and reviewers for their support and guidance with this project. And finally, we thank our spouses and families for their support and understanding during this extensive endeavor.

The famous French physiologist Claude Bernard said: "It is what we know already that often prevents us from learning." With this in mind, enjoy the insights of leading experts in hip and knee pain disorders.

We hope you are inspired by this book!

Benoy Mathew
London, UK 2022

Carol A. Courtney
Chicago, USA 2022

César Fernández-de-las-Peñas
Madrid, Spain 2022

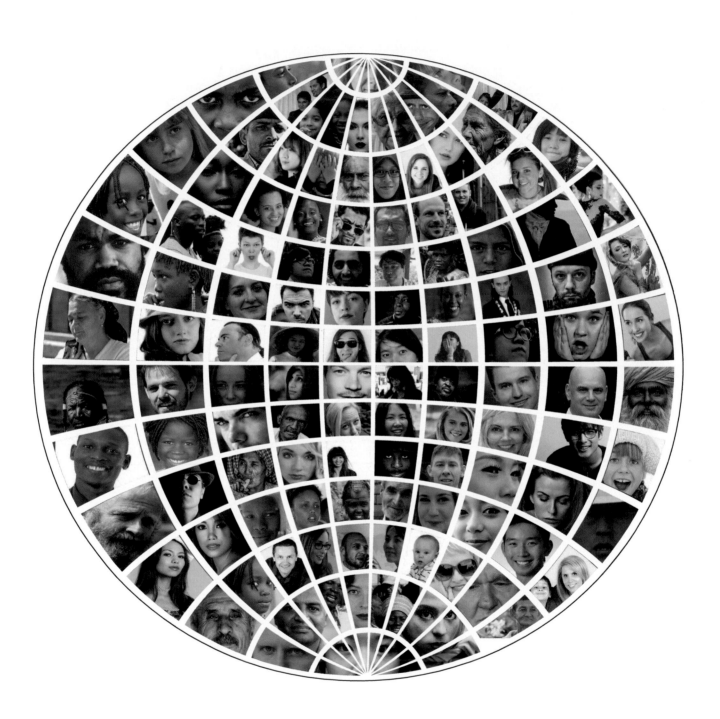

Our stories: Living with hip and knee pain

Benoy Mathew, Carol A. Courtney, César Fernández-de-las-Peñas

Alleviation of pain is a key aim of therapy intervention, yet pain can remain a puzzle, since it is not always related to a specific pathology. The experience of pain lies at the intersection of biology and culture. Affirming a patient's experience of their symptoms and allowing an empathetic interpretation of their story is integral to effective care. Central to gaining therapeutic relationship is the recognition of the patient as a person, whose life can be deeply changed by their pain experience.

Hip and knee pain disorders accounts for a significant portion of workload in most musculo-skeletal settings. Pain and especially chronic pain, involves a significant burden on an individual and societal level. Psychosocial factors have been shown to play a major role in the development of disability in both acute and persistent musculoskeletal pain. Early identification of psychological distress from the initial consultation can enable the therapist to target specific intervention, to reduce pain-related disability in our patients.

Active listening with empathy, validation of their pain experience, reassurance and encouragement are powerful professional tools that the therapist can utilize in helping our patients to overcome the challenges, while recovering from hip and knee pain. Chapter 8 is devoted to communicating with a person seeking care who is experiencing hip and knee pain.

In this section, three people with hip and knee pain relate their individual journeys through the health system, highlighting their unique experience, concerns, and frustrations. Each personal story highlights a certain dilemma and struggle for meaning and certainty, during their individual pain experience. To maintain authenticity, editing has been kept to a minimum to ensure it is the patient's voices and experiences that we are hearing.

We would like to thank all the patients for sharing their personal story while dealing with their hip and knee pain.

A Patient's Journey: Bilateral Developmental Dysplasia of the Hips

This is the account of 36-year-old M-J Sharp's experience of the condition and of being diagnosed with hip dysplasia.

I have bilateral hip dysplasia. My left hip was diagnosed as a newborn and treated for a short period before being discharged, and it being pain-free as I was growing up. Symptoms started up again in both hips at 22. It took four years to be referred for an X-ray and receive a diagnosis for my left hip, and another four years for my right hip to be diagnosed. I have had seven surgeries, which have included a diagnostic arthroscopy, pelvic osteotomies on both sides, and their related metalwork removals.

My Symptoms

The symptoms I experienced were similar to what many of my peers with hip dysplasia seemed to have experienced. They began as what felt like a very mild muscular groin strain and gradually progressed over a number of years. At first, they only occurred with sport or running, so I stopped those activities. This progressed to having pain with brisk walking or standing for long periods. Eventually, they deteriorated quite suddenly over the space of about three months to significantly affecting my mobility. At this point, I was struggling to walk 5 minutes down the street or even stand to cook a meal for myself. I had some horrendous pain flares in which I would not be able to find any position to take the weight off my hips to be free from pain, apart from crook lying in bed.

Other varying signs and symptoms I experienced along my route to diagnosis included:

- Clicking, catching, and occasional joint locking
- Pain deep inside the hip joint
- Gluteal tendinopathy
- Sacroiliac joint pain
- Generalized pelvic pain, which felt very mechanical in nature
- At times my hip would give way, and I would have to catch myself from falling over
- Sometimes I experience pain much later after activity; my hip is fine walking around during the day, but if I don't use a crutch, I then experience a flare of symptoms in the evening and struggle standing up
- On particularly fatiguing days, I experience spasming in some muscles, as they would be compensating for the abnormal anatomy underneath
- I have a small tibial torsion in my left leg (the lower part of my leg appears rotated outwards) as a result of that hip not developing properly from birth. This has caused intermittent flares of knee pain.
- I also have some mild joint hypermobility which I am aware can commonly go hand in hand with dysplastic hips.

My Route to Diagnosis

The hip pain began when I had been trying to get back into hockey after having played it in school. When I first went to my GP, I was referred to physiotherapy and was given an exercise program that included pelvic floor exercises and general hip strengthening. These exercises helped a little, but the symptoms still re-occur when running. I didn't understand why physical therapy did not really solve the problem, so I resolved to just refrain from running activities and hockey and was discharged from physical therapy.

Four years later, when I returned to my GP with worsening symptoms in both hips and my left knee, I was referred for an X-ray at my local hospital and saw an orthopedic consultant. When my left hip was diagnosed, I was informed I could have a pelvic osteotomy on that side to correct the hip socket. I knew that I had had the "clicky hip" as a newborn. However, I had no idea that this was called "hip dysplasia" and that it could be a longer-lasting issue. Unfortunately, I found the communication on my initial diagnosis quite poor, and I struggled to find clear information myself about the condition, surgery, and long-term prognosis. However, I was informed that this surgery had good outcomes and so decided to go ahead with it. The recovery was long, but symptoms initially seemed to improve afterward.

After that, there began to be a lot of to-ing and fro-ing, to different health professionals and consultants, as there was a lack of decisiveness about my right hip. I underwent a diagnostic arthroscopy at one point and was informed I had "borderline" dysplasia in this side, but in the to-ing and fro-ing, I continued to be confused about a definitive diagnosis. I was told by three different physios that I had femoroacetabular impingement. By this time, I had begun training as my experience rehabilitating from my first surgery had sparked an interest in the profession. However, I was continuing to have intermittent issues with both hips, pelvic pain, and flares of sacroiliac joint pain, and I was having a hard time knowing if this was what I was meant to expect or if I should be pain-free by now. It had not at any point been explained to me what the long-term prognosis should be in terms of my pain and function.

It was the fourth orthopedic hip consultant I saw who was able to definitively diagnose both hips with dysplasia. For the first time, I was able to discuss the diagnosis fully and gain a clear understanding of the long-term prognosis. I had my questions answered about particular symptoms and was able to lay out all my options of treatment going forwards – and the consequences of those options. Unfortunately, it became apparent that my previous left pelvic osteotomy had not been performed correctly, so I had to undergo pelvic osteotomies on both hips in the coming two years, the right hip and the redo osteotomy on the left. These surgeries went a lot more smoothly and have had much more successful outcomes.

My Frustrations

The frustrations through my experiences have firstly been related to the circuitous route to diagnosis. Having to re-iterate my story and symptoms to multiple health professionals became quite wearing. These professionals included my GP, orthopedic surgeons, physical therapists, and a podiatrist. At one point, on being referred back to physio, I felt treated like a malingerer, and I didn't feel comfortable with the looks I saw on people's faces when seeing me back there (yes, patients pick up on this!). I felt treated like I was a problem at times, and the onus was placed on me that I wasn't doing enough strengthening, despite the fact that I had been continuing to keep up with physio exercises and Pilates classes regularly.

What I had wanted to do more than once was to just sit down with a health professional and have the condition and prognosis explained to me fully, lay all my options out and ask questions that I needed to – even silly-sounding ones. But there never seemed to be the chance to in appointments. I got the impression from things I read that hip dysplasia can significantly affect a person's mobility, and that for some, they did end up needing to use a wheelchair for some activities. I wanted to ask if I would need to use a wheelchair in the future, but I feared that this would be interpreted as

me being dramatic. However, I genuinely didn't know as the information had been so poor.

There didn't seem to be an understanding from all health professionals that hip dysplasia is a degenerative condition that worsens over time, causing osteoarthritis and poor mobility – or at least, not one which was discussed with me. I, at times, felt that to speak about that was considered catastrophizing. This was exacerbated by messages we receive as student physical therapists that structural abnormalities aren't always important. I felt confused, as everything I was finding out about hip dysplasia seemed to suggest that, in this case, the structure *is* important!

Some exercises I was given at times, I found unhelpful and worsened my symptoms. Single leg dips are one example of this. I discovered later on that doing this would have been putting more load on the acetabular labrum – which in my case was already sore. I have a mild tibial torsion in the left leg due to the way that the hip has developed. Attempting to keep my knee in line with my toes during this exercise is not possible, but I was encouraged by more than one physio that this was due to my weak gluteal muscles. Physios who did listen and helped me adapt to things like this were a godsend.

I felt there was a lack of awareness of how my pain and symptoms were affecting day to day life. A 5-minute walk to the shops, standing up to cook a meal, and having to consider leaving my job were all things that became a difficult factor when my mobility worsened. These are things that aren't always seen in a clinic room and were sometimes hard to describe in appointments. Perhaps it is the reserved nature of our society and formality of those kinds of appointments, or perhaps it was because I didn't like sounding like a hypochondriac.

Lastly, the fact that under one surgeon I had to undergo a diagnostic arthroscopy in my right hip, when a more experienced hip specialist could diagnose the dysplasia just from looking at an X-ray, is something that will always infuriate me. That was an unnecessary surgery, and I feel that with some simple training, any orthopedic who treats patients with hip problems should be able to diagnose dysplasia from an X-ray.

The Emotional Journey

The long route I had to diagnosis with hip dysplasia, being overlooked or misdiagnosed by more than one clinician, caused me to become angry with health professionals in general. This meant that I wasn't always trusting of advice given to me. It also meant that by the time I was correctly diagnosed and informed, I would benefit from the pelvic osteotomy surgery, which required a long period of recovery and rehab.

I was already exasperated and with significantly reduced exercise tolerance. This is a hard place to start from mentally and physically when facing this kind of challenge, as rehab after a pelvic osteotomy is no mean feat.

The emotional rollercoaster of those multiple surgeries had a huge effect on my mental health and resolve. I had one very understanding physio who was non-judgmental as I sat and ugly-cried my way through one or two outpatient appointments. They also understood that I am not a rehab machine, and at times encouraged normal activity and exercise for the fun of it.

I found that it took me time to come to terms with the diagnosis of hip dysplasia and what it means for me for the rest of my life. This was not helped by the lack of definitive information given to me about the condition. I found it difficult to get my head around the fact that without treatment, it would significantly affect my mobility and that even after the corrective surgeries, I could still have some limitations in certain activities, and my hips still may deteriorate at a later point in my life. Once I had started to feel clearer about that, I felt happier and able to consider how I could manage my hips in the long run. But it would have been a lot more helpful if these kinds of conversations would have happened with health professionals earlier on, as these things had a huge impact on my decisions about life choices, particularly in whether to continue to pursue my career in an active job as a physiotherapist.

These days both hips are doing much better. I am working full-time as a physiotherapist, which is a pretty active job where I'm on my feet all day. I have been able to start doing very short runs, and I have returned to hockey training. I have not been quite able to join in on matches but can hit a ball about and have a bit of a run-around, which feels fantastic in itself, and I walked and ran a 10 km race too. I have to pace myself, and I would say I'm prone to fatiguing at times. I find certain positions, such as deep squatting, can cause pain flares, mostly in my left hip, so I have to adapt these movements. I am aware that at some point, one or both hips may deteriorate and will require a total hip replacement, but I have come to terms with that, and overall, I am living life with minimal restrictions.

M-J Sharp
United Kingdom, June 2021

A Patient's Journey: Femoroacetabular Impingement Syndrome (FAIS)

This is the account of 31-year-old Daniel Harris's experience of the condition and of being diagnosed and managing FAIS.

My Symptoms

The onset of groin pain in my left hip started approximately four years ago, at the age of 27. I first experienced discomfort of my left hip, following an increase in the volume of lunges and squats at the gym. At the time, I was studying for a Pre-registration Physiotherapy MSc, so I was well placed to be examined by my peers. A few student physiotherapists from my cohort collectively performed an assessment of my hip and nothing reproduced my groin pain. My hip was less irritable after a month and it wasn't affecting my quality of life, so I continued to play recreational sport and exercised as I had done previously. However, the symptoms were not fully resolved and I would occasionally experience mild discomfort after playing sports such as football and squash. The symptoms gradually worsened over time. Static positions such as sitting for long periods with my knees above my hips or crouching down to speak to patients at work began to aggravate my hip too. I started to become very concerned that my hip pain would have a negative impact on my work, as it can be very physical in nature working as a physiotherapist, so I began to explore my options to seek help from musculoskeletal specialists.

Previous Injuries

Whilst visiting family in Spain in 2020, I arranged to see a family friend, who is an experienced osteopath, regarding my hip pain. He gained a comprehensive subjective history from me, dating back to when I first started playing sport as a child. Between the ages of 10 and 12, when I was playing competitive football, I suffered with Osgood Schlatter's disease in both my knees, my left being worse than my right, presumably as I am predominantly left-footed. I recall having debilitating knee pain for days following high-impact activities involving running and jumping, especially after playing football on concrete all day with my friends. After my experience of Osgood Schlatter's until the age of 21, I had only suffered minor repetitive strain injuries from resistance training.

Chronic Low Back Pain and Surgery

At 21 years old, I began to experience a deep dull ache in my right gluteal region. During this time, I was completing a strength training programme at the gym, comprising compound lifts such as squats and deadlifts 3 times a week. In addition to this, I was practicing Olympic lifts for my UKSCA accreditation and working part-time in furniture removals. The intensity of pain in my right buttock progressively worsened and I started to experience radicular pain down the posterolateral of my calf and into my foot. For approximately 5 years, the sciatic pain was present daily, although some days were worse than others. I was treated conservatively by various NHS and private physiotherapists, however this proved to be unsuccessful in managing my pain and my quality of life was reduced significantly. I was unable to sit for long periods, sleep undisrupted or participate in the type of sports and resistance training I enjoyed. When the pain became unbearable after a few years, I requested to be sent for a scan during an appointment with my general practitioner. The MRI scan showed disc herniations at L4/5 and L5/S1. Out of desperation to relieve the pain after 3 years of conservative management, I opted to self-fund a minimally invasive surgery called Disc-FX. This combined a thermal procedure to reduce the volume by evaporating disc tissue and removal of protruding disc tissue. At the time, I was informed the success rate was approximately 65% and it was a risk I was willing to take to resolve my pain. Unfortunately, my pain levels had not improved 18 months post-surgery and I began to experience new radicular pain down my left leg, as well as the long-standing pain down my right leg. Consequently, I attended a consultation with an orthopedic spinal surgeon through NHS England to discuss undergoing a more invasive procedure, known as a micro-discectomy. I eventually went ahead with the procedure, which has proven to be successful in resolving the radicular pain to date, however I am still required to manage residual lumbar spine stiffness and hamstring tightness on a daily basis.

Diagnosis of FAI Syndrome

Following the osteopath gaining a history from me about my physical activity and previous injuries, he performed an objective assessment which highlighted limited flexion and rotation of my hips and a positive impingement test. I was sent for an X-ray the next day, reporting bilateral CAM morphology that was more pronounced in my left hip. I received three treatment sessions from the osteopath whilst in Spain, consisting of spinal manipulations and hip mobilizations. My pain and function improved slightly following each session, however due to having limited time I was unable to observe any longer-term changes.

Clarity and Moving Forward

On my return to England, my goal was to continue learning about my condition and self-manage my problem going forward. Therefore, I decided to book an appointment with Benoy Mathew, a hip specialist physiotherapist I have followed with interest on Twitter and podcasts for years. Prior to my initial appointment, I was required to complete an outcome measure for patients living with hip pain. During the appointment, Benoy performed a detailed subjective and objective assessment, in addition to discussing my outcome measure score of 86%, which highlighted my quality of life and function were still at a good level, with surgical referral not typically being indicated, unless my score fell below 70%. Furthermore, he reassured me that surgery could be avoided with lifestyle changes and a periodized rehabilitation programme. Benoy Mathew explained the relationship between FAI and exercises in young athletes and how this can affect an individual as an adult in later life. He also hypothesized my spinal issues could be attributed to excessive movement and loading of my lumbar spine in order to compensate for my lack of hip rotation and flexion. Following the session, I felt extremely relieved to have clarity on my injury, with a clear short- to long-term term plan of how to manage my pain.

My Rehabilitation

The aim of the first phase of rehab was to minimize irritability of the left hip. It consisted of limiting 90 degrees of hip flexion, excessive adduction and internal rotation where possible, as well as adjusting my technique of gym-based exercises. In addition to this, I completed hip mobility and glutei activation exercises 5 days a week. Benoy was very clear on exercise dosage, demonstrated each exercise on video and ensured that I was able to perform the exercises. During the initial 6 weeks, I felt significantly more aware of the lifestyle modifications required to avoid aggravating my hip, which was extremely important going forward to minimize pain and improve quality of life. Phase two of rehab comprised strengthening the hip flexors, adductors and musculature related to the pelvis and spine, four times a week. This was in addition to integrating phase one exercises into my resistance training preparation.

I was provided with an extensive vocabulary of exercise videos to add variety to my rehabilitation and given clear instructions on daily selection and dosage. Benoy also outlined a "flare up" plan to manage my pain in moments when my hip is highly aggravated, which included recommendations on analgesics and exercises to assist with relieving the pain. Lastly, I was advised on which exercises would be most appropriate to incorporate into my warm up routine for leg day at the gym and playing golf. Following the appointment, I felt well-equipped to progress my rehab, prepare for exercise effectively and manage future flare ups correctly. In the near future with the guidance of Benoy, I plan to progress my rehabilitation to functional exercises and to start to run again.

I feel extremely positive and confident that I can manage my hip pain long-term with the knowledge and tools I have gained thus far, knowing that Benoy is available to answer any questions regarding my condition.

Daniel Harris
United Kingdom, June 2021

A Patient's Journey: When Knee Pain is Not Just Knee Pain – Recognizing Spine-Related Lower Extremity Pain

This is the account of 68-year-old Mary Smith's experience of knee pain symptoms associated with lumbar spine involvement.

My Symptoms

My main complaint was left knee pain and stiffness. I experienced a twisting event in my knee when walking, with subsequent intermittent left knee symptoms. The symptoms were worse in the morning, with an occasional feeling of swelling in the left knee and ankle. I felt the knee pain deep and I thought that I had a "trick knee" with intermittent catching and giving way. I was unable to lay my leg flat on the bed at night and often I woke with a decreased ability to fully straighten out the left knee. Pain intensity was highly variable, 1/10 at rest, 2/10 with activity and 7/10 at worst. Aggravating factors for my knee pain include walking, stairs, squatting, and getting out of the bed in the morning. Relieving factors include rest, movement, hot baths and change of position.

I visited the medical doctor for consultation. An osteoporosis DEXA scan was negative. I have a past medical history including hypertension, gastroesophageal reflux disease with hiatal hernia, asthma, allergic rhinitis, universal ulcerative colitis (chronic), diverticulosis of colon and vitamin D imbalance. After taking medication for months but without clear improvement, I asked to be referred to a physical therapist. My primary care physician did not order imaging prior to physical therapy referral.

Clinical Examination

Christine, my physical therapist, conducted an exhaustive interview and clinical examination. She asked for the presence of low back, hip, or ankle pain, and other issues in the right lower extremity, which I denied. I explained to her that I did not experience numbness, tingling, weakness or paresthesia in either the upper or lower extremities. I commented to Christine that I did have an increased right anterior shoulder pain that started after attempting to reposition my 90-year-old mother in bed. In fact, I explained that I related stress and poor sleep due to my caregiver responsibilities with my elderly mother.

During my physical examination, it was clear that my main problem was a limited extension range of motion in both knees, more pronounced in the left one. I experienced more pain with the knee extended. The physical therapist explained to me that I was ambulating with decreased knee extension during mid-stance on the left and decreased stance time on the left and that I exhibit bilateral toeing-in and increased pelvic rotation while walking. In general, I did not feel loss of strength in my lower extremity; however, I experienced pain when descending stairs. Christine explained to me that she considered that I exhibited poor neuromuscular control during lower extremity exercises such as lunges and squats. Palpation and other passive tests were not conclusive.

Initial Clinical Impression

At this point, the working hypothesis was a left tibiofemoral and patellofemoral joint condition, probably secondary to a potential diagnosis of osteoarthritis (OA) of the knee. The physical therapist explained to me that I met several of the criteria for diagnosis of knee OA such as knee pain with weight-bearing activities that improve with rest, marked decreased knee extension, and morning stiffness. While imaging would have helped confirm the presence of knee OA, the therapist explained to me the discordance between radiographs and clinical signs and symptoms of knee OA. We agreed to a potential intervention based on this hypothesis.

Initial Rehabilitation Intervention

I received a treatment plan of 12 visits with physical therapy interventions aimed at reducing knee impairment and improving function. I received several manual therapy interventions and strengthening of relevant hip and knee muscles. Admittedly, I was inconsistent in attending my physical therapy appointments which may have hampered my overall progress and also lengthened my episode of care. I did experience a reduction in pain and improvement in function after 12 treatment sessions. I recovered some but not full knee extension during the mid-stance phase of gait. However, I still felt knee irritation in the morning especially when the sheets in bed touched it when I woke up. In addition, I continued to experience fluctuating changes in knee extension range of motion and knee pain. In fact, objective range of motion assessment in supine revealed a 10-degree deficit in knee extension.

Lumbar Spine Hypothesis Involvement

I also continued experiencing intense pain levels during palpation of my knee. At that point, Christine conducted an exhaustive palpation of the knee area and revealed that my hamstring musculature was extremely tight and painful. Further, hamstring strength was also decreased. High pain intensity with hamstring contraction and the high rating of pain with palpation led her to reconsider the lumbar spine as a potential source of these findings; therefore, she again conducted a lumbar spine screening. She also noted an increased lumbar lordosis and anterior pelvic tilt.

The lumbar spine examination revealed a reduced range of motion in extension and left lateral flexion, although no knee symptoms were reproduced. The physical therapist applied some "neural provocation tests," e.g., straight leg raise test and the slump test. I explained to her that although these tests did not reproduce my concordant pain, they were extremely painful on the left side and not on the right side. Based on these findings, Christine hypothesized that maybe it was the lumbar spine and not the knee that was the source of my knee pain symptoms. Accordingly, she applied mobilizations on my lumbar spine, and to be honest, I felt an increase in knee extension range of motion and less pain at the end of that treatment session.

Additional Interventions

Lumbar spine interventions were incorporated into my plan of care. Lumbar spine manual therapies and "nerve slider maneuvers" were applied. The therapist explained to me that the objective of these interventions was to decrease lumbar spine involvement into my lower extremity. All these lumbar spine interventions were integrated into an exercise home program for the lower extremity musculature.

General Opinion from the Patient

After lumbar spine interventions were incorporated into the plan of care, I experienced an improvement in my general status. I could sleep, I could wake without pain, although I should remark that I continued to exhibit a decrease in knee extension range of motion. Probably, I have a knee problem that I will need to manage with the physician, but today I have better function thanks to my physical therapist. I did not have imaging to confirm the suspected knee OA so I do not know the degree of degenerative joint changes that may be found in my knee. However, I now clearly understand that radiographs are just one diagnostic piece that contributes to the overall clinical presentation of OA, and that I fit several other criteria of the diagnosis of knee OA. In retrospect, I was surprised that my lumbar spine could cause knee symptoms. Understanding this has been a great help to the self-management of my condition.

Mary Smith

Hip and Knee Pain Disorders

1

Epidemiology of hip and knee pain

1

Alison H. Chang, Andrea Mosler, Joanne Kemp

Introduction

Hip and knee pain are highly prevalent across the age spectrum and a leading reason for seeking musculoskeletal care. This chapter sets the stage by providing an overview of the prevalence, incidence, disease burden, and risk factors of common knee and hip pathologies and relevant classification systems. Primary knee pathologies discussed are knee osteoarthritis and arthroplasty, anterior cruciate ligament injury and reconstruction, meniscal injury, patellofemoral pain, and patellar tendinopathy. Based on recently expanded understanding of the hip and groin pain, three consensus agreements to classify, define, and diagnose hip-related pain will also be summarized. Epidemiology of hip and groin pain in the athletic population and intra-articular hip conditions in young and middle-aged adults are reviewed.

Knee Osteoarthritis

Osteoarthritis (OA) of the knee represents a continuum of disease, characterized by progressive pathologies involving the whole joint, including cartilage degradation, osteophyte formation, bone remodeling, meniscal damage, and synovial inflammation (Osteoarthritis Research Society International, 2016; Hunter & Bierma-Zeinstra, 2019; Kolasinski et al., 2020). One or more of the three compartments of medial tibiofemoral, lateral tibiofemoral, and patellofemoral may be affected, resulting in pain, swelling, stiffness, function loss, and disability. Typical clinical presentations include crepitus, bony enlargement, bone margin or joint line tenderness, and limited range of motion. Disease severity is classified by Kellgren Lawrence grade (Kellgren & Lawrence, 1957). Knee joint replacement is reserved for individuals with end-stage disease, severe pain, and substantially compromised activities of daily living. Readers are referred to Chapter 4 of this textbook for further information on knee OA.

Prevalence and Incidence

Knee OA accounts for nearly 80% of the burden of OA worldwide and its impact will likely escalate with the growing aging population and obesity epidemic (GBD 2015 Disease and Injury Incidence and Prevalence Collaborators, 2016). The estimated incidence and prevalence of knee OA depends on the definition used (symptomatic vs. radiographic vs. doctor-diagnosed by self-report). Prevalence estimates for symptomatic OA tend to be lower than radiographic OA because its presence is defined by a combination of symptoms in addition to radiographic disease. Similar to the discordant structure–symptom relationship observed in low back pain, the presence of radiographic knee OA does not correlate with symptoms and symptomatic knees do not necessarily have radiographic findings (see Chapter 4 for further discussion). In a recent systematic review and meta-analysis of 88 studies, including any of the three aforementioned definitions of knee OA, the pooled global prevalence of knee OA was 22.9% (95%CI 19.8% to 26.1%) in adults aged 40 or older, equivalent to approximately 645 million people internationally (Cui et al., 2020). The prevalence is higher in women than in men and increases with age. The global inci dence was 203 per 10,000 person-years (95%CI 106 to 331) in individuals aged 20 and older (Cui et al., 2020).

Disability, Morbidity, and Economic Burdens

Difficulty with walking, stair negotiation, and exercise participation due to chronic joint symptoms leads to functional impairments and disability. OA at the knee or hip was ranked as the 11th highest contributor to global disability (Cross et al., 2014). Based on the 2017 Global Burden of Disease Study, knee OA is responsible for 6.1% of years lived with disability (YLDs) among musculoskeletal disorders and about 1% in all causes (GBD 2017 Disease and Injury Incidence and Prevalence Collaborators, 2018). Given that knee OA is more common in older adults, and it shares some of the risk factors (e.g., obesity, aging, inflammation) for other diseases, many men and women with knee OA also have other medical comorbidities. Compared to those without OA, individuals with OA are 1.2 times more likely to have any comorbidity and 2.5 times more likely to have at least three medical comorbidities (Swain et al., 2020), such as cardiovascular disease, hypertension, diabetes, peptic ulcer, and depression (Louati et al., 2015; Calvet et al., 2016; Swain et al., 2020).

Older adults with cardiovascular and/or metabolic conditions are often advised to exercise and lose weight.

Those with moderate-to-advanced knee OA are trapped in a vicious cycle of physical inactivity due to joint complaints and worsening cardiometabolic profiles (e.g., obesity and systemic inflammation), which further exacerbate knee symptoms and walking difficulties. Knee or hip OA is linked to a greater risk of future all-cause and cardiovascular mortality; this relationship was largely explained by OA-related walking difficulties (Nüesch et al., 2011; Hawker et al., 2014; Kendzerska et al., 2017). These data underscore that knee OA is a serious disease, and that preventive and therapeutic strategies are needed to address impaired/painful walking and insufficient physical activity or exercise and ultimately halt the downward spiral toward disability and mortality.

The high prevalence of knee OA manifests in enormous economic and societal costs. The United States Bone and Joint Initiative highlights the impact of OA in its *Burden of Musculoskeletal Diseases Report* (United States Bone and Joint Initative). In 2013, 20.78 million ambulatory care visits and 2.95 million hospitalizations (the second most costly health conditions treated in hospitals) were attributed to OA and related disorders (United States Bone and Joint Initative). Annual per-person medical costs for OA averaged $11,052 between 2008 and 2014 (United States Bone and Joint Initative). It is estimated that total lost wages due to arthritis were $164 billion, or $4,040 less per American with arthritis versus without (Centers for Disease Control and Prevention [CDC], 2020). In Australia, retiring early due to arthritis contributes to $9 billion loss in gross domestic product; reduced work productivity while employed adds to further societal costs (Ackerman et al., 2015).

Risk Factors

Overweight/obesity, increasing age, female sex, prior knee injury or surgery, demanding physical occupational load, and malalignment are associated with increased risk for knee OA.

High BMI is a strong predictor for the development and progression of knee OA. In a 2015 systematic review and meta-analysis, being overweight was associated with a pooled odds ratio (OR) of 1.98 (95%CI 1.57 to 2.20) and obesity with a pooled OR of 2.66 (95%CI 2.15 to 3.28) (Silverwood et al., 2015). Obesity influences the disease course through two primary mechanisms of increased joint loading and adipose tissue low-grade inflammation

(Thijssen et al., 2015). With increasing age, the likelihood of knee OA accelerates. There is a sharp rise in disease incidence between the ages of 50 and 75, which levels off after 75 or 80 years of age (Silverwood et al., 2015). Women had 1.68 times (95%CI 1.37 to 2.07) higher risk of knee OA than men (Silverwood et al., 2015). This sex difference remains unclear; it could be related to genetics, hormones, and other unknown factors.

Knee injury and/or resulting surgeries is a potent risk factor for the development of knee OA not only in middle-aged or older adults (Muthuri et al., 2011; Silverwood et al., 2015; Khan et al., 2019), but also in adolescents and young adults (Muthuri et al., 2011; Whittaker et al., 2018; Snoeker et al., 2020). The estimated risk increased by a range of 3 to 10 fold (Muthuri et al., 2011; Silverwood et al., 2015; Whittaker et al., 2018; Khan et al., 2019; Snoeker et al., 2020). Young adults in their late 20s and early 30s, who sustained a knee injury, had a six times greater likelihood of diagnosed knee OA than their uninjured counterparts during an 11-year follow-up period (Snoeker et al., 2020). Cruciate ligament injuries, meniscal tears, and intra-articular fractures had the greatest elevated risk (Snoeker et al., 2020). There is no cure for knee OA, and arthroplasty is reserved for those with advanced disease. An "old" knee in a relatively young person presents a considerable challenge in disease management. Research efforts on understanding and managing post-traumatic knee OA have been on the rise, since early stage of knee OA could present a window of opportunity to slow and/or stop disease progression when joint symptoms are frequently minimal or mild and tissue damage is not yet widespread.

Repetitive knee bending (e.g., kneeling and squatting) in daily working activities has been linked to an increased risk of developing knee symptoms (Yucesoy et al., 2015). Agricultural and construction sectors, which typically involve lifting, kneeling, climbing, squatting, and standing, had increased odds of knee OA (OR 1.52, 95%CI 1.37 to 1.69) (Wang et al., 2020). Frontal-plane knee malalignment has been shown to elevate the likelihood of tibiofemoral OA progression in a compartment-specific pattern: varus malalignment to medial compartment disease and valgus to lateral (Tanamas et al., 2009; Moisio et al., 2011; Felson et al., 2013; Sharma et al., 2013). Dynamic varus thrust observed during gait is common in persons with knee OA (Chang et al., 2010; Lo et al., 2012) and is an independent risk factor for medial disease worsening (Chang et al.,

2004; Sharma et al., 2017). Visual gait observation is a simple, low-cost, quick, yet informative assessment of probable loading patterns and the impact of pain on movement during ambulation and is recommended as part of the core evaluation of knee OA.

Knee Arthroplasty

Total knee arthroplasty (TKA), the most frequently performed elective orthopedic procedure, aims to treat refractory pain and function limitation and disability associated with end-stage knee OA. It is estimated that 54% of patients with knee OA will receive TKA during their lifetime (Losina et al., 2015); they nonetheless spent an average of 13 years after exhausting non-surgical managements before undergoing surgery (Losina et al., 2015).

The 2010 prevalence of TKA was 1.52% in the total population in the United States, with a higher prevalence in women and older adults (Kremers et al., 2015). The prevalence peaked at 1 in every 10 adults ≥80 years of age (Kremers et al., 2015). Over 658,000 American adults undergo TKA annually (Agency for Healthcare Research and Quality, 2010; Bhandari et al., 2012). The utilization of TKA continues to rise at an alarming pace. The projected TKA utilization will jump by 182% from the year 2014 to 2030, with a predicted volume of 1,921,000 (95%CI 1,530,000 to 2,410,000) in the year 2030 (Singh et al., 2019). In Australia, the incidence of TKA is estimated to rise by 276% by the year 2030 (Ackerman et al., 2019b).

A notable trend of younger patients receiving surgery is also concerning. By the year 2030, 55% of TKAs are projected to be implanted in patients younger than 65 years, with the steepest increase in patients aged 45–55 years (Kurtz et al., 2009; Schreurs & Hannink, 2017). These younger patients will consequentially require a revision surgery during their lifetime. Patients aged 50–55 years at the time of primary TKA had a 35% (95%CI 30.9 to 39.1) lifetime risk for revision, in contrast to a risk ranging from 1% to 6% observed in those older than 70 years at the time of primary TKA (Bayliss et al., 2017). Rising obesity rates in the general population and increased post-traumatic knee OA in active individuals have been theorized to contribute to the downward shift toward younger patients.

TKA imposes overwhelming societal and economic burdens. During the fiscal year 2011, the United States Medicare program reimbursed hospitals $3.5 billion for knee joint replacement, which is the program's largest expenditure for a single procedure (Culler et al., 2015). For perspective, the second largest expense was for heart failure at $3.4 billion annually. In 2013, the average cost for primary TKA in the US was $20,293 and for revision TKA $26,388 (Losina et al., 2015).

The average disease duration of symptomatic knee OA spans over 28.4 years (Losina et al., 2015), starting from initial diagnosis, undergoing bouts of conservative treatments, injections, and arthroscopy, to the eventual TKA. This chronic condition substantially impacts activity engagement, physical function, and mobility in patients seeking physical therapy care. Manual therapy and exercise regimes to manage this high-burden condition will be discussed in ensuing chapters.

Anterior Cruciate Ligament Injury and Reconstruction

The anterior cruciate ligament (ACL) is a primary stabilizing structure of the knee, restraining excessive anterior translation and internal rotation of the tibia on the femur and knee hyperextension. ACL tear may occur via contact (e.g., blow to the lateral knee) or non-contact (e.g., downhill skiing, cutting, and pivoting) mechanisms. Most involve a non-contact injury sustained during athletic activities (Yu & Garrett, 2007; Boden et al., 2010).

Incidence and Economic Burdens

ACL tear accounts for more than half of knee injuries (Musahl & Karlsson, 2019) and could have a devastating impact on patients' athletic careers, activity levels, and quality of life. Between 100,000 to 200,000 ACL tears occur each year in the United States, with an estimated annual incidence rate ranging from 30 to 78 per 100,000 persons in the general population (Bollen, 2000; Gans et al., 2018; Padua et al., 2018). These estimates are derived from injury registries by US college and high school athletes. The actual incidence may be higher due to the absence of a standardized national surveillance system in the general population. ACL injuries are frequently accompanied by other knee structural damage, including damage to menisci, articular cartilage, subchondral bone, and collateral ligaments.

CHAPTER ONE

ACL injuries can be managed operatively or non-operatively. The decision to have surgery is based upon the patient's age, activity level, functional demand during sports or occupation, and presence of concomitant injuries. The rate of ACL reconstructions was 73.6 per 100,000 person-years (Herzog et al., 2018). Trend analysis showed a concerning rise in the reconstruction rate in adolescents aged 13 to 17 years (Herzog et al., 2018), who may experience a less favorable long-term outcome. A physeal sparing procedure is indicated for skeletally immature patients. The risk of re-injury is twice as high as it is in adults (Dekker et al., 2018). Reconstruction at an early age may also shift the eventual progression to knee OA at an earlier age, complicating management options and strategies.

Irrespective of the management approach (conservative vs. surgical), ACL tear, particularly when associated with meniscal damage, increases the lifetime risk of knee OA. Compared with the non-injured knee, the injured knee was 3.89 (95%CI 2.72 to 5.57) times more likely to develop radiographic knee OA during a mean follow-up of 10 years (Ajuied et al., 2014). Approximately 16% (95%CI 7% to 34%) of subjects with isolated ACL reconstruction had subsequent radiographic knee OA; the frequency increased to 50% (95%CI 27% to 73%) in those with both ACL reconstruction and partial/complete meniscectomies (Ruano et al., 2017). The path from ACL tears to post-traumatic knee OA has substantial repercussions, contributing an annual increment of 30,000 to 38,000 patients with knee OA and 25,000 to 30,000 TKAs. Only 60% of non-elite and 80% of elite athletes returned to their pre-injury level of sport after ACL reconstruction and rehabilitation (Ardern et al., 2014; Lai et al., 2018). Realistic goals and expectations should be discussed with patients prior to surgical repairs.

Risk Factors

A number of potential risk factors for non-contact ACL injuries have been identified, including anatomic, physiological, neuromuscular, biomechanical, and environmental factors.

Female athletes are more likely to sustain injury than their male counterparts participating in the same sport or activity, possibly due to disparity in anatomy, physiology, neuromechanics, and biomechanics discussed below. Anatomically, greater knee valgus alignment and narrower femoral intercondylar notch lead to increased risk of ACL stress and impingement. Physiologically, fluctuating serum estrogen and relaxin may influence connective tissue strength and elasticity; however, the definitive role of hormones remains debatable. Key neuromuscular and biomechanical factors are dynamic knee valgus during landing or change of direction, reduced knee flexion during landing, quadriceps dominance, under-utilization of hamstrings or hip external rotators, and weak core stabilization. Unlike anatomical and physiological factors, these deficits can be mitigated with neuromuscular training programs.

Imbalanced activation of weaker hamstrings but stronger quadriceps and a stiffer landing knee place the ACL at risk. Medial collapse movement patterns of hip adduction, femoral internal rotation, and knee valgus are associated with an increased risk of injury. Pre-puberty, no measurable sex differences in lower limb motor control exist. After puberty, females exhibit quadriceps dominance, greater dynamic knee valgus, increased femoral internal rotation, lower gluteal muscle activation, and less trunk mediolateral stability, compared to their male counterparts. Clinicians may assess these risk factors by simple visual observation of movement patterns during single-leg squat, vertical drop jump landing, or cutting/pivoting tasks, augmented by 2D video recordings, although more high-quality research to assess measurement reliability, validity, and clinical utility is needed (Parks et al., 2019). Neuromuscular training to reduce the risk of non-contact ACL injury has been supported in a variety of programs and implemented in many high school, collegiate, and professional sports organizations (Hewett et al., 2016; Padua et al., 2018; Petushek et al., 2019). These programs are especially beneficial to female and younger athletes. Briefly, these programs focus on maintaining proper hip and knee alignment during landing (e.g., knees over toes) and improving shock absorption during landing (e.g., landing softly) during an array of landing stabilization drills as well as strengthening of ACL agonists (e.g., hamstrings and calves) and gluteal muscles (Petushek et al., 2019). Adherence and delivery by trained personnel (e.g., coaches, trainers) are critical to the success of these programs.

Lastly, external/environmental factors, coupled with individual predispositions, could potentially be responsible for ACL injury. Increased friction of synthetic playing surface increased the rate of ACL injury in American football, but not in soccer (Balazs et al., 2015). The impact of footwear is less clear, and there is currently no consensus regarding the role of shoe-surface interface in ACL injury (Alentorn-Geli et al., 2014). Neuromuscular and cognitive fatigue toward the end of a game or after consecutive games may compromise the athlete's ability to control, absorb, and transfer force, thus placing greater stress on the ACL and increasing the risk of injury; however, experimentally induced muscle fatigue did not consistently impair lower limb neuromuscular control during planned or reactive tasks of drop jump, single-leg hop, or cutting maneuvers in lab settings (Barber-Westin & Noyes, 2017).

Meniscal Injury

The second most commonly injured knee structure, the meniscus, plays a critical protective role in the knee by absorbing shock, distributing load, and improving joint congruency and stability (Chang et al., 2011). Meniscal injury can be dichotomized as either traumatic tears that occur in younger patients or degenerative damages that are frequently seen in older adults. The predominant mechanism of injury is a combination of axial loading and rotational forces on the meniscus, although older adults may develop degenerative tears with minimal or no trauma. There is no universally accepted system to classify meniscal tears. Full or partial thickness characterizes the vertical depth of a tear; anterior horn, body, or posterior horn indicates the location of a tear; vertical longitudinal, radial, horizontal, parrot beak, bucket handle, or complex degenerative describes the morphology of a tear. Depending on the magnitude and direction of the traumatic stress, meniscal tear may occur in isolation or with an associated ACL injury, MCL injury, or bone contusion/fracture.

Prevalence and Incidence

The pooled prevalence of MRI-assessed meniscal tears in 3761 asymptomatic uninjured knees was 10% (95%CI 7% to 13%) and more prevalent in adults aged 40 and older (19% vs. 4% in those under 40 years of age) (Culvenor et al., 2019). The incidence rates varied widely depending on the population studied. An injury surveillance study of US high school athletes reported 0.05 injuries per 1000 athletic exposures (Rauh et al., 2000). There were 8.27 cases per 1000 active-duty US military service personnel and those aged 40 or older were 4.25 times more likely to experience injuries than those under 20 years of age (Jones et al., 2012). Professional

basketball players had the highest injury incidence of 82 tears per 1000 athletes (Yeh et al., 2012). In the Netherlands, the incidence was 2 per 1000 patients (Snoeker et al., 2013).

Based on 7-year (year 2005–2011) private medical insurance claim data, representing roughly 9% of the US population under 65 years of age, 387,833 meniscectomies and 23,640 meniscal repairs were performed in the US (Abrams et al., 2013). The overall incidence of meniscectomy was between 0.21% to 0.24%. After meniscal repair incidence rose from 0.01% to 0.02%. ACL reconstruction with meniscal repair incidence was consistent at 0.01%. The majority of meniscal repairs were performed in a younger population, whereas most meniscectomies were performed in adults over 45 years of age. In a Danish study spanning 12 years (year 2000–2011), the number of yearly meniscus surgeries doubled from 8750 to 17,368 with a 3-fold increase in patients older than 55 years and a 2-fold increase in patients between 35 and 55 years of age (Thorlund et al., 2014).

The benefit of surgery for patients aged 40 years or older with degenerative tears has been challenged by recent evidence (Thorlund et al., 2019). Exercise therapy is considered the treatment of choice for improving pain, function, and strength. For those younger than 40 years of age who have sustained a traumatic tear, conservative exercise intervention is recommended, unless the patient has painful mechanical symptoms of locking.

Risk Factors

A systematic review and meta-analysis of 10 studies identified a number of risk factors for degenerative meniscal tears, including increased age (older than 60 years), male sex, work-related kneeling and squatting greater than 1 hour per day, standing or walking more than 2 hours per day, walking greater than 2 miles per day, climbing more than 30 flights of stairs daily, and lifting or carrying more than 10-kg objects at least 10 times per week (Snoeker et al., 2013). Sitting more than 2 hours per day reduced the likelihood of degenerative tears. For acute meniscal tears, playing soccer, playing rugby, and swimming each elevated the risk (soccer: OR 3.58, 95%CI 1.87 to 6.86 and rugby: OR 2.84, 95%CI 1.48 to 5.45 and swimming: OR 1.54, 95%CI 1.09 to 2.17) (Snoeker et al., 2013). Lastly, delaying ACL reconstruction greater than 12 months was a risk factor for medial meniscal tears with knee laxity (Snoeker et al., 2013).

In occupational settings, meniscal tears are among the frequently diagnosed work-related knee pathologies. Risk factors were kneeling >1 hour per day, squatting or crouching >1 hour per day, crawling, stair or ladder climbing (>30 flights per day), lifting/carrying/moving, standing up from a kneeling or squatting position (>30 times daily), and sitting while driving >4 hours daily (Reid et al., 2010). Given frequent and prolonged kneeling or squatting performed in their job, coal miners and carpet layers are particularly susceptible to meniscal disorders and subsequent knee OA (McMillan & Nichols, 2005; Snoeker et al., 2013).

Patellofemoral Pain

Patellofemoral pain (PFP) is a frequent complaint in adolescents, adults, and those with a high level of activity, such as elite athletes and the military population. It is characterized by an insidious onset of poorly defined peri- or retro-patellar pain that is aggravated when the knee is flexed during weight-bearing activities, such as squatting, prolonged sitting, ascending/descending stairs, jumping, or running. An accurate diagnosis and definitive underlying etiologies remain elusive because the exact patho-mechanics and/or pathophysiology are not well understood and a diagnostic gold standard does not exist (Willy et al., 2019). The diagnosis of PFP is usually made after excluding other potential intra-articular or peri-articular pathologies.

Prevalence and Incidence

Reported prevalence and incidence of PFP are vastly variable, likely due to inconsistent diagnostic criteria and differing populations analyzed. A systematic review and meta-analysis summarized the following epidemiological data (Smith et al., 2018). Annual prevalence was 22.7% in the general population, with 29.2% in females and 15.5% in males. The point prevalence in females was 12%–13%. For adolescents, the pooled point prevalence was 7.2% (95%CI 6.3% to 8.3%) for both sexes, but 22.7% (95%CI 17.4% to 28.0%) in females only. Among elite athletes, professional male cyclists had an annual prevalence of 6.4% with symptoms lasting ≥30 days; female Olympians who had symptoms greater than 3 months had a point prevalence of 16.7%. In a mixed female and male military recruit group, the point prevalence was 13.5%. Despite the broad range of prevalence, females are consistently twice as likely to experience PFP.

The incidence rate of PFP among amateur runners in the general population was 1080.5/1000 person-years; in adolescent amateur athletes 5.1%–14.9% over 1 season, and in military recruits ranging from 9.7 to 571.4 per 1000 person-years (Smith et al., 2018). Symptoms tend to persist in over 50% of the patients (Rathleff et al., 2016), some lasting more than a decade (Stathopulu & Baildam, 2003).

Is PFP a precursor for patellofemoral osteoarthritis (PFOA)? These two conditions share several risk factors and clinical characteristics, such as female sex, retro- or peri-patellar pain, knee crepitus, weak quadriceps, pain aggravated by squats or stair negotiation. Furthermore, the traditional view of PFP as a self-limiting condition has been refuted by recent evidence that symptoms persisted in more than 50% of patients at long-term follow-ups (Stathopulu & Baildam, 2003; Rathleff et al., 2016). It is plausible that focal compressive and shear stresses on the cartilage and the presence of synovitis and inflammatory cytokines may contribute to gradual articular tissue degradation and the eventual development of PFOA. Currently, high-quality longitudinal evidence is not available to answer this question. Only a few studies have investigated the longitudinal link between PFP and PFOA and yielded conflicting findings (Utting et al., 2005; Schiphof et al., 2014; Conchie et al., 2016; Willy et al., 2019). Inconsistent definitions of PFOA (e.g., by radiographic evidence, MRI assessment, or unicompartmental PF arthroplasty) and self-reported biases when recalling the history of PFP may lead to contrasting results among these studies. Future large-scale prospective studies are needed to elucidate this potential connection and further our understanding of the disease course of PFOA.

Risk Factors

Management of PFP is challenging, because the etiology is likely multifactorial and the exact source of nociceptive input for PFP is poorly understood and may be person-specific. Plausible anatomical sources include subchondral bone, synovial membrane, infrapatellar fat pad, and retinacular structures. Patients with chronic symptoms may also experience pain sensitization confirmed by quantitative sensory testing (De Oliveira Silva et al., 2019). Understanding potential risk factors may inform evidence-based multimodal intervention and prevent symptom development or worsening. Development and persistence of symptoms have been attributed to anthropometrics, overuse, and proximal, local, and distal factors that elevate load or stress on the patellofemoral joint.

Body anthropometrics and demographic characteristics are often considered contributing factors to incident PFP. Three systematic reviews have demonstrated that age, body weight, body height, BMI, and percent body fat are not associated with PFP (Lankhorst et al., 2012; Pappas & Wong-Tom, 2012; Neal et al., 2019). Sex and the mode of sports participation also can influence the development of PFP. Physically active women were more likely to develop PFP than physically active men (Boling et al., 2010). Among 546 female adolescent athletes, specializing in a single sport, compared to multiple sports, increased the likelihood of having PFP by 1.5 fold (Hall et al., 2015).

The proximal factors of hip and/or trunk kinematics/alignment and weak hip musculature have been postulated to contribute to PFP. Individuals with PFP have weak hip posterolateral muscles, including abductors, extensors, and external rotators. A systematic review with meta-analysis of 21 cross-sectional and 3 prospective longitudinal studies confirmed that men and women with PFP had lower isometric hip strength compared to pain-free individuals, but decreased hip strength did not predict the subsequent onset of PFP (Rathleff et al., 2014). Therefore, hip weakness is likely a consequence of PFP, rather than a cause.

Local factors, such as Q angle, frontal plane projection angle (i.e., dynamic knee valgus), quadriceps strength, knee extensor flexibility, and patellofemoral bony geometry, have been hypothesized to increase the risk of PFP. The current literature does not support the role of Q angle (assessed in either non-weight-bearing or weight-bearing) or frontal plane projection angle in predicting the development of PFP (Lankhorst et al., 2012; Pappas & Wong-Tom, 2012; Neal et al. 2019). Knee extensor strength deficits have consistently been linked to incident PFP (Lankhorst et al., 2012; Pappas & Wong-Tom, 2012; Neal et al., 2019); this association is particularly pronounced when strength was normalized to BMI (Neal et al., 2019). One small prospective study of 282 college students followed for two years reported an association between decreased quadriceps flexibility and future PFP (Witvrouw et al., 2000). There was no relationship of PFP with patellar mobility or MRI-assessed patellofemoral bony geometry (e.g., trochlear sulcus angle and ratio of patellar tendon length to patella length) (Willy et al., 2019).

Distal factors may include static foot posture, dynamic foot movement, and calf muscle flexibility. Prescribing foot orthotics for managing PFP is premised on the assumption that excessive or prolonged pronation during weight-bearing activities could lead to anterior knee pain. However, current evidence is conflicting and inconclusive regarding the relationship between altered foot alignment and mechanics and the development or presence of PFP (Neal et al., 2019; Willy et al., 2019). In some systematic reviews, arch height index and foot alignment dichotomized as pes cavus vs. pes planus were not associated with PFP; in others, increased amount of rearfoot eversion at initial contact during walking and greater navicular drop distance were each linked to the presence of PFP.

Taken together, the underlying contributing factors to PFP are probably highly heterogeneous and person-specific. Intervention should be tailored to target individual anatomical, mechanical, and psychosocial profiles. Exercise therapy is recommended as the cornerstone of conservative management (Willy et al., 2019); its target muscles, strengthening mode, delivery methods, and dosing could be individualized. Adjunct strategies, such as taping, foot orthotics, manual therapy and neuromuscular stimulation, could be incorporated based on patient-specific examination findings, movement observations, activity demands, and psychosocial considerations.

Patellar Tendinopathy

Patellar tendinopathy (PT), also known as "jumper's knee," is an overuse injury of the knee extensor mechanism due to repetitive tensile stress during activities of jumping, landing, cutting, and rapid acceleration/deceleration. Microtears and degenerative changes occur when the volume of repetitive load to which the tendon is exposed exceeds its capacity in a single session or over multiple bouts of activities with insufficient rest in between. The most common site of symptoms is at the inferior pole of the patella, where the patella tendon inserts. Patellar tendinopathy is prevalent in sports requiring frequent jumps, including basketball, volleyball, and handball. It could potentially be a debilitating condition for athletes. Around 33% of athletes seen in an Australian sports medicine clinic for patellar tendinopathy were unable to return to sports within six months (Cook et al., 1997).

Prevalence and Incidence

In a cohort of 2229 elite European male soccer club players observed during the period 2001 to 2009, the prevalence of patellar tendinopathy (diagnosed by clinical examinations performed by team medical staff) was 2.4% in each season; the incidence rate was 0.12 injuries per 1000 hours of play (Hägglund et al., 2011). Notably, around 20% of tendinopathies were recurrent complaints (Hägglund et al., 2011). Retrospective analysis of 8-season injury medical reports among soccer, basketball, handball, roller hockey, and futsal players in Spain found an overall 11.7% prevalence rate (95%CI 10.0 to 13.5) (Florit et al., 2019). Subgroup analyses showed the highest prevalence of 22.7% in professional basketball players and 11.4% in youth basketball players; men were three times more likely to sustain patellar tendinopathy than women (Florit et al., 2019). Prevalence of self-reported jumper's knee in Dutch non-elite athletes ranged from 14.4% (volleyball) to 2.5% (soccer); male athletes had a 2-fold increased risk when compared to their female counterparts (Zwerver et al., 2011).

Defined by pain with palpation and the presence of a hypoechoic region on an ultrasonographic image, patellar tendinopathy was identified in 21% (20 out of 95) of US male collegiate basketball players before the start of the season. Interestingly, 34% (32 out of 95) of the players displayed ultrasonographic abnormalities but were asymptomatic (Hutchison et al., 2019). Following 106 US collegiate female volleyball players over a 4-month season, 21% (22/106) had ultrasonographic evidence of patellar tendon abnormalities at baseline; the incidence was 0.26 (95%CI 0.04 to 0.85) per 1000 athletic exposures (Hutchison et al., 2020).

Risk Factors

A multitude of potential risk factors for patellar tendinopathy has been proposed, but high quality evidence is unavailable, as elucidated in several systematic reviews (van der Worp et al., 2011; Sprague et al., 2018) and case–control investigations (Janssen et al., 2015; Morton et al., 2017). Most studies were small and involved cross-sectional comparisons between individuals with vs. without patellar tendinopathy; hence causal inference cannot be made. There was limited evidence for the following demographic, body anthropometric, musculoskeletal health, and training factors. Being male, experiencing previous knee injury, and having a family history of tendon problems are linked to increased risk. Elevated body weight or BMI, higher waist-to-hip ratio, more pronounced leg length discrepancy, and lower foot arch may place an individual at greater risk for patellar tendinopathy. Compared to healthy controls, athletes with patellar tendinopathy were more likely to have reduced ankle dorsiflexion range of motion, diminished quadriceps and hamstring flexibility, weaker quadriceps, and back pain. Training variables associated with the presence of patellar tendinopathy included greater total activity time, higher jump training volume, and larger counter-movement jump height.

Similar to the management of PFP, a comprehensive plan of care for patellar tendinopathy needs to address hypothesized contributing factors and focuses on progressively developing load tolerance of the tendon with emphasis on eccentric-concentric loading.

Hip and Groin Pain: Terminology and Consensus Agreements

The hip and groin region is described as the "Bermuda triangle of sports medicine" (Bizzini, 2011) due to its complex anatomy and reported difficulty in diagnosing and managing pain presentations (Hölmich, 2017). The etiology of hip and groin pain is multifactorial, with coexisting pathological processes often observed in different tissues within the anatomical region of the groin (Thorborg & Hölmich, 2013; Weir et al., 2015). Further, a high prevalence of what has traditionally been considered as "structural pathology" has been reported in asymptomatic people, adding to the complexity of diagnosis, management and prevention of groin pain (Weir et al., 2015). Recently, an enhanced understanding of the relevance of hip-related pathologies as a source of groin pain has made the diagnosis and classification of hip and groin pain even more complicated (Thorborg & Hölmich, 2013).

Widespread variability in diagnostic terminology and classification systems for hip and groin pain is apparent in published literature. Heterogeneity in operational definitions and nomenclature used in hip and groin injury research has made it difficult to synthesize clinical research findings. This clear need for standardized terminology and definitions for hip and groin pain diagnosis has resulted in three recent consensus agreements on the terminology and definitions for hip and groin pain: the Doha agreement

(Weir et al., 2015), the Warwick agreement on femoroacetabular impingement (FAI) syndrome (Griffin et al., 2016), and the Zurich consensus on the classification, definition and diagnostic criteria of hip-related pain (Reiman et al., 2020).

Doha Agreement

In November 2014, an agreement meeting was held in Doha, Qatar where consensus was reached on standardized taxonomy and terminology to describe hip and groin pain in athletes, providing recommendations for clinicians and researchers (Weir et al., 2015). The agreed-upon classification system (Table 1.1) includes the four defined clinical entities of adductor-, iliopsoas-, inguinal- and pubic-related groin pain, and two additional categories of hip-related and "other" causes of groin pain.

The Doha agreement groin pain classification system is based on the clinical examination of people with groin pain where their recognizable pain is reproduced on pain-provocation testing, and tenderness on palpation

TABLE 1.1 Current Classification System of Hip and Groin Pain, Adapted from Recent Consensus Meetings			
Defined clinical entities*	Symptoms	Definition	More likely if patient presents with
Adductor-related groin pain*	Pain around the insertion of the adductor longus tendon at the pubic bone. Pain may radiate distally along the medial thigh	Adductor tenderness **AND** pain on resisted adduction testing	
Iliopsoas-related groin pain*	Pain in the anterior part of the proximal thigh, more laterally located than adductor-related groin pain	Iliopsoas tenderness (either supra- or infra-inguinal)	Pain reproduced on resisted hip flexion and/or pain on hip flexor stretching
Inguinal-related groin pain*	Pain in the inguinal region which worsens on activity. If pain is severe, often have inguinal pain when cough or sneeze, or sit up in bed	Pain in the inguinal canal and inguinal canal tenderness, or pain with: Valsalva, cough and/or sneeze. No palpable inguinal hernia found, including on invagination of the scrotum to palpate the inguinal canal	Pain reproduced on resisted abdominal muscle testing
Pubic-related groin pain*	Pain in the region of the symphysis joint and the immediately adjacent bone	Local tenderness of the pubic symphysis and the immediately adjacent bone	No particular resistance test, but more likely if pain reproduced by resisted abdominal and adduction testing
Additional Categories*			
Other*	Clinical suspicion if symptoms cannot be easily classified into one of the commonly defined clinical entities	Any other orthopedic, neurological, rheumatological, urological, gastrointestinal, dermatological, oncological or surgical condition causing pain in the groin region	

(Continued)

TABLE 1.1 *(Continued)*

Defined clinical entities*	Symptoms	Definition	More likely if patient presents with
Hip-related groin pain*		Clinical suspicion that the hip joint is the source of groin pain, either through history or clinical examination	Mechanical symptoms present, such as catching, locking, clicking or giving way
After imaging, hip-related pain may be further delineated into¥:			
FAI syndrome†¥	Motion- or position-related pain in the hip or groin. Pain may also be felt in the back, buttock or thigh. Patients may also describe clicking, catching, locking, stiffness, restricted range of motion, or giving way	Motion-related clinical disorder of the hip with a triad of symptoms, clinical signs and imaging findings. Cam and or/pincer morphology must be present on imaging	Pain reproduced with FADIR test. Often a limited range of hip motion, more likely if Hip IR <15 degrees and evidence of labral or chondral injury on imaging
Acetabular dysplasia and/or hip instability¥			
Other conditions causing hip-related pain (including chondral, labral, ligamentum teres) without specific bony morphology¥			

*Doha agreement (Weir et al., 2015).

†Warwick agreement (Griffin et al., 2016).

¥Zurich hip consensus (Reiman et al., 2020).

(Adapted from Weir et al., 2015; Griffin et al., 2016; Thorborg et al., 2018; Reiman et al., 2020.)

(Holmich et al., 2004; Hölmich, 2007; Weir et al., 2015). Good intra- and inter-observer agreement has been demonstrated with this approach (kappa values ≥0.70) (Holmich et al., 2004). The category of hip-related pain was only vaguely defined in this consensus paper, creating the impetus for the next two consensus meetings in the hip and groin pain area.

The Zurich and Warwick Consensus Meetings on Hip Pain

Building on the Doha agreement for groin pain, the International Hip-related Pain Research Network (IHPRN) consensus in Zurich made more specific recommendations on the classification of hip-related pain, or pain originating from the hip joint (Reiman et al., 2020). The three classifications that were agreed on were: (1) femoroacetabular impingement (FAI) syndrome; (2) acetabular dysplasia/ hip instability; and (3) other intra-articular sources of pain (e.g., labral, cartilage or ligamentum teres), with no bony morphological variant present.

The Warwick Agreement (Griffin et al., 2016) had previously defined FAI syndrome as having three key components: (1) pain and symptoms; (2) signs typically seen in FAI syndrome; and (3) positive imaging findings which are typically either cam morphology, pincer morphology or a combination of both. Between these three consensus statements, a framework of classification of hip and groin pain for future epidemiological studies is provided and an improved ability to synthesize study findings.

Hip and Groin Pain Epidemiology

Hip and groin pain is particularly problematic in athletes, especially in sports which require high loads of running, change of direction, and kicking; such as the various football codes (Ryan et al., 2014; Walden et al., 2015; Whittaker et al., 2015; Mosler et al., 2018a; Kerbel et al., 2018; Werner et al., 2019). A recent systematic review synthesized the epidemiology of hip and groin pain reported in prospective studies of senior football players (Walden et al., 2015). Hip/ groin pain was found to be the third most common injury experienced by male professional football players, accounting for around 13% of all time-loss injuries sustained each season, with reported frequencies varying from 4% to 19% (Walden et al., 2015). Groin injuries are less prevalent in elite female football players (Orchard, 2015), where they represent only 7% (range: 2%–11%) of all reported injuries (Walden et al., 2015). Similarly, across various collegiate sports played in the United States, sex-related differences in hip and groin injury incidence rates were found with male athletes experiencing higher rates of hip and groin pain than comparable female athletes (Kerbel et al., 2018).

Incidence rates for time-loss groin injury vary from 0.6 to 1.1/1000hrs (Esteve et al., 2020; Walden et al., 2015; Mosler et al., 2018a; Werner et al., 2019) and prevalence rates are high with 21% of professional male football players experiencing a time-loss hip/groin injury each season (Werner et al., 2009; Mosler et al., 2018a). Most groin injuries are of gradual onset (Werner et al., 2009; Mosler et al., 2018a; Kerbel et al., 2018), and result in less than one week's absence from the sport, but the risk of recurrence is high (Mosler et al., 2018a; Werner et al., 2019). Furthermore, symptoms may persist following return to play, and be carried into the following season (Thorborg et al., 2017; Langhout et al., 2019). While the predominance of epidemiological data is published from male football populations, hip and groin pain is also frequently experienced in other football codes such as rugby union and league, Australian rules, American and Gaelic football (Ryan et al., 2014; Whittaker et al., 2015; Roe et al., 2018), and in other sports such as ice hockey, basketball, cricket, baseball, and in professional dancing (Orchard 2015; Dalton et al., 2016; Mlynarek & Coleman, 2018).

Sports injury surveillance studies have traditionally used a time-loss injury definition. However, hip and groin pain commonly causes symptoms and reduced performance, without forcing time-loss from training and/or match play (Esteve et al., 2020; Langhout et al., 2019). Therefore, the use of the time-loss injury definition is likely to underestimate the true hindrance of this injury in athletes (Kerbel et al., 2018). Studies of groin symptoms in male football players (with and without time-loss) report prevalence rates as high as 59% (Esteve et al., 2020; Harøy et al., 2017), with 20%–30% of players experiencing some form of groin problem during any given week (Harøy et al., 2017, 2019).

In epidemiological studies published since the Doha agreement, adductor-related groin pain is the most common entity experienced across a variety of sports (Kerbel et al., 2018). In professional male football players, adductor-related groin pain accounts for at least two-thirds of groin injuries (Mosler et al., 2018a; Werner et al., 2019). The next most common entity categorized is iliopsoas-related groin pain followed by inguinal- and pubic-related groin pain (Mosler et al., 2018a; Werner et al., 2019). Hip-related groin pain was categorized in less than 5% of time-loss groin injuries in professional male football players (Werner et al., 2009, 2019; Mosler et al., 2018a). Similarly, across various collegiate sports, adductor strain was the most commonly reported injury accounting for 25% of all hip/groin injuries, while intra-articular hip conditions only constituted 3% of these injuries (Kerbel et al., 2018). Conversely, hip pathology was cited as the most common condition diagnosed in two large case series involving consecutive athletes presenting to the clinic (Bradshaw et al., 2008;

Rankin et al., 2015). These findings have been contradicted in other case series (Hölmich 2007; Taylor et al., 2018), and in population-based epidemiological studies (Werner et al., 2009, 2019; Mosler et al., 2018a; Kerbel et al., 2018a). These inconsistencies in epidemiological patterns of hip and groin pain mostly likely exemplify the lack of standardization in diagnostic categorization that has been present in the field until very recently.

Intra-articular Hip Conditions

Bony Hip Morphology

Bony hip morphology refers to the surface shape of the bones that form the hip joint, specifically the femoral head and neck, and the acetabulum. The bony hip morphological variants most commonly associated with hip pathology are

cam morphology, pincer morphology and acetabular dysplasia (Figure 1.1).

The word "cam" is a mechanical term referring to a rotating piece with an irregular shape and, when applied to the hip, refers to an aspherical or oval-shaped femoral head (Ito et al., 2001). Cam morphology is characterized by excessive bone formation at the anterolateral aspect of the femoral head/neck junction, creating an aspherical femoral head (Figure 1.1) (Ito et al., 2001; Leunig et al., 2008). Pincer morphology describes acetabular over-coverage, while acetabular dysplasia is under-coverage of the femoral head (Figure 1.1) (Agricola et al., 2013a).

While acetabular morphology is mostly determined at birth (Hogervorst et al., 2012; Goldstein et al., 2014), much of the recent research on bony hip morphology has

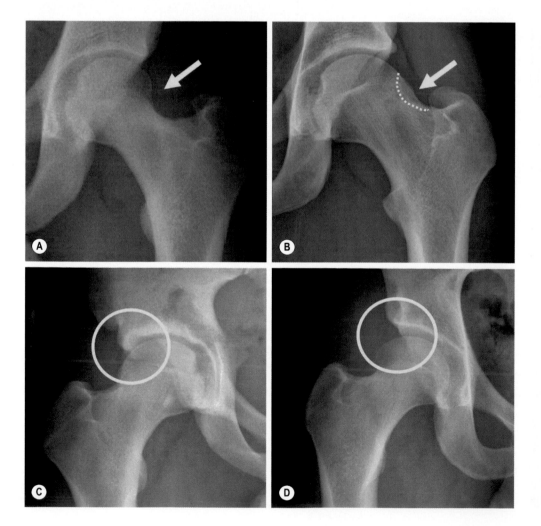

FIGURE 1.1
Bony hip morphology. (A) Normal shaped femur. (B) Cam morphology. (C) Pincer morphology. (D) Acetabular dysplasia. Reproduced with permission from Mosler et al., 2018b.

been aimed at determining the prevalence, etiology, and clinical significance of cam morphology, which is further delineated into primary and secondary cam morphology. While the cause of primary cam morphology is not known definitively, it is likely to develop gradually during maturation as a result of high impact load on the femoral capital physis with athletic activity (Siebenrock et al., 2011, 2013; Agricola et al., 2014; Tak et al., 2015; Palmer et al., 2018; van Klij et al., 2018). Conversely, secondary cam morphology is caused by pre-existing hip disease or trauma, including Perthes disease, slipped capital femoral epiphysis (SCFE), healed proximal femoral fractures, avascular necrosis or osteophytes (Agricola et al., 2013b; van Klij et al., 2018).

With the etiology of primary cam morphology most likely due to participation in vigorous sporting activities during maturation, the prevalence of cam morphology is observed to be higher in athletes than in less athletic controls (Frank et al., 2015; Nepple et al., 2015; Dickenson et al., 2016; Mascarenhas et al., 2016). Cam morphology prevalence in athletes participating in high-impact sports ranges from 55% to 92%, compared to ranges reported in the general population of 12%–68% (Frank et al., 2015; Nepple et al., 2015; Dickenson et al., 2016; Mascarenhas et al., 2016; Kopec et al., 2020). Pincer morphology prevalence is difficult to ascertain due to the poorly defined characteristics of this morphology and poor reliability of radiographic parameters, such as the crossover sign, existing in current literature (Zaltz et al., 2013; Frank et al., 2015; Mascarenhas et al., 2016). Consequently, pincer morphology prevalence ranges from 18% to 67% across both athletic and general populations, depending on definition (Frank et al., 2015; Mascarenhas et al., 2016).

In three large population studies in Scandinavia, the prevalence of radiologic signs of acetabular dysplasia ranged from 1.7% to 20% (Jacobsen et al., 2005; Gosvig et al., 2010; Engesæter et al., 2013). Broadly, the prevalence of acetabular dysplasia appears to be similar in people with and without symptoms, and there are minimal differences in prevalence between sexes (Jacobsen & Sonne-Holm, 2005; Gosvig et al., 2010; Engesæter et al., 2013). Acetabular dysplasia prevalence has rarely been reported in athletic populations, but the range reported is 1.9%–37%, with variance found between studies and across sports (Harris et al., 2016; Mosler et al., 2016).

Prevalence of Intra-articular Hip Conditions

It is difficult to ascertain the true prevalence of hip-related pain in young and middle-aged adults due to the overlap with extra-articular causes of pain. The point prevalence of hip pain at a population level suggests that approximately 5% of younger adults will have hip-related pain at any point in time (Picavet & Schouten, 2003). In general populations with long-standing groin pain presenting to tertiary care clinics, it appears that half will have hip-related pain as opposed to extra-articular groin pain (Larson et al., 2018; Pålsson et al., 2019).

Recent work has suggested that the prevalence of hip joint findings on imaging is similar in people with hip-related pain compared to healthy controls. A recent systematic review showed that the prevalence of labral tears was the same in individuals with and without pain (62% and 54%, respectively) but there was a higher prevalence of cartilage lesions in people with pain (64%) compared to those without (12%) (Heerey et al., 2018). Heerey et al. (2020) recently examined a large cohort of sub-elite soccer and Australian football players. They reported a similar prevalence of cam morphology in players with (71%) and without (63%) hip and groin pain (Heerey et al., 2020). In the same cohort, there was no difference between football players with and those without hip and groin pain for labral tears and cartilage lesions, except for full-thickness cartilage lesions which were more common in those with hip pain (Heerey et al., 2021). These findings suggest that intra-articular findings such as cartilage lesions only become symptomatic when more advanced. While the prevalence of intra-articular hip findings on imaging is now well established, the relationship between these findings and the presence of pain is still uncertain.

Etiology of Intra-articular Hip Conditions

Hip-related pain may represent early-stage osteoarthritis on the continuum of hip disease. Middle-aged and older adults with cam morphology are more likely to develop end-stage hip OA and undergo hip replacement surgery (Agricola et al., 2012; Kowalczuk et al., 2015; Shapira et al., 2020). Early changes to cartilage and labrum are thought to represent osteoarthritis in its early stages (Pritzker et al., 2006; Pollard et al., 2008). People with osteoarthritic changes such as full-thickness cartilage lesions at arthroscopy progress to a total hip replacement within two years

(Kemp et al., 2015). The mechanisms by which some people with hip-related pain progress to hip osteoarthritis is not yet known, but it is most likely due to a number of intrinsic (such as body mass, genetics, cartilage quality, inflammatory profile) and extrinsic factors (such as a history of loading and activity, past injury).

Occupational activity is considered to be a risk factor for the development of hip OA, where people exposed to heavy manual labor are at increased risk of hip OA in later life (Juhakoski et al., 2009). Similarly, elite athletes are at increased risk of hip OA and total hip replacement in later life (Vigdorchik et al., 2017; Petrillo et al., 2018), suggesting that the type and volume of joint load in younger adulthood may increase the risk of hip OA later. Our work has also shown that people suffering a sports injury are 4 times more likely than those without to have a hip replacement within 15 years (Ackerman et al., 2019a). However, moderate leisure-time exercise does not increase the risk of hip OA, and may actually protect against hip OA (Wang et al., 2011; Ageberg et al., 2012).

The Burden of Intra-articular Hip Conditions

Hip-related pain and hip OA are one of a number of musculoskeletal conditions that are a leading cause of pain and disability, and the second-largest global contributor to years lived with disability (Vos et al., 2020). The economic burden of hip-related pain is unclear; however, the individual burden on younger adults is high and occurs at a time of many work, sporting, and family commitments. Younger adults with hip-related pain have pain (Hinman et al., 2013; Freke et al., 2019), sporting participation and quality of life outcomes that are as bad, or worse, than those seen in older adults with hip osteoarthritis (Olsen et al., 2020).

These outcomes remain considerably worse than those seen in healthy age-matched peers even after hip arthroscopy surgery (Kemp et al., 2014). As a result, they have daily pain impairing sleep, and preventing participation in work, sport and exercise, and social activities. The resultant effects of reduced participation in physical activity (Jones et al., 2020) and subsequent sedentary lifestyles place these individuals at risk of comorbidities including mental health conditions (Rhon et al., 2019) and possible increased mortality (Ekelund et al., 2020).

The burden of hip OA is better established. One in four people will develop hip OA in their lifetime (Murphy et al., 2010). Over time, they stop enjoying physical activities, put on weight and become less fit – increasing their risk of other chronic diseases (e.g., diabetes and cardiovascular disease) (Williams et al., 2018). Few effective treatments exist, forcing people to wait for hip replacement surgery. Annual hip replacement rates in Australia will rise to 80,000 by 2030, reaching an unsustainable cost of $2 billion annually (Ackerman et al., 2019b). Joint replacement costs contribute to total annual healthcare/lost productivity costs of osteoarthritis in Australia of $24 billion (Australian Bureau of Statistics, 2009). By 2030, the economic burden of OA on the Australian healthcare system is predicted to rise by 38% (Ackerman et al., 2016), mostly because of escalating joint replacement surgery rates. It is also expected that over $9 billion in gross domestic product in Australia will be lost from people withdrawing from the workforce because of arthritis (Schofield et al., 2016). The personal burden of hip OA includes living with substantial pain, physical inactivity, elevated body mass index (BMI), greater comorbidity risk (e.g., diabetes, cardiovascular disease), social disengagement, psychological distress, and poor quality of life (Williams et al., 2018).

References

Abrams GD, Frank RM, Gupta AK, et al. Trends in meniscus repair and meniscectomy in the United States, 2005-2011. Am J Sports Med. 2013;41:2333–9.

Ackerman IN, Bucknill A, Page RS, et al. The substantial personal burden experienced by younger people with hip or knee osteoarthritis. Osteoarthritis Cartilage. 2015;23:1276–84.

Ackerman I, Bohensky M, Pratt C, et al. Counting the Cost Part 1: Healthcare Costs: The Current and Future Burden of Arthritis. Sydney, Australia: Arthritis Australia; 2016.

Ackerman IN, Bohensky MA, Kemp JL, De Steiger R. Quantifying the likelihood and costs of hip replacement surgery after sports injury: a population-level analysis. Phys Ther Sport. 2019a;41:9–15.

Ackerman IN, Bohensky MA, Zomer E, et al. The projected burden of primary total knee and hip replacement for osteoarthritis in Australia to the year 2030. BMC Musculoskelet Disord. 2019b;20:90.

Ageberg E, Engstrom G, Gerhardsson de Verdier M, et al. Effect of leisure time physical activity on severe knee or hip osteoarthritis leading to total joint replacement: a population-based prospective cohort study. BMC Musculoskelet Disord. 2012;13:73.

Agency for Healthcare Research and Quality. Healthcare Cost and Utilization Project. [Internet]. 2010. Available from: https://www.ahrq.gov/data/hcup/index.html

Agricola R, Heijboer MP, Bierma-Zeinstra SMA, et al. Cam impingement causes osteoarthritis of the hip: a nationwide prospective cohort study (CHECK). Ann Rheum Dis. 2012;72:918–23.

Agricola R, Heijboer MP, Roze RH, et al. Pincer deformity does not lead to osteoarthritis of the hip whereas acetabular dysplasia does: acetabular coverage and development of osteoarthritis in a nationwide prospective cohort study (CHECK). Osteoarthritis Cartilage. 2013a;21:1514–21.

Agricola R, Waarsing JH, Arden NK, et al. Cam impingement of the hip: a risk factor for hip osteoarthritis. Nat Rev Rheumatol. 2013b;9:630-4.

Agricola R, Heijboer MP, Ginai AZ, et al. A CAM deformity is gradually acquired during skeletal maturation in adolescent and young male soccer players: a prospective study with minimum 2-year follow-up. Am J Sports Med. 2014;42:798–806

Ajuied A, Wong F, Smith C, et al. Anterior cruciate ligament injury and radiologic progression of knee osteoarthritis: a systematic review and meta-analysis. Am J Sports Med. 2014;42(9):2242–52.

Alentorn-Geli E, Mendiguchía J, Samuelsson K, et al. Prevention of anterior cruciate ligament injuries in sports. Part I: systematic review of risk factors in male athletes. Knee Surg Sports Traumatol Arthrosc. 2014;22:3–15.

Ardern CL, Taylor NF, Feller JA, Webster KE. Fifty-five per cent return to competitive sport following anterior cruciate ligament reconstruction surgery: an updated systematic review and meta-analysis including aspects of physical functioning and contextual factors. Br J Sports Med. 2014;48:1543–52.

Australian Bureau of Statistics. National Health Survey: Summary of Results 2007–2008 (Reissue). Canberra; 2009.

Balazs GC, Pavey GJ, Brelin AM, et al. Risk of anterior cruciate ligament injury in athletes on synthetic playing surfaces: a systematic review. Am J Sports Med. 2015;43:1798–804.

Barber-Westin SD, Noyes FR. Effect of fatigue protocols on lower limb neuromuscular function and implications for anterior cruciate ligament injury prevention training: a systematic review. Am J Sports Med. 2017;45:3388–96.

Bayliss LE, Culliford D, Monk AP, et al. The effect of patient age at intervention on risk of implant revision after total replacement of the hip or knee: a population-based cohort study. Lancet. 2017;389:1424–30.

Bhandari M, Smith J, Miller LE, Block JE. Clinical and economic burden of revision knee arthroplasty. Clin Med Insights Arthritis Musculoskelet Disord. 2012;5:89–94.

Bizzini M. The groin area: the Bermuda triangle of sports medicine? Br J Sports Med. 2011;45:1.

Boden BP, Sheehan FT, Torg JS, Hewett TE. Non-contact anterior cruciate ligament injuries: mechanisms and risk factors. J Am Acad Orthop Surg. 2010;18:520–7.

Boling M, Padua D, Marshall S, et al. Gender differences in the incidence and prevalence of patellofemoral pain syndrome. Scand J Med Sci Sports. 2010;20:725–30.

Bollen S. Epidemiology of knee injuries: diagnosis and triage. Br J Sports Med. 2000;34:227–8.

Bradshaw CJ, Bundy M, Falvey E. The diagnosis of longstanding groin pain: a prospective clinical cohort study. Br J Sports Med. 2008;42:551–4.

Calvet J, Orellana C, Larrosa M, et al. High prevalence of cardiovascular co-morbidities in patients with symptomatic knee or hand osteoarthritis. Scand J Rheumatol. 2016;45:41–4.

Centers for Disease Control and Prevention (CDC). Arthritis Cost Statistics [Internet]. 2020 [cited 2021 Feb 23]. Available from: https://www.cdc.gov/arthritis/data_statistics/cost.htm

Chang A, Hayes K, Dunlop D, et al. Thrust during ambulation and the progression of knee osteoarthritis. Arthritis Rheum. 2004;50:3897–903.

Chang A, Hochberg M, Song J, et al. Frequency of varus and valgus thrust and factors associated with thrust presence in persons with or at higher risk of developing knee osteoarthritis. Arthritis Rheum. 2010;62:1403–11.

Chang A, Moisio K, Chmiel JS, et al. Subregional effects of meniscal tears on cartilage loss over 2 years in knee osteoarthritis. Ann Rheum Dis. 2011;70:74–9.

Conchie H, Clark D, Metcalfe A, et al. Adolescent knee pain and patellar dislocations are associated with patellofemoral osteoarthritis in adulthood: a case control study. The Knee. 2016;23:708–11.

Cook JL, Khan KM, Harcourt PR, et al. A cross sectional study of 100 athletes with jumper's knee managed conservatively and surgically. The Victorian Institute of Sport Tendon Study Group. Br J Sports Med. 1997;31:332–6.

Cross M, Smith E, Hoy D, et al. The global burden of hip and knee osteoarthritis: estimates from the Global Burden of Disease 2010 study. Ann Rheum Dis. 2014;73:1323–30.

Cui A, Li H, Wang D, et al. Global, regional prevalence, incidence and risk factors of knee osteoarthritis in population-based studies. EClinicalMedicine [Internet]. 2020 Dec 1 [cited 2021 Feb 21];29.

Culler SD, Jevsevar DS, Shea KG, et al. The incremental hospital cost and length-of-stay associated with treating adverse events among Medicare beneficiaries undergoing TKA. J Arthroplasty. 2015;30:19–25.

Culvenor AG, Øiestad BE, Hart HF, et al. Prevalence of knee osteoarthritis features on magnetic resonance imaging in asymptomatic uninjured adults: a systematic review and meta-analysis. Br J Sports Med. 2019;53:1268–78.

Dalton SL, Zupon AB, Gardner EC, et al. The Epidemiology of Hip/Groin Injuries in National Collegiate Athletic Association Mens and Womens Ice Hockey: 2009-2010 Through 2014-2015 Academic Years. Orthop J Sports Med. 2016;4:2325967116632692.

De Oliveira Silva D, Rathleff MS, Petersen K, et al. Manifestations of pain sensitization across different painful knee disorders: a systematic review including meta-analysis and metaregression. Pain Med Malden Mass. 2019;20:335–58.

Dekker TJ, Rush JK, Schmitz MR. What's new in pediatric and adolescent anterior cruciate ligament injuries? J Pediatr Orthop. 2018;38:185–92.

Dickenson E, Wall PDH, Robinson B, et al. Prevalence of cam hip shape morphology: a systematic review. Osteoarthritis Cartilage. 2016;24:949–61.

Ekelund U, Dalene KE, Tarp J, Lee IM. Physical activity and mortality: what is the dose response and how big is the effect? Br J Sports Med. 2020;54:1125–6.

Engesæter IØ, Laborie LB, Lehmann TG, et al. Prevalence of radiographic findings associated with hip dysplasia in a population-based cohort of 2081 19-year-old Norwegians. Bone Jt J. 2013;95:279–85.

Esteve E, Clausen MB, Rathleff MS, et al. Prevalence and severity of groin problems in Spanish football: a prospective study beyond the time-loss approach. Scand J Med Sci Sports. 2020;30:914–21.

Felson DT, Niu J, Gross KD, et al. Valgus malalignment is a risk factor for lateral knee osteoarthritis incidence and progression: findings from the Multicenter Osteoarthritis Study and the Osteoarthritis Initiative. Arthritis Rheum. 2013;65:355–62.

Florit D, Pedret C, Casals M, et al. Incidence of tendinopathy in team sports in a multidisciplinary sports club over 8 seasons. J Sports Sci Med. 2019;18:780–8.

Frank JM, Harris JD, Erickson BJ, et al. Prevalence of femoroacetabular impingement imaging findings in asymptomatic volunteers: a systematic review. Arthrosc J Arthrosc Relat Surg. 2015;31:1199–204.

Freke MD, Crossley KM, Russell T, et al. Associations between type and severity of hip pathology with pre-operative patient reported outcome measures. Braz J Phys Ther. 2019;23:402–11.

Gans I, Retzky JS, Jones LC, Tanaka MJ. Epidemiology of recurrent anterior cruciate ligament injuries in National Collegiate Athletic Association Sports: The Injury Surveillance Program, 2004-2014. Orthop J Sports Med. 2018;6:2325967118777823.

GBD 2015 Disease and Injury Incidence and Prevalence Collaborators. Global, regional, and national incidence, prevalence, and years lived with disability for 310 diseases and injuries, 1990-2015: a systematic analysis for the Global Burden of Disease Study 2015. Lancet 2016;388:1545–602.

GBD 2017 Disease and Injury Incidence and Prevalence Collaborators. Global, regional, and national incidence, prevalence, and years lived with disability for 354 diseases and injuries for 195 countries and territories, 1990-2017: a systematic analysis for the Global Burden of Disease Study 2017. Lancet 2018;392:1789–858.

Goldstein RY, Kaye ID, Slover J, Feldman D. Hip dysplasia in the skeletally mature patient. Bull Hosp Jt Dis. 2014;72:28–42.

Gosvig KK, Jacobsen S, Sonne-Holm S, et al. Prevalence of malformations of the hip joint and their relationship to sex, groin pain, and risk of osteoarthritis: a population-based survey. J Bone Jt Surg-Am 2010;92:1162–9.

Griffin DR, Dickenson EJ, O'Donnell J, et al. The Warwick Agreement on femoroacetabular impingement syndrome (FAI syndrome): an international consensus statement. Br J Sports Med. 2016;50:1169–76.

Hägglund M, Zwerver J, Ekstrand J. Epidemiology of patellar tendinopathy in elite male soccer players. Am J Sports Med. 2011;39:1906–11.

Hall R, Barber Foss K, Hewett TE, Myer GD. Sport specialization's association with an increased risk of developing anterior knee pain in adolescent female athletes. J Sport Rehabil. 2015;24:31–5.

Harøy J, Clarsen B, Thorborg K, et al. Groin problems in male soccer players are more common than previously reported. Am J Sports Med. 2017;45:1304–8.

Harøy J, Clarsen B, Wiger EG, et al. The Adductor Strengthening Programme prevents groin problems among male football players: a cluster-randomised controlled trial. Br J Sports Med. 2019;53:150–7.

Harris JD, Gerrie BJ, Varner KE, et al. Radiographic prevalence of dysplasia, cam, and pincer deformities in elite ballet. Am J Sports Med. 2016;44:20–7.

Hawker GA, Croxford R, Bierman AS, et al. All-cause mortality and serious cardiovascular events in people with hip and knee osteoarthritis: a population based cohort study. PloS One. 2014;9:e91286.

Heerey JJ, Kemp JL, Mosler AB, et al. What is the prevalence of imaging-defined intra-articular hip pathologies in people with and without pain? A systematic review and meta-analysis. Br J Sports Med. 2018;52:581–93.

Heerey J, Agricola R, Smith R, et al. Is self-reported hip and groin pain alongside a positive FADIR related to the size and prevalence of bony hip morphology in football players? J Orthop Sports Phys Ther. 2020; In Press.

Heerey JJ, Srinivasan R, Agricola R, et al. Prevalence of early hip OA features on MRI in high-impact athletes. The femoroacetabular impingement and hip osteoarthritis cohort (FORCe) study. Osteoarthritis Cartilage. 2021;29:323–34.

Herzog MM, Marshall SW, Lund JL, et al. Trends in incidence of ACL reconstruction and concomitant procedures among commercially insured individuals in the United States, 2002-2014. Sports Health. 2018;10:523–31.

Hewett TE, Myer GD, Ford KR, et al. Mechanisms, prediction, and prevention of ACL injuries: cut risk with three sharpened and validated tools. J Orthop Res Off Publ Orthop Res Soc. 2016;34:1843–55.

Hinman RS, Dobson F, Takla A, et al. Which is the most useful patient-reported outcome in femoroacetabular impingement? Test-retest reliability of six questionnaires. Br J Sports Med. 2013;48:458–63.

Hogervorst T, Eilander W, Fikkers JT, Meulenbelt I. Hip ontogenesis: how evolution, genes, and load history shape hip morphotype and cartilotype. Clin Orthop. 2012;470:3284–96.

Hölmich P. Long-standing groin pain in sportspeople falls into three primary patterns, a "clinical entity" approach: a prospective study of 207 patients. Br J Sports Med. 2007;41:247–52.

Hölmich P. Groin injuries in athletes: new stepping stones. Sports Orthop Traumatol. 2017;33:106–12.

Holmich P, Holmich L, Bjerg A. Clinical examination of athletes with groin pain: an intraobserver and interobserver reliability study. Br J Sports Med. 2004;38:446–51.

Hunter DJ, Bierma-Zeinstra S. Osteoarthritis. Lancet 2019;393:1745–59.

Hutchison MK, Houck J, Cuddeford T, et al. Prevalence of patellar tendinopathy and patellar tendon abnormality in male collegiate basketball players: a cross-sectional study. J Athl Train. 2019;54:953–8.

Hutchison MK, Patterson C, Cuddeford T, et al. Low prevalence of patellar tendon abnormality and low incidence of patellar tendinopathy in female collegiate volleyball players. Res Sports Med Print. 2020;28:155–67.

Ito K, Minka-ii M-A, Leunig M, et al. Femoroacetabular impingement and the cam-effect. Bone Jt J. 2001;83:171–6.

Jacobsen S, Sonne-Holm S. Hip dysplasia: a significant risk factor for the development of hip osteoarthritis. A cross-sectional survey. Rheumatol 2005;44:211–8.

Jacobsen S, Sonne-holm S, Søballe K, et al. Hip dysplasia and osteoarthrosis: a survey of 4 151 subjects from the osteoarthrosis substudy of the Copenhagen city heart study. Acta Orthop. 2005;76:149–58.

Janssen I, Steele JR, Munro BJ, Brown NT. Previously identified patellar tendinopathy risk factors differ between elite and sub-elite volleyball players. Scand J Med Sci Sports. 2015;25:308–14.

Jones DM, Crossley KM, Ackerman IN, et al. Physical activity following hip arthroscopy in young and middle-aged adults: a systematic review. Sports Med – Open. 2020;6:7.

Jones JC, Burks R, Owens BD, et al. Incidence and risk factors associated with meniscal injuries among active-duty US military service members. J Athl Train. 2012;47:67–73.

Juhakoski R, Heliovaara M, Impivaara O, et al. Risk factors for the development of hip osteoarthritis: a population-based prospective study. Rheumatology. 2009;48:83–7.

Kellgren JH, Lawrence JS. Radiological assessment of osteo-arthrosis. Ann Rheum Dis. 1957;16:494–502.

Kemp JL, Collins NJ, Roos EM, Crossley KM. Psychometric properties of patient-reported outcome measures for hip arthroscopy. Am J Sports Med. 2013;41:2065–73.

Kemp JL, Makdissi M, Pritchard MG, et al. Chondropathy of the hip at arthroscopy: prevalence and relationship to labral pathology, femoro-acetabular impingement and patient-reported outcomes. Br J Sports Med. 2014;48:1102–7.

Kemp JL, MacDonald D, Collins NJ, et al. Hip arthroscopy in the setting of hip osteoarthritis: systematic review of outcomes and progression to hip arthroplasty. Clin Orthop Relat Res. 2015;473:1055–73.

Kendzerska T, Jüni P, King LK, et al. The longitudinal relationship between hand, hip and knee osteoarthritis and cardiovascular events: a population-based cohort study. Osteoarthritis Cartilage. 2017;25:1771–80.

Kerbel YE, Smith CM, Prodromo JP, et al. Epidemiology of hip and groin injuries in collegiate athletes in the United States. Orthop J Sports Med. 2018;6:2325967118771676.

Khan T, Alvand A, Prieto-Alhambra D, et al. ACL and meniscal injuries increase the risk of primary total knee replacement for osteoarthritis: a matched case-control study using the Clinical Practice Research Datalink (CPRD). Br J Sports Med. 2019;53:965–8.

Kolasinski SL, Neogi T, Hochberg MC, et al. 2019 American College of Rheumatology/Arthritis Foundation Guideline for the Management of Osteoarthritis of the Hand, Hip, and Knee. Arthritis Care Res. 2020;72:149–62.

Kopec JA, Hong Q, Wong H, et al. Prevalence of femoroacetabular impingement syndrome among young and middle-aged white adults. J Rheumatol. 2020;47:1440–5.

Kowalczuk M, Yeung M, Simunovic N, Ayeni O. Does femoroacetabular impingement contribute to the development of hip osteoarthritis? A systematic review. Sports Med Arthrosc Rev. 2015;23:174–9.

Kremers HM, Larson DR, Crowson CS, et al. Prevalence of total hip and knee replacement in the United States. J Bone Joint Surg Am. 2015;97:1386–97.

Kurtz SM, Lau E, Ong K, et al. Future young patient demand for primary and revision joint replacement: national projections from 2010 to 2030. Clin Orthop. 2009; 467:2606–12.

Lai CCH, Ardern CL, Feller JA, Webster KE. Eighty-three per cent of elite athletes return to preinjury sport after anterior cruciate ligament reconstruction: a systematic review with meta-analysis of return to sport rates, graft rupture rates and performance outcomes. Br J Sports Med. 2018;52:128–38.

Langhout R, Weir A, Litjes WG, et al. Hip and groin injury is the most common non-time-loss injury in female amateur football. Knee Surg Sports Traumatol Arthrosc. 2019;27:3133–41.

Lankhorst NE, Bierma-Zeinstra SMA, van Middelkoop M. Risk factors for patellofemoral pain syndrome: a systematic review. J Orthop Sports Phys Ther. 2012;42:81–94.

Larson CM, Safran MR, Brcka DA, et al. Predictors of clinically suspected intra-articular hip symptoms and prevalence of hip pathomorphologies presenting to sports medicine and hip preservation orthopaedic surgeons. Arthrosc J Arthrosc Relat Surg. 2018;34:825–31.

Leunig M, Beaulé PE, Ganz R. The concept of femoroacetabular impingement: current status and future perspectives. Clin Orthop. 2008;467:616–22.

Lo GH, Harvey WF, McAlindon TE. Associations of varus thrust and alignment with pain in knee osteoarthritis. Arthritis Rheum. 2012;64:2252–9.

Losina E, Paltiel AD, Weinstein A, et al. Lifetime medical costs of knee osteoarthritis management in the United States: impact of extending indications for total knee arthroplasty. Arthritis Care Res. 2015;67:203 15.

Louati K, Vidal C, Berenbaum F, Sellam J. Association between diabetes mellitus and osteoarthritis: systematic literature review and meta-analysis. RMD Open. 2015;1:e000077.

Mascarenhas VV, Rego P, Dantas P, et al. Imaging prevalence of femoroacetabular impingement in symptomatic patients, athletes, and asymptomatic individuals: a systematic review. Eur J Radiol. 2016;85:73–95.

McMillan G, Nichols L. Osteoarthritis and meniscus disorders of the knee as occupational diseases of miners. Occup Environ Med. 2005;62:567–75.

Mlynarek RA, Coleman SH. Hip and groin injuries in baseball players. Curr Rev Musculoskelet Med. 2018;11:19–25.

Moisio K, Chang A, Eckstein F, et al. Varus-valgus alignment: reduced risk of subsequent cartilage loss in the less loaded compartment. Arthritis Rheum. 2011;63:1002–9.

Morton S, Williams S, Valle X, et al. Patellar tendinopathy and potential risk factors: an International Database of Cases and Controls. Clin J Sport Med Off J Can Acad Sport Med. 2017;27:468–74.

Mosler AB, Crossley KM, Waarsing JH, et al. Ethnic differences in bony hip morphology in a cohort of 445 professional male soccer players. Am J Sports Med. 2016;44:2967–74.

Mosler AB, Weir A, Eirale C et al. Epidemiology of time loss groin injuries in a men's professional football league: a 2-year prospective study of 17 clubs and 606 players. Br J Sports Med. 2018a;52:292–7.

Mosler AB, Agricola R, Thorborg K, et al. Is bony hip morphology associated with range of motion and strength in asymptomatic male soccer players? J Orthop Sports Phys Ther. 2018b;48:250–9.

Murphy LB, Helmick CG, Schwartz TA, et al. One in four people may develop symptomatic hip osteoarthritis in his or her lifetime. Osteoarthr Cartil OARS Osteoarthr Res Soc. 2010;18:1372–9.

Musahl V, Karlsson J. Anterior cruciate ligament tear. N Engl J Med. 2019;380:2341–8.

Muthuri SG, McWilliams DF, Doherty M, Zhang W. History of knee injuries and knee osteoarthritis: a meta-analysis of observational studies. Osteoarthritis Cartilage. 2011;19:1286–93.

Neal BS, Lack SD, Lankhorst NE, et al. Risk factors for patellofemoral pain: a systematic review and meta-analysis. Br J Sports Med. 2019;53:270–81.

Nepple JJ, Vigdorchik JM, Clohisy JC. What is the association between sports participation and the development of proximal femoral cam deformity?: A systematic review and meta-analysis. Am J Sports Med. 2015;43:2833–40.

Nüesch E, Dieppe P, Reichenbach S, et al. All cause and disease specific mortality in patients with knee or hip osteoarthritis: population based cohort study. BMJ. 2011;342:d1165.

Olsen AL, Magnussen LH, Skjaerven LH, et al. Movement quality evaluation and its correlation with recommended functional measures in hip osteoarthritis. Physiother Res Int. 2020;25:e1848

Orchard JW. Men at higher risk of groin injuries in elite team sports: a systematic review. Br J Sports Med. 2015;49:798–802.

Osteoarthritis Research Society International. Osteoarthritis: a serious disease. Osteoarthritis Cartilage. 2016;1–103.

Padua DA, DiStefano LJ, Hewett TE, et al. National Athletic Trainers' Association Position Statement: Prevention of Anterior Cruciate Ligament Injury. J Athl Train. 2018;53:5–19.

Palmer A, Fernquest S, Gimpel M, et al. Physical activity during adolescence and the development of cam morphology: a cross-sectional cohort study of 210 individuals. Br J Sports Med. 2018;52:601–10.

Pálsson A, Kostogiannis I, Lindvall H, Ageberg E. Hip-related groin pain, patient characteristics and patient-reported outcomes in patients referred to tertiary care due to longstanding hip and groin pain: a cross-sectional study. BMC Musculoskelet Disord. 2019;14;20:432.

Pappas E, Wong-Tom WM. Prospective predictors of patellofemoral pain syndrome: a systematic review with meta-analysis. Sports Health. 2012;4:115–20.

Parks MT, Wang Z, Siu KC. Current low-cost video-based motion analysis options for clinical rehabilitation: a systematic review. Phys Ther. 2019;99:1405–25.

Petrillo S, Papalia R, Maffulli N, et al. Osteoarthritis of the hip and knee in former male professional soccer players. Br Med Bull. 2018;125:121–30.

Petushek EJ, Sugimoto D, Stoolmiller M, et al. Evidence-based best-practice guidelines for preventing anterior cruciate ligament injuries in young female athletes: a systematic review and meta-analysis. Am J Sports Med. 2019;47:1744–53.

Picavet HSJ, Schouten JSAG. Musculoskeletal pain in the Netherlands: prevalences, consequences and risk groups, the DMC3-study. Pain. 2003;102:167–78.

Pollard TCB, Gwilym SE, Carr A. The assessment of early osteoarthritis. J Bone Jt Surg Br. 2008;90B:411–21.

Pritzker KPH, Gay S, Jimenez SA, et al. Osteoarthritis cartilage histopathology: grading and staging. Osteoarthritis Cartilage. 2006;14:13–29.

Rankin AT, Bleakley CM, Cullen M. Hip joint pathology as a leading cause of groin pain in the sporting population: a 6-year review of 894 cases. Am J Sports Med. 2015;43:1698–703.

Rathleff MS, Rathleff CR, Crossley KM, Barton CJ. Is hip strength a risk factor for patellofemoral pain? A systematic review and meta-analysis. Br J Sports Med. 2014;48:1088.

Rathleff MS, Rathleff CR, Olesen JL, et al. Is knee pain during adolescence a self-limiting condition? Prognosis of patellofemoral pain and other types of knee pain. Am J Sports Med. 2016;44:1165–71.

Rauh MJ, Margherita AJ, Rice SG, et al. High school cross country running injuries: a longitudinal study. Clin J Sport Med Off J Can Acad Sport Med. 2000;10:110–16.

Reid CR, Bush PM, Cummings NH, et al. A review of occupational knee disorders. J Occup Rehabil. 2010;20:489–501.

Reiman MP, Agricola R, Kemp JL, et al. Consensus recommendations on the classification, definition and diagnostic criteria of hip-related pain in young and middle-aged active adults from the International Hip-related Pain Research Network, Zurich 2018. Br J Sports Med. 2020;54:631–41.

Rhon DI, Greenlee TA, Marchant BG, et al. Comorbidities in the first 2 years after arthroscopic hip surgery: substantial increases in mental health disorders, chronic pain, substance abuse and cardiometabolic conditions. Br J Sports Med. 2019;53:547–53.

Roe M, Murphy JC, Gissane C, Blake C. Lower limb injuries in men's elite Gaelic football: a prospective investigation among division one teams from 2008 to 2015. J Sci Med Sport. 2018;21:155–9.

Ruano JS, Sitler MR, Driban JB. Prevalence of radiographic knee osteoarthritis after anterior cruciate ligament reconstruction, with or without meniscectomy: an evidence-based practice article. J Athl Train. 2017;52:606–9.

Ryan J, DeBurca N, McCreesh K. Risk factors for groin/hip injuries in field-based sports: a systematic review. Br J Sports Med. 2014;48:1089–96.

Schiphof D, van Middelkoop M, de Klerk BM, et al. Crepitus is a first indication of patellofemoral osteoarthritis (and not of tibiofemoral osteoarthritis). Osteoarthritis Cartilage. 2014;22:631–8.

Schofield D, Schrestha R, Cunich M. Counting the Cost Part 2: Economic Costs: The Current and Future Burden of Arthritis [Internet]. Sydney, Australia: Arthritis Australia; 2016.

Schreurs BW, Hannink G. Total joint arthroplasty in younger patients: heading for trouble? Lancet. 2017;389:1374–5.

Shapira J, Chen JW, Bheem R, et al. Radiographic factors associated with hip osteoarthritis: a systematic review. J Hip Preserv Surg. 2020;7:4-13.

Sharma L, Chmiel JS, Almagor O, et al. The role of varus and valgus alignment in the initial development of knee cartilage damage by MRI: the MOST study. Ann Rheum Dis. 2013;72:235–40.

Sharma L, Chang AH, Jackson RD, et al. Varus thrust and incident and progressive knee osteoarthritis. Arthritis Rheumatol. 2017;69:2136–43.

Siebenrock KA, Ferner F, Noble PC, et al. The cam-type deformity of the proximal femur arises in childhood in response to vigorous sporting activity. Clin Orthop Relat Res. 2011;469:3229–40.

Siebenrock KA, Kaschka I, Frauchiger L, et al. Prevalence of cam-type deformity and hip pain in elite ice hockey players before and after the end of growth. Am J Sports Med. 2013;41:2308–13.

Silverwood V, Blagojevic-Bucknall M, Jinks C, et al. Current evidence on risk factors for knee osteoarthritis in older adults: a systematic review and meta-analysis. Osteoarthritis Cartilage. 2015;23:507–15.

Singh JA, Yu S, Chen L, Cleveland JD. Rates of total joint replacement in the united states: future projections to 2020-2040 Using the National Inpatient Sample. J Rheumatol. 2019;46:1134–40.

Smith BE, Selfe J, Thacker D, et al. Incidence and prevalence of patellofemoral pain: a systematic review and meta-analysis. PLoS One 2018;13:e0190892.

Snoeker BAM, Bakker EWP, Kegel CAT, Lucas C. Risk factors for meniscal tears: a systematic review including meta-analysis. J Orthop Sports Phys Ther. 2013;43:352–67.

Snoeker B, Turkiewicz A, Magnusson K, et al. Risk of knee osteoarthritis after different types of knee injuries in young adults: a population-based cohort study. Br J Sports Med. 2020;54:725–30.

Sprague AL, Smith AH, Knox P, et al. Modifiable risk factors for patellar tendinopathy in athletes: a systematic review and meta-analysis. Br J Sports Med. 2018;52:1575–85.

Stathopulu E, Baildam E. Anterior knee pain: a long-term follow-up. Rheumatol 2003;42:380–2.

Swain S, Sarmanova A, Coupland C, et al. Comorbidities in osteoarthritis: a systematic review and meta-analysis of observational studies. Arthritis Care Res. 2020;72:991–1000.

Tak I, Weir A, Langhout R, et al. The relationship between the frequency of football practice during skeletal growth and the presence of a cam deformity in adult elite football players. Br J Sports Med. 2015;49:630–4.

Tanamas S, Hanna FS, Cicuttini FM, et al. Does knee malalignment increase the risk of development and progression of knee osteoarthritis? A systematic review. Arthritis Rheum. 2009;61:459–67.

Taylor R, Vuckovic Z, Mosler A, et al. Multidisciplinary assessment of 100 athletes with groin pain using the Doha Agreement: high prevalence of adductor-related groin pain in conjunction with multiple causes. Clin J Sport Med. 2018;28:364–9.

Thijssen E, van Caam A, van der Kraan PM. Obesity and osteoarthritis, more than just wear and tear: pivotal roles for inflamed adipose tissue and dyslipidaemia in obesity-induced osteoarthritis. Rheumatology. 2015;54:588–600.

Thorborg K, Hölmich P. Advancing hip and groin injury management: from eminence to evidence. Br J Sports Med. 2013;47:602–5.

Thorborg K, Rathleff MS, Petersen P, et al. Prevalence and severity of hip and groin pain in sub-elite male football: a cross-sectional cohort study of 695 players. Scand J Med Sci Sports. 2017;27:107–14.

Thorborg K, Reiman MP, Weir A, et al. Clinical examination, diagnostic imaging, and testing of athletes with groin pain: an evidence-based approach to effective management. J Orthop Sports Phys Ther. 2018;48: 239–49.

Thorlund JB, Hare KB, Lohmander LS. Large increase in arthroscopic meniscus surgery in the middle-aged and older population in Denmark from 2000 to 2011. Acta Orthop. 2014;85:287–92.

Thorlund JB, Rodriguez Palomino J, Juhl CB, et al. Infographic. Exercise therapy for meniscal tears: evidence and recommendations. Br J Sports Med. 2019;53:315–16.

United States Bone and Joint Initative. The Burden of Musculoskeletal Diseases in the United States (BMUS) [2021 Feb 23]. Available from: https://www.boneandjointburden.org/fourth-edition/iiib10/osteoarthritis

Utting MR, Davies G, Newman JH. Is anterior knee pain a predisposing factor to patellofemoral osteoarthritis? Knee. 2005;12:362–5.

van Klij P, Heerey J, Waarsing JH, Agricola R. The prevalence of cam and pincer morphology and its association with development of hip osteoarthritis. J Orthop Sports Phys Ther. 2018;48:230–8.

Vigdorchik JM, Nepple JJ, Eftekhary N, et al. What is the association of elite sporting activities with the development of hip osteoarthritis? Am J Sports Med. 2017;45:961–4.

Vos T, Lim SS, Abbafati C, et al. Global burden of 369 diseases and injuries in 204 countries and territories, 1990–2019: a systematic analysis for the Global Burden of Disease Study 2019. Lancet. 2020;396:1204–22.

Walden M, Hagglund M, Ekstrand J. The epidemiology of groin injury in senior football: a systematic review of prospective studies. Br J Sports Med. 2015;49:792–7.

Wang X, Perry TA, Arden N, et al. Occupational risk in knee osteoarthritis: a systematic review and meta-analysis of observational studies. Arthritis Care Res. 2020;72:1213–23.

Wang Yuanyuan, Simpson JA, Wluka AE, et al. Is physical activity a risk factor for primary knee or hip replacement due to osteoarthritis? A prospective cohort study. J Rheumatol. 2011;38:350–7.

Weir A, Brukner P, Delahunt E, et al. Doha agreement meeting on terminology and definitions in groin pain in athletes. Br J Sports Med. 2015;49:768–74.

Werner J, Hagglund M, Walden M, Ekstrand J. UEFA injury study: a prospective study of hip and groin injuries in professional football over seven consecutive seasons. Br J Sports Med. 2009;43:1036–40.

Werner J, Hägglund M, Ekstrand J, Waldén M. Hip and groin time-loss injuries decreased slightly but injury burden remained constant in men's professional football: the 15-year prospective UEFA Elite Club Injury Study. Br J Sports Med. 2019;53:539–46.

Whittaker JL, Small C, Maffey L, Emery CA. Risk factors for groin injury in sport: an updated systematic review. Br J Sports Med. 2015;49:803–9.

Whittaker JL, Toomey CM, Woodhouse LJ, et al. Association between MRI-defined osteoarthritis, pain, function and strength 3–10 years following knee joint injury in youth sport. Br J Sports Med. 2018;52:934–9.

Williams A, Kamper SJ, Wiggers JH, et al. Musculoskeletal conditions may increase the risk of chronic disease: a systematic review and meta-analysis of cohort studies. BMC Med. 2018;16:167.

Willy RW, Hoglund LT, Barton CJ, et al. Patellofemoral pain. J Orthop Sports Phys Ther. 2019;49:CPG1–95.

Witvrouw E, Lysens R, Bellemans J, et al. Intrinsic risk factors for the development of anterior knee pain in an athletic population. A two-year prospective study. Am J Sports Med. 2000;28:480–9.

van der Worp H, van Ark M, Roerink S, et al. Risk factors for patellar tendinopathy: a systematic review of the literature. Br J Sports Med. 2011;45:446–52.

Yeh PC, Starkey C, Lombardo S, et al. Epidemiology of isolated meniscal injury and its effect on performance in athletes from the National Basketball Association. Am J Sports Med. 2012;40:589–94.

Yu B, Garrett WE. Mechanisms of non-contact ACL injuries. Br J Sports Med. 2007;41:S47-51.

Yucesoy B, Charles LE, Baker B, Burchfiel CM. Occupational and genetic risk factors for osteoarthritis: a review. Work Read Mass. 2015;50:261–73.

Zaltz I, Kelly BT, Hetsroni I, Bedi A. The crossover sign overestimates acetabular retroversion. Clin Orthop. 2013;471:2463–70.

Zwerver J, Bredeweg SW, van den Akker-Scheek I. Prevalence of jumper's knee among nonelite athletes from different sports: a cross-sectional survey. Am J Sports Med. 2011;39:1984–8.

Clinical reasoning for hip and knee tendinopathies

2

Ebonie Rio, Susan Mayes, Katia Ferrar, Craig Purdam, Michael Freeman, Jill Cook

Introduction

Tendinopathy is the clinical presentation of pain and dysfunction within a tendon. Tendon pathology is usually present; however, tendon pathology can exist without symptoms. Tendon pathology results in disruption of the structure of the tendon matrix and a change in the cells and matrix proteins. The transition of a tendon from normal to a degenerative pathology is a progressive change. The continuum of tendon pathology is a conceptual model of four stages of pathology to describe this transition: reactive tendon pathology, tendon dysrepair, degenerative tendinopathy, and reactive on degenerative (Cook & Purdam, 2009; Cook et al., 2016). Tendon structure can be normalized in the early stages but is not possible in the latter stages of the continuum.

The model aims to assist clinicians in understanding tendinopathy presentations and direct their management (Cook & Purdam 2009). The primary focus at every stage is improving pain and function. Recent reflections on the model support its usefulness as a clinical reasoning framework to enhance clinician understanding and guide diagnosis and management of tendinopathy (Cook et al., 2016). Specifically, the ability to integrate tendon structure with pain, dysfunction and load capacity may allow clinicians to target treatment at the critical limiting factors. The aim of treatment is to reduce load-related pain and improve function; these are closely connected.

Clinical Reasoning for Tendon Interventions

Interventions Targeting Structure

The reactive stage provides a possible opportunity to influence tendon structure with interventions such as reducing provocative loads and identifying dysfunction. In the degenerative stage, interventions targeting structural change reversal are unsuccessful (Drew et al., 2014). There is evidence in the patellar and Achilles tendons that a degenerative tendon appears to adapt through an increase in cross-sectional area to maintain sufficient volumes of load-bearing tissue (Docking & Cook, 2016). However, this may differ between tendons. For example, it does not appear to be the case for the gluteus medius or tibialis posterior tendon. The goal is to always improve function and the mechanisms may differ between tendons.

Interventions Targeting Pain

Clinically, tendon pain occurs in the reactive pathology stages (1) reactive tendon and (2) reactive-on-degenerative tendon pathology; both can occur following acute or persistent overload (Cook & Purdam, 2009; Cook et al., 2016). This strongly suggests that reactive tendon pathology has an unidentified local nociceptive driver.

The nerve supply of tendons is mainly in the peritendon structures. It is important to remember that interventions directed solely at pain will not result in a positive outcome as they do not address dysfunction, such as motor inhibition, strength and power deficits, or tendon load capacity. Low to moderate evidence supports the use of non-exercise-based interventions such as non-steroidal anti-inflammatory drugs, corticosteroid injections, extracorporeal shockwave therapy, low-level laser therapy, and minimally invasive surgical procedures for pain relief. Long-term effectiveness is variable and long-term use is contraindicated in some interventions (e.g., non-steroidal anti-inflammatories) (Irby et al., 2020). Isometric exercise may be an exercise-based short-term analgesic option, with the approach supported by evidence in the lower limb for patellar tendinopathy (Rio et al., 2015; Van Ark et al., 2016; Rio et al., 2019) and gluteal tendinopathy (Clifford et al., 2019), and clinical experience of the authors for other tendons.

Interventions Targeting Function and Load Capacity

Research has looked at different contraction types, in different scenarios (for example in-season or rehabilitation) and for different periods of time (Lim & Wong, 2018). No single contraction type will be sufficient for long-term clinical improvement and evidence-based management should include progressive load specific to the individual (Breda et al., 2021). There are also situations where certain contraction types are to be avoided; for example, the original research in eccentric exercise and patellar tendinopathy supported its use; however, when eccentric exercises have been used in athletes participating in-season, they have been provocative (Visnes et al., 2006). The tensile load and loading rate of the Achilles and patellar tendons in the athletic pursuits of running and jumping are far greater than during normal ambulation. This often requires a staged approach to progression of tensile loads, rate of loading and volume of these activities for a successful and sustained return to sport (Breda et al., 2021).

Diagnostic Considerations

Clinical Features of Tendinopathy

Tendinopathies can present with similar clinical features, regardless of the body location. These clinical features are useful for clinicians as they assist with the diagnosis and consideration of differential diagnoses. There are common clinical features consistent across (almost all) hip and knee tendinopathies (Table 2.1).

Imaging and Tendinopathy

As our understanding of tendinopathy improves, the clinical utility of imaging modalities such as ultrasound and magnetic resonance imaging (MRI) is questioned. Ultrasound and MRI have been used to diagnose and monitor tendinopathy

TABLE 2.1 Common Tendinopathy: Clinical Findings	
Subjective Clinical Findings	
Body chart	Localized pain in the tendon that does not refer. The exception is gluteus medius, which can have a wider distribution (usually not past the knee). Generally, in lower limb tendinopathy larger or spreading distribution of pain should raise the possibility of a different diagnosis.
Pain behavior	Present with "warm-up phenomenon." The tendon may be sore to start activity, respond variably to warm-up (from completely relieving symptoms to little improvement) and will then be worse the next day, which can persist for several days. Tendon pain occurs with loading and eases when the load is removed.
Palpation	Localized pain on tendon palpation is diagnostically useful for few lower limb tendinopathies (see tendon-specific sections).
Inflammatory symptoms	Night pain and morning stiffness are rarely reported, unless the symptoms are severe (again gluteus medius is the exception due to compression).
Aggravating activities	Pain during tendon-loading tasks. Energy storage and release and compressive loads are the most provocative. Combination loads can be especially aggravating.
History	Identification of the tendon overload. If there is no identifiable change in load history, an alternative diagnosis may be considered.
Objective Clinical Findings	
Observation	Muscle wasting in tendon-associated muscle and anti-gravity muscles below the level of the tendinopathy.
Pain provocation	Localized tendon pain reproduced with specific tendon-loading activities, especially energy storage and release and compression. Tendinopathy pain increases with higher rate of application of tendon load e.g., faster running (Achilles) or decelerations/landing (patellar tendon).
Function	Kinetic chain function is often affected, and deficits are apparent.

and tendon pathology. However, like other musculoskeletal conditions such as osteoarthritis and non-specific low back pain, there is no direct link between tendon abnormality on imaging and symptoms (Docking et al., 2015).

Clinical Reasoning Key Points

- Tendon abnormalities on imaging do not confirm that the pain and dysfunction are necessarily related to the tendon.

- Clinical history, pain localization and examination including load provocation provide the most robust determination of a diagnosis of tendinopathy.

- A normal tendon (on imaging) rules out the tendon as a source of pain and dysfunction.

- Imaging does not provide the entire clinical picture in tendinopathy and should not be used as a sole diagnostic criterion.

- Structural disorganization identified on imaging should be considered as part of a risk profile for tendinopathy, like that of load, genetics and anthropometric factors (Malliaras & O'Neill, 2017).

- There are no consistent relationships (intervention study results) between changes in tendon structure and changes in function and pain in tendinopathy (Docking et al., 2015). Imaging to monitor treatment efficacy is not recommended or supported by high-level evidence.

- Imaging may be useful in the differential diagnosis.

Stages of Tendon Rehabilitation

A four-stage progressive rehabilitation program for tendinopathy is proposed, based on available evidence and the clinical experience of the authors (Figure 2.1). The functional requirements of the patient, whether that be elite sport or recreational hobbies, dictate the start and end point of the plan.

Stage 1: Isometric Exercise, Education and Tendon Response Monitoring

Isometric exercises are indicated to reduce and manage tendon pain and initiate loading of the muscle–tendon unit or

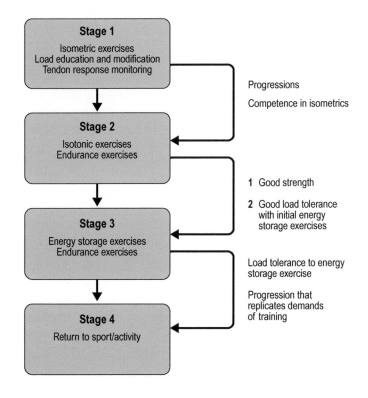

FIGURE 2.1
Stages of tendon rehabilitation. Note: progression criteria are tailored to the individual patient based on pain, function and strength.

fear may limit the ability to perform isotonic exercises. A good prognostic sign for isometrics is an immediate reduction in pain with loading tests after isometric exercise. It is important that there be good muscle control during the isometric exercises; the load must be high but not exceed muscle capacity (for example, no shaking during the contraction).

This stage should be the priority when managing individuals with a high level of irritability. Other exercises, such as to address other strength deficits (Stage 2) throughout the lower extremity, can also be initiated during Stage 1.

Load education and modification. Education is essential to ensure the patient understands how tendons respond to load, how their condition developed and the proposed tendinopathy management plan. When a patient embraces an understanding that tendon pain increases with excessive tendon loading, this may provide a basis to then modify loading to reduce symptoms.

Tendon response monitoring. Tendon rehabilitation may be uncomfortable at times, but the authors do not advocate painful rehabilitation. The tendon response in the 24 hours after activity subjectively and on an objective test (e.g., decline squat for patellar tendinopathy) is the most important gauge of progression. If pain increases, the loading (or diagnosis) is wrong. It is acceptable if the pain response stays the same while load increases. The ideal scenario is a reduction of pain with increasing load. Listening to the tendon is critical for exercise prescription and progression, and to enable the patient to self-monitor and modify activity to minimize pain.

Stage 2: Isotonic Exercises

Loaded isotonic exercise is initiated when isometric exercises are well controlled. Isotonic load is important to restore muscle bulk strength and endurance through functional ranges. Stage 1 exercises can be continued to manage pain. A positive response to regular reassessment of pain with load tests continues to be important.

Stage 3: Energy Storage Exercises

Reintroduction of energy-storage loads on the myotendinous unit and kinetic chain is critical to increase load tolerance and improve power as a progression to return to sport and activity. Initiating this stage is based on the following strength and pain criteria: (1) good strength and endurance as necessary; and (2) good load tolerance with initial energy-storage exercises, defined as minimal pain while performing the exercises, and return to baseline pain (if there was an initial increase) during 24-hour load tests, such as the single-leg decline squat.

As with the other stages, individualization and clinical reasoning are necessary. In addition, progression should be developed based on the individual's sport or activity-specific load requirements.

Stage 4: Return to Sport/Activity

Progression back to sport or activity-specific training can be commenced when the individual has completed energy-storage progressions that replicate the demands of their sport or activity. At that time, Stage 3 exercises are replaced by a graded return to activity (i.e., volume and intensity of relevant energy-storage functions) or training and

eventually competition (for sportspeople). Stage 2 exercises should be continued throughout rehabilitation and return to sport/activity.

Return to sport is recommened when full training is tolerated without symptom provocation (24-hour response on load test, such as the single-leg decline squat) and any existing strength, endurance, and power deficits have been resolved.

In-season Rehabilitation

Managing tendinopathy during the sporting or elite performing season can be very challenging for the clinician and the patient. The demands of training and competitions can make conventional load reduction and rehabilitation programs unsuitable. Management strategies that control pain and maintain performance are required.

Load Management: The most common in-season tendinopathy presentation would be reactive on degenerative tendinopathy. The key intervention should be to reduce the activation and/or sensitization of the tenocytes by reducing high loads. The total load and contribution of different load types need to be considered when managing in-season tendinopathy. Excessive or rapid increases in tensile load need to be avoided. Compressive loads, which are greater in outer muscle ranges, can be detrimental, particularly in combination with high tensile loads. Reduction in compressive loads while maintaining tensile loading can be useful. This can be achieved by reducing loads in outer muscle ranges, which reduces compression of the tendon against the proximal bone. Reduction of the volume of these provocative activities as well as avoidance of stretching related muscles can also reduce overall compressive loads (Cook & Purdam, 2012).

Loading to manage pain should occur early in management. Isometric loading, as described in Stage 1 of conventional tendinopathy rehabilitation, can be used to trigger analgesia (see Stage 1: Isometric Exercise, Education and Tendon Response Monitoring). Moderate to heavy loads with machine-based weights rarely provoke pain (Stage 2). These exercises should be completed in the mid to inner range of the muscle–tendon unit to reduce compression load. In-season eccentric loading programs (e.g., decline board program) can irritate tendinopathy (Visnes et al., 2006 Fredberg et al., 2008) and should be avoided.

Greater Trochanteric Pain Syndrome (GTPS)/Gluteal Tendinopathy

Pathology in the gluteus medius and minimus enthesis that causes lateral hip pain has several clinical names, none of which reflect the condition well. These terms include trochanteric bursitis, gluteus medius tendinopathy and gluteal tendon pain syndrome. The pathology occurs in the gluteal tendons (both gluteus medius and gluteal minimus) in the area of the attachment of the tendon to the greater trochanter. As with most entheseal attachments the tendons pass over a bony prominence (the trochanter) to attach just below. The tendons appose the trochanter and there are adaptations in and around the tendon to ameliorate this contact, including fibrocartilage in the tendon, extensive bursae and cartilage on the bone surface (Benjamin et al., 2004). Excess apposition due to poor pelvic control, excessive hip adduction in walking or running and direct compression (side-lying) can cause pathology in the tendon and bursa; these changes occur simultaneously and isolated changes in one structure only are rare. Because women have a greater femoral neck to shaft angle (termed Q angle) they are more susceptible to GTPS than men and the greater this angle the more likelihood of progressed pathology (Fearon et al., 2012). Extensive pathology can result in complete tears of some or all of the tendons.

Clinical Presentation

Post-menopausal women most often present with symptoms. It can present in older men and in younger active people, but it is less common and seems not to be as disabling or chronic. The presentation can be variable, depending on length of symptoms, age, body weight, comorbidities and activity levels (Table 2.2).

Examination

Most examination can be done in standing with simple functional tests. Testing for function, strength and pain can be done with a double or single leg sit to stand, heel raise test and hip hitch test.

If needed, supine clinical tests such as the external derotation test, the same test started in a position of flexion/adduction (modified external derotation test), the flexion, abduction, external rotation (FABER) test, palpation over the greater trochanter and the Trendelenburg test (standing on one leg for 30 seconds) have been shown to be sensitive tests for this condition (Ganderton et al., 2017; Lequesne et al., 2008).

The Victorian Institute of Sports Assessment for Gluteal Tendinopathy (VISA-G) documents pain, dysfunction and exercise tolerance (Fearon et al., 2015) and has been shown to be sensitive for this condition.

Differential Diagnosis

Because of their age and comorbidities, differential diagnosis is critical in this age group and often difficult as there may be more than one source of pain. Hip joint osteoarthritis is common and can cause pain in the same region, but specific questioning about pain and aggravating activities can be helpful to decide how much pain is from the tendons and how much from the joint. Clinical examination that shows deficits in the range of hip joint movement and/or pain on movement generally indicates joint involvement, as this is not found in those with pain in the gluteal tendons. Caution is advised, however, as pain provoked by hip joint examination may not necessarily be the pain they are experiencing, so careful questioning and accurate examination is important.

Similarly, low back pain can refer to the same area as in GTPS and hip joint arthritis. Again, low back pain is prevalent in this age group, but is more difficult to differentiate as signs and symptoms of low back pain are less clearly defined. These three main differential diagnoses can be present together, requiring excellent clinical skills for diagnosis, and management of all pain sources is important for a positive outcome.

Patients may present with a diagnosis of trochanteric bursitis, often previously treated with corticosteroid injection. As with all entheseal pathology and pain, the bursa cannot solely be the source of pain: the enthesis organ (the tendon, the bursa and other structures) is involved and management must include all structures. Solely managing the bursa results in short term benefits with poor longer-term outcomes.

Rehabilitation

Treatment is directed at improving strength, endurance and power in the affected gluteal muscle–tendon unit but

TABLE 2.2 Clinical Findings of Greater Trochanteric Pain Syndrome (GTPS)/Gluteal Tendinopathy	
Subjective Clinical Findings	
Body chart	The pain is mostly felt in the region of the greater trochanter but can spread down the lateral side of the thigh because of bursal involvement.
Pain behavior	Sufferers report night pain as their biggest symptom. Sleeping on their side can cause them to wake often and prevent getting to sleep (due to compression). Sleeping on the back can assist but rolling to one side can wake them again.
Aggravating activities	Sleeping on their side and rolling over.
	They dislike single-leg stance, getting up from a chair and stair climbing. They are also wary of slopes, all these activities can be painful, and difficult because of progressive dysfunction. This pain and dysfunction can be severe enough to affect activities of daily living such as shopping, gardening and housework, and they are as disabled as someone with severe osteoarthritis of the hip waiting for hip replacement surgery (Fearon et al., 2014).
History	Older women, mostly post-menopausal, present with this condition, usually after change in activity (a walking holiday after retirement) or circumstance (after a knee or hip replacement). Increased loading either from a stable base (a holiday) or from a position of dysfunction (long term hip pain that reduces capacity for walking until a joint replacement makes walking easier and less painful) are common presentations. The condition can be bilateral but often one hip is worse, it can also shift from hip to hip as unloading strategies relieve one hip only to overload the other.
Objective Clinical Findings	
Observation	Muscle wasting in gluteal muscles, and often in quadriceps and calf muscles.
	Trendelenburg gait.
Palpation	Localized pain on tendon palpation (Ganderton et al., 2017).
Pain provocation	Localized tendon pain reproduced with tendon loading activities such as stairs, single-leg stance and rising from a chair.
Function	The most severely affected have gait changes (most commonly a Trendelenburg gait).
Imaging	Imaging of the hip can show pathology in several structures and may not help determine the source of pain (see Imaging and Tendinopathy). Tendons accumulate pathology over the lifespan and the gluteal tendons are no exception, a normal tendon is rare in women older than 60 (Ganderton et al., 2017). Hence findings of pathology in the gluteal tendons does not mean they are the source of pain as many women with pathology have no symptoms. Importantly serial imaging to determine if pathology is resolving is pointless, tendon/entheseal improvements on imaging are absent or minimal and not related to changes in symptoms.

also the kinetic chain (particularly the quadriceps and calf muscles). All exercises must be performed without compressive loads at the enthesis; persistent attention to pelvic positioning to avoid adduction of the leg on the pelvis is essential. Although single-leg exercises are essential for most tendon rehabilitation, this is a case for bilateral exercises early as it reduces the potential for compressive loads on the gluteal tendons.

Gluteal rehabilitation can start with isometric exercises (see Stages of Tendon Rehabilitation), simply lifting the unaffected leg off the ground a minimal amount and holding for a reasonable time (30–45 seconds repeated 5 times) can begin the strength process and relieve pain. This is a simple strategy that can be performed before aggravating activities, e.g., before bed, shopping, stairs.

Once isometrics are performed reasonably, then adding exercises that further challenge the gluteals (Stage 2) such as lifting the unaffected leg higher, hip hitches (Figure 2.2), swinging the unaffected leg (i.e., hip flexion/extension swing) or beginning a stair-climbing exercise can be commenced (Ganderton et al., 2018). Attention to the required strength and endurance endpoint is critical, rehabilitating beyond required capacity is pointless as gains in strength are lost once exercise stops.

Kinetic chain rehabilitation of the quads and calf is essential and can be started early in rehabilitation as load on the gluteal tendon is low and not provocative. Simple sit to stand exercises from a higher chair and heel raise exercises are a good place to start especially in those with low levels of strength. Wall slides can be added when quadriceps

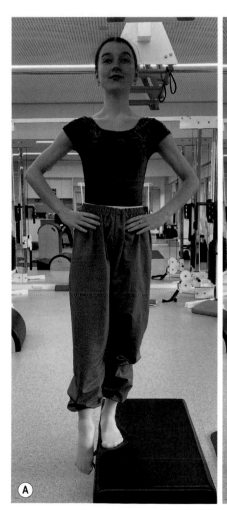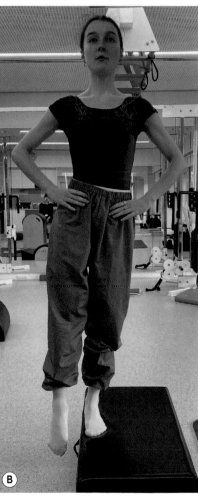

FIGURE 2.2
Hip hitches.

strength improves and increasing the number of calf raises to improve their strength endurance is also beneficial. If the person is more active or requires rehabilitation to return to higher level activities, then a gym program that includes heavy slow resistance training of all muscles will accelerate strength gains to the required level.

Rehabilitation of faster loads is rarely required because of the population with this condition; again this is specific to the person. Simple jumping and hopping exercises (Stage 3) are sufficient to recover enough power and endurance for most; this is extended if demands are high.

Education is essential and can be sufficient to get clinical improvement. Avoiding compressive loads such as crossing legs in sitting, sitting in low chairs, standing with a hip drop on one side, and lying on the side in bed can make a marked difference to symptoms. Further education on the role of imaging, the need for passive interventions and the disconnect between pathology and pain is always helpful.

Adductor-related Groin Pain/Adductor Tendinopathy

Clinical Presentation

Adductor tendinopathy is a common overuse injury seen in athletes participating in sports involving running, sprinting, change of direction and kicking. The Doha agreement (Weir et al., 2015) recommends using the term adductor-related groin pain instead of adductor tendinopathy. The adductor longus is the most common adductor muscle prone to adductor-related groin pain. Table 2.3 summarizes clinical presentation of adductor-related groin pain.

Examination

Contraction and strength assessment are critical in determining the severity of the injury and degree of impairment. Pain on contraction testing should be felt in the adductor muscles, whereas pain felt in other areas of the hip or groin are more suggestive of other possible causes (Weir et al., 2015). Adductor contraction tests for groin pain are both reliable and reproducible (Hölmich et al., 2004). Contraction and strength tests include squeeze tests at varying degrees of hip flexion (usually 0, 45 and 90 degrees), resisted adduction at 0 degrees hip flexion (both from a neutral and

abducted hip position), and resisted adduction at 45 degrees hip flexion (both from a neutral and abducted hip position). Typically, the patient will have symptoms with stretching the adductor muscle with passive hip abduction in both hip neutral and hip flexed positions. A comprehensive strength assessment of the patient with adductor-related groin pain should also involve the abdominals, quadriceps, hamstrings, calf, and foot intrinsics.

The Hip and Groin Outcome Score (HAGOS) is a recommended patient-reported outcome measure for young to middle-aged individuals with groin pain (Thorborg et al., 2011, 2015).

Differential Diagnosis

Groin pain is complex and involves a large number of different anatomical structures within a small area. The Doha agreement (Weir et al., 2011) categorizes groin pain into three main subheadings:

1. Defined clinical entities (including adductor-related, iliopsoas-related, pubic-related and inguinal-related)

2. Hip joint-related

3. Other causes of groin pain in athletes.

These subheadings should be considered with respect to diagnosis and it is important to remember that multiple entities can be present. Other causes of groin pain, such as referred pain from the lumbar spine or sacroiliac joint, nerve entrapment, stress fracture, osteoarthritis and red flags such as tumors, should be ruled out. In children and adolescents, apophysitis, slipped capital femoral epiphysis and Perthes disease should be considered.

Rehabilitation

Load management involves modification of running activities such as total volume, speed, acceleration, and change of direction. Modification in the type and amount of jumping, kicking and other skills-based training may be indicated. In more severe cases early load management may involve a short period of complete rest from activity to settle pain levels.

There is moderate evidence for exercise-based rehabilitation for adductor-related groin pain compared with passive interventions (Serner et al., 2015). In the early stages

TABLE 2.3 Clinical Presentation of Adductor-related Groin Pain/Adductor Tendinopathy

Subjective Clinical Findings

Body chart	The pain is usually quite specific to the proximal adductor region of the medial thigh, most commonly the adductor longus tendon. The anatomical crossover with other structures in the groin can cause more diffuse symptoms, particularly distal into the medial thigh (Thorborg et al., 2018).
Pain behavior	Present with "warm-up phenomenon." Symptoms are strongly related to the intensity of activity, i.e., amount of sprinting, change of direction, and kicking.
Aggravating activities	Exercise, most commonly running (especially sprinting and change of direction) and kicking, aggravate symptoms.
History	Pain generally presents insidiously during exercise. A specific incident resulting in acute pain may be an acute adductor muscle strain. An acute spike in training load in the preceding weeks leading up to the injury is a common presentation, e.g., pre-season training or after a long layoff from exercise. This can include increases in volume or intensity or introduction of a new type of activity.

Objective Clinical Findings

Observation	Muscle wasting of the adductors and gluteals on the same side may be present. Muscle guarding of the affected adductors may also be present.
Palpation	Specific palpation is important given the number of anatomical structures present in the groin. There will be tenderness at the proximal adductor region of the medial thigh, most commonly at the adductor longus tendon, and this assessment technique has been shown to be both reliable and reproducible (Hölmich et al., 2004). Tenderness upon palpation should be the pain the individual identifies as their injury pain.
Pain provocation	Pain on adductor palpation and adductor pain on contraction testing are both required for adductor-related groin pain diagnosis (Weir et al., 2015). Individuals with groin pain will usually present with some level of functional impairment. There are no current evidence-based standardized functional assessments for adductor-related groin pain (Thorborg et al., 2018); however, common provocative functional activities include squatting, lunging, hopping, running, change of direction running and kicking.
Function	Reduced speed and a loss of power with accelerating, sprinting, jumping and kicking are often present. Trendelenburg sign and dynamic knee valgus during the stance phase of running are common presentations. Weak or pain inhibited adductor muscles on resisted testing (Thorborg et al., 2014).
Imaging	There is poor correlation between imaging findings and clinical signs and symptoms of adductor-related groin pain (Branci et al., 2015) and pathological findings on imaging in asymptomatic individuals are common. Therefore, imaging findings should not be used in isolation when diagnosing adductor-related groin pain. Imaging is more commonly utilized to identify alternate diagnoses.

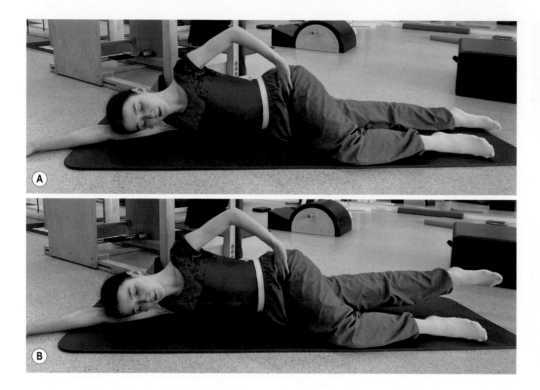

FIGURE 2.3
Copenhagen adductor strengthening exercise level 1. (**A**) Starting position. (**B**) Lifting the lower extremity.

of rehabilitation, the focus is on reducing pain with Stage 1–2 exercises and addressing deficits in other lower limb muscle groups. Examples of specific Stage 1 adductor exercises include adductor squeeze isometrics (see Chapter 19), standing hip adductor slide isometrics, and side-lying adductor isometrics (Copenhagen level 1, Figure 2.3).

Strength and endurance (Stage 2) are added as the patient progresses. The focus needs to be on all muscular groups, but specific adductor exercises commonly include Copenhagen adductor exercises (Figures 2.4–2.5) and standing hip adduction with resistance band or cable. The Copenhagen adductor strength program has been shown to both improve eccentric adductor strength (Pérez-Gómez et al., 2020) and reduce risk of onset of groin pain in male football players (Harøy et al., 2019).

Following strength and endurance-based rehabilitation the individual progresses towards more power-based (Stage 3) and functional exercises in preparation for full and unrestricted return to sport or other activities (Stage 4). This should be specifically tailored to the individual and can include plyometric exercises such as jump and land practice, running-based drills including acceleration, deceleration, change of direction and high-speed running building

up towards maximal sprinting, and sport-specific drills. In sports involving kicking, loads need to be appropriately progressed in terms of distance and intensity of kicking given the load placed on the adductor longus during maximal kicking efforts as the hip flexes from a maximally hip-extended position (Charnock et al., 2009).

Manual therapy particularly of hypertonic muscles may be of benefit for symptom management and return to sport (Serner et al., 2015) but should only be used as an adjunct to a high-quality rehabilitation program.

Patellar Tendinopathy

Patellar tendinopathy, or "jumper's knee," is the diagnosis of dysfunction and pain in the patellar tendon. Patellar tendinopathy is a condition seen in young highly loaded athletes, specifically those who play fast jumping and change of direction sports such as volleyball and basketball. Patellar tendinopathy can affect quality of life, limiting sporting participation and activities of daily living (e.g., stairs and stand to sit). Patellar tendinopathy is a small sub-group of anterior knee pain even in sports such as basketball where high prevalence of patellofemoral pain is seen (Hannington et al., 2020).

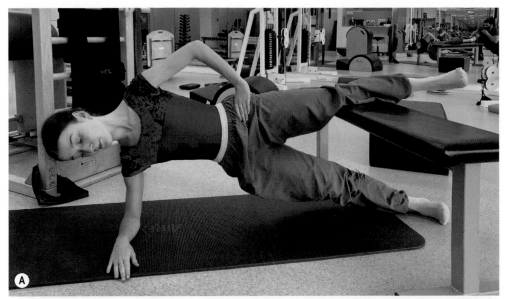

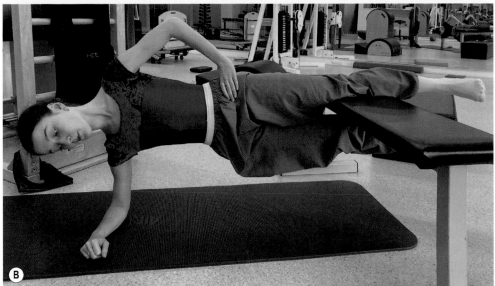

FIGURE 2.4
Copenhagen adductor strengthening exercise level 2. (A) Starting position. (B) Lifting the lower extremity.

That is, even in a jumping sport, one should not assume it is "jumper's knee."

Clinical Presentation

The clinical presentation of patellar tendinopathy refers to localized pain at the inferior pole of the patella during high patellar tendon loads (Coombes et al., 2020; Malliaras et al., 2015) (Table 2.4). The athlete with patellar tendinopathy is most commonly young, elite and male as they are capable of generating high patellar tendon loads in their sport (even accounting for muscle mass), and have greater volume of these loads during their training week (male volleyball athletes have been shown to jump more than women) (Lian et al., 2003, 2005; van der Worp et al., 2012).

Examples of high patellar tendon load include maximal jumping, particularly counter movement jump seen in volleyball or a "pull up jump shot" in basketball (though patellar tendinopathy is more common in volleyball) (van der Worp et al., 2012). Fast lunging as a strategy for change of direction where the tibia goes forward of the ankle and the

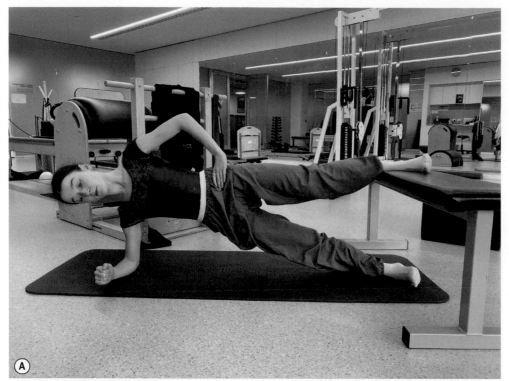

FIGURE 2.5
Copenhagen adductor
strengthening exercise
level 3. (A) Starting position.
(B) Lifting the lower
extremity.

(A)

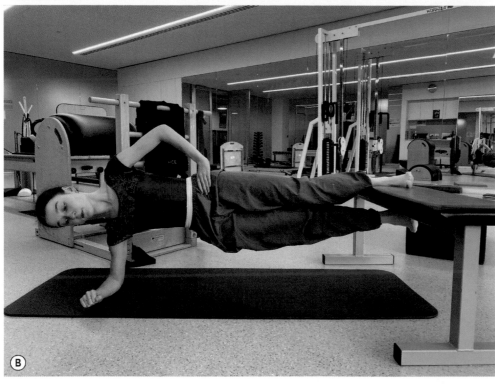

(B)

TABLE 2.4 Clinical Findings of Patellar Tendinopathy	
Subjective Clinical Findings	
Body chart	Pain location remains at the inferior pole during testing. There is no mid-portion patellar tendinopathy.
Pain behavior	The pain is localized and does not move or spread with loading. Pain increases with loaded activities that place demand on the knee extensors, particularly in activities that store and release energy in the patellar tendon. The "warm-up phenomenon" is distinctive in patellar tendinopathy.
Aggravating activities	Pain is reported with activities with demand on the knee extensors and patellar tendon-related energy-storage activities, e.g., jump/landing and changing directions. Pain with prolonged sitting, squatting, and stairs, may be present. Sustained end of range extension and sustained knee flexion (sitting) may be uncomfortable. Pain at rest or during low tendon loads (such as cycling, walking) is uncommon and suggests another diagnosis.
History	Individuals will report tendon overload such as an increase of load from a stable base (e.g., participation in a high-volume competition, tournament or performance) or returning to normal training/activity after a significant period of rest or downtime (e.g., return to training after injury or off-season).
Objective Clinical Findings	
Observation	Wasting of quadriceps and calf muscles (especially gastrocnemius) on the same side.
Palpation	Tenderness on palpation is a poor diagnostic criterion and should not be used as an outcome measure (Cook et al., 2001). The patellar tendon is known to be sensitive in other knee conditions including patellofemoral pain and even osteoarthritis thus tenderness can be misleading and result in a false positive diagnosis of tendinopathy.
Pain provocation	Single-leg decline squat (SLDS) test at 25° (see Figure 2.6) is used for diagnosis and to monitor response to interventions. Other types of anterior knee pain can be provoked with the SLDS test so pain location and pain behavior must also be considered.
Function	Poor leg spring function with knee stiffness and poor energy absorption in the ankle and hip. Deficits in squatting, lunging, and cutting/changing direction may also be evident.
Imaging	Imaging can also be misleading in diagnosis as changes in the patellar tendon likely represent loading history in jump–land sports, particularly during the athlete's pubertal growth years (Ducher et al., 2010; Rudavsky et al., 2018). Repeat imaging is not indicated in tendinopathy as changes in pain do not correlate with changes on imaging (van Ark et al., 2018). A normal tendon essentially rules out tendinopathy. Imaging is therefore not required to make a diagnosis and the potential negative impact of imaging should be carefully considered.

athlete springs back in another direction using their patellar tendon as a key spring in the movement is also high patellar tendon load, and can be seen in net play in tennis, lunging, deceleration, and change of direction in basketball. Importantly, activities such as cycling and jogging are not high loads for the patellar tendon (but are for the Achilles tendon and patellofemoral joint) (Willy et al., 2016). This is clinically helpful to assist consideration in how likely patellar tendinopathy is as a diagnosis based on the sport or activity the individual participates in, their gender, and age.

Examination

A key test is the single-leg decline squat (SLDS) (Figure 2.6). While standing on the affected leg on a 25° decline board, the patient is asked to maintain an upright trunk and squat up to 90° knee flexion if possible. The test is conducted on the unaffected leg also for comparison. Maximum knee flexion achieved (degrees) is recorded, at which point pain score is recorded on a visual analog scale. The pain should remain localized to the tendon and should replicate the individual's pain. It is the authors' experience that while the SLDS provokes many different types of anterior knee pain including patellar tendinopathy and patellofemoral pain, there are differences between these presentations. Clinicians must observe the degrees/depth achieved before pain provocation; it is frequently shallow in patellar tendinopathy and deeper in patellofemoral joint pain and secondly, patellar tendinopathy pain location remains focal at the inferior pole during SLDS, whereas patellofemoral joint pain can move and be diffuse depending on joint compression.

Kinetic chain functional tests based on the patient history and aggravating activities include single-leg hop tests, jumping tests, landing techniques and change in direction tasks. Evidence (Bisseling et al., 2008; Van der Worp et al., 2014) and the clinical experience of the authors suggests athletes with patellar tendinopathy and pain tend to reduce the amount of knee flexion and appear stiff in their landing or jumps and hops. Video/biomechanical analysis can help with more nuanced analysis of elite athletes' movement patterns. Foot posture/alignment (Crossley et al., 2007), quadriceps and hamstring flexibility (Witvrouw et al., 2001) as well as weight-bearing ankle dorsiflexion range of motion (Malliaras et al., 2006) have been associated with patellar tendinopathy and should also be assessed.

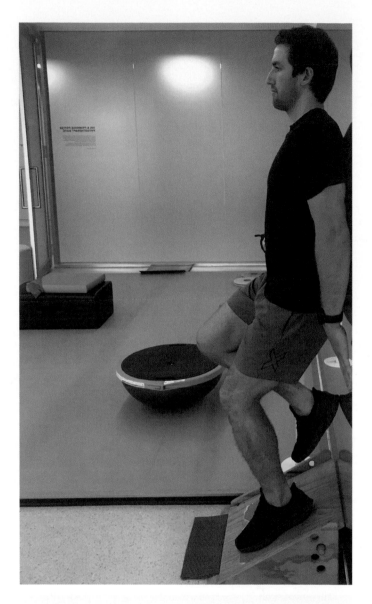

FIGURE 2.6
Single-leg decline squat (SLDS).

Other sport-specific testing may include progressive change of direction at speed, deceleration, jumping and hopping and will be tailored to the individual and their stage of rehabilitation. The Victorian Institute of Sport Assessment patella (VISA-P) questionnaire (Visentini et al., 1998) is a validated pain and function outcome measure that can also be used to assess severity of symptoms as well as to monitor outcomes (Korakakis et al., 2021).

Differential Diagnosis

In runners, older athletes, low patellar tendon load activities and females, the evidence suggests patellofemoral pain is far more common in the patient with atraumatic anterior knee pain (Zwerver et al., 2011). Specific questions to ascertain what loads and what activities cause pain are critical as there are similarities in provocative activities for patellofemoral pain and patellar tendinopathy (for example stairs can be uncomfortable for both conditions). Palpation pain alone is misleading in patellar tendinopathy (Cook et al., 2001) as the patellar tendon can be sensitive in other anterior knee conditions including patellofemoral pain, osteoarthritis, and indeed even athletes without symptoms have been shown to be sensitive.

The single-leg decline squat board at 25° is a pain provocation test for the anterior knee, and athletes must be questioned where their pain is during this test as this will also provoke other anterior knee pain such as patellofemoral pain (Purdam et al., 2003). The ability to squat deeper during this test is also likely to indicate a patellofemoral pain diagnosis. To assist differential diagnosis, it may be useful to trial a bolus of low tendon load such as isometric or isotonic leg extension for the quadriceps and reassess pain response on decline board as heavy weights can irritate the patellofemoral joint but do not excessively provoke the patellar tendon.

Athletes who display a knee valgus/hip adduction position during hopping are also more likely to have patellofemoral pain (Herrington, 2014). Other objective assessment may include a check for knee joint effusion as the patellar tendon is extra-articular; knee swelling indicates internal articular or structural injury. A history of trauma or a specific incident points to other diagnoses. Other anterior knee pain producing conditions such as plica irritation, chondral surface pathology and Osgood–Schlatter syndrome (young and adolescent individuals) should also be considered.

Rehabilitation

For athletes or other populations in rehabilitation (i.e., not in-season), removing high patellar tendon load is the first step. High tendon load energy storage activities such as jumping, rapid change of direction and plyometrics should be removed while continuing with the first two stages of rehabilitation (Stages of Tendon Rehabilitation).

Stage 1 exercise will include isometric leg extension exercises to reduce pain (Rio et al., 2015). Sustained holds of 45 seconds, 4–5 repetitions, can be repeated during the day or several times per week. In the authors' experience, using a leg extension machine (isolated) and working in mid-range knee flexion (where the quadriceps can generate the most torque) is ideal. Resistance is relative to the individual and can be heavy because this is well tolerated and not high load for the tendon, aiming for 70% maximal voluntary contraction. Pain during this exercise strongly implicates the patellofemoral joint, which is compressed in this position. The Spanish squat (Figure 2.7) is an alternative if gym equipment is not available, for example the traveling athlete.

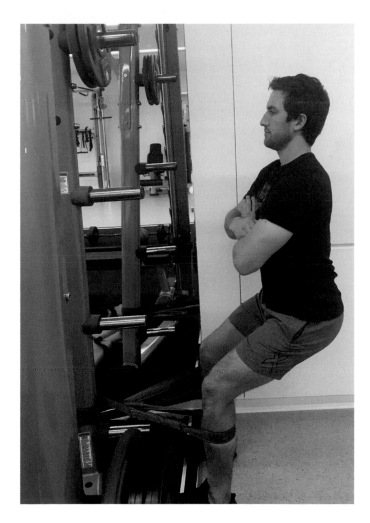

FIGURE 2.7
Spanish squat.

For the patellar tendon, exercise programs should be single leg as asymmetries exist (Gaida et al., 2004). Addressing deficits in calf (both seated and standing, strength and strength endurance) as well as the gluteals/pelvic stabilizers and any other muscle group identified in the objective assessment is recommended. The calf, particularly soleus, is critical for deceleration and unloading the anterior knee.

In Stage 2, isotonic (concentric/eccentric) work is commenced. This is also known as heavy slow resistance (Kongsgaard et al., 2009) and where possible should be single-leg and isolated to address any deficits (for example, single-leg extension for quadriceps should be included). Other exercises can be added such as unilateral concentric/eccentric Bulgarian squats, hack squats, and leg press. The recommended prescription for each exercise is 4 sets of 6–8 repetitions every second day. The calf is critical in terms of load distribution and must be included in both seated (Figure 2.8) and standing positions as well as endurance and strength doses depending on the individual demands.

The focus should be on improving strength measures sufficient to the athletic or daily demands and not just to be symmetrical with the other leg that may also be deconditioned. Cross-education is the concept of strength training one side and transferring strength onto the other side (Manca et al., 2017) and is another justification for unilateral loading. There are changes in the way the brain and spinal cord control the leg extensors in people with patellar tendinopathy and the use of a metronome to provide external cueing is one method in the early stages that seeks to restore this (Rio et al., 2016).

As the individual improves their functional capacity and strength, they should transition to higher patellar tendon loads (energy storage, Stage 3), for example a deceleration activity, progressing to split squat non-continuous jumps and then into continuous jumps as they demonstrate tolerance with load and do not experience an increase in pain the day after loading.

Stage 4 rehabilitation will see Stage 3 exercises replaced by a graded return to loads used in training and eventually return to training and competition. Return to sport is recommended when full training is tolerated without symptom provocation (single-leg decline squat 24 hours later) and any existing strength, endurance and power deficits have been resolved. The authors use the triple hop test for distance (Hamilton et al., 2008) or maximal vertical hop height for that purpose.

Education is critical. Teaching athletes which activities are high tendon load and what activities to avoid will assist with reducing symptoms. We commonly observe athletes ceasing all lower leg gym activities, which is unnecessary (and further reduces capacity) – in the early stages the loads to remove are fast lunging or jumping but static and slow loads can and should be completed. Education should also include when to "listen to their tendon," that is, assess response to load and what outcome measures are valuable (single-leg decline squat in the short term and VISA-P in the longer term), but not palpation pain or repeat imaging.

Iliopsoas-related Groin Pain/Iliopsoas Tendinopathy

Iliopsoas tendinopathy is a less common injury, and little is known of the mechanism of injury or outcomes of rehabilitation. The condition typically presents in athletes and dancers who generate high hip flexion forces in activities such as kicking, sprinting and change of direction or cutting actions, as well as during high ranges of hip flexion and

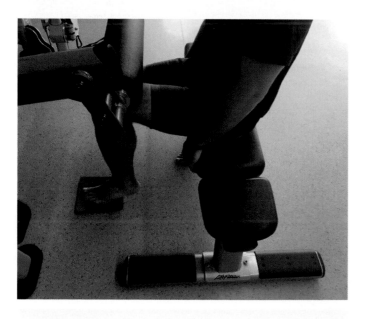

FIGURE 2.8
Seated single-leg calf raise strengthening exercise.

eccentric control of hip extension. Iliopsoas tendon injury can also result from internal snapping hip syndrome, impingement post total hip replacement, and can be a complication of hip arthroscopy (Adib et al., 2018; Nazal et al., 2019). Iliopsoas tendinopathy is rarely an isolated finding and often coexists with other hip and groin pathologies (Thorborg et al., 2018).

The deep surface of the iliopsoas tendon is exposed to compressive forces as it crosses the anterior femoral head and provides anterior hip joint stability in low flexion angles and in late swing phase of gait (Hirase et al., 2020). The tendon translates laterally across the femoral head when the hip moves from combined hip flexion, abduction and external rotation to neutral and can snap during this maneuver and can cause pain (Audenaert et al., 2020). The iliopsoas bursa protects the iliopsoas from friction between the femoral head and the tendon and bursitis can become a source of symptoms. The bursa communicates with the hip joint and an enlarged bursa may be secondary to hip joint synovitis or effusion, and underlying hip joint pathology should be considered.

Clinical Presentation

Marked reduction of pain within an hour following local anesthetic injection with imaging guidance into the tendon sheath supports the diagnosis. Arthroscopy can diagnose tendinopathy and anterior hip joint capsular fibrosis, a potential consequence of previous hip surgery (Nazal et al., 2019). Table 2.5 summarizes clinical presentation of iliopsoas-related groin pain.

Examination

Key tests to assist diagnosis include the Thomas test, passive hip flexion and the FADIR test (see Chapter 12 of this textbook). The Thomas test stretches the iliopsoas and compresses the tendon against the femoral head and can reveal loss of range of motion and reproduce symptoms. Passive hip flexion and the FADIR test may impinge the iliopsoas tendon and reproduce pain.

Isometric hip flexion strength and endurance testing should be done in hip flexion above 90° in supine or sitting and compared to the contralateral side. Pain and weakness are usually worse when resisting an active straight leg raise due to the longer lever arm.

The HAGOS (Thorborg et al., 2011) should be used to objectively assess and monitor hip symptoms.

Differential Diagnosis

The Doha agreement (Weir et al., 2011) can be used to guide differential diagnosis with groin pain categorized into three main subheadings:

1. Defined clinical entities (including adductor-related, iliopsoas-related, pubic-related and inguinal-related)

2. Hip joint-related

3. Other causes.

Hip joint-related pain is the most common entity and often coexists with iliopsoas conditions. A negative FADIR test can rule out the hip joint as a source of symptoms, but the test can be positive with iliopsoas tendinopathy. Marked reduction of pain within an hour following local anesthetic injection with imaging guidance into the hip joint supports the diagnosis of hip joint-related pain.

Iliopsoas bursitis can coexist with tendinopathy or be an isolated entity. They present similarly, with pain on palpation, pain with stretch, isometric contraction of iliopsoas, hip flexion and the FADIR test. Bursitis often responds better than a tendinopathy to anti-inflammatory medication. Imaging, such as ultrasound or MRI, is usually required to differentiate between these conditions. Marked reduction of pain within an hour following local anesthetic injection into the bursa with imaging guidance supports the diagnosis of bursitis.

Iliopsoas tendon snapping can be asymptomatic and, based on the authors' experience, symptoms can develop in athletes who are typically adolescent, more often female and young dancers. The mechanism of the snap remains unclear, but dynamic ultrasound has shown that in most cases the tendon suddenly flips off the iliacus belly onto the pubic bone as the leg is moved from flexion, abduction and external rotation to neutral (Deslandes et al., 2008). An acute tear of iliopsoas requires MRI to accurately diagnose as clinical testing has been shown to be unreliable (Serner et al., 2016).

A study on acute groin injuries found that clinical examination cannot differentiate between rectus femoris and iliopsoas injury (Serner et al., 2016). Both iliopsoas and rectus

TABLE 2.5 Clinical Presentation of Iliopsoas-related Groin Pain/Iliopsoas Tendinopathy

Subjective Clinical Findings

Body chart	The pain is felt anterior to the hip joint within the femoral triangle but can refer proximally into the lower abdomen and distally into the thigh. It can be difficult to differentiate from rectus femoris musculotendinous pain or pain from the underlying hip joint and bursa.
Pain behavior	Pain and stiffness generally improve with activity, pain can worsen with higher levels of loading, faster speeds and as a training session or game progresses, and individuals often report anterior hip stiffness when they cool down and in the morning.
Aggravating activities	Individuals report pain with kicking, sprinting and change of direction or cutting actions, sustained high ranges of hip flexion and ballistic hip extension. Stair and hill running, standing up from prolonged sitting and swinging the leg in and out of a car can also be problematic. Anterior hip stretching and prolonged hip flexion can be provocative.
History	Onset is either acute or insidious and generally follows a sudden unaccustomed increase in hip flexor loading. Iliopsoas tendinopathy can be a secondary overload injury due to compensation for other weak or injured hip flexors such as rectus femoris or adductor longus. Hip joint instability due to acetabular dysplasia or femoral anteversion can lead to an insidious onset of iliopsoas tendinopathy.

Objective Clinical Findings

Observation	Individuals may stand with excessive posterior pelvic tilt that chronically compresses the tendon against the femoral head. During gait there may be a lack of hip extension at the end of a stride and excessive anterior or posterior pelvic tilt throughout stance. There may be less ankle plantarflexion at toe off resulting in hip flexor overload during the swing phase to compensate for a weak calf and lack of propulsion. A lack of hip flexion may be noted when walking or ascending stairs. Poor lumbopelvic stability may be noted in dynamic activities.
Palpation	The psoas belly may have high tone and the tendon can be tender at the anterior hip joint, although palpation of the anterior hip joint can be unreliable due to the proximity of numerous structures. Lack of pain on palpation can rule out this diagnosis (Serner et al., 2016).
Pain provocation	Pain can be reproduced with a Thomas stretch and/or a hip flexion isometric contraction either at length or at inner range. Pain may be reproduced with passive hip flexion and the FADIR test. A painful snap of the iliopsoas can occur as the leg is returned to neutral from a flexed, abducted, and externally rotated position in standing or supine.
Function	Pain or weakness in standing hip flexion, especially above 90˚ of hip flexion or with a long lever such as flexing a straight leg. Symptoms are often worse if the leg is flexed in an abducted and externally rotated position. Endurance of sustaining high hip flexion may be lacking. Speed may be compromised in sprinting and agility may be affected in cutting or change of direction tasks. Deceleration of the extending hip may be difficult in ballistic tasks.
Imaging	Imaging should never be used in isolation to diagnose hip pain, as iliopsoas abnormalities and other hip joint findings are common in asymptomatic individuals and imaging cannot accurately determine the source of the symptom. Imaging can reveal peritendinous or intra-tendinous signal changes and bursitis. Dynamic ultrasound can reveal a snapping iliopsoas tendon. An X-ray should be taken to rule out acetabular dysplasia, hip osteoarthritis and impingement by the components of a total hip replacement.

femoris injury can be implicated if pain and weakness are experienced with a resisted straight leg raise test. Iliopsoas is a more effective hip flexor in higher ranges of hip flexion, and therefore, strength testing of hip flexion between 90° and maximum hip flexion is less symptomatic with rectus femoris than with iliopsoas tendinopathy due to the muscles' different length–tension relationships.

An acute avulsion of the lesser trochanter is rare but can occur in adolescents. An X-ray or MRI is required to rule out this injury if the individual has difficulty actively flexing the hip or walking.

Femoral neck or shaft stress fractures are usually not symptomatic in the morning, but present with night pain, easing of pain with rest, and increasing pain with activity. A hop test or countermovement jump can generally reproduce bony symptoms, whereas iliopsoas is generally asymptomatic with vertical loading. The patellar–pubic percussion and the fulcrum test can rule out femoral neck and shaft stress fractures respectively (Reiman & Thorborg, 2014). A femoral stress reaction or fracture could be diagnosed with MRI.

The lumbar spine can refer to the anterior hip and dysfunction of psoas can be a consequence of lumbar pain. Less common presentations include pubic stress fracture, ankylosing spondylitis, inflammatory conditions, and neuropathy/nerve entrapment. Infection, tumor, gynecological disorders, slipped capital femoral epiphysis, Perthes and femoral head avascular necrosis should also be considered.

Rehabilitation

There is currently no high-level evidence for or against non-surgical management of iliopsoas-related hip pain; therefore, management should aim at addressing the functional deficits (Philippon et al., 2011) and incorporate principles of managing tendinopathy.

Initially, iliopsoas should be strengthened in positions that avoid tendon compression such as hip extension and maximal hip flexion. An active straight leg raise in supine is considered reasonably high load due to the long lever arm and should not be incorporated too early. Mid-range hip flexion strengthening can be achieved in prone kneeling or supine with the hips at 90° of hip flexion and progressed to standing to achieve a larger range of motion. The exercise could start as an isometric action against external loading (Stage 1) such as an elastic band or cable, and progress to isotonic (Stage 2) through gradually increasing range of motion (Figure 2.9). The load applied can increase during these slow contractions and finally speed can be applied to

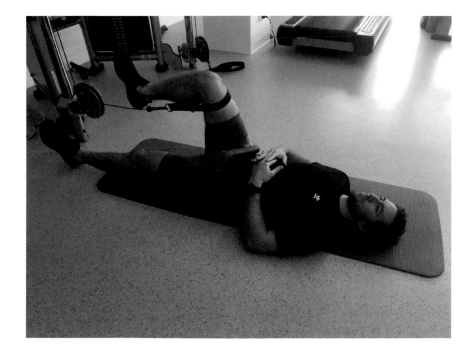

FIGURE 2.9
Isotonic through range hip flexion with pulley resistance.

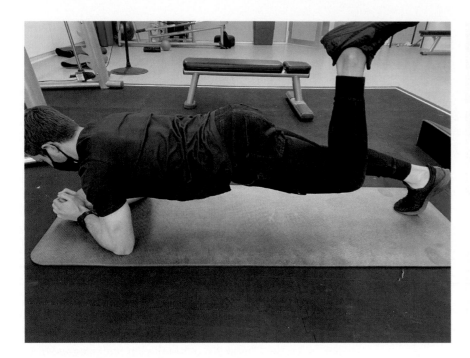

FIGURE 2.10
Plank with single-leg hip extension.

improve power and eccentric control at end-range extension. Significantly improved hip flexor strength has been demonstrated with external loading using elastic bands in a 6-week RCT (Thorborg et al., 2016). Stage 3 and 4 functional training should commence in the sagittal plane and then add change of direction progressions and finally speed. Stage 3 rehabilitation can include plyometric exercises such as box jumps to target power and promote hip flexion.

As the iliopsoas is a trunk and hip flexor, assuming a plank position can effectively target the muscle. Progressing the plank from four-point contact to adding a single-leg hip extension (Figure 2.10) can further challenge iliopsoas on the supporting hip.

Rehabilitation of the kinetic chain should include lumbopelvic stability exercises, strengthening of all hip flexors, especially adductor longus and calf and foot intrinsic muscles. Gluteus medius and minimus weakness may overload iliopsoas (Philippon et al., 2011), and may need specific attention. The posterior chain should be assessed and addressed if anterior pelvic tilt and pelvic/hip stability are concerns.

To prevent compression of the tendon, stretching of the hip into hip extension should be avoided, at least in the initial phase. Prolonged stretching of the hip in hip extension could increase anterior hip joint contact forces, and lead to capsular insufficiency that may predispose the joint to instability and injury. Although a weak iliopsoas may lead to loss of hip extension and a feeling of tension, strengthening the iliopsoas can alleviate these issues.

Proximal Hamstring Tendinopathy (PHT)

Pathology in the tendons of origin of the semimembranosus or the common tendon of the long head biceps femoris and semitendinosus may present with pain, generally localized to the ischial region. These entheseal changes are concordant with histological findings in other tendinopathies (Benazzo et al., 2013; Lempainen et al., 2009). Onset is common following an increase in combined tensile and compressive load on the region, provoked in dynamic positions of hip flexion in higher load athletic activities (Goom et al., 2016). The condition paradoxically is also seen in the sedentary population, where compressive overload through sitting on a hard chair appears to provoke symptoms.

Clinical Presentation

The condition is most seen in football and hockey players who have frequent lunging or squatting demands, yet is also prevalent in distance running athletes and race walkers where the hamstring group may be a dominant contributor. A significant change in the training load pattern may be identified as an extrinsic factor (Goom et al., 2016).

The presentation can be variable, depending on length of symptoms, age, body weight, comorbidities and activity levels (Table 2.6).

Examination

Posterior observation (with the patient in shorts) allows determination of side-to-side differences in muscle bulk of hamstring, gluteal, adductor magnus, and triceps surae muscle groups. It is useful for the patient to carefully identify their region of pain during the load testing.

Functional tests of double-leg squat, single-leg lunge (slow then fast), and arabesque are undertaken to determine any reproduction and consistency of pain site. Single-leg stance in standing or on a decline board and even hopping can be useful to determine lateral pelvic stability. Assessment of standing lumbar movements is useful.

TABLE 2.6 Clinical Presentation of Proximal Hamstring Tendinopathy	
Subjective Clinical Findings	
Body chart	The pain is mostly felt in the region of the lateral or central inferior ischium but can radiate a few centimeters distally.
Pain behavior	Patients report localized pain on sitting or lunging activities. Pain may improve with running, whereas sitting over longer periods makes it worse. More pain with increased running speed is common.
Aggravating activities	Lunging, deep weighted squats, overzealous hamstring stretching and uphill running can aggravate the condition.
History	Insidious onset after increase in loaded hip flexion (squats, lunges or change of direction activity). Often follows a period of reduced activity. Alternatively, prolonged sitting such as a long flight or car trip or unaccustomed/prolonged hamstring stretching.
Objective Clinical Findings	
Observation	Muscle wasting in the hamstring group, often with gluteals (maximus and medius).
Palpation	Localized pain at the lateral (semimembranosus origin) or inferomedial (biceps femoris long head) facet of the ischium and proximal tendon. Care should be taken not to confuse with the adjacent ischiogluteal bursa, sciatic nerve, or adductor magnus.
Pain provocation	Localized pain is reproduced with tendon tensile and compression loading such as bent knee hamstring bridges, lunging, arabesques or sitting on a hard chair. Cacchio provocation tests 2 and 3 (Cacchio et al., 2012) are generally positive, with greater pain on test 3.
Function	More severely affected patients have pain with squatting and sitting.
Imaging	Imaging of the ischial region can reflect pathology in several structures including the tendons. Peritendinous entheseal and intratendinous signal reflects tendinopathic change, also a breakdown in the normally sharp definition of the entheseal cartilage. Ischial bone edema may be variably present (Zissen et al., 2010). The "sickle sign" signal at the deeper aspect of the origin on coronal views may reflect partial tears or delamination (Degen, 2019). MRI is favored as it can identify many of the alternative diagnoses.
	However, imaging does not determine the source of pain. In an MRI study of 236 hemipelves (age range 4–87 years), 90% of those with signal change in the proximal hamstring tendon region were asymptomatic (De Smet et al., 2012). Thus, it is important to rationalize imaging against the signs determined in the physical examination (see Imaging and Tendinopathy).

Exclusion or inclusion of peripheral sciatic nerve sensitization in the deep gluteal space may comprise use of the Puranen–Orava test (Puranen & Orava, 1988). Sitting slump tests and seated piriformis test (Martin et al., 2014) further assist determination of sciatic involvement at spinal or gluteal interfaces.

With the patient supine, hip flexion and rotation ranges are assessed as the hip may be a contributing factor (Gerhardt, 2019). Performing a maximal hip flexion active knee extension (Whiteley et al., 2018) provides a good reflection of general hamstring flexibility. This may be progressed to the use of Cacchio tests 2 and 3 (Cacchio et al., 2012) that provide moderate to high validity and high sensitivity and specificity for PHT.

Hamstring strength measures with hand-held dynamometer (Thorborg et al., 2010), bridges (Freckleton et al., 2014) or hamstring curls (Goom et al., 2016) quantify hamstring function and are useful in reassessment in ongoing management.

Differential Diagnosis

The ischial region is poorly represented in the sensory cortex, leading to difficulty in localization of structures. Thus, quite a few conditions may mimic PHT. Sciatic and other neuritides, deep external rotator or adductor magnus muscle strain, ischial bursitis, posterior hip pain, bony and seronegative conditions may all be alternative diagnoses or comorbidities. Sciatic neuritis is the most common, due to its close proximity to the semimembranosus tendon origin. Not uncommonly a PHT and sciatic neuritis may coexist, confusing the examination and requiring management of both structures.

Sacroiliac and lumbar referral should also be considered, although the pain distribution is generally less well localized and the specific pain on loading is lacking. Sacroiliac joint-specific testing described by Laslett (2008) may be useful if required (see Chapter 13 of this textbook). Hip joint dysfunction is not uncommon and may contribute to dysfunction in the region but only rarely appears to refer pain to the ischium (Gerhardt, 2019). Ankylosing spondylitis may present primarily as a PHT, with associated stiffness and pain in the hips and lumbar spine. Awareness of this possibility and medical consultation is recommended.

Rehabilitation

Management consists of initial settling of acute symptoms through load modification; reducing combined tensile and compressive loads at the ischium through abstinence or reduction of lunge, change of direction and squat lifts in the gym. This is followed by improving strength, endurance and, later, power in the affected hamstring muscle–tendon unit. Other synergists are also addressed as required, in particular gluteus maximus and adductor magnus.

All exercises are initially performed avoiding compressive loads at the ischium through working the hamstring and gluteus maximus in a hip neutral position. For the hamstring group, useful examples are the double-leg, long leg bridge (Figure 2.11) or prone hamstring curls in hip neutral or slight hip flexion (Figure 2.12) (Stage 1). Initially these are performed as isometric exercises (30–45 seconds repeated 5 times, 4 times daily) to assist hamstring muscle activation and relieve pain (Rio et al., 2015). Nordic hamstring curls may be performed limiting hip flexion in

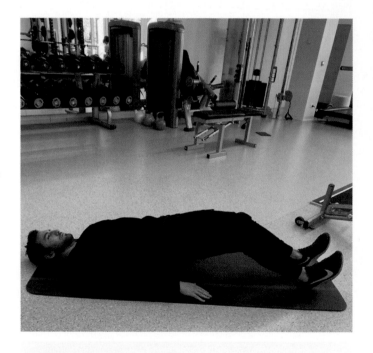

FIGURE 2.11
Double-leg long leg bridge.

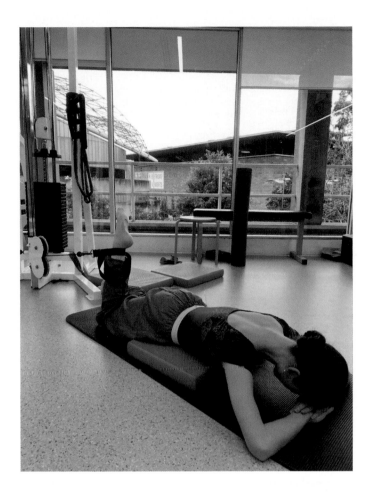

FIGURE 2.12
Prone hamstring curls in slight hip flexion.

Once isometrics have settled symptoms, hamstring loading is progressed with slowly increasing hip range, slow resisted isotonic or eccentrics if tolerated (Stage 2). Posterior chain work, utilizing sled push, is progressed with increases in volume, weight and graduating hip flexion range (Goom et al., 2016). Attention to the required strength and endurance endpoint is critical, as is 24-hour pain monitoring of ischial pain on testing. Continued emphasis on higher-level kinetic chain rehabilitation, addressing the gluteus maximus and medius, is important in many cases. Maintenance of other major groups – core, quads and calf – are essential for most levels of athlete.

Later stage rehabilitation for many sports requires progression into deeper ranges of hip–knee flexion, which must be quantified and monitored as this may provoke a recurrence in symptoms. If so, reduction in range for a week or two (while maintaining strength work) then revisiting at lower volumes often assists this transition. Athletes may encounter higher tendon loads through accelerations, lunging and change of direction (Stage 3). A structured approach to prepare for this element is required, through limiting this to two sessions per week, separated by 2 days. Activities such as bounding, stair running, weaving and easy change of direction are quantified and progressed over weeks to the higher-level demands such as lunging and change of direction to ultimately meet the demands of the sport (Stage 4 – return to sport). Importantly, to reduce overload, Stage 3 exercises are dropped as higher-level (Stage 4) challenges are gradually introduced but strength work (Stage 2) is always continued.

Education is essential and can be sufficient to get clinical improvement. Avoiding compressive loads, such as sitting on hard chairs, exercises into trunk/hip flexion in the gym (such as deadlifts and squats), running or accelerating with an anteriorly rotated pelvis, can make a marked difference to symptoms. Further education on the limited role of imaging to direct management (and even in diagnosis or reassessment due to the disconnect between pathology and pain) and the limited need for passive interventions is always helpful.

the earlier stage in higher level athletes (see Chapter 6 of this textbook). Gluteus maximus strengthening can commence early with double-leg to single-leg gluteal bridges (see Chapter 19 of this textbook). Similarly, gluteus medius exercises can be introduced early as indicated. Where an athlete may exhibit poor pelvic control in the frontal plane within their sport, e.g., racewalking, re-education may also be required to further reduce compression loading of the semimembranosus origin.

References

Adib F, Johnson AJ, Hennrikus WL, et al. Iliopsoas tendonitis after hip arthroscopy: Prevalence, risk factors and treatment algorithm. J Hip Preserv Surg. 2018;5:362–9.

Audenaert EA, Khanduja V, Claes P, et al. Mechanics of psoas tendon snapping. A virtual population study. Front Bioeng Biotechnol. 2020;8.

Benazzo F, Marullo M, Zanon G, et al. Surgical management of chronic proximal hamstring tendinopathy in athletes: A 2 to 11 years of follow-up. J Orthopaed Traumatol. 2013;14:83–9.

Benjamin M, Moriggl B, Brenner E, et al. The "enthesis organ" concept: Why enthesopathies may not present as focal insertional disorders. Arthritis Rheum. 2004;50:3306–13.

Bisseling RW, Hof AL, Bredeweg SW, et al. Are the take-off and landing phase dynamics of the volleyball spike jump related to patellar tendinopathy? Br J Sports Med. 2008;42:483–9.

Branci S, Thorborg K, Bech BH, et al. MRI findings in soccer players with long-standing adductor-related groin pain and asymptomatic controls. Br J Sports Med. 2015;49:681–91.

Breda SJ, Oei EH, Zwerver J, et al. Effectiveness of progressive tendon-loading exercise therapy in patients with patellar tendinopathy: A randomised clinical trial. Br J Sports Med. 2021;55:501–9.

Cacchio A, Borra F, Severini G, et al. Reliability and validity of three pain provocation tests used for the diagnosis of chronic proximal hamstring tendinopathy. Br J Sports Med. 2012;46:883–7.

Charnock BL, Lewis CL, Garrett Jr WE, Queen RM. Adductor longus mechanics during the maximal effort soccer kick. Sports Biomech. 2009;8:223–34.

Clifford C, Paul L, Syme G, Millar NL. Isometric versus isotonic exercise for greater trochanteric pain syndrome: A randomised controlled pilot study. BMJ Open Sport Exerc Med. 2019;5:e000558.

Cook J, Purdam CR. Is tendon pathology a continuum? A pathology model to explain the clinical presentation of load-induced tendinopathy. Br J Sports Med. 2009;43:409–16.

Cook J, Rio E, Purdam C, Docking S. Revisiting the continuum model of tendon pathology: What is its merit in clinical practice and research? Br J Sports Med. 2016;50:1187–91.

Cook JL, Khan K, Kiss ZS, et al. Reproducibility and clinical utility of tendon palpation to detect patellar tendinopathy in young basketball players. Br J Sports Med. 2001;35:65–9.

Cook JL, Purdam C. Is compressive load a factor in the development of tendinopathy? Br J Sports Med. 2012;46:163–8.

Coombes BK, Mendis MD, Hides JA. Evaluation of patellar tendinopathy using the single leg decline squat test: Is pain location important? Phys Ther Sport. 2020;46:254–9.

Crossley KM, Thancanamootoo K, Metcalf BR, et al. Clinical features of patellar tendinopathy and their implications for rehabilitation. J Orthop Res. 2007;25:1164–75.

De Smet AA, Blankenbaker DG, Alsheik NH, Lindstrom MJ. MRI appearance of the proximal hamstring tendons in patients with and without symptomatic proximal hamstring tendinopathy. AJR Am J Roentgenol. 2012;198:418–22.

Degen RM. Proximal hamstring injuries: Management of tendinopathy and avulsion injuries. Curr Rev Musculoskelet Med. 2019;12:138–46.

Deslandes M, Guillin R, Cardinal É, et al. The snapping iliopsoas tendon: New mechanisms using dynamic sonography. AJR Am J Roentgenol. 2008;190:576–81.

Docking S, Cook J. Pathological tendons maintain sufficient aligned fibrillar structure on ultrasound tissue characterization (UTC). Scand J Med Sci Sports. 2016;26:675–83.

Docking SI, Ooi CC, Connell D. Tendinopathy: Is imaging telling us the entire story? J Orthop Sports Phys Ther. 2015;45:842–52.

Drew BT, Smith TO, Littlewood C, Sturrock B. Do structural changes (e.g., collagen/matrix) explain the response to therapeutic exercises in tendinopathy: A systematic review. Br J Sports Med. 2014;48:966–72.

Ducher G, Cook J, Spurrier D, et al. Ultrasound imaging of the patellar tendon attachment to the tibia during puberty: A 12-month follow-up in tennis players. Scand J Med Sci Sports. 2010;20:e35–e40.

Fearon A, Stephens S, Cook JL, et al. The relationship of femoral neck shaft angle and adiposity to greater trochanteric pain syndrome in women. A case control morphology and anthropometric study. Br J Sports Med. 2012;46:888–92.

Fearon AM, Cook JL, Scarvell JM, et al. Greater trochanteric pain syndrome negatively affects work, physical activity and quality of life: A case control study. J Arthroplasty. 2014;29:383–6.

Fearon A, Ganderton C, Scarvell JM, et al. Development and validation of a visa tendinopathy questionnaire for greater trochanteric pain syndrome, the visa-G. Man Ther. 2015;20:805–13.

Freckleton G, Cook J, Pizzari T. The predictive validity of a single leg bridge test for hamstring injuries in Australian rules football players. Br J Sports Med. 2014;48:713–17.

Fredberg U, Bolvig L, Andersen NT. Prophylactic training in asymptomatic soccer players with ultrasonographic abnormalities in Achilles and patellar tendons: The Danish Super League Study. Am J Sports Med. 2008;36:451–60.

Gaida JE, Cook JL, Bass S, et al. Are unilateral and bilateral patellar tendinopathy distinguished by differences in anthropometry, body composition, or muscle strength in elite female basketball players? Br J Sports Med. 2004;38:581–5.

Ganderton C, Semciw A, Cook J, Pizzari T. Demystifying the clinical diagnosis of greater trochanteric pain syndrome in women. J Womens Health. 2017;26:633–43.

Ganderton C, Semciw A, Cook J, et al. Gluteal loading versus sham exercises to improve pain and dysfunction in postmenopausal women with greater trochanteric pain syndrome: A randomized controlled trial. J Womens Health. 2018;27:815–29.

Gerhardt M. Editorial Commentary: Proximal hamstring injuries – is the hip to blame? Arthroscopy. 2019;35:1403–5.

Goom TS, Malliaras P, Reiman MP, Purdam CR. Proximal hamstring tendinopathy: Clinical aspects of assessment and management. J Orthop Sports Phys Ther. 2016;46:483–93.

Hamilton RT, Shultz SJ, Schmitz RJ, Perrin DH. Triple-hop distance as a valid predictor of lower limb strength and power. J Athl Train. 2008;43:144–51.

Hannington M, Docking S, Cook J, et al. Self-reported jumpers' knee is common in elite basketball athletes–but is it all patellar tendinopathy? Phys Ther Sport. 2020;43:58–64.

Harøy J, Clarsen B, Wiger EG, et al. The adductor strengthening programme prevents groin problems among male football players: A cluster-randomised controlled trial. Br J Sports Med. 2019;53:150–7.

Herrington L. Knee valgus angle during single leg squat and landing in patellofemoral pain patients and controls. Knee. 2014;21:514–17.

Hirase T, Mallett J, Barter LE, et al. Is the iliopsoas a femoral head stabilizer? A systematic review. Arthrosc Sports Med Rehabil. 2020;2:e847–e853.

Hölmich P, Hölmich L, Bjerg A. Clinical examination of athletes with groin pain: An intraobserver and interobserver reliability study. Br J Sports Med. 2004;38:446–51.

Irby A, Gutierrez J, Chamberlin C, et al. Clinical management of tendinopathy: A systematic review of systematic reviews evaluating the effectiveness of tendinopathy treatments. Scand J Med Sci Sports. 2020;30:1810–26.

Kongsgaard M, Kovanen V, Aagaard P, et al. Corticosteroid injections, eccentric decline squat training and heavy slow resistance training in patellar tendinopathy. Scand J Med Sci Sports. 2009;19:790–802.

Korakakis V, Whiteley R, Kotsifaki A, et al. A systematic review evaluating the clinimetric properties of the Victorian Institute of Sport Assessment (VISA) questionnaires for lower limb tendinopathy shows moderate to high-quality evidence for sufficient reliability, validity and responsiveness: Part II. Knee Surg Sports Traumatol Arthrosc. 2021;1–24.

Laslett M. Evidence-based diagnosis and treatment of the painful sacroiliac joint. J Man Manip Ther. 2008;16:142–52.

Lempainen L, Sarimo J, Mattila K, et al. Proximal hamstring tendinopathy: Results of surgical management and histopathologic findings. Am J Sports Med. 2009;37:727–34.

Lequesne M, Mathieu P, Vuillemin-Bodaghi V, et al. Gluteal tendinopathy in refractory greater trochanter pain syndrome: Diagnostic value of two clinical tests. Arthritis Rheum. 2008;59:241-6.

Lian Ø, Refsnes P-E, Engebretsen L, Bahr R. Performance characteristics of volleyball players with patellar tendinopathy. Am J Sports Med. 2003;31:408–13.

Lian ØB, Engebretsen L, Bahr R. Prevalence of jumper's knee among elite athletes from different sports: A cross-sectional study. Am J Sports Med. 2005;33:561–7.

Lim HY, Wong SH. Effects of isometric, eccentric, or heavy slow resistance exercises on pain and function in individuals with patellar tendinopathy: A systematic review. Physiother Res Int. 2018;23:e1721.

Malliaras P, Cook JL, Kent P. Reduced ankle dorsiflexion range may increase the risk of patellar tendon injury among volleyball players. J Sci Med Sport. 2006;9:304–9.

Malliaras P, Cook J, Purdam C, Rio E. Patellar tendinopathy: Clinical diagnosis, load management, and advice for challenging case presentations. J Orthop Sports Phys Ther. 2015;45:887–98.

Malliaras P, O'Neill S. Potential risk factors leading to tendinopathy. Apunts. Medicina de l'Esport. 2017;52:71–7.

Manca A, Dragone D, Dvir Z, Deriu F. Cross-education of muscular strength following unilateral resistance training: A meta-analysis. Eur J Appl Physiol. 2017;117:2335–54.

Martin HD, Kivlan BR, Palmer IJ, Martin RL. Diagnostic accuracy of clinical tests for sciatic nerve entrapment in the gluteal region. Knee Surg Sports Traumatol Arthrosc. 2014;22:882–8.

Nazal MR, Parsa A, Martin SD. Arthroscopic diagnosis and treatment of chronic hip pain after total hip arthroplasty and the role of anterior capsule disruption in iliopsoas tendinopathy. Orthop J Sports Med. 2019;7:2325967119854362.

Pérez-Gómez J, Villafaina S, Adsuar JC, et al. Copenhagen adduction exercise to increase eccentric strength: A systematic review and meta-analysis. Appl Sci. 2020;10:2863.

Philippon MJ, Decker MJ, Giphart JE, et al. Rehabilitation exercise progression for the gluteus medius muscle with consideration for iliopsoas tendinitis: An in vivo electromyography study. Am J Sports Med. 2011;39:1777–86.

Puranen J, Orava S. The hamstring syndrome: A new diagnosis of gluteal sciatic pain. Am J Sports Med. 1988;16:517–21.

Purdam CR, Cook JL, Hopper DM, et al. Discriminative ability of functional loading tests for adolescent jumper's knee. Phys Ther Sport. 2003;4:3–9.

Reiman MP, Thorborg K. Clinical examination and physical assessment of hip joint-related pain in athletes. Int J Sports Phys Ther. 2014;9:737.

Rio E, Kidgell D, Purdam C, et al. Isometric exercise induces analgesia and reduces inhibition in patellar tendinopathy. Br J Sports Med. 2015;49:1277–83.

Rio E, Kidgell D, Moseley G, Cook J. Elevated corticospinal excitability in patellar tendinopathy compared with other anterior knee pain or no pain. Scand J Med Sci Sports. 2016;26:1072–9.

Rio E, Purdam C, Girdwood M, Cook J. Isometric exercise to reduce pain in patellar tendinopathy in-season: Is it effective "on the road"? Clin J Sport Med. 2019;29:188–92.

Rudavsky A, Cook J, Docking S. Proximal patellar tendon pathology can develop during adolescence in young ballet dancers: A 2-year longitudinal study. Scand J Med Sci Sports. 2018;28:2035–41.

Serner A, van Eijck CH, Beumer BR, et al. Study quality on groin injury management remains low: A systematic review on treatment of groin pain in athletes. Br J Sports Med. 2015;49:813.

Serner A, Weir A, Tol JL, et al. Can standardised clinical examination of athletes with acute groin injuries predict the presence and location of MRI findings? Br J Sports Med. 2016;50:1541–7.

Thorborg K, Petersen J, Magnusson SP, Hölmich P. Clinical assessment of hip strength using a hand-held dynamometer is reliable. Scand J Med Sci Sports. 2010;20:493–501.

Thorborg K, Hölmich P, Christensen R, et al. The Copenhagen Hip and Groin Outcome Score (HAGOS): Development and validation according to the COSMIN checklist. Br J Sports Med. 2011;45:478–91.

Thorborg K, Branci S, Nielsen MP, et al. Eccentric and isometric hip adduction strength in male soccer players with and without adductor-related groin pain: An assessor-blinded comparison. Orthop J Sports Med. 2014;2:2325967114521778.

Thorborg K, Tijssen M, Habets B, et al. Patient-reported outcome (PRO) questionnaires for young to middle-aged adults with hip and groin disability: A systematic review of the clinimetric evidence. Br J Sports Med. 2015;49:812.

Thorborg K, Bandholm T, Zebis M, et al. Large strengthening effect of a hip-flexor training programme: A randomized controlled trial. Knee Surg Sports Traumatol Arthrosc. 2016;24:2346–52.

Thorborg K, Reiman MP, Weir A, et al. Clinical examination, diagnostic imaging, and testing of athletes with groin pain: An evidence-based approach to effective management. J Orthop Sports Phys Ther. 2018;48:239–49.

van Ark M, Cook JL, Docking SI, et al. Do isometric and isotonic exercise programs reduce pain in athletes with patellar tendinopathy in-season? A randomised clinical trial. J Sci Med Sport. 2016;19:702–6.

van Ark M, Rio E, Cook J, et al. improvements are not explained by changes in tendon structure on UTC following an exercise program for patellar tendinopathy. Am J Phys Med Rehabil. 2018;97:708–14.

van der Worp H, van Ark M, Zwerver J, van den Akker-Scheek I. Risk factors for patellar tendinopathy in basketball and volleyball players: A cross-sectional study. Scand J Med Sci Sports. 2012;22:783–90.

van der Worp H, de Poel HJ, Diercks RL, et al. Jumper's knee or lander's knee? A systematic review of the relation between jump biomechanics and patellar tendinopathy. Int J Sports Med. 2014;35:714–22.

Visentini PJ, Khan KM, Cook JL, et al. The VISA score: An index of severity of symptoms in patients with jumper's knee (patellar tendinosis). J Sci Med Sport. 1998;1:22–8.

Visnes H, Hoksrud A, Cook J, Bahr R. No effect of eccentric training on jumper's knee in volleyball players during the competitive season: A randomized clinical trial. Scand J Med Sci Sports. 2006;16:215.

Weir A, Jansen J, Van de Port I, et al. Manual or exercise therapy for long-standing adductor-related groin pain: A randomised controlled clinical trial. Man Ther. 2011;16:148–54.

Weir A, Brukner P, Delahunt E, et al. Doha agreement meeting on terminology and definitions in groin pain in athletes. Br J Sports Med. 2015;49:768–74.

Whiteley R, van Dyk N, Wangensteen A, Hansen C. Clinical implications from daily physiotherapy examination of 131 acute hamstring injuries and their association with running speed and rehabilitation progression. Br J Sports Med. 2018;52:303–10.

Willy RW, Halsey L, Hayek A, et al. Patellofemoral joint and Achilles tendon loads during overground and treadmill running. J Orthop Sports Phys Ther. 2016;46:664–72.

Witvrouw E, Bellemans J, Lysens R, et al. Intrinsic risk factors for the development of patellar tendinitis in an athletic population: A two-year prospective study. Am J Sports Med. 2001;29:190–5.

Zissen MH, Wallace G, Stevens KJ, et al. High hamstring tendinopathy: MRI and ultrasound imaging and therapeutic efficacy of percutaneous corticosteroid injection. AJR Am J Roentgenol. 2010;195:993–8.

Zwerver J, Bredeweg SW, van den Akker-Scheek I. Prevalence of jumper's knee among nonelite athletes from different sports: A cross-sectional survey. Am J Sports Med. 2011;39:1984–8.

Patellofemoral pain

3

Dhinu J. Jayaseelan, Derek Griffin, Gregory J. Lehman

Introduction

Patellofemoral pain (PFP) is one of the most common health conditions seen in orthopedic and sports settings. Studies have reported a prevalence up to 40%, although a systematic review notes a general population annual prevalence of 22.7% and 28.9% in adolescents (Smith et al., 2018b). High-volume runners seem to have a high incidence, with a point prevalence of 13.5% reported in the military population. While high loads may increase the likelihood of developing an overuse condition, numerous factors play a role in the development of PFP. For example, females are twice as likely to have the condition as compared to males (Boling et al., 2010).

Despite the high proportion of individuals experiencing PFP, a considerable number of persons with PFP have persistent symptoms and functional decline, despite treatment. One study noted 57% of responding participants with PFP reported an unfavorable outcome at 5–8 years post-assessment (Lankhorst et al., 2016). In another study tracking children with anterior knee pain, 91% of respondents at a 4–18-year follow-up reported ongoing knee pain (Stathopulu & Baildam, 2003). While not all of these adolescents had PFP, these statistics remain alarming. The poor outcomes with PFP highlight the complexity of PFP and the need for ongoing research into managing this challenging condition.

To date there has been extensive research into the evaluation and management of PFP. A quick search in medical electronic databases retrieves thousands of studies on this condition, with an upward trend in the last decade. In fact, clinical practice guidelines and expert consensus statements have been developed to guide management of this challenging condition (Barton et al., 2015; Collins et al., 2018; Willy et al., 2019). For in-depth descriptions of current and best practice treatment guidance, readers are encouraged to refer to these guidelines. Although guidelines are being implemented into practice by many clinicians, guidelines are not sufficient to steer the management of challenging cases. Additionally, several other factors exist and probably are not properly understood; therefore, it is important to continue to investigate optimal management of individuals with PFP.

To this end, rather than strictly reviewing available evidence, this chapter will attempt to analyze commonly accepted models for the evaluation and management of PFP. Relevant research, strengths and areas for development will be highlighted. Contemporary trends and implications related to pain science and psychosocial variables will also be presented with the intent of narrowing the gap between the laboratory and the clinic. We do not propose that one specific model is correct or incorrect, but rather that emerging evidence suggests previously held beliefs should be questioned and contemporary evidence should be incorporated into clinical practice. While continued investigation is suggested, we contend that an integration of the ideas discussed is likely more effective in the management of PFP than individual theories or principles. It is our hope that by understanding where PFP research has been and where it seems to be going, researchers, clinicians, and all other stakeholders can appreciate the high complexity of PFP and improve the clinical reasoning process in its management.

Kinesiopathological and Impairment-driven Model of Patellofemoral Pain

The contemporary model of physiotherapy for the treatment of PFP and most musculoskeletal injuries is premised upon the relationship of applied loads and the ability of the person to tolerate those loads. Injuries or pain are proposed to exist when load exceeds the capacity of the person (Dye, 2005; McGill, 1997). Treatment involves both the manipulation of those applied stressors and the person's response to those stressors as outlined by Meuller and Maluf in the Physical Stress Theory (Mueller & Maluf, 2002).

Within this simple framework is the impairment driven and *kinesiopathological* model for the treatment of PFP. The basic assumption behind the kinesiopathological and impairment driven model of PFP is that deviations from an assumed "normal" or "ideal" lead to increased loading on the patella that exceeds the current capacity or tolerance and causes or perpetuates pain/injury (Sahrmann et al., 2017). Examples of assumed dysfunctions in movement or motor control in PFP include: (1) alterations in VMO muscle timing; (2) increased hip adduction or internal rotation; and (3) knee and hip muscle deficits.

CHAPTER THREE

The purpose of this section is to briefly summarize and debate the research on specific proposed examples of the kinesiopathological model while highlighting the current gaps in our knowledge on the most common theories. A practical critical analysis will be performed that will lead to a reframing of the movement impairment model.

By examining common theories about the development and continuation of PFP, clinicians will be better equipped to consider different treatment modalities. Without reframing or considering different explanations for the mechanisms of therapy we could possibly miss out on other potentially helpful explanations. The following section aims to reframe some of the common theories behind PFP which will allow clinicians to consider alternative treatment approaches.

Proposed Risk Factor: Vastus Medialis Obliquus (VMO)-related Patellar Mal-tracking

Delays in the onset of VMO excitation relative to the vastus lateralis (VL) have been proposed as a mechanism of PFP. It is proposed that delayed VMO force production leads to a quadriceps force imbalance causing lateral tracking of the patella and subsequently greater stress on the PF joint (Pal et al., 2019). For this proposal, the basic premise insinuates that an optimal position of the patella relative to the femur to tolerate joint stress exists. In theory, deviations from this optimal position or range are due to proposed alterations in the function of the VMO leading to mal-tracking and increases in patellofemoral joint (PFJ) area-specific stress that might ultimately cause pain, injury, or future degeneration (Pal et al., 2011).

A meta-analysis by Grant et al. (2021) found that in subjects with PFP there was a difference in the patellofemoral kinematics (lateral shift and lateral tilt) when measured during quadriceps activation compared with pain-free controls (Grant et al., 2021). This analysis highlights that differences may exist in patellar kinematics when pain is present; however, caution into causation should be considered. Individual studies show that differences in kinematics may be related to altered onset in VMO versus VL muscle excitation (Pal et al., 2011). Pal et al. (2011) found a relationship between VMO activation delay and patellar mal-tracking in a subset of PFP patients. VMO activation delay was correlated with what the authors deemed "abnormal" patellar tilt and bisect offset in a subset of those with pain. Abnormal tracking was defined as those being in the highest 25% for

patella tilt or bisect offset. However, in the pain-free control group and in the PFP group as a whole there was no relationship between VMO onset timing and patellar kinematics. In effect, the authors suggested that a subset of participants exists (those with the most extreme patellofemoral kinematics) where VMO timing is associated with patellar kinematics. Conversely, the study also demonstrated that there are individuals with delays in VMO timing who have no differences in patellofemoral kinematics and no pain. Thus, the strength of VMO timing delays can be questioned as a risk factor for PFP.

There are two primary criticisms of the VMO-related patellar mal-tracking/malalignment paradigm for PFP. The first flaw would be related to the fact that patellar malalignment cannot be adequately and reliably assessed in the clinical environment (Wilson, 2007). While more potentially accurate measures of alignment and patellar kinematics might exist with the use of diagnostic imaging modalities, its clinical utility is currently unknown, which is the primary idea behind the second criticism of the VMO:VL-related patellar mal-tracking theory. The second criticism is more of a pragmatic reframing of current clinical research to date. The argument is essentially based on the fact that specific VMO timing retraining is not just necessary for a good clinical outcome in these patients (Crossley & Cowan, 2019). Crossley and Cowan note general quadricep resistance training or hip muscle exercise are equally as effective as VMO retraining studies, and suggest a reframing of the patellar mal-tracking clinical research (Crossley & Cowan, 2019). These authors acknowledged that there is biomechanical plausibility behind the concept since cadaveric and modeling studies have demonstrated that alterations in VMO and VL muscular forces can influence PFJ stresses; however, the electromyographic research is less clear. They highlighted that VMO onset delay is not present in all cases, and also that there is no evidence that altered muscle onset timing changes muscle forces and PFJ forces.

The strongest argument for a reframing of the VMO retraining paradigm can also be used as a model for the critique and reframing of the entire kinesiopathological or impairment driven framework for PFP. The authors (Crossley & Cowan, 2019) argued that the strongest criticism of the VMO retraining paradigm is the strong evidence that supports basic exercise without VMO retraining emphasis for PFP. The authors go on to suggest that their clinical VMO onset retraining program could be viewed through a progressive loading lens. Where initial exercises are dosed and chosen according to current tolerances and progressed through a rehabilitation program where some pain is allowed may even influence a person's negative belief about their knee (e.g., pain means exercise and stress is off-limits). The program is progressed to build tolerance to more demanding activities and is specific to the person's activity goals (e.g., sport specific). Readers are referred to Chapter 19 for examples of strengthening exercises and the rationale for progression.

Proposed Risk Factor: Movement Coordination Deficits

Movement coordination deficits (Willy et al., 2019) are colloquially termed "faulty movement patterns" (Davis et al., 2020) and are an example of the pathoanatomical (Powers et al., 2017) or kinesiopathological framework where deviations from an assumed ideal movement pattern predispose one to injury and pain (Sahrmann et al., 2017). Again, the underlying assumption is that certain mechanics of movement lead to increased or abnormal PFJ loading beyond the ability of the person to adapt. Therefore, movement coordination deficits would be one manifestation of the load versus capacity injury framework. This concept assumes that specific movement patterns increase the load on the PFJ to such an extent that the organism cannot tolerate (i.e., does not have the capacity) or adapt to the applied loads, and pain or injury emerge.

Powers et al. (2017) offered an excellent overview of the potential mechanical contributors to increased PFJ stress. Those potential and proposed mechanical contributors included:

1. Impaired quadriceps function
2. Excessive femur rotation
3. Impaired soft tissue restraints
4. Abnormal PFJ anatomy
5. Altered hip kinematics
6. Altered foot kinematics
7. Altered ground reaction forces
8. Altered trunk kinematics

In-depth exploration of mechanical pathoanatomical mechanical contributors to the kinesiopathological model are beyond the scope of the current chapter. For the purposes of this chapter, we will focus on the proposed mechanical contributor described as a Movement Coordination Deficit in the Clinical Practice Guideline (CPG) for PFP developed by the Academy of Orthopaedic Physical Therapy (Willy et al., 2019). The PFP CPG proposed a classification system for PFP consisting of four sub-categories:

1. Overload without impairment
2. Muscle performance deficit
3. Movement coordination deficit
4. Mobility impairments

The subclassification of "movement coordination deficit" posits that increased hip adduction, hip internal rotation and knee abduction lead to increases in PFJ stress and therefore the movement coordination deficits are a potential cause and mediating variable for the pain. Thus, changing those specific movement patterns may be helpful for rehabilitation. The case for movement coordination deficits being a contributor or cause of PFP is made via a number of different research pathways, which will be explored individually:

1. Biomechanical modeling of joint stress
2. Biomechanical cross-sectional and prospective studies
3. Movement retraining intervention studies

Biomechanical modeling of joint stress

Biomechanical modeling was used to investigate the influence of kinematics on patellar cartilage stress with varying results. Liao et al. modeled the influence of changing femoral kinematics on patellar joint stress during a bilateral squat to 45 degrees (Liao et al., 2018). The authors estimated joint stress at this degree of knee flexion via a finite element model of the knee. The model allowed the authors to investigate how changes in the amount of hip adduction or femoral rotation between 2 and 10 degrees would influence estimates of PFJ stress. They found that 6–10 degrees of increased femoral internal rotation (beyond that of the participant's natural rotation) increased joint stress between 41% and 77%. Additionally, only increases of hip adduction of 10 degrees led to statistically significant increases in joint stress. In a later study, investigators modeled the medial and lateral patella femoral joint stress in runners with and without PFP (Liao & Powers, 2019). They found no between-group differences in joint stress but did find tibiofemoral rotation was a variable that influenced the location of the joint stress. Increases in femoral internal rotation (relative to the tibia) were associated with greater lateral joint stress but tibiofemoral rotation in the frontal plane (e.g., femur adduction/abduction relative to the tibia) was not considered a significant variable in lateral patellar joint stress. Increased external rotation of the femur relative to the tibia (or increased internal rotation of the tibia relative to the femur) and increased adduction of the tibia relative to the femur were associated with increased medial patellar joint stress. In terms of biomechanical modeling studies there is some evidence that lower limb kinematics can influence both the magnitude and location of patellar femoral joint stress. Whether this is an important variable for incidence or maintenance of PFP is currently unknown.

Biomechanical cross-sectional and prospective studies

Few prospective studies have examined the link between hip kinematics and future PFP development. Two specific studies (albeit investigating different populations they find conflicting results) prospectively evaluated whether 3-dimensional lower limb kinematics were related to future PFP. Noehren et al. (2013) found that those who went on to develop PFP had on average 12.1 degrees of hip adduction at contact during running gait, while the non-injured control group had 8.1 degrees. The authors found no difference between the two groups in hip internal rotation. Boling et al. (2009) assessed the relationship between lower limb kinematics found during a drop jump and future PFP in a military population. As stand-alone measures there were no differences in hip adduction or hip internal rotation between the injured and non-injured groups. However, when the authors compared injuries between those that had the greatest and the least hip internal rotation (90th versus 10th percentile), they concluded that hip internal rotation, when combined with other variables in their statistical model, was associated with PFP development.

While there are few prospective studies examining whether hip kinematics are a risk factor for future PFP there are a number of retrospective cross-sectional studies that assess whether differences exist in hip kinematics in those with pain and uninjured controls. In general, there is moderate evidence that both hip adduction and hip internal rotation angles are greater during stance in those with PFP. A systematic review suggests these variations are seen during both running and squatting/jumping tasks (Neal et al., 2016).

Movement Retraining

Increased hip adduction and internal rotation have been a target of gait retraining studies in those with PFP. Two well-cited and well-conducted studies are often used to argue that certain kinematics are relevant to the maintenance of PFP. Both Willy et al. (2012) and Noehren et al. (2011) attempted to change hip mechanics during running with different types of feedback (mirror and monitor displayed measured joint kinematics, respectively). Both studies had an inclusion criterion where individuals with PFP must have had 20 degrees or more of hip adduction during running. This value was considered to be "abnormal" and was 1 standard deviation above average hip adduction found in their research laboratory database.

Both studies were successful in changing both hip adduction and pain. Willy et al. (2012) reported a decrease in hip adduction from 20.7–14.8 degrees following 8 weeks of gait retraining. At 3-month follow-up, hip adduction was still reduced compared to baseline but increased to 16.4 degrees. Significant reductions in hip internal rotation were not seen in this gait retraining study (Willy et al., 2012). In a separate study, Noehren et al. (2011) demonstrated a reduction in hip adduction from 22.0 to 16.5 degrees after 8 weeks of gait retraining. While neither study reported statistically significant changes in hip internal rotation during running, both studies reported significant reductions in pain.

Proposed Risk Factor: Hip Kinematics

Cross-sectional studies have reported that increased hip adduction and hip internal rotation are sometimes found in individuals with PFP (Neal et al., 2016). Fewer prospective studies have been performed, with conflicting results found. Intervention studies (Noehren et al., 2011; Willy et al., 2012) have shown that changing hip kinematics can be associated with decreases in hip adduction, but also importantly can reduce pain.

In clinical practice, clinicians are interested in whether variables increase one's risk of developing PFP or if variables exist that maintain or mediate PFP. To determine whether a variable increases the risk of developing PFP prospective data are needed. Some have suggested following the van Mechelen (1992) "sequence of prevention" model to assess whether a variable is related to development of PFP (Neal et al., 2019; van Mechelen et al., 1992). This model requires that a prospective association between the potential variable (e.g., hip kinematics) and PFP exist and that prevention strategies designed to change that variable lead to reductions in PFP. Currently, we do not have the prospective or prevention intervention studies to make these claims.

While it remains unclear if higher range of motion in hip adduction or hip internal rotation increase the risk of developing PFP, those mechanical factors might still be involved as mediators of recovery. Hip adduction may not cause PFP but having increased amounts of PFP might be a barrier to recovery and, unless these movement kinematics are changed, it may be difficult to recover and run without symptoms. Despite there being research that shows decreases in pain and decreases in hip adduction following gait retraining (Noehren et al., 2011; Willy et al., 2012), clinicians cannot currently conclude that the mechanism of this pain reduction is mediated via hip adduction. These studies are small (n=10) and they do not have control groups (Noehren et al., 2011; Willy et al., 2012). Other variables could explain the mechanisms of pain reduction and this area requires additional investigation.

A mechanical argument against proposed movement coordination deficits being a mediator of pain can also be made in gait retraining studies (Noehren et al., 2011; Willy et al., 2012). The rationale for decreasing hip adduction or hip internal rotation is to decrease PFJ stress. This is based on previous studies already described in this chapter. Yet, in those experimental models it was shown that increases of 10 degrees of hip adduction (beyond the participant's normal movement) was required to statistically increase joint stress. Yet, in the Willy study, peak decreases of only 5 and then after 3 months only 3 degrees of decreased hip adduction were demonstrated, yet a successful recovery (in terms of pain) was maintained (Willy et al., 2012). While it is difficult to compare kinematic measurements across studies due to different methods and measurements, it may not be a reduction in PFJ joint stress that mediates recovery.

This concept can be more simply explained by observing the functional recovery of these individuals in the gait retraining studies (Noehren et al., 2011; Willy et al., 2012). Joint stress is assumed to have increased beyond what a person can tolerate. So, it is considered beneficial to decrease joint stress a small amount (e.g., 10%–20%) per step. Yet, we need to juxtapose this with the massive increases in cumulative load we see when athletes recover and during these successful gait retraining studies. The time running in these experiments was increased from 15 minutes to 30 minutes over a 2-week period. Hence, we have quite large increases in the cumulative load yet individuals are able to recover. This would question whether small changes in joint stress or load is the true mediating variable for a successful return to running. A caveat here could be that it is the joint stress per step that might be the mediating factor rather than cumulative load. Perhaps there is a certain transient per step threshold that an individual can tolerate and when this is exceeded after a specific number of steps the pain inhibits performance.

An extension of this reframing might also encompass the modifications of painful movements. Rather than viewing these movements as inherently "faulty," they are viewed as merely sensitive where there might be value in avoiding these difficult movements temporarily (fear avoidance) and then reintroducing them as rehabilitation progresses. In Table 3.1 we present examples of interactions that are supportive and avoid excessive biomedical discussion. Because it is pain that drives which movements are temporarily avoided, it would be symptom modification that could drive clinical decision-making rather than using a biomechanical reasoning framework (i.e., more load occurs with a certain movement strategy, therefore those movements should be avoided). This reasoning may be difficult for some because it assumes that a number of movements and associated kinetics and kinematics are acceptable and safe.

There are numerous options for exercising in less painful ways. The presented figures offer some options, although the specific prescription will be patient-specific and

TABLE 3.1 Phrasing Options to Reframe Exercise Participation in Patellofemoral Pain

"These are movements you have had trouble with so we will temporarily avoid or modify them based on your symptoms."

"You've avoided some of these movements as they have been difficult and painful. Now it's time to start re-introducing these movements to build up your tolerance."

"No movement is inherently faulty but sometimes we become sensitized to them. Since these are movements that you have to perform in your goal activities, let's slowly build up your capacity to tolerate them."

"These movement modifications may be helping because they shift the stress or emphasis of the exercise. We can make it harder or easier but the main goal is to keep you active. Movement and activity seem particularly useful with most patellofemoral related pain."

dependent on their symptoms and activity-specific needs (see Chapter 19). Figure 3.1 shows modifications in the sagittal plane where (A) the patient can use increased trunk flexion or (B) the patient can elevate their heels and add resistance during a common squat exercise. As can be seen in Figure 3.2, the patient can change movement patterns in the transverse plane with (A) increased hip external rotation or (B) increased hip internal rotation. Figure 3.3 shows a single-leg squat with an emphasis on the frontal plane where (A) shows a neutral stance limb, (B) shows excessive hip adduction, and (C) shows a compensatory contralateral trunk flexion. Again, while some of these movement patterns may not be "normal," continued participation in exercise in less provocative positions, even if "abnormal," can be useful in some cases. In fact, it may actually be advantageous to use these movement adaptations to increase the stress on other regions to catalyze adaptation. Perhaps we are not just avoiding a sensitive movement with adaptation, but we may actually be "building up" other regions. Clinicians should be able to program an exercise protocol personally adapted to each individual according to particular demands.

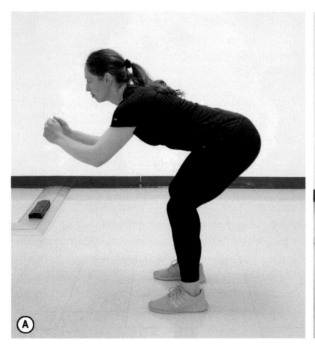 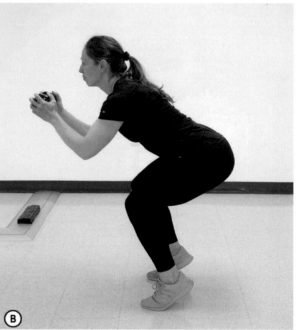

FIGURE 3.1
Modifications in the sagittal plane of regular squat exercise. (A) The patient can use increased trunk flexion. (B) The patient can elevate their heels and add resistance with a kettlebell.

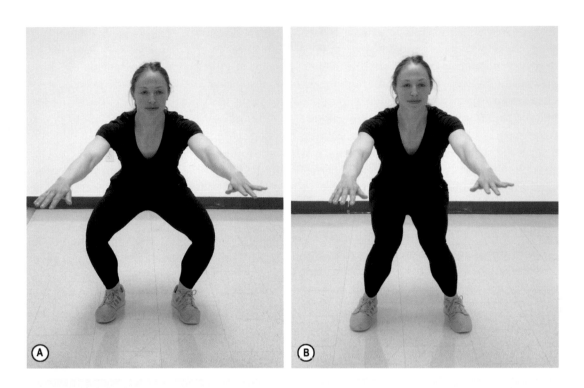

FIGURE 3.2
Changes in movement patterns in the transverse plane of regular squat exercise with (A) an increased hip external rotation and (B) an increased hip internal rotation.

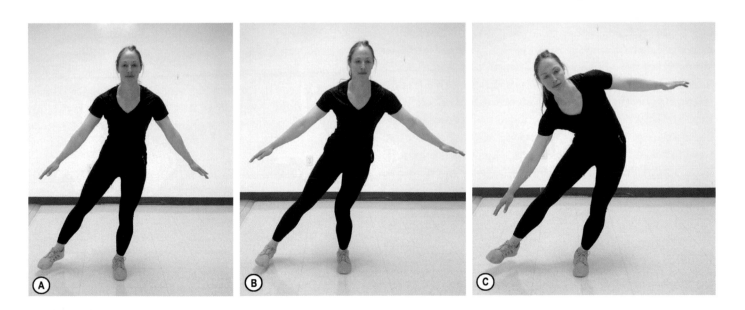

FIGURE 3.3
Single-leg squat with an emphasis on corrections in the frontal plane: (A) neutral stance; (B) excessive hip adduction; (C) a compensatory contralateral trunk flexion.

Muscle performance deficits (e.g., muscle weakness) have also been proposed to be a relevant mediator and cause of PFP in a subcategory of individuals (Willy et al., 2019). While only documented in the military population, thigh extension weakness has been prospectively associated with future development of knee pain (Neal et al., 2019). Hip weakness has been associated with PFP but has not been prospectively linked (Neal et al., 2019). More studies are needed, but it can be suggested that hip weakness may be a potential consequence of PFP and a potential mediator of ongoing pain.

Clinical Relevance of these Deficits

Both hip and quadriceps strengthening regimes are recommended in the treatment of PFP with hip combined with knee strengthening programs considered superior to knee exercises alone (Lack et al., 2015). Readers are referred to Chapters 15 and 19 of this textbook summarizing current evidence of exercises and other therapies for people with PFP. However, while strength deficits have been suggested to be a mediator of knee pain, it is unknown if these exercise regimes work through an increase in the ability to produce force. While there is some research that suggests there are individuals who respond to strengthening regimes (Bolgla et al., 2016) it is unclear if we can identify which individuals are more likely to respond to treatment based on their pre-treatment levels of strength. While strength increased to a greater extent for some movements (hip and knee extension strength but not hip abduction strength across both sexes) in the responder category, we cannot conclude that it is the strength gains that mediate this recovery. Rather, similar to how hip weakness may be a consequence of pain, changes in muscle strength may occur via reductions in pain that were initiated by other mechanisms (e.g., exercise-induced hypoalgesia). For example, Willy and Meira (2016) suggested that the process of strengthening may mediate recovery via increasing the load tolerance of the PFJ and associated structures. In other words, strength changes could be considered as an epiphenomenon that parallels treatment success rather than driving this clinical outcome success.

Summarizing the Kinesiopathological Model of Patellofemoral Pain

Broadly, the kinesiopathological model suggests that deviations from normal movement, when performed enough to exceed tissue capacity, can lead to the development of, and perpetuate the existence of pain and functional limitation in the knee. To this end, a priority of evaluation and management of PFP should be to "normalize" kinematics: reduce excessive hip internal rotation and adduction, optimize foot position to avoid tibial deflection in the frontal plane, etc. While this does make sense theoretically, and small intervention studies have managed to reduce PFP through gait retraining, there are likely additional mechanisms involved in the development, mediation, and recovery of PFP. These additional variables should be examined, since conflicting evidence exists regarding the influence of altered kinematics in PFP, and few large prospective cohort trials outside of the military exist to confirm or refute the relevance of these principles. Next, we will present some of those variables.

Contemporary Pain Science and Considerations for Patellofemoral Pain

While prevalent, PFP can be a challenging condition to effectively manage. In fact, poor clinical outcomes can be linked to a wide variety of factors, such as biomechanical variables; therefore, complexity of pain should be considered in the management of this condition. Individuals with PFP will most commonly present with diffuse pain localized to the anterior knee, exacerbated with joint loading particularly in positions of knee flexion. While PFP classically is reported in a specific region, contemporary pain science suggests factors beyond the knee may play an important role in the development and persistence of PFP. In this section, research related to pain neurophysiology associated with PFP will be presented, and clinical implications will be explored.

For many years, altered patellar and general lower limb kinematics and kinetics have been suggested as a causal mechanism underlying the development of PFP. The premise, as previously described, has been that such altered kinematics result in knee pain via increased mechanical stress on the PFJ structures and the subsequent activation and/or sensitization of peripheral nociceptors. Recent developments in understanding of the complex neuroimmune mechanisms underlying persistent pain states challenge the viewpoint that non-traumatic PFP can be understood solely through a kinesiopathological or biomechanical lens. While pain is often associated with the activation of peripheral nociceptors, pain is not synonymous with nociception.

In 1965 Melzack and Wall published their seminal work which for the first time hypothesized that peripheral nociception could be modulated by the spinal cord neuronal circuitry (Melzack & Wall, 1965). It is now well established that in the presence of ongoing peripheral nociception, neurons in the dorsal horn of the spinal cord can become sensitized and increase their responsiveness to peripheral input, a phenomenon termed central sensitization (Woolf, 2011). Furthermore, processing in the dorsal horn is influenced by facilitatory and/or inhibitory descending control mechanisms (Bannister & Dickenson, 2017). In such a scenario, nociceptive pain processing is influenced by a number of factors including tissue-related/pathological factors, cognitive factors, psychosocial factors, comorbidities, general health and lifestyle (Goffaux et al., 2007; Sawicki et al., 2021). This complexity can underlie the mismatch between the state of the tissue and pain.

More recently, the important role of prior experiences and expectations in pain perception has also been examined (Tracey, 2010). In other words, peripheral sensory input can be "weighted" in the context of an individual's prior experiences and predictions about their condition and recovery (Lim et al., 2020; Tabor & Burr, 2019; Wiech, 2016). Pain therefore is ultimately a highly context-specific experience where the state of the peripheral tissues (and associated nociceptive input), while relevant, cannot fully account for the experience itself. The nociceptive circuitry can undergo significant plastic changes following an injury or peripheral event and the neuroimmune mechanisms underlying these changes have been the focus of research in recent times (Grace et al., 2021; Jain et al., 2020; Price & Gold, 2018; Price & Ray, 2019). In 2020 the International Association for the Study of Pain announced a revised definition of pain which was accompanied by six specific notes (Raja et al., 2020). The task force specified that "pain and nociception are different phenomena," going on to state that "pain cannot be inferred solely from activity in sensory neurons." The important distinction between peripheral tissue nociception and pain has important implications for our patients' interpretation of pain. That pain intensity (1) is influenced by a range of non-tissue factors, (2) does not provide an accurate measure of the health of the tissue(s) and therefore (3) does not by default imply damage or further injury forms the basis of modern approaches to rehabilitation for the patient experiencing persistent pain.

Pain Mechanisms Involved in Patellofemoral Pain

Strictly considering biomedical or biomechanical constructs of PFP can offer a strong foundation for managing of PFP in some patients, e.g., sport players with a clear biomechanical component, but it is important to consider numerous factors play a role in pain. In recent years, a variety of studies investigating different body regions have reported a high prevalence of pathology detected on imaging of asymptomatic individuals (Brinjikji et al., 2015; Girish et al., 2011; Horga et al., 2020). The knee is no different. Perhaps because of the clinical diagnostic challenges with PFP, studies have attempted to identify structural abnormalities causing or contributing to PFP. While altered PFJ morphology, alignment and shape may be linked to some persons with PFP, these abnormalities are infrequently linked to symptoms (Collins et al., 2021; Drew et al., 2017; Fick et al., 2020; Macri et al., 2020; van der Heijden et al., 2016; van Middelkoop et al., 2018). Because of the disconnect between structural abnormality and symptoms, it is important clinicians consider the impact of nociceptive input and processing, perhaps independent of a target tissue.

One way to identify contributing factors to an individual's symptoms is to identify primary pain mechanisms at fault. There are a number of mechanisms for pain, generally divided into nociceptive, neuropathic, and nociplastic presentations (Raja et al., 2020). Often in an individual's pain experience there is a primary pain mechanism (peripherally mediated drive) contributing to symptoms but it is common to have multiple mechanisms involved (centrally mediated drivers). Although interventions do not singularly target a specific mechanism, the presence of certain mechanisms may guide the clinician's development of an effective plan of care (Chimenti et al., 2018).

As PFP is typically localized to the anterior knee, aggravated with activities involving the knee and generally alleviated with rest, it is considered to be driven by a primary peripheral nociceptive mechanism. With peripheral nociceptive pain mechanisms, interventions will typically be directed towards building capacity of the relevant musculoskeletal structures to accept the imposed loads through activities such as progressive strengthening, and/or stretching, etc. Similarly, strategies to modify activity to match the load to the capacity will be completed through progressive training programs which may include altering running frequency, intensity, duration, etc.

Interestingly, in addition to its peripheral manifestation, recent investigations have linked PFP to altered central nervous system sensitization. Systematic reviews including meta-analysis have reported the presence of signs of altered central nervous system sensitization, including widespread pain hyperalgesia, impaired conditioned pain modulation and temporal summation in people with PFP as compared to pain-free controls (Bartholomew et al., 2019; De Oliveira Silva et al., 2019; Sigmund et al., 2021). Results also suggest a higher proportion of altered pain processing in females and younger individuals, suggesting particular effort should be made to consider the presence of nociplastic presentations in these populations (Bartholomew et al., 2019). Chronic musculoskeletal pain rarely presents at a single site (Carnes et al., 2007) and more pain sites reported in persons with PFP may be predictive of worse outcomes (Hott et al., 2020). While additional investigations can elucidate the usefulness of various interventions to mitigate the effect of altered central nervous system sensitization on individuals with PFP, evaluation and treatment beyond local factors at and around the knee are warranted.

Table 3.2 offers characteristics of nociceptive and nociplastic dominant presentations. However, more frequently individuals will present with a mixed presentation, where multiple mechanisms are involved to some extent, so persons with PFP may not sit completely on one side of the spectrum, just peripheral or just central. Mixed presentations relate to the overlap of mechanisms but also the complexity of pain which includes contextual, social, and psychological factors.

Psychosocial Variables and Patellofemoral Pain

It is well established that the experience associated with pain is individual – two different people with the same condition will not have the same pain experience. A variety of factors play a role in the interpretation of pain and the impact it has on one's life. Some of the variables associated with pain may in fact be related to specific tissues but it is essential to identify the contextual factors involved in an individual's life that contribute to the perception, persistence and effect of pain (Courtney et al., 2017). Perhaps less effectively captured at initial examination are the individual psychological variables that may mediate pain in persons with PFP (Nicholas et al., 2011).

In recent years, a number of studies have investigated the role of psychosocial factors in people with PFP. Specifically, and not dissimilar to findings from the broader musculoskeletal pain literature, a higher level of fear avoidance, anxiety, depression and catastrophizing is associated with a higher level of pain intensity and disability among individuals with PFP (Maclachlan et al., 2017). For example, in a prevalence study in the United Kingdom, depression and anxiety were found to be more common in individuals with PFP as compared to the general population (Wride & Bannigan, 2019). The negative impact of psychological variables on PFP has also been replicated among the adolescent population (Selhorst et al., 2020). In a recent cross-sectional study, those with PFP as the primary symptom were at a 55% increased risk of having kinesiophobia as compared to those in the control group (Maclachlan et al., 2020). Furthermore, a recent investigation showed that pain and disability were more related to kinesiophobia than PFJ loading variables (De Oliveira Silva et al., 2020). Together, this body of research points to a complex etiology of PFP, that cannot be explained solely by joint- or tissue-specific factors. The important role of psychosocial factors in the transition from acute to persistent pain and as determinants of patient outcomes has been extensively investigated in other musculoskeletal pain problems, most notably low back pain (Flink et al., 2020). There is no reason why such findings are not applicable to people with PFP, but considering particular features of the knee. The effect of psychosocial factors on pain may be mediated via direct neuroimmune mechanisms or alternatively via altered movement and behavioral responses to pain. To illustrate the latter, a study by De Oliveira Silva et al. showed that kinesiophobia and not muscle strength was related to cadence and peak knee flexion angle during stair descent among individuals with PFP (De Oliveira Silva et al., 2020).

While a correlational relationship has been detected between these psychological variables and PFP, addressing psychological variables does not automatically reduce function. For example, while kinesiophobia and pain catastrophizing were elevated in females with PFP, these variables were not correlated to performance on objective functional tasks (Priore et al., 2019). While negative psychological factors may play a role in PFP, additional investigation into its prognostic effect are warranted.

TABLE 3.2 Possible Clinical Presentations of Nociceptive and Nociplastic Dominant Mechanisms of Patellofemoral Pain

Clinical Characteristic	Nociceptive Pain	Nociplastic Pain
Subjective Examination		
Reported Pain Location	Diffuse, anterior knee	Diffuse, anterior knee; bilateral pain; multiple pain sites frequently reported
Aggravating Activities	Running, jumping, stairs, kneeling, squatting	Running, jumping, stairs, kneeling, squatting; seemingly innocuous activity
Alleviating Activities	Rest, not performing aggravating activities	May not report activities offering relief
Mechanism of Injury	Insidious, overuse	Insidious, overuse
Symptom Severity	Low to high	High
Symptom Irritability	Low to high	High: takes little activity to create substantial symptoms, which take a long time to subside
Psychological Involvement	Minimal	Higher levels of stress or anxiety, presence of depression, low self-efficacy
Physical Examination		
Palpation	Localized tenderness	Hyperalgesia locally and at remote sites; possible allodynia
Functional Movements	Typical symptom reproduction; movement variables frequently detected	Typical symptom reproduction; fear-avoidance present; willingness to move is reduced
Strength	Resisted knee extension strong but painful	Resisted knee extension painful limiting strength
Mobility	Soft tissue or joint restrictions at the knee	Soft tissue or joint restrictions at the knee

Clinical Application of Patellofemoral Pain Science

PFP is most commonly and effectively managed with appropriate exercise (Willy et al., 2019). However, a substantial proportion (greater than 50% in some cases) of individuals with the condition do not attain positive outcomes, particularly those with the condition for longer durations and higher self-reported disability at baseline (Lankhorst et al., 2016). The poor outcomes in a large group of individuals suggests continued research is needed to guide effective evaluation and treatment processes.

Altered central nervous system sensitization may help explain the persistent nature of PFP. If individuals with PFP and nervous system sensitization are treated primarily based on physical impairments, it is possible that nociceptive pathways may go unaddressed, and sensitivity may remain heightened. Importantly, elevated pain reports or sensitivity may be predictive of a worse prognosis at intermediate and long-term follow-up for peripheral pain conditions (Collins et al., 2010; Mills et al., 2019; Roh et al., 2019). Quantitative sensory testing and psychological factors may predict sensitivity to physical activity (Wideman et al., 2014), and may be helpful in the clinical examination and exercise prescription for persons with PFP. Quantitative sensory testing may also discriminate scores on the Central Sensitization Inventory (Zafereo et al., 2021), which is a self-reported questionnaire that has convergent validity in identifying psychological-related factors associated with central sensitization (van Wilgen et al., 2018). While preliminary evidence exists related to physical examination tools and outcome measures detecting nociplastic conditions, limitations in the generalizability of these tools exist, and a thorough subjective history should guide the use of assessments.

As previously discussed, PFJ morphology, alignment and structural alterations are not directly related to pain. Despite this, it is common for people with PFP to attribute their pain to structural or anatomical reasons (Smith et al., 2018a). Among individuals with shoulder pain, attributing pain solely to anatomy and structure appears to have a negative impact on individuals' expectations of recovery and likelihood to engage in rehabilitation programs (Cuff & Littlewood, 2018). Similarly, individuals with persistent low back pain and who cite a specific pathoanatomical cause of their pain report higher pain and disability levels (Briggs et al., 2010). The dominant, kinesiopathic model of PFP, with its emphasis on biomechanical or movement "faults" (e.g., mal-tracking, Q-angle, patellar position, etc.) could potentially present similar problems and is something clinicians should consider in their interaction with patients. Of interest, a number of interventions which do not explicitly address biomechanical or anatomical factors have been shown to be effective for people with PFP (Esculier et al., 2018; Kooiker et al., 2014; Rathleff et al., 2019). While the mediators of change are largely unknown, changing biomechanical or kinematic variables does not appear to be a prerequisite to reduce pain and improve function in PFP.

The emerging data on the role of psychosocial factors among people with PFP highlights the inadequacy of a biomedical/biomechanical model to capture the individual experience of pain. Contemporary models of care in the musculoskeletal domain center on a biopsychosocial framework that is person-centered. Importantly, the biopsychosocial model of pain does not discount or downplay the role of biomechanical factors, anatomical factors, or local tissue alterations in the experience of pain. Instead it emphasizes that an individual's symptoms, the resulting behavioral response and disability level will be influenced by many factors across social, psychological, lifestyle, and work-related domains in addition to one's previous experiences, expectations, general health, and overall wellbeing. The need to adopt a biopsychosocial approach for those with PFP was emphasized in a recent editorial (Vicenzino et al., 2019). The authors of this editorial, among others (Crossley et al., 2019), highlight the unfavorable outcome for a substantial portion of individuals who engage in rehabilitation, which in the most part has been based on a biomechanical paradigm. There is therefore a need to develop more effective interventions for this cohort of patients and biopsychosocial approaches to care seem an obvious choice to further evaluate.

Bridging the Knowledge Gap – Implications for PFP Management

We presented plausible biomechanical mechanisms for PFP, which have been extensively used and integrated in clinical practice. We also provided conflicting evidence related to biomechanical variables in PFP as well as recent developments in pain science which should at minimum lead readers to question the relevance of previous research efforts in current patient management. This process of questioning evidence does not mean disregarding evidence but rather deepening our understanding of how evidence guides our practice. However, when numerous studies suggest biomechanical abnormalities are present in persons without symptoms, or that we have normal movement abnormality, clinicians should re-evaluate the importance of theoretical models in some cases. Biomechanical "abnormality" may have a role to play in the development and persistence of PFP, and it may not be as relevant as previously thought. Thorough subjective and objective information (see Chapter 12 of this textbook) gathering using a person-centric method, evaluating for relevant pain mechanisms and contextual factors will likely lead to the most positive outcomes in the highest percentage of individuals.

So, if biomechanics do not guide our evaluation and treatment of PFP completely, what should we do? An interesting perspective to this answer comes from the work of Rathleff et al. (2019). Whether biomechanical "faults" exist or not, appropriate load management and activity modification may lead to substantial self-reported improvement and immediate and 1-year follow-up. In their study, researchers found that pain with activity can be present, if tolerable, and certain "abnormal" movements do not need to be directly addressed and normalized to improve symptomatic and functional reports. It is possible that training individuals in activities that are less sensitive or irritable for a period of time, and then progressively improving load capacity to match task necessity is more important than prescriptions based on specific kinematic and kinetic principles. This graduated load progression even with pain has been supported by other experts for PFP (Crossley & Cowan, 2019) and has demonstrated effectiveness for Achilles tendinopathy, another peripheral overuse soft-tissue condition (Silbernagel et al., 2007). We should not "throw the baby out with the bathwater," but we should realize that there are numerous "roads to Rome" when it comes to managing PFP.

Pain is complex, and human beings are even more complex. Clinicians should not overcomplicate the management of either. Current PFP outcomes are not ideal, and we need to continue investigating optimal management of individuals with this pain condition. We suggest understanding the biomechanical variables associated with PFP, understanding the pain mechanisms at fault, addressing psychosocial factors limiting recovery, being supportive along the path of recovery, and progressively improving load – be it through ideal movement strategies or not.

Conclusion

PFP is a common yet challenging condition seen in musculoskeletal and sports settings. Despite substantial research efforts to unravel most effective evaluation and management strategies, outcomes of PFP remain poor for many individuals, suggesting additional research is necessary. In addition to more research, current evidence needs to be critically appraised. Biomechanical variables play an important role in PFP; however, studies suggest it is unclear if biomechanics are intimately related to pain or outcomes as strongly as has been previously believed. Recent reports have suggested altered central nervous system sensitization, kinesiophobia and psychological variables may play an important role in PFP, which would imply that treating the knee or associated body regions may not be sufficient. The authors suggest an integration of available kinematic studies and pain science in a person-centric management strategy, using a dynamic clinical reasoning process in order to optimize outcomes.

References

Bannister K, Dickenson AH. The plasticity of descending controls in pain: translational probing. J Physiol. 2017;595:4159–66.

Bartholomew C, Lack S, Neal B. Altered pain processing and sensitisation is evident in adults with patellofemoral pain: a systematic review including meta-analysis and meta-regression. Scand J Pain. 2019;20:11–27.

Barton CJ, Lack S, Hemmings S, et al. The 'Best Practice Guide to Conservative Management of Patellofemoral Pain': Incorporating level 1 evidence with expert clinical reasoning. Br J Sports Med. 2015;49:923–34.

Bolgla LA, Earl-Boehm J, Emery C, et al. Pain, function, and strength outcomes for males and females with patellofemoral pain who participate in either a hip/core- or knee-based rehabilitation program. Int J Sports Phys Ther. 2016;11:926–35.

Boling MC, Padua DA, Marshall SW, et al. A prospective investigation of biomechanical risk factors for patellofemoral pain syndrome: the Joint Undertaking to Monitor and Prevent ACL Injury (JUMP-ACL) cohort. Am J Sports Med. 2009;37:2108–16.

Boling M, Padua D, Marshall S, et al. Gender differences in the incidence and prevalence of patellofemoral pain syndrome. Scand J Med Sci Sports. 2010;20:725–30.

Briggs AM, Jordan JE, Buchbinder R, et al. Health literacy and beliefs among a community cohort with and without chronic low back pain. Pain. 2010;150:275–83.

Brinjikji W, Luetmer PH, Comstock B, et al. Systematic literature review of imaging features of spinal degeneration in asymptomatic populations. AJNR Am J Neuroradiol. 2015;36:811–16.

Carnes D, Parsons S, Ashby D, et al. Chronic musculoskeletal pain rarely presents in a single body site: Results from a UK population study. Rheumatology. 2007;46:1168–70.

Chimenti RL, Frey-Law LA, Sluka KA. A mechanism-based approach to physical therapist management of pain. Phys Ther. 2018;98:302–14.

Collins NJ, Crossley KM, Darnell R, Vicenzino B. Predictors of short and long term outcome in patellofemoral pain syndrome: a prospective longitudinal study. BMC Musculoskelet Disord. 2010;11:11.

Collins NJ, Barton CJ, van Middelkoop M, et al. Consensus statement on exercise therapy and physical interventions (orthoses, taping and manual therapy) to treat patellofemoral pain: recommendations from the 5th International Patellofemoral Pain Research Retreat, Gold Coast, Australia, 2017. Br J Sports Med. 2018;52:1170–8.

Collins NJ, van der Heijden, RA, Macri EM, et al. Patellofemoral alignment, morphology and structural features are not related to sitting pain in individuals with patellofemoral pain. Knee. 2021;28:104–9.

Courtney CA, Fernandez-de-las-Penas C, Bond S. Mechanisms of chronic pain: key considerations for appropriate physical therapy management. J Man Manip Ther. 2017;25:118–27.

Crossley KM, Cowan SM. Vastus medialis obliquus (VMO) retraining or graduated loading programme for patellofemoral pain: Different paradigm with similar results? Br J Sports Med. 2019;53:917-098736.

Crossley KM, van Middelkoop M, Barton CJ, Culvenor AG. Rethinking patellofemoral pain: Prevention, management and long-term consequences. Best Pract Res Clin Rheumatol. 2019;33:48–65.

Cuff A, Littlewood C. Subacromial impingement syndrome - What does this mean to and for the patient? A qualitative study. Musculoskelet Sci Pract. 2018;33:24–8.

Davis IS, Tenforde AS, Neal BS, et al. Gait retraining as an intervention for patellofemoral pain. Curr Rev Musculoskelet Med. 2020;13:103–14.

De Oliveira Silva D, Rathleff MS, Petersen K, et al. Manifestations of pain sensitization across different painful knee disorders: a systematic review including meta-analysis and metaregression. Pain Med. 2019;20:335–58.

De Oliveira Silva D, Willy RW, Barton CJ, et al. Pain and disability in women with patellofemoral pain relate to kinesiophobia, but not to patellofemoral joint loading variables. Scand J Med Sci Sports. 2020;30:2215–21.

Drew BT, Bowes MA, Redmond AC, et al. Patellofemoral morphology is not related to pain using three-dimensional quantitative analysis in an older population: data from the Osteoarthritis Initiative. Rheumatology (Oxford). 2017;56:2135–44.

Dye SF. The pathophysiology of patellofemoral pain: a tissue homeostasis perspective. Clin Orthop Relat Res. 2005;436:100–10.

Esculier JF, Bouyer LJ, Dubois B, et al. Is combining gait retraining or an exercise programme with education better than education alone in treating runners with patellofemoral pain? A randomised clinical trial. Br J Sports Med. 2018;52:659–66.

Fick CN, Grant C, Sheehan FT. Patellofemoral pain in adolescents: understanding patellofemoral morphology and its relationship to maltracking. Am J Sports Med. 2020;48:341–50.

Flink IK, Reme S, Jacobsen HB, et al. Pain psychology in the 21st century: lessons learned and moving forward. Scand J Pain. 2020;20:229–38.

Girish G, Lobo LG, Jacobson JA, et al. Ultrasound of the shoulder: Asymptomatic findings in men. Am J Roentgenol. 2011;197:W713–19.

Goffaux P, Redmond WJ, Rainville P, Marchand S. Descending analgesia – when the spine echoes what the brain expects. Pain. 2007;130:137–43.

Grace PM, Tawfik VL, Svensson CI, et al. The neuroimmunology of chronic pain: From rodents to humans. J Neurosci. 2021;41:855–65.

Grant C, Fick CN, Welsh J, et al. A word of caution for future studies in patellofemoral pain: a systematic review with meta-analysis. Am J Sports Med. 2021;49:538–51.

Horga LM, Hirschmann AC, Henckel J et al. Prevalence of abnormal findings in 230 knees of asymptomatic adults using 3.0 T MRI. Skeletal Radiol. 2020;49:1099–107.

Hott A, Brox JI, Pripp AH, et al. Predictors of pain, function, and change in patellofemoral pain. Am J Sports Med. 2020;48:351–8.

Jain A, Hakim S, Woolf CJ. Unraveling the plastic peripheral neuroimmune interactome. J Immunol. 2020;204:257–63.

Kooiker L, Van De Port IG, Weir A, Moen MH. Effects of physical therapist-guided quadriceps-strengthening exercises for the treatment of patellofemoral pain syndrome: a systematic review. J Orthop Sports Phys Ther. 2014;44:391–402, B1.

Lack S, Barton C, Sohan O, et al. Proximal muscle rehabilitation is effective for patellofemoral pain: a systematic review with meta-analysis. Br J Sports Med. 2015;49:1365–76.

Lankhorst NE, van Middelkoop M, Crossley KM, et al. Factors that predict a poor outcome 5-8 years after the diagnosis of patellofemoral pain: a multicentre observational analysis. Br J Sports Med. 2016;50:881–6.

Liao TC, Powers CM. Tibiofemoral kinematics in the transverse and frontal planes influence the location and magnitude of peak patella cartilage stress: An investigation of runners with and without patellofemoral pain. Clin Biomech. 2019;62:72–8.

Liao TC, Yin L, Powers CM. The influence of isolated femur and tibia rotations on patella cartilage stress: a sensitivity analysis. Clin Biomech. 2018;54:125–31.

Lim M, O'Grady C, Cane D, et al. Threat prediction from schemas as a source of bias in pain perception. J Neurosci. 2020;40:1538–48.

Maclachlan LR, Collins NJ, Matthews MLG, et al. The psychological features of patellofemoral pain: a systematic review. Br J Sports Med. 2017;51:732–42.

Maclachlan LR, Collins NJ, Hodges PW, Vicenzino B. Psychological and pain profiles in persons with patellofemoral pain as the primary symptom. Eur J Pain. 2020;24:1182–96.

Macri EM, Neogi T, Tolstykh I, et al. Relation of patellofemoral joint alignment, morphology, and radiographic osteoarthritis to frequent anterior knee pain: data from the Multicenter Osteoarthritis Study. Arthritis Care Res 2020;72:1066–73.

McGill SM. The biomechanics of low back injury: implications on current practice in industry and the clinic. J Biomech. 1997;30:465–75.

Melzack R, Wall PD. Pain mechanisms: a new theory. Science. 1965;150:971–9.

Mills K, Eyles JP, Martin MA, et al. Exploratory study of 6-month pain trajectories in individuals with predominant patellofemoral osteoarthritis: A cohort study. J Orthop Sports Phys Ther. 2019;49:5–16.

Mueller MJ, Maluf KS. Tissue adaptation to physical stress: a proposed "Physical Stress Theory" to guide physical therapist practice, education, and research. Phys Ther. 2002;82:383-403.

Neal BS, Barton CJ, Gallie R, O'Halloran P, Morrissey D. Runners with patellofemoral pain have altered biomechanics which targeted interventions can modify: A systematic review and meta-analysis. Gait Posture. 2016;45:69–82.

Neal BS, Lack SD, Lankhorst NE, et al. Risk factors for patellofemoral pain: a systematic review and meta-analysis. Br J Sports Med. 2019;53:270–81.

Nicholas MK, Linton SJ, Watson PJ, Main CJ, the "Decade of the Flags", Working Group. Early identification and management of psychological risk factors ("yellow flags") in patients with low back pain: A reappraisal. Phys Ther. 2011;91:737-53.

Noehren B, Scholz J, Davis I. The effect of real-time gait retraining on hip kinematics, pain and function in subjects with patellofemoral pain syndrome. Br J Sports Med. 2011;45:691–6.

Noehren B, Hamill J, Davis I. Prospective evidence for a hip etiology in patellofemoral pain. Med Sci Sports Exerc. 2013;45:1120–4.

Pal S, Draper CE, Fredericson M, et al. Patellar maltracking correlates with vastus medialis activation delay in patellofemoral pain patients. Am J Sports Med. 2011;39:590–8.

Pal S, Besier TF, Gold GE, et al. Patellofemoral cartilage stresses are most sensitive to variations in vastus medialis muscle forces. Comput Methods Biomech Biomed Engin. 2019;22:20616.

Powers CM, Witvrouw E, Davis IS, Crossley K. Evidence-based framework for a pathomechanical model of patellofemoral pain: 2017 patellofemoral pain consensus statement from the 4th International Patellofemoral Pain Research Retreat, Manchester, UK: part 3. Br J Sports Med. 2017;51:1713–23.

Price TJ, Gold MS. From mechanism to cure: Renewing the goal to eliminate the disease of pain. Pain Med. 2018;19:1525–49.

Price TJ, Ray PR. Recent advances toward understanding the mysteries of the acute to chronic pain transition. Curr Opin Physiol. 2019;11:42–50.

Priore LB, Azevedo FM, Pazzinatto MF, et al. Influence of kinesiophobia and pain catastrophism on objective function in women with patellofemoral pain. Phys Ther Sport. 2019;35:116–21.

Raja SN, Carr DB, Cohen M, et al. The revised International Association for the Study of Pain definition of pain: concepts, challenges, and compromises. Pain. 2020;161:1976–82.

Rathleff MS, Graven-Nielsen T, Hölmich P, et al. Activity modification and load management of adolescents with patellofemoral pain: A prospective intervention study including 151 adolescents. Am J Sports Med. 2019;47:1629–37.

Roh YH, Gong HS, Baek GH. The prognostic value of pain sensitization in patients with lateral epicondylitis. J Hand Surg Am. 2019;44:250. e1–e7.

Sahrmann S, Azevedo DC, Dillen LV. Diagnosis and treatment of movement system impairment syndromes. Braz J Phys Ther. 2017;21:391–9.

Sawicki CM, Humeidan ML, Sheridan JF. Neuroimmune interactions in pain and stress: An interdisciplinary approach. Neuroscientist. 2021;27:113–28.

Selhorst M, Fernandez-Fernandez A, Schmitt L, Hoehn J. Adolescent psychological beliefs, but not parent beliefs, associated with pain and function in adolescents with patellofemoral pain. Phys Ther Sport. 2020;45:155–60.

Sigmund KJ, Hoeger Bement MK, Earl-Boehm JE. Exploring the pain in patellofemoral pain: A systematic review and meta-analysis examining signs of central sensitization. J Athl Train. 2021;56:887–901.

Silbernagel KG, Thomee R, Eriksson BI, Karlsson J. Continued sports activity, using a pain-monitoring model, during rehabilitation in patients with Achilles tendinopathy: a randomized controlled study. Am J Sports Med. 2007;35:897–906.

Smith BE, Moffatt F, Hendrick P, et al. The experience of living with patellofemoral pain-loss, confusion and fear-avoidance: a UK qualitative study. BMJ Open. 2018a;8:e018624.

Smith BE, Selfe J, Thacker D, et al. Incidence and prevalence of patellofemoral pain: A systematic review and meta-analysis. PLoS One. 2018b;13:e0190892.

Stathopulu E, Baildam E. Anterior knee pain: a long-term follow-up. Rheumatology (Oxford). 2003;42:380–2.

Tabor A, Burr C. Bayesian learning models of pain: a call to action. Curr Opin Behav Sci. 2019;26:54–61.

Tracey I. Getting the pain you expect: mechanisms of placebo, nocebo and reappraisal effects in humans. Nat Med. 2010;16:1277–83.

van der Heijden RA., de Kanter JL, Bierma-Zeinstra S, et al. Structural abnormalities on magnetic resonance imaging in patients with patellofemoral pain: A cross-sectional case-control study. Am J Sports Med. 2016;44:2339–46.

van Mechelen W, Hlobil H, Kemper HC. Incidence, severity, aetiology and prevention of sports injuries. A review of concepts. Sports Med. 1992;14:82–99.

van Middelkoop M, Macri EM, Eijkenboom JF, et al. Are patellofemoral joint alignment and shape associated with structural magnetic resonance imaging abnormalities and symptoms among people with patellofemoral pain? Am J Sports Med. 2018;46:3217–226.

van Wilgen CP, Vuijk PJ, Kregel J, et al. Psychological distress and widespread pain contribute to the variance of the Central Sensitization Inventory: A cross-sectional study in patients with chronic pain. Pain Pract. 2018;18:239–46.

Vicenzino B, Maclachlan L, Rathleff MS. Taking the pain out of the patellofemoral joint: articulating a bone of contention. Br J Sports Med. 2019;53:268–9.

Wideman TH, Finan PH, Edwards RR, et al. Increased sensitivity to physical activity among individuals with knee osteoarthritis: relation to pain outcomes, psychological factors, and responses to quantitative sensory testing. Pain. 2014;155:703–11.

Wiech K. Deconstructing the sensation of pain: The influence of cognitive processes on pain perception. Science. 2016;354:584–7.

Willy RW, Meira EP. Current concepts in biomechanical interventions for patellofemoral pain. Int J Sports Phys Ther. 2016;11:877–90.

Willy RW, Scholz JP, Davis IS. Mirror gait retraining for the treatment of patellofemoral pain in female runners. Clin Biomech (Bristol, Avon). 2012;27:1045–51.

Willy RW, Hoglund LT, Barton CJ et al. Patellofemoral pain. J Orthop Sports Phys Ther. 2019;49:CPG1–95.

Wilson T. The measurement of patellar alignment in patellofemoral pain syndrome: are we confusing assumptions with evidence? J Orthop Sports Phys Ther. 2007;37:330–41.

Woolf CJ. Central sensitization: implications for the diagnosis and treatment of pain. Pain. 2011;152:2.

Wride J, Bannigan K. Investigating the prevalence of anxiety and depression in people living with patellofemoral pain in the UK: the Dep-Pf Study. Scand J Pain. 2019;19:375–82.

Zafereo J, Wang-Price S, Kandil E. Quantitative sensory testing discriminates Central Sensitization Inventory scores in participants with chronic musculoskeletal pain: An exploratory study. Pain Pract. 2021;21(5):547–56

Hip and knee osteoarthritis

4

Kristian Kjær Petersen, Henrik Bjarke Vægter, Lars Arendt-Nielsen

Introduction to Pain in Osteoarthritis

Global Burden of Disease studies estimate that the highest prevalence of osteoarthritis (OA) is found in North America, Africa, the Middle East, and Australia (Safiri et al., 2020) with an estimated prevalence of 3754 per 100,000 capita. It is well-known that the prevalence of OA increases with increasing age (Berenbaum et al., 2018) and thus the global change in demographics will increase the prevalence of OA in future.

Obesity – as a result of lifestyle changes – is a growing clinical issue (Stanaway et al., 2018) and studies suggest that the future proportion of obese subjects will continue rise (Jaacks et al., 2019). Increased prevalence in obesity will increase the prevalence of OA and cause a faster progression in weight-bearing and non-weight-bearing joints (Reyes et al., 2016). Kurtz et al. (2007) developed a projection model which estimated an increase in total knee arthroplasty (the end-stage treatment of knee OA) by six fold in the time span from 2005 to 2030 in the United States, and similar predictions have been published for Australia (Ackerman et al., 2019). The Australian study calls for action as the burden of total joint arthroplasties (TJAs) will have a major impact on the healthcare budget (Ackerman et al., 2019). As such, OA is a prevalent disease in the world, and it will continue to rise in the future.

OA is characterized by cartilage generation, joint stiffness, and pain. Joint degeneration is assessed using X-ray imaging and the degree of degeneration can be classified using, e.g., the Kellgren and Lawrence (KL) scale (Kellgren & Lawrence, 1957). Under normal conditions cartilage is aneural and not innervated by nociceptors (Felson, 2005). Therefore, degeneration of the cartilage in itself cannot produce pain, but changes in the joint environment due to OA can promote nerve innervation which can lead to nociception and pain (Grässel, 2014). It is evident that the extent of cartilage degeneration does not correspond well with the pain intensity and disability reported by patients (Hannan et al., 2000; Dieppe & Lohmander, 2005; Felson, 2005) since a person with severely degenerated knees can experience minor pain complaints while a person with minor cartilage degeneration can experience major pain issues (Finan et al., 2013; Arendt-Nielsen et al., 2015a). The pain

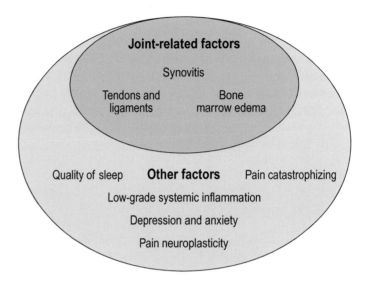

FIGURE 4.1
Multiple factors affect pain in osteoarthritis, and these can be divided into two categories: factors directly associated with the joint and other factors. The list presented here is not exhaustive.

manifestations in OA are complicated with multiple factors that may increase or decrease the clinical pain intensity and its manifestations (Arendt-Nielsen et al., 2015b; Petersen & Arendt-Nielsen, 2016a). These factors can roughly be divided into factors directly and not directly associated with the joint. This will be described in the following sections; see Figure 4.1 for overview.

Pain Mechanisms in the Joint

Nociceptors are found in, e.g., the synovium membrane, Hoffa's fat pad, and subchondral bone (Felson, 2005; Grässel, 2014). Synovitis is present in more than 50% of patients with OA (Hunter et al., 2013) and can be assessed using, e.g., MRI technologies with (Riis et al., 2017) and without (Hunter et al., 2008) the use of contrast. Synovitis is often located at the Hoffa's fat pad (Petersen et al., 2016b; Riis et al., 2017), and most studies find an association between severe synovitis and severe pain intensity (Baker et al., 2010) although contradicting literature does exist (Petersen et al., 2016b). Pro-inflammatory cytokines released from nerve terminals or immune cells are known to sensitize the peripheral nerves leading to increased firing of peripheral nociceptors (Schaible, 2014), which is most likely one link between increased severity of synovitis and severe pain.

Bone marrow edema as assessed by MRI and not X-ray (Manara and Varenna, 2014) has consistently been shown to be related to pain intensity in OA (Yusuf et al., 2011; Driban et al., 2013) and a decrease in bone marrow edema may lead to a decrease in pain intensity (Driban et al., 2013) although conflicting evidence exists (Felson et al., 2001).

Pain Mechanisms not Directly Associated with the Joint

Factors not directly linked to the joint itself may directly or indirectly influence pain in patients with OA (Arendt-Nielsen et al., 2015a; Petersen & Arendt-Nielsen, 2016a). The following sections will discuss some of these factors.

Systemic Low-Grade Inflammation

Inflammatory mediators (e.g., cytokines and chemokines) may sensitize nerve endings leading to amplification of nociceptive signaling (Schaible, 2004, 2014). Therefore, systemic inflammation might trigger widespread effects. Synovitis is a local inflammatory issue, but it seems evident that a subset of patients with OA experience systemic low-grade inflammation directly or indirectly related to joint-related inflammatory processes (Siebuhr et al., 2014). The degree of systemic inflammation might be associated with the degree of synovitis (Petersen et al., 2016b), but multiple other factors may also affect systemic inflammatory processes in OA. Obesity is more prevalent among patients with OA (Reyes et al., 2016) as compared with healthy subjects and obesity in itself is associated with systemic low grade inflammation (Saltiel & Olefsky, 2017) resulting in lower pain thresholds (McKendall & Haier, 1983). Additionally, obesity increases the risk of diabetes, and patients with OA and diabetes patients demonstrate higher synovial levels of interleukin (IL)-6 and higher clinical pain intensities than patients with OA without diabetes (Eitner et al., 2017). Guideline-based patient education and exercise therapy for 12 weeks targeting knee and hip OA have been implemented in, e.g., Denmark, Australia, and Canada. This therapy provides OA-related pain relief for almost 50% of the referred patients with knee and hip OA (Roos et al., 2021). The effect of exercise and diet on pain and function in patients with knee OA has recently been shown to be partially mediated by changes in inflammatory factors (Runhaar et al., 2019).

More recently, studies have assessed epigenetic factors possibly associated with pain in OA. MicroRNA has been suggested to act as the "master-shift" of the inflammatory cascades (Sommer et al., 2018) and microRNAs are dysregulated in multiple chronic pain conditions when compared with healthy subjects (Orlova et al., 2011; Andersen et al., 2016; Leinders et al., 2016). Other studies have demonstrated an association between elevated levels of systemic preoperative microRNA-146 a (presumably associated with expression of IL-1β and tumor necrosis factor α (TNF α) (Nakasa et al., 2008; Churov et al., 2015)) and chronic postoperative pain following total knee arthroplasty (Giordano et al., 2018), which could indicate the importance of understanding the role of microRNAs in OA pain.

Sensitization of Central Pain Pathways

Sensitization is a phenomenon in which the peripheral and central nervous system amplify incoming nociceptive information. Central sensitization is only defined for animals as it requires assessments of, e.g., activity in dorsal horn neurons (Woolf & Salter, 2000; Woolf, 2011), but the term has often been used in a clinical context as different proxies have been used to probe what is assumed to reflect central mechanisms. Multiple studies have used quantitative sensory testing (QST) in individuals with OA, and these studies often rely on pressure pain thresholds (PPTs), temporal summation of pain, and conditioned pain modulation (CPM). The assessment of temporal summation of pain is believed to be a proxy for the wind-up process in dorsal horn neurons, which is assessed in animals (Arendt-Nielsen & Graven-Nielsen, 2011). CPM is believed to be a proxy for diffuse noxious inhibitory control, which assesses the balance between activity in descending pain inhibitory and facilitatory mechanisms from the brain towards the dorsal horn in animals (Yarnitsky 2010; Cummins et al., 2020).

PPTs are assessed using a handheld algometer, and assessments at, e.g., the knee mainly reflect localized pressure pain sensitivity whereas an assessment at an extra-segmental site to the knee may reflect widespread pressure pain sensitivity (Figure 4.2A). Temporal summation of pain is assessed by fast repetitive stimuli with the same intensity while the subject is instructed to either rate the level of pain to the first and the last stimuli (Petersen et al., 2015a) or to rate each of the individual stimuli (Petersen et al., 2019a) (Figure 4.2B). CPM can be assessed using a number of different painful modalities (Imai et al., 2016), but common to all the paradigms is that the assessment requires a test stimulus and a conditioning stimulus and that the CPM effect is calculated as the difference in the test stimulus with and without the conditioning stimulus (Figure 4.2C).

Many patients with OA have lowered PPTs at the OA-affected joint and at extra-segmental sites (e.g., the arm) compared with healthy subjects (Arendt-Nielsen et al., 2010, 2015a). This seems to be more noticeable as clinical pain and pain duration increases (Arendt-Nielsen et al., 2010, 2015a). Facilitated temporal summation of pain and

impaired CPM can be seen in patients with severe knee OA compared with healthy subjects (Arendt-Nielsen et al., 2015b), although this does not seem to be true for all patients with knee OA (Petersen et al., 2016b). Some patients with knee OA seem to be more sensitive to painful stimulation than others; for example, patients with high clinical pain intensity and low KL classification seem to be a specific subgroup with facilitated temporal summation of pain and impaired CPM compared with other patients with knee OA (Arendt-Nielsen et al., 2015b).

The assessment of QST has gained interest since studies have found associations between preoperative QST and chronic postoperative pain (Wylde et al., 2013, 2015; Petersen et al., 2015b, 2016a; Izumi et al., 2017; Petersen et al., 2018b; Larsen et al., 2020), pre-treatment QST and analgesic effect of non-steroidal anti-inflammatory drugs (NSAIDs) and

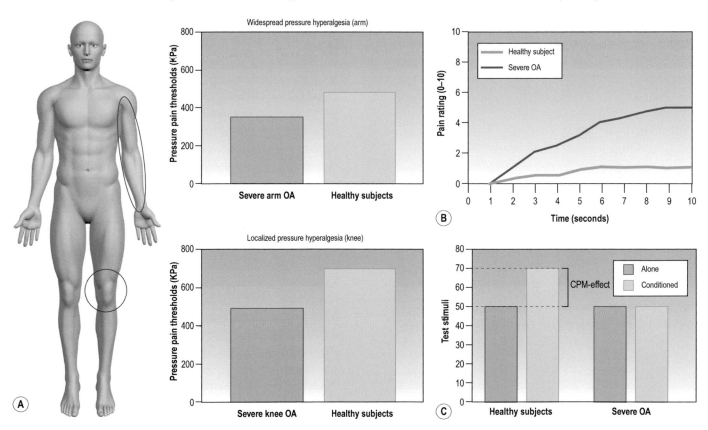

FIGURE 4.2
Assessment of (A) pressure pain thresholds, (B) temporal summation of pain, and (C) conditioned pain modulation (CPM) and a comparison between healthy subjects and patients with severe osteoarthritis (OA).
(Modified from Arendt-Nielsen et al., 2015a.)

paracetamol (Edwards et al., 2016; Petersen et al., 2019a, 2019b), and pre-treatment QST and response to exercise therapy (O'Leary et al., 2018; Hansen et al., 2020). This indicates potential clinically relevant differences in pain sensitivity among patients with OA and that these differences might guide therapy in the future. Despite these interesting findings, a recent systematic review (Petersen et al., 2021) highlights that QST parameters might be associated with treatment outcomes. However, the predictive value remains low and therefore these results should be interpreted with caution.

Duloxetine is an anti-depressive drug (serotonin–noradrenaline re-uptake inhibitor) and has recently been conditionally recommended by the Osteoarthritis Research Society International (OARSI) for treatment of patients with knee OA, widespread pain, and/or depression (Bannuru et al., 2019). Patients with depression often report concurrent pain and it has been hypothesized that duloxetine might treat the subset of patients with OA also suffering from depression. However, animal data suggest that serotonin and noradrenalin are important neurotransmitters for the descending pain inhibitory systems (Bannister et al., 2017; Lockwood et al., 2019) and duloxetine has been reported to improve CPM in patients with diabetic neuropathies (Yarnitsky et al., 2012). Further, it has been hypothesized that duloxetine will be beneficial for the subset of patients with OA who have reported impaired CPM. A recent study recruited patients with knee OA who, based on the "Central Sensitization Inventory," were classified as "central pain sensitized" (although not validated, it relates to any central neuronal mechanisms) and who were scheduled for total knee arthroplasty. The study found that preoperative and 6-week postoperative administration of duloxetine was associated with lower pain scores in the first 12 postoperative weeks compared with placebo (Koh et al., 2019). These findings could suggest that a subset of patients might benefit from administration of duloxetine in a surgical setting. However, these data must be confirmed in future trials.

Psychological Distress

Chronic pain is prevalent in patients with depression, patients with chronic pain are frequently diagnosed with depressive symptoms, and depressive symptoms and chronic pain seem to enhance each other (Bair et al., 2003). Depression as a diagnosis requires assessment by a psychiatrist, but several questionnaires are available to screen for depressive symptoms. Mood disorders, anxiety, depression, and psychological distress are prevalent in a subset of patients with OA (Lingard & Riddle 2007; Marks, 2009), and these factors can amplify the clinical pain manifestations in OA (Edwards et al., 2011). Preoperative depressive symptoms have been associated with chronic postoperative pain after total knee arthroplasty (Brander et al., 2007; Petersen et al., 2018b), indicating the clinical importance of depressive symptoms in OA pain.

Pain catastrophizing is described as a maladaptive approach to (1) coping with pain, (2) rumination about pain, and (3) helplessness in coping with pain (Petrini & Arendt-Nielsen, 2020). These three aspects can be assessed using, e.g., the Pain Catastrophizing Scale (Sullivan et al., 1995). High levels of pain catastrophizing are observed in a subset of patients with OA (Edwards et al., 2011) and increased levels of pain catastrophizing are associated with increased clinical pain in OA (Campbell et al., 2015). Pain catastrophizing is a well-known preoperative risk factor for chronic postoperative pain following TJA (Riddle et al., 2010, 2011, 2019) and studies indicate a link between pain catastrophizing and pain sensitivity in OA (Campbell et al., 2015). A recent study found that the combination of preoperatively impaired CPM and high levels of pain catastrophizing predicted the chronic postoperative pain intensity better than each of the preoperative factors alone (Larsen et al., 2020) indicating that a combined battery of preoperative risk factors might improve our understanding of high-risk OA pain patients.

Cognitive behavioral therapy can reduce pain catastrophizing, and studies suggest that cognitive behavioral therapy is pain alleviating for a subset of patients with OA (Foo et al., 2020). Recent randomized controlled trials have reduced preoperative pain catastrophizing using cognitive behavioral therapy prior to total knee arthroplasty. However, this has not resulted in a reduction of the chronic postoperative pain intensity when compared with placebo (Riddle et al., 2019; Birch et al., 2020) indicating that a modulation of preoperative pain catastrophizing alone is not sufficient to reduce the risk of chronic postoperative pain.

Poor Sleep Quality

High clinical pain results in poor quality of sleep and poor quality of sleep results in increased clinical pain (Choy, 2015).

In addition, poor quality of sleep assessed in healthy subjects is associated with the development of chronic widespread pain later in life (Youngstedt & Kline, 2006; Mork & Nilsen, 2012; McBeth et al., 2015). Quality of sleep can be assessed using, e.g., the Pittsburgh Sleep Quality Index (Beaudreau et al., 2012), sleep labs using polysomnography, or by use of wearables such as motion-tracking watches (de Zambotti et al., 2018).

A recent study characterized patients with OA as good and poor sleepers based on the Pittsburgh Sleep Quality Index. The study found that the poor sleepers had higher clinical pain intensities, higher levels of pain catastrophizing, higher levels of anxiety, and higher levels of depression compared with the good sleepers (Larsen et al., 2021a). High levels of pain catastrophizing, anxiety, and depression are known to elevate clinical pain intensities (Edwards et al., 2009) and poor quality of sleep is likely to promote clinical pain through these mechanisms. However, other mechanisms might also affect clinical pain manifestations.

Irwin et al. (2016) reviewed the literature on sleep disturbances and inflammation and in a meta-analysis concluded that sleep disturbances enhance systemic elevation of IL-6. Studies have also demonstrated an association between poor quality of sleep or lack of sleep and decreases in pain thresholds and impaired CPM in both healthy subjects (Staffe et al., 2019) and patients with OA (Campbell et al., 2015). Finally, poor quality of sleep is linked to a range of diseases such as cardiovascular problems (Kwok et al., 2018) or diabetes (Shan et al., 2015), which are known comorbidities to increase clinical pain.

Limited evidence suggests that improving sleep quality through cognitive behavioral therapy in patients with knee OA and insomnia can improve movement-related/activity-related knee pain (e.g., pain when getting out of bed), function and decrease IL-6 compared to no treatment (Heffner et al., 2018), but more studies are needed to confirm this.

Chronic Postoperative Pain

Total joint arthroplasty is the end-stage treatment of OA with implant survivability being high and surgical technical errors remaining low. However, approximately 10–20% of patients experience chronic postoperative pain (Beswick et al., 2012). The underlying reasons for chronic postoperative pain are largely unknown and it remains unsolved why pain arises after surgical removal of the OA damaged tissue. Evidence suggests that patients with chronic postoperative pain after total knee arthroplasty will report worse physical function compared with patients with knee OA scheduled for total knee arthroplasty (Larsen et al., 2021b). Kurien et al. (2018) found higher levels of synovitis and tibial bone marrow lesions in patients with chronic postoperative pain when compared with patients without chronic postoperative pain following total knee arthroplasty and argued that these remaining peripheral mechanisms might be drivers of the postoperative pain. Skou et al. (2014) found facilitated temporal summation of pain in patients with knee OA with chronic postoperative pain compared with patients with chronic postoperative pain indicating that the pain sensitization might remain elevated despite removal of the OA-affected tissue. Recently, Skrejborg et al. (2021) assessed patients 5 years after total knee arthroplasty and found higher levels of systemic hsCRP in patients with chronic postoperative pain compared with patients without chronic postoperative pain indicating elevated levels of systemic inflammation in patients with chronic postoperative pain.

In 80–90% of patients, revision joint arthroplasty (re-TJA) surgery is based on the indication of infection, aseptic loosening, instability or stiffness of the joint or pain (Roberts et al., 2007; Lidgren et al., 2010; Robertsson et al., 2010). Studies suggest that the proportion of chronic postoperative pain following joint arthroplasty revision is higher, quality of life is lower and joint function is decreased when compared with primary total knee arthroplasty (Petersen et al., 2015b). Patients with chronic postoperative pain after re-TJA demonstrate widespread pressure hyperalgesia, facilitated temporal summation of pain, and impaired CPM compared with patients with no or limited pain after re-TJA (Skou et al., 2013). This could indicate that sensitization is maintaining the chronic postoperative pain state or that chronic postoperative pain continues to interfere with central pain mechanisms.

Intensive daily multimodal exercise and pain neuroscience education for three weeks has been associated with a decrease in pain and improved function in patients with chronic postoperative pain following primary and revision total knee arthroplasty (Larsen et al., 2020). However, standardized evidence-based treatment for chronic postoperative pain after joint arthroplasty is largely missing and needs to gain focus in future due to the rising number of

CHAPTER FOUR

total joint arthroplasties and thereby the rising number of patients with chronic postoperative pain.

Conclusion

This chapter has reviewed factors associated with pain in OA. Synovitis and bone marrow edema are localized joint factors associated with nociceptive input from the joint while low-grade systemic inflammation, pain hypersensitivity, psychological distress, and poor quality of sleep are central and cortical factors not directly associated with the joint but involved in the modulation of OA-related pain. Our understanding of chronic postoperative pain after total joint arthroplasty is limited and standardized evidence-based treatments are largely missing.

References

Ackerman IN, Bohensky MA, Zomer E, et al. The projected burden of primary total knee and hip replacement for osteoarthritis in Australia to the year 2030. BMC Musculoskelet Disord. 2019;20:90–9.

Andersen HH, Duroux M, Gazerani P. Serum MicroRNA signatures in migraineurs during attacks and in pain-free periods. Mol Neurobiol. 2016;53:1494–500.

Arendt-Nielsen L, Graven-Nielsen T. Translational musculoskeletal pain research. Best Pract Res Rheumatol. 2011;25:209–26.

Arendt-Nielsen L, Nie H, Laursen MB, et al. Sensitization in patients with painful knee osteoarthritis. Pain. 2010;149:573–81.

Arendt-Nielsen L, Egsgaard LL, Petersen KK, et al. A mechanism-based pain sensitivity index to characterize knee osteoarthritis patients with different disease stages and pain levels. Eur J Pain. 2015a;19:1406–17.

Arendt-Nielsen L, Skou ST, Nielsen TA, et al. Altered central sensitization and pain modulation in the CNS in chronic joint pain. Curr Osteoporos Rep. 2015b;13:225–34.

Bair MJ, Robinson RL, Katon W, et al. Depression and pain comorbidity. Arch Intern Med. 2003;163:2433.

Baker K, Grainger A, Niu J, et al. Relation of synovitis to knee pain using contrast-enhanced MRIs. Ann Rheum Dis. 2010;69:1779–83.

Bannister K, Lockwood S, Goncalves L, et al. An investigation into the inhibitory function of serotonin in diffuse noxious inhibitory controls in the neuropathic rat. Eur J Pain. 2017;21:750–60.

Bannuru RR, Osani MC, Vaysbrot EE, et al. OARSI guidelines for the non-surgical management of knee, hip, and polyarticular osteoarthritis. Osteoarthr Cartil. 2019;27:1578–89.

Beaudreau SA, Spira AP, Stewart A, et al. Validation of the Pittsburgh Sleep Quality Index and the Epworth Sleepiness Scale in older black and white women. Sleep Med. 2012;13:36–42.

Berenbaum F, Wallace IJ, Lieberman DE, et al. Modern-day environmental factors in the pathogenesis of osteoarthritis. Nat Rev Rheumatol. 2018;14:674–81.

Beswick AD, Wylde V, Gooberman-Hill R, et al. What proportion of patients report long-term pain after total hip or knee replacement for osteoarthritis? A systematic review of prospective studies in unselected patients. BMJ Open. 2012;2:e000435.

Bie Larsen J, Arendt-Nielsen L, Simonsen O, et al. Pain, sensitization and physical performances in patients with chronic painful knee osteoarthritis or chronic pain following total knee arthroplasty: An explorative study. Eur J Pain. 2021;25:213–24.

Birch S, Stilling M, Mechlenburg I, et al. No effect of cognitive behavioral patient education for patients with pain catastrophizing before total knee arthroplasty: a randomized controlled trial. Acta Orthop. 2020;91:98–103.

Brander V, Gondek S, Martin E, et al. Pain and depression influence outcome 5 years after knee replacement surgery. Clin Orthop Relat Res. 2007;464:21–6.

Campbell CM, Buenaver LF, Finan P, et al. Sleep, pain catastrophizing, and central sensitization in knee osteoarthritis patients with and without insomnia. Arthritis Care Res. 2015;67:1387–96.

Choy EHS. The role of sleep in pain and fibromyalgia. Nat Rev Rheumatol. 2015;11:513–20.

Churov A V, Oleinik EK, Knip M. MicroRNAs in rheumatoid arthritis: Altered expression and diagnostic potential. Autoimmun Rev. 2015;14:1029–37.

Cummins TM, Kucharczyk M, Graven-Nielsen T, et al. Activation of the descending pain modulatory system using cuff pressure algometry: Back translation from man to rat. Eur J Pain. 2020;24:1330–8.

de Zambotti M, Goldstone A, Claudatos S, et al. A validation study of Fitbit Charge 2TM compared with polysomnography in adults. Chronobiol Int. 2018;35:465–76.

Dieppe P, Lohmander L. Pathogenesis and management of pain in osteoarthritis. Lancet. 2005;365:965–73.

Driban JB, Price L, Lo GH, et al. Evaluation of bone marrow lesion volume as a knee osteoarthritis biomarker - longitudinal relationships with pain and structural changes: data from the Osteoarthritis Initiative. Arthritis Res Ther. 2013;15:R112.

Edwards RR, Haythornthwaite JA, Smith MT, et al. Catastrophizing and depressive symptoms as prospective predictors of outcomes following total knee replacement. Pain Res Manag. 2009;14:307–11.

Edwards RR, Cahalan C, Mensing G, et al. Pain, catastrophizing, and depression in the rheumatic diseases. Nat Rev Rheumatol. 2011;7:216–24.

Edwards RR, Dolman AJ, Martel MO, et al. Variability in conditioned pain modulation predicts response to NSAID treatment in patients with knee osteoarthritis. BMC Musculoskelet Disord. 2016;17:284–92.

Eitner A, Pester J, Vogel F, et al. Pain sensation in human osteoarthritic knee joints is strongly enhanced by diabetes mellitus. Pain. 2017;158:1743–53.

Felson DT. The sources of pain in knee osteoarthritis. Curr Opin Rheumatol. 2005;17:624–8.

Felson DT, Chaisson CE, Hill CL, et al. The association of bone marrow lesions with pain in knee osteoarthritis. Ann Intern Med. 2001;134:541.

Finan PH, Buenaver LF, Bounds SC, et al. Discordance between pain and radiographic severity in knee osteoarthritis: Findings from quantitative sensory testing of central sensitization. Arthritis Rheum. 2013;65:363–72.

Foo CN, Arumugam M, Lekhraj R, et al. Effectiveness of health-led cognitive behavioral-based group therapy on pain, functional disability and psychological outcomes among knee osteoarthritis patients in malaysia. Int J Environ Res Public Health. 2020;17:6179.

Giordano R, Petersen KK, Andersen HH, et al. MicroRNAs expression as circulating genomic biomarkers in patients with chronic postoperative pain after total knee replacement. 17th World Congress on Pain, IASP 2018 - Boston, MA, USA, 2018.

Grässel S. The role of peripheral nerve fibers and their neurotransmitters in cartilage and bone physiology and pathophysiology. Arthritis Res Ther. 2014;16:485–97.

Hannan MT, Felson DT, Pincus T. Analysis of the discordance between radiographic changes and knee pain in osteoarthritis of the knee. J Rheumatol. 2000;27:1513–17.

Hansen S, Vaegter HB, Petersen KK. Pretreatment exercise-induced hypoalgesia is associated with change in pain and function after standardized exercise therapy in painful knee osteoarthritis. Clin J Pain. 2020;36:16–24.

Heffner KL, France CR, Ashrafioun L, et al. Clinical pain-related outcomes and inflammatory cytokine response to pain following insomnia improvement in adults with knee osteoarthritis. Clin J Pain. 2018;34:1133–40.

Hunter DJ, Lo GH, Gale D, et al. The reliability of a new scoring system for knee osteoarthritis MRI and the validity of bone marrow lesion assessment: BLOKS (Boston Leeds Osteoarthritis Knee Score). Ann Rheum Dis. 2008;67:206–11.

Hunter DJ, Guermazi A, Roemer F, et al. Structural correlates of pain in joints with osteoarthritis. Osteoarthr Cartil. 2013;21:1170–8.

Imai Y, Petersen KK, Mørch CD, et al. Comparing test–retest reliability and magnitude of conditioned pain modulation using different combinations of test and conditioning stimuli. Somatosens Mot Res. 2016;33:169–77.

Irwin MR, Olmstead R, Carroll JE. Sleep disturbance, sleep duration, and inflammation: A systematic review and meta-analysis of cohort studies and experimental sleep deprivation. Biol Psychiatry. 2016;80:40–52.

Izumi M, Petersen KK, Laursen MB, et al. Facilitated temporal summation of pain correlates with clinical pain intensity after hip arthroplasty. Pain. 2017;158:323–32.

Jaacks LM, Vandevijvere S, Pan A, et al. The obesity transition: stages of the global epidemic. Lancet Diabetes Endocrinol. 2019;7:231–40.

Kellgren JH, Lawrence JS. Radiological assessment of osteo-arthrosis. Ann Rheum Dis. 1957;16:494–502.

Koh IJ, Kim MS, Sohn S, et al. Duloxetine reduces pain and improves quality of recovery following total knee arthroplasty in centrally sensitized patients. J Bone Joint Surg. 2019;101:64–73.

Kurien T, Iwabuchi S, Petersen KK, et al. Chronic postoperative pain after total knee arthroplasty is associated with a functional MRI signature of facilitated temporal summation of pain. Boston: World Conference on Pain, 2018.

Kurtz S, Ong K, Lau E, et al. Projections of primary and revision hip and knee arthroplasty in the United States from 2005 to 2030. J Bone J Surg. 2007;89:780–5.

Kwok CS, Kontopantelis E, Kuligowski G, et al. Self-reported sleep duration and quality and cardiovascular disease and mortality: A dose-response meta-analysis. J Am Heart Assoc. 2018;7:e008552.

Larsen JB, Mogensen L, Arendt-Nielsen L, et al. Intensive, personalized multimodal rehabilitation in patients with primary or revision total knee arthroplasty: a retrospective cohort study. BMC Sport Sci Med Rehabil. 2020;12:5.

Larsen DB, Laursen MB, Simonsen OH, et al. The association between sleep quality, preoperative risk factors for chronic postoperative pain, and postoperative pain intensity 12 months after knee and hip arthroplasty. Br J Pain. 2021a. In press.

Larsen DB, Mogens L, Edwards RR, et al. The combination of preoperative pain, conditioned pain modulation, and pain catastrophizing predicts postoperative pain 12 months after total knee arthroplasty. Pain Med. 2021b;22(7):1583-90.

Leinders M, Doppler K, Klein T, et al. Increased cutaneous miR-let-7d expression correlates with small nerve fiber pathology in patients with fibromyalgia syndrome. Pain. 2016;157:2493–503.

Lidgren L, Sundberg M, Dahl AW, et al. Swedish Knee Arthroplasty Register, Annual report 2010.

Lingard EA, Riddle DL. Impact of psychological distress on pain and function following knee arthroplasty. J Bone Joint Surg Am. 2007;89:1161–9.

Lockwood SM, Bannister K, Dickenson AH. An investigation into the noradrenergic and serotonergic contributions of diffuse noxious inhibitory controls in a monoiodoacetate model of osteoarthritis. J Neurophysiol. 2019;121:96–104.

Manara M, Varenna M. A clinical overview of bone marrow edema. Reumatismo. 2014;66:184.

Marks R. Comorbid depression and anxiety impact hip osteoarthritis disability. Disabil Health J. 2009;2:27–35.

McBeth J, Wilkie R, Bedson J, et al. Sleep disturbance and chronic widespread pain. Curr Rheumatol Rep 2015;17:469.

McKendall MJ, Haier RJ. Pain sensitivity and obesity. Psychiatry Res. 1983;8:119–25.

Mork PJ, Nilsen TIL. Sleep problems and risk of fibromyalgia: Longitudinal data on an adult female population in Norway. Arthritis Rheum. 2012;64:281–4.

Nakasa T, Miyaki S, Okubo A, et al. Expression of microRNA-146 in rheumatoid arthritis synovial tissue. Arthritis Rheum. 2008;58:1284-92.

Orlova IA, Alexander GM, Qureshi RA, et al. MicroRNA modulation in complex regional pain syndrome. J Transl Med. 2011;9:195.

O'Leary H, Smart KM, Moloney NA, et al. Pain sensitization associated with nonresponse after physiotherapy in people with knee osteoarthritis. Pain. 2018;159:1877–86.

Petersen KK, Arendt-Nielsen L. Chapter 11: Chronic pain after joint surgery. In: Arendt-Nielsen L, Perrot S, editors. Pain in the Joints. IASP press, 2016a.

Petersen KK, Arendt-Nielsen L. Chronic postoperative pain after joint replacement. Pain Clin Updat. 2016b;24.

Petersen KK, Arendt-Nielsen L, Simonsen O, et al. Presurgical assessment of temporal summation of pain predicts the development of chronic postoperative pain 12 months after total knee replacement. Pain. 2015a;156:55–61.

Petersen KK, Simonsen O, Laursen MB, et al. Chronic postoperative pain after primary and revision total knee arthroplasty. Clin J Pain. 2015b;31:1–6.

Petersen KK, Graven-Nielsen T, Simonsen O, et al. Preoperative pain mechanisms assessed by cuff algometry are associated with chronic postoperative pain relief after total knee replacement. Pain. 2016a;157:1400–6.

Petersen KK, Siebuhr AS, Graven-Nielsen T, et al. Sensitization and serological biomarkers in knee osteoarthritis patients with different degrees of synovitis. Clin J Pain. 2016b;32:841–8.

Petersen KK, Lunn TH, Husted H, et al. The influence of pre- and perioperative administration of gabapentin on pain 3-4 years after total knee arthroplasty. Scand J Pain. 2018a;18:237–45.

Petersen KK, Simonsen O, Laursen MB, et al. The role of preoperative radiologic severity, sensory testing, and temporal summation on chronic postoperative pain following total knee arthroplasty. Clin J Pain. 2018b;34:193–7.

Petersen KK, Olesen AE, Simonsen O, et al. Mechanistic pain profiling as a tool to predict the efficacy of 3-week nonsteroidal anti-inflammatory drugs plus paracetamol in patients with painful knee osteoarthritis. Pain. 2019a;160:486–92.

Petersen KK, Simonsen O, Olesen AE, et al. Pain inhibitory mechanisms and response to weak analgesics in patients with knee osteoarthritis. Eur J Pain. 2019b;23:1904–12.

Petersen KK, Vaegter HB, Stubhaug A, et al. The predictive value of quantitative sensory testing. Pain. 2021;162:31–44.

Petrini L, Arendt-Nielsen L. Understanding pain catastrophizing: putting pieces together. Front Psychol. 2020;11:603420.

Reyes C, Leyland KM, Peat G, et al. Association between overweight and obesity and risk of clinically diagnosed knee, hip, and hand osteoarthritis: A population-based cohort study. Arthritis Rheumatol. 2016;68:1869–75.

Riddle D, Keefe F, Nay W, et al. Pain coping skills training for patients with elevated pain catastrophizing who are scheduled for knee arthroplasty: A quasi-experimental study. Natl Inst Heal. 2011;92:859–65.

Riddle DL, Keefe FJ, Ang DC, et al. Pain coping skills training for patients who catastrophize about pain prior to knee arthroplasty: A multisite randomized clinical trial. J Bone Joint Surg Am. 2019;101:218–27.

Riddle DL, Wade JB, Jiranek WA, et al. Preoperative pain catastrophizing predicts pain outcome after knee arthroplasty. Clin Orthop Relat Res. 2010;468:798–806.

Riis RGC, Gudbergsen H, Simonsen O, et al. The association between histological, macroscopic and magnetic resonance imaging assessed synovitis in end-stage knee osteoarthritis: a cross-sectional study. Osteoarthr Cartil. 2017;25:272–80.

Roberts VI, Esler CNA, Harper WM. A 15-year follow-up study of 4606 primary total knee replacements. J Bone Joint Surg Br. 2007;89:1452–6.

Robertsson O, Bizjajeva S, Fenstad AM, et al. Knee arthroplasty in Denmark, Norway and Sweden. Acta Orthop. 2010;81:82–9.

Roos EM, Grønne DT, Skou ST, et al. Immediate outcomes following the GLA:D® program in Denmark, Canada and Australia. A longitudinal analysis including 28,370 patients with symptomatic knee or hip osteoarthritis. Osteoarthr Cartil. 2021;29(4):502–6.

Runhaar J, Beavers DP, Miller GD, et al. Inflammatory cytokines mediate the effects of diet and exercise on pain and function in knee osteoarthritis independent of BMI. Osteoarthr Cartil. 2019;27:1118–23.

Safiri S, Kolahi A-A, Smith E, et al. Global, regional and national burden of osteoarthritis 1990-2017: a systematic analysis of the Global Burden of Disease Study 2017. Ann Rheum Dis. 2020;79:819–28.

Saltiel AR, Olefsky JM. Inflammatory mechanisms linking obesity and metabolic disease. J Clin Invest. 2017;127:1–4.

Schaible H-G. Spinal mechanisms contributing to joint pain. Novartis Found Symp. 2004;260:4–22.

Schaible H-G. Nociceptive neurons detect cytokines in arthritis. Arthritis Res Ther. 2014;16:470–8.

Shan Z, Ma H, Xie M, et al. Sleep duration and risk of type 2 diabetes: a meta-analysis of prospective studies. Diabetes Care. 2015;38:529–37.

Siebuhr AS, Petersen KK, Arendt-Nielsen L, et al. Identification and characterisation of osteoarthritis patients with inflammation derived tissue turnover. Osteoarthr Cartil. 2014;22:44–50.

Skou ST, Graven-Nielsen T, Rasmussen S, et al. Widespread sensitization in patients with chronic pain after revision total knee arthroplasty. Pain. 2013;154:1588–94.

Skou ST, Graven-Nielsen T, Rasmussen S, et al. Facilitation of pain sensitization in knee osteoarthritis and persistent post-operative pain: a cross-sectional study. Eur J Pain. 2014;18:1024–31.

Skrejborg P, Petersen KK, Kold S, et al. Patients with high chronic postoperative knee pain 5 years after total knee replacement demonstrate low-grad inflammation, impairment of function, and high levels of pain catastrophizing. Clin J Pain. 2021;37:161–7.

Sommer C, Leinders M, Üçeyler N. Inflammation in the pathophysiology of neuropathic pain. Pain. 2018;159:595–602.

Staffe AT, Bech MW, Clemmensen SLK, et al. Total sleep deprivation increases pain sensitivity, impairs conditioned pain modulation and facilitates temporal summation of pain in healthy participants. PLoS One. 2019;14:e0225849.

Stanaway JD, Afshin A, Gakidou E, et al. Global, regional, and national comparative risk assessment of 84 behavioural, environmental and occupational, and metabolic risks or clusters of risks for 195 countries and territories, 1990–2017: a systematic analysis for the Global Burden of Disease Study. Lancet. 2018;392:1923–94.

Sullivan MJL, Bishop SR, Pivik J. The pain catastrophizing scale: development and validation. Psychol Assess. 1995;7:524–32.

Woolf CJ. Central sensitization: Implications for the diagnosis and treatment of pain. Pain. 2011;152:S2–15.

Woolf CJ, Salter MW. Neuronal plasticity: increasing the gain in pain. Science. 2000;288:1765–9.

Wylde V, Palmer S, Learmonth ID, et al. The association between pre-operative pain sensitisation and chronic pain after knee replacement: An exploratory study. Osteoarthr Cartil. 2013;21:1253–6.

Wylde V, Sayers A, Lenguerrand E, et al. Preoperative widespread pain sensitization and chronic pain after hip and knee replacement. Pain. 2015;156:47–54.

Yarnitsky D. Conditioned pain modulation (the diffuse noxious inhibitory control-like effect): its relevance for acute and chronic pain states. Curr Opin Anaesthesiol. 2010;23:611–15.

Yarnitsky D, Granot M, Nahman-Averbuch H, et al. Conditioned pain modulation predicts duloxetine efficacy in painful diabetic neuropathy. Pain. 2012;153:1193–8.

Youngstedt SD, Kline CE. Epidemiology of exercise and sleep. Sleep Biol Rhythms. 2006;4:215–21.

Yusuf E, Kortekaas MC, Watt I, et al. Do knee abnormalities visualised on MRI explain knee pain in knee osteoarthritis? A systematic review. Ann Rheum Dis. 2011;70:60–7.

Femoroacetabular Impingement Syndrome

Introduction

Chronic hip pain can be challenging to diagnose and treat because of the potential multiple sources of pain and dysfunction. Patients with intra-articular hip pathology see an average of four clinicians before establishing an accurate diagnosis (Kahlenberg et al., 2014). A well-recognized cause of hip pain in active individuals is femoroacetabular impingement (FAI) (Keogh & Batt, 2008). In fact, it is the most common cause of intra-articular hip pain and the prevalence of FAI has been reported to be 61.3% in patients with hip pain who do not have osteoarthritis (Jauregui et al., 2020).

FAI is a clinical syndrome in which morphological abnormalities of the femoral head and/or the acetabulum result in an abnormal contact between the femur and acetabulum during hip motion, leading to cartilage and/or labral damage and hip pain (Nakano & Khanduja, 2018). FAI has gained significant importance in the recent past and an important reason for this interest is because it has been considered a precursor to hip osteoarthritis (Aliprandi et al., 2014).

FAI was first reported by Smith-Petersen in 1936, as a source of hip pain and disability by the impact mechanism of the femoral neck against the acetabular rim (Hernigou, 2014). As a self-standing pathology, it was described by Ganz (2003) as a risk factor for hip osteoarthritis, due to the pathological contact between the acetabular rim and the femur that can derive from both anatomical and functional discrepancies. The actual prevalence of intra-articular hip disorders such as FAI may have been underestimated over the years and FAI is considered by many as the greatest discovery in hip pathologies in recent times (Matsumoto et al., 2020).

The aims of this section are to provide clinicians with information regarding the pathogenesis of FAI, describe the clinical history and physical exam elements, and introduce rehabilitation strategies for patients with FAI syndrome.

Prevalence

Radiographic findings consistent with FAI morphology are common in asymptomatic patients (Hack et al., 2010).

A systematic review by Frank et al. (2015) found the prevalence of cam and pincer deformity to be 37% and 67% in asymptomatic individuals, respectively. The prevalence of radiographic findings consistent with FAI has been shown to be 60.5% in patients presenting with hip pain (Zhou et al., 2020). In a large cohort study of 716 patients diagnosed with FAI syndrome, female patients had a higher incidence of FAI than male patients (67%) and the mean age was around 27.2 ± 8.4 years (Hale et al., 2021).

Pathophysiology

FAI presents in three main forms: the cam, pincer and mixed type (Figure 5.1). Cam morphology is an osteochondral prominence at the femoral head–neck junction leading to loss of the normal femoral head–neck offset (Genovese et al., 2013). Cam lesions are most commonly anterolateral and affect the anterosuperior chondrolabral junction. Pincer morphology involves over-coverage of the femoral head by the acetabulum due to focal rim lesions or cephalad retroversion (Hadeed et al., 2016).

Table 5.1 compares the characteristics of the two types of FAI. Interestingly, the most common form of FAI is the combined-type impingement, where there are features of both cam and pincer morphology (Beck et al., 2005). In cross-sectional and longitudinal natural history studies of FAI, cam-type FAI has consistently shown an association with developing hip osteoarthritis (Wylie & Kim, 2019), whereas pincer-type FAI was not associated with development of hip osteoarthritis (Agricola et al., 2013). A case–control study of 952 patients had shown that BMI greater than 29, male sex, and increased age at the time of presentation with hip pain were risk factors for hip OA (Melugin et al., 2020).

The etiology of FAI is not fully understood, but appears to be associated with the developmental changes in the growing hip. Participation in high-intensity sporting activities during adolescence is associated with an increased risk of the cam morphology (Siebenrock et al., 2011). Cam morphology is more common in adolescent populations who participate in sporting activities like soccer before the age of 14 and therefore could be considered as a developmental adaptation triggered by intense sporting activity during the closure of the femoral head growth plate (Agricola et al., 2012).

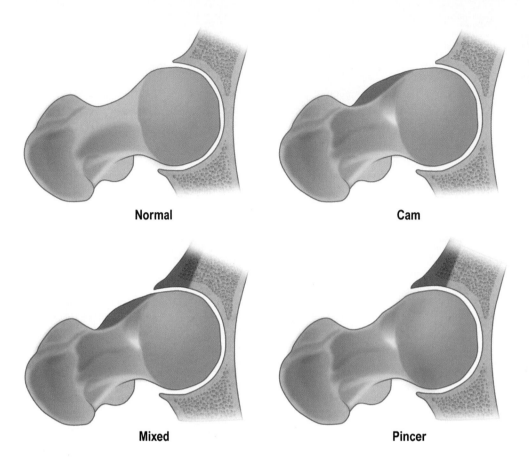

Normal

Cam

Mixed

Pincer

FIGURE 5.1
FAI morphology: cam, pincer and mixed.

Patients with FAI morphology who do not participate in activities requiring significant ROM in specific planes or who do not participate in repetitive, intense activity are less likely to develop FAI syndrome (Register et al., 2012).

Clinical Presentation

In a large multi-center, prospective, longitudinal cohort of 1076 patients, FAI occurred predominantly in young, white patients with a normal BMI (Clohisy et al., 2013). In the athletic population, FAI is primarily seen in individuals who are involved in sports which involve cutting and pivoting activities, rapid lateral motion, acceleration, and deceleration (Knapik & Salata, 2019). Soccer, basketball, rugby, ice hockey and Australian rules football have a proportionally high incidence of FAI (Nawabi et al., 2014). Patients typically present with symptoms of gradually increasing activity-related hip or groin pain (Table 5.2). The classical presentation of FAI is normally anterior or anterolateral hip/groin pain, which can radiate down the anterior or anterolateral aspect of the thigh. However, location of pain with FAI patients can be variable as shown by Clohisy et al., 2009, with 88% of patients having groin pain, 67% having lateral hip pain, 35% having anterior thigh pain, 29% having buttock pain, and 27% having knee pain.

Patients often grasp the affected hip with their hand, demonstrating the classical "C-sign" (Byrd, 2007). Patients may note specific positions within sports, or even activities such as extended sitting and stairs, appear to trigger and exacerbate their hip pain. Almost 45% of patients with FAI report having pain when transitioning from a seated to standing position (Philippon et al., 2007).

The majority of patients cannot recall when the specific injury occurred, and most patients will have modified their competitive level of activity by the time of evaluation (Philippon et al., 2007). In FAI syndrome, the symptoms are usually aggravated by activities that involve deep hip flexion, squatting, internal rotation, twisting of the hip and are alleviated by rest or modification of the activity.

TABLE 5.1 Characteristics of the Two Types of FAI		
Criteria	**CAM Impingement**	**Pincer Impingement**
Average age (range) (y)	32 (21–51)	40 (40–57)
Sex distribution (M:F)	14:1	1:3
Osseous morphology	Aspherical bump at the femoral head–neck junction, decreased femoral head–neck offset	Focal or global acetabular over-coverage; acetabular retroversion
Radiographic predictors	Pistol grip deformity; alpha angle >60 degrees	LCEA >40 degrees, posterior wall sign
Injury mechanism	Jamming of aspherical head into acetabulum Primarily affects cartilage with repeated flexion The labrum gets damaged secondarily	Linear contact between over-covering rim and head–neck junction Affects labrum primarily; with damage patterns located on the peripheral acetabulum Associated with contrecoup lesions
Typical location of cartilage damage	11- to 3-o'clock position	Circumferential with contrecoup
Average depth of cartilage damage (mm)	11	4
(Adapted from Tannast et al., 2007.)		

It is also not uncommon for patients to report mechanical symptoms such as clicking, snapping, popping and subjective stiffness of the hip (Egger et al., 2016). Patients may note specific positions within sports, or even activities such as extended sitting, stairs or incline walking, appear to trigger and exacerbate their hip pain. Further, patients may complain of decreased function and inability to continue their current level of sporting activity due to their symptoms (Tranovich et al., 2014).

There are distinct, sex-dependent disease patterns in FAI patients as outlined in Table 5.3. Generally females have more profound symptomatology and milder morphologic abnormalities, while males have a higher activity level, larger morphologic abnormalities and more extensive intra-articular disease (Halim et al., 2015).

FAI and Core Muscle Injury/Athletic Pubalgia

There is often overlap between intra-articular and extra-articular pathology for patients presenting with chronic hip and groin pain. Due to the loss of functional hip range of motion, FAI can contribute to compensatory extra-articular injuries and lead to increased motion and stress through the lumbar spine, sacroiliac joints, pubic symphysis, and core muscles (Padaki et al., 2021).

A significant subset of FAI patients will also have symptoms of core muscle injury/athletic pubalgia (Ross et al., 2015). Direct evidence between athletic pubalgia and FAI was first described by Larson et al. (2011). Most athletes require 30 degrees of hip internal rotation to be functional, during sporting activities (Roach & Miles, 1991). It is

TABLE 5.2 Clinical Characteristics of Patients with FAI Syndrome

Profile	Age: 18–40, F>M, normal BMI
	Active individuals involved in regular sporting activities
Clinical history	Insidious onset of activity-related hip and groin pain and stiffness, demonstrates "C sign", mechanical symptoms of clicking, catching, popping
	Aggravated by deep hip flexion, sitting, squatting, twisting, pivoting and cutting activities
Hip joint ROM	Decreased hip flexion and internal rotation
Hip muscle strength	Reduced strength of trunk and hip muscles, especially hip abductors, adductors and rotators, and less consistently hip extensors
Function	Limited motion with bilateral squats, limitation with motions that cause hip flexion, adduction and internal rotation
	Impaired dynamic single-leg balance
Special testing	Positive impingement tests, pain on end-range flexion and internal rotation
Diagnostic imaging	*Radiographs:*
	Cam-type FAI includes an alpha-angle >60 degrees and head–neck offset less than 8 mm
	Pincer-type FAI includes a lateral center edge angle >40 degrees and acetabular index (Tonnis angle) of less than 0 degrees

TABLE 5.3 Sexual Dimorphisms Associated with Femoro-acetabular Impingement

Males
Males are more likely than females to have radiographic cam-type FAI
Hip flexor strength seems to be associated with cam morphology severity in men
Males are more likely than females to have bilateral FAI presentation
Males are significantly more likely to have advanced cartilage lesions and larger labral tears
Males are more likely to progress to hip osteoarthritis than females

Females
Alpha angles are significantly smaller in females than in males
Female patients have greater hip motion than males
Hip anteversion is significantly more in females than in males
Hip abductor strength seems to be associated with the extent of hip symptoms in women
Female patients have significantly greater disability at presentation and hip function scores are significantly lower for females than in males

plausible that the range of motion limitations associated with FAI could lead to compensatory patterns, overloading of the trunk and pelvic muscles, and may lead to athletic pubalgia (Strosberg et al., 2016).

Physical Examination

A thorough history will provide the clinician with a focused differential that will guide subsequent physical examination and diagnostic tests and imaging. Comprehensive evaluation and physical examination of an adult with hip pain is covered in Chapter 12 of this textbook.

Patients with FAI usually exhibit hip and groin pain with end-range hip flexion and internal rotation of the hip, and may also experience limited hip internal rotation and abduction on examination (DiSilvestro et al., 2020). It is recommended that range of motion at the hip should always be compared to the contralateral hip.

An imaging study by Kubiak-Langer et al. (2007) has shown that hips with FAI have decreased flexion, internal rotation and abduction. Further, FAI patients have significant restriction in internal rotation while comparing with asymptomatic individuals (Audenaert et al., 2012). Also, the internal rotation decreased with increased hip flexion and adduction and loss of internal rotation becomes profound, when the hip is flexed to 90 degrees.

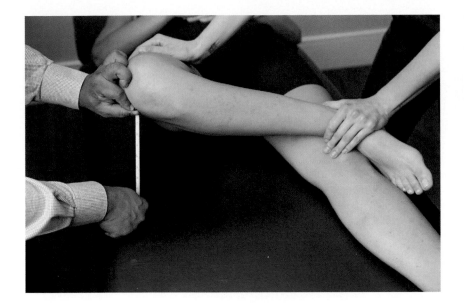

FIGURE 5.2
FABER distance test (FDT). FABER distance testing on a right hip, in the supine position. With the pelvis in neutral rotation, the hip is flexed, abducted, and externally rotated, with the foot resting proximal to the contralateral knee. Measurements are taken from the inferior aspect of the knee to the examination table and compared with the contralateral side.

While there are multiple provocative maneuvers that can be used to evaluate for FAI, only two tests have demonstrated clinical efficacy. The first maneuver involves flexion, adduction, and internal rotation (FADIR) and is also referred to as the anterior impingement sign and the second maneuver uses flexion, abduction, and external rotation (FABER) to assume a figure 4-like position. While these tests are largely non-specific, both the FADIR and FABER have demonstrated excellent sensitivity (Tijssen et al., 2017) and a negative FADIR test helps to rule out intra-articular hip disease (Reiman et al., 2020).

Another useful test is the FABER distance test (FDT), a variation of the FABER, where the affected leg is flexed and its heel positioned on the contralateral knee, above the patella and the distance from the lateral epicondyle is measured while stabilizing the pelvis (Bagwell, 2016; Figure 5.2). A positive FDT (defined as a difference of 4 cm or more between hips) is a reliable diagnostic exam for cam-type FAI (Trindade et al., 2019).

Reliable strength assessment of hip muscle groups, can be undertaken using hand-held dynamometry (HHD; Figure 5.3). The clinician should be aware that in hip strength assessments using HHD, systematic bias exists between testers of different sex, which could be explained by differences in upper-extremity strength (Thorborg et al., 2013). Inter-tester reliability can be improved using external fixation, while performing strength testing using HHD (Byrne et al., 2020).

Imaging

If suspecting underlying FAI in a patient with chronic hip pain, plain radiographs should be performed to evaluate pathology and the femoral head–neck junction and acetabulum. Initial radiographic evaluation should include a well-aligned anteroposterior (AP) pelvis and lateral hip radiographs to identify cam or pincer lesions, as well as to rule out other causes of hip pain such as dysplasia and osteoarthritis (Mascarenhas et al., 2020).

The alpha angle, or the angle between the femoral neck axis and a line through a point where the contour of the femoral head–neck junction exceeds the radius of the femoral head, is considered diagnostic of cam morphology when greater than 60 degrees (van Klij et al., 2020). The lateral center edge angle (LCEA) is one of the most commonly utilized measurements to define the amount of acetabular coverage. A normal LCEA is typically between 20 and 39 degrees, whereas <20 degrees represents acetabular dysplasia and >40 degrees is defined as global over-coverage (Lim & Park, 2015).

In addition, magnetic resonance imaging (MRI) may be obtained to evaluate for the presence of labral pathology, chondral injury, soft tissue lesions, and to rule out red flags such as avascular necrosis or stress fractures, which may be missed on plain radiographs (Riley et al., 2015).

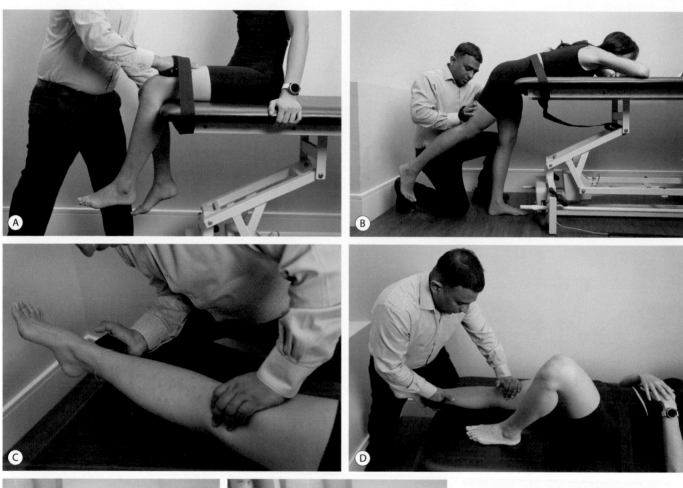

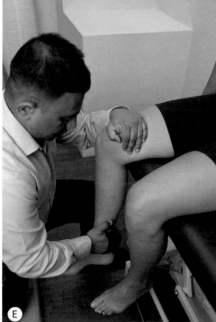

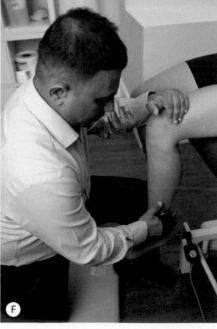

FIGURE 5.3
Strength testing using hand-held dynamometry: (A) hip flexors; (B) hip extensors; (C) hip abductors; (D) hip adductors; (E) hip external rotators; (F) hip internal rotators.

Diagnostic Intra-articular Hip Injection

Many patients with long-standing history of hip and groin pain may undergo a diagnostic hip injection to differentiate between intra-articular and extra-articular sources of pain. Although intra-articular injections with glucocorticoids have not shown long-lasting pain-relief effect in FAI patients, intra-articular injection with local anesthetic can be a valuable tool in the diagnostic process (Khan et al., 2015).

If the pain is markedly improved or disappears following the injection of local anesthetic or steroid, it is confirmed that the patient has intra-articular pathology. In addition, it has been shown that pain relief from intra-articular injections was not affected by coexisting intra-articular pathologies such as adductor, iliopsoas, or gluteal muscle pathologies (Kivlan et al., 2011). This study also highlighted those patients with an eventual FAI diagnosis experienced 85% relief from an intra-articular steroid injection compared with 64% mean relief in patients without an eventual FAI diagnosis. Further, a negative result has been proved to be a strong predictor of a poor postoperative outcome in FAI patients (Ayeni et al., 2014).

Clinical Diagnosis of FAI Syndrome

The diagnosis of FAI syndrome can be challenging to make, given its insidious onset and variable physical exam findings. It is important to highlight that the radiographic presence of a cam or pincer deformity does not equate to a clinical diagnosis of FAI.

In 2016, the Warwick Agreement established guidelines with regard to clinical diagnosis of FAI syndrome (Table 5.4). It defined FAI as "a clinical entity in which a pathological mechanical process causes hip pain when morphological abnormalities of the acetabulum and/or femur, combined with vigorous hip motion (especially at the extremes), lead to repetitive collisions that damage the soft-tissue structures within the joint itself" (Griffin et al., 2016). As per the consensus, FAI syndrome can be diagnosed only in the presence of a triad comprising symptoms, clinical signs, and radiographic findings.

Confirmation of diagnosis is usually achieved in combination with imaging such as radiographs, computed tomography (CT), and magnetic resonance imaging (MRI). As per the Warwick Agreement, the term FAI syndrome (FAIS) is the recommended term for patients with symptoms, clinical signs, and the relevant imaging findings, and terminologies such as FAI morphology, cam or pincer lesions should be avoided.

Non-surgical Management of FAI Syndrome

The treatment of FAIS is an evolving science. A systematic review of non-operative treatment for FAIS by Wall et al. (2013) showed improvement ranging from 44% to 72% with conservative management, and this improvement was maintained for up to 2 years in a long-term study (Emara et al., 2011). Two landmark RCTs have shown hip arthroscopy to be superior to non-operative treatment of FAI (Griffin et al., 2018; Palmer et al., 2019). However, it should be noted that the treatment programs of the non-operative branches of these RCTs did not address the underlying individual impairments and were too short in duration (Kemp et al., 2019).

In a recent metanalysis of five randomized controlled trials, it was observed that conservative management was an effective initial option for managing FAIS patients (Hoit et al., 2020). Further, a review showed that supervised physiotherapy programs focusing on active strengthening are more effective than unsupervised and passive programs. Conservative management of non-arthritic hip pain should focus on addressing neuromuscular deficits through rehabilitation of the hip and lumbopelvic regions and should include patient education, activity modification and cessation of provocative movements and implementation of an individualized impairment-based rehabilitation (McGovern et al., 2019).

Patient Education

Modifying activity levels and avoiding provocative positions is paramount in the management of FAIS. Pain during sitting is common in FAIS patients. Sitting in low chairs where the knees are higher than the hips can be very provocative in these patients. Avoiding prolonged sitting (>30 minutes), taking frequent postural breaks, keeping the hips more elevated than the knees, should be discussed with FAIS patients to minimize symptoms. Also, frequent sitting with legs crossed should be discouraged, as it combines hip flexion and adduction. Oral anti-inflammatory medications can be used to alleviate pain and enable the patient to better participate in physical therapy.

TABLE 5.4 2016 Warwick Consensus Statement Questions

Questions	Consensus
What is FAI syndrome?	FAI syndrome is a motion-related clinical disorder of the hip with a triad of symptoms, clinical signs and imaging findings. It represents symptomatic premature contact between the proximal femur and the acetabulum.
How should FAI syndrome be diagnosed?	Symptoms, clinical signs, and imaging findings must be present to diagnose FAI syndrome.
Symptoms	FAI syndrome commonly has motion-related or position-related pain in the hip or groin. Patients also may describe clicking, catching, locking, stiffness, restricted range of motion, or giving way.
Clinical signs	The diagnosis of FAI syndrome does not depend on a single clinical sign. The FADIR test is sensitive but not specific for FAI syndrome. Internal rotation of the hip is commonly restricted.
Diagnostic imaging	Obtain an AP radiograph of the pelvis and a lateral femoral neck view of the symptomatic hip. Advanced imaging can be considered to further assess the morphological changes of the hip and the surrounding soft tissue.
Treatment of FAI syndrome	FAI syndrome can be treated by conservative care, rehabilitation or surgery. Conservative care may involve education, watchful waiting, lifestyle and activity modification. Physiotherapy-led rehabilitation aims to improve hip stability, neuromuscular control, strength, range of motion and movement patterns. Surgery, either open or arthroscopic, aims to improve the hip morphology and repair damaged tissue.
Prognosis of FAI syndrome	Most patients can return to full activity, including sports, with treatment. OA appears to be a long-term outcome of cam morphology. However, it is currently unknown whether treatment for FAI syndrome prevents hip osteoarthritis.

Another common complaint among patients with FAS is pain during squatting, especially with increasing depth or narrow stance. Exercises such as hip thruster or split-squat could be discussed as alternatives with the client. Reducing the squat depth to less than 60 degrees and performing the squat in an abducted and externally rotated position can decrease impingement symptoms and avoid aggravating the hip. These recommendations can also be applied to other exercises such as the leg press, lunge, hack or goblet squat. As a general rule, it is beneficial to avoid/limit exercises that impinge the hip (i.e., hip flexion >90 degrees), such as deep squats, incline leg press or high step-ups. Extreme trunk rotation towards the symptomatic side should be limited, since this can be provocative for individuals with FAIS, as it places the hip in excessive internal rotation. Cycling should be restricted during the initial stages. If unavoidable, elevation of the cycle seat and slightly abducting the legs can help in avoiding impingement symptoms.

Manual Therapy and Soft Tissue Techniques

From a mobility perspective, hip flexion, adduction and internal rotation are restricted in FAIS patients (Samora et al., 2011).

It is important to address range of motion deficits which can be improved. Manual therapy interventions to improve global hip mobility and for decreasing symptoms can be beneficial, especially if the patient has high pain levels affecting participation in rehabilitation (Lebeau et al., 2014). Readers seeking a more detailed discussion of hip manual therapy techniques are encouraged to read Chapter 16. To allow carry-over of the manual techniques, a home-based hip self-mobilization program can help in promoting patient independence in the management of their mobility deficits (Reiman et al., 2013). Soft tissue and dry needling treatment, to reduce pain and overactivity of hip stabilizer musculature, can also be utilized if clinically indicated (see Chapter 17 of this textbook).

Individualized Impairment-based Rehabilitation

Common physical impairments in FAI include reduced trunk muscle strength and pelvic control, reduced strength of hip muscles, especially hip abductors and rotators, impaired dynamic single-leg balance and reduced functional impairments (Freke et al., 2016). Evidence suggests that exercise therapy is beneficial in the majority of patients with FAIS, particularly in the initial stages (Wall et al., 2013). For optimal benefits, the strengthening programs should be administered for a minimum of 3 months (Kemp et al., 2020).

Exercise therapy aims to reduce pain and improve hip function. This can be achieved by decreasing hip loads by reducing/minimizing the provocative activities and progressively strengthening the hip and trunk muscles. In addition, treatment should also include strategies on increasing the mobility and strength of the surrounding links of the kinetic chain to make up for limited hip motion. At this stage, there is a paucity of research trials to support what might be considered the ideal rehabilitation strategy for patients with FAIS. Following on from a comprehensive objective assessment, a specific rehab program can be implemented in FAIS patients to address their individual impairment (Figure 5.4).

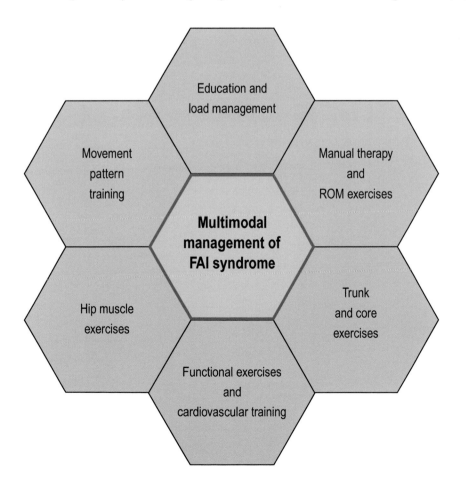

FIGURE 5.4
Key components of rehabilitation of FAI syndrome.
(Adapted from Heerey et al., 2018; Short et al., 2021.)

Essential Elements of Exercise Program

Initial exercise selection will be highly dependent on the patient's symptom severity and level of function at the time of presentation, as outlined in Table 5.5.

Postural and Movement-Pattern Training

Postural training is often overlooked in these patients. Pelvic tilt can either increase or decrease the point to impingement between the femoral neck and the acetabulum and is a target for rehabilitation (Azevedo et al., 2016). Increased anterior tilt at the pelvis reduces hip flexion, adduction and internal rotation, which may increase hip and groin symptoms in patients with FAIS (Ross et al., 2014). Further, Reynolds et al. (1999) have shown that as the pelvis rotates anteriorly, the functional retroversion of the acetabulum is increased, which could lead to an increased likelihood of impingement occurring at the acetabular rim, with hip flexion activities. Given the

relationship between hip impingement and an exaggerated anterior pelvic tilt, it is reasonable to promote a more natural posture in these patients. Therefore, exercises aimed at altering the tilt of the pelvis may reduce the frequency of impingement and could limit further joint damage (Patel et al., 2020).

Altered movement patterns such as excessive hip adduction during functional tasks have been observed in patients with intra-articular hip pathology (Austin et al., 2008). These may alter mechanical forces on the joint and increased strain on intra-articular structures such as the cartilage and the acetabular labrum. A randomized controlled trial by Harris-Hayes et al. (2016) has shown rehabilitation using movement-pattern training can yield positive outcomes in the young adult population with chronic hip pain. However, we cannot conclude that this form of training is superior to other treatment strategies in the management of FAIS. Further trials are needed to compare this approach to a standard rehabilitation approach.

TABLE 5.5 FAI Symptom Rating Scale			
Stage	Activity of Daily Living	Sporting Activity	Night Pain
1	No pain during daily activities	Pain or stiffness only following sporting activities. Symptoms usually resolve within 24 hours. Able to continue sports without major modification.	No
2	Symptoms felt during certain daily activities It usually involves deep hip flexion, internal rotation or twisting activities.	Pain or stiffness during sporting activities, which need modification. Symptoms can persist beyond 24 hours, following cessation of provocative activities.	No
3	Pain that is present during most daily activities Symptoms interfere with daily life on a regular basis	Unable to participate in sporting activities at the desired level, due to increasing symptoms.	Intermittent rest pain that does not disturb sleep regularly
4	Pain that is present during all activities and adversely affecting activities of daily living. Unable to tolerate prolonged seated position. May report episodes of limping during flare-up.	Not participating in sporting activities.	Constant rest pain that disturbs sleep regularly

Deep Hip Rotator Muscle Strengthening

The majority of prescribed therapeutic exercises in FAI are uniplanar, mainly involving the sagittal and frontal planes (Wright et al., 2021). Exercise design should incorporate exercises reflecting the contributing patho-mechanics associated with FAIS. Lack of control in the transverse plane has been implicated as a factor related to increased pain in FAIS (Austin et al., 2008). The deep external rotators (quadratus femoris, obturator internus and externus and the gemelli) have been proposed as key active stabilizers of the hip (Ward et al., 2010). These muscles have a short lever arm and therefore have the potential to act as deep stabilizers, to steady the femoral head in the acetabulum. Along with the hip abductors, they are called "hip joint rotating sleeves" which control hip stability and fine joint movement (Hu et al., 2021). Strengthening the deep hip external rotators (Figure 5.5) has the potential to improve dynamic stability of the hip joint in the transverse plane (Retchford et al., 2013). Extremes of hip rotation, especially in combination with hip flexion, should be avoided to minimize exacerbation of symptoms.

Hip Muscle Strengthening

Progressive resistance training for individuals with FAIS should focus on strengthening the hip abductors, adductors, external rotators, and extensors. These muscles play a crucial role in providing dynamic hip stability during activities like squatting, running, and jumping and also maintain good alignment to reduce excessive adduction and internal rotation (Kolber et al., 2015). Overzealous or end-range strengthening of hip flexors, adductors and internal rotators should be avoided to prevent flare-up of FAIS symptoms, especially in the early stages. Examples of a progressive hip strength program are outlined in Figure 5.6 (early stage) and Figure 5.7 (mid to late stage).

A common muscle group which has shown to have weakness in FAIS patients is the hip abductors. Hip abductor strength seems to be associated to the extent of hip symptoms, especially in women (Maffiuletti et al., 2020). Hip adductor strength is also an important target, since greater adductor strength is associated with better hip-related quality of life, following hip arthroscopy (Kemp et al., 2016a).

Closed-chain exercises should be incorporated to model functional activities. Gradually, more global exercises should be introduced with reducing the focus on isolated strengthening exercises. Functional exercises should be implemented to fit the patient's goals and specific demands of the sport (Enseki et al., 2010). These exercises may include advanced strength and neuromuscular control such as

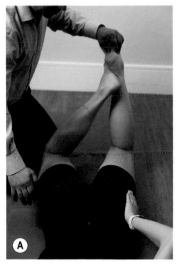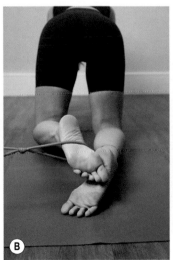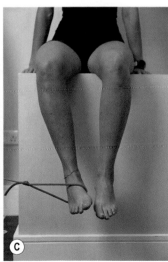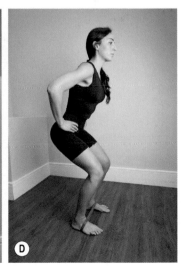

FIGURE 5.5
Progressive deep hip rotator muscle strengthening examples: (A) prone isometric heel squeeze; (B) 4-point hip rotation; (C) seated hip rotation; (D) midfoot crab walks.

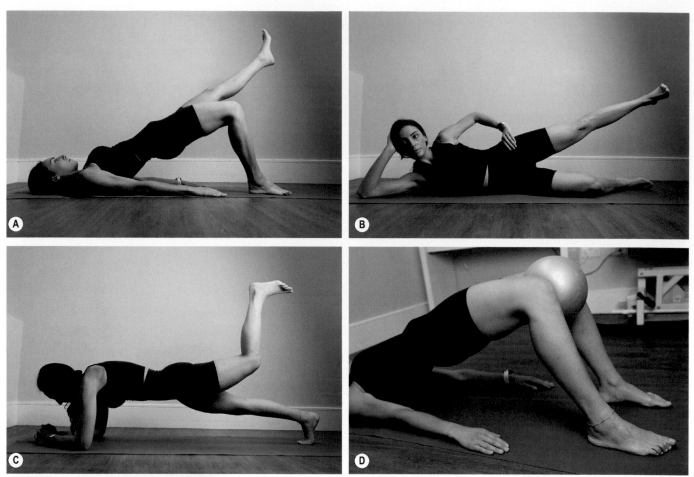

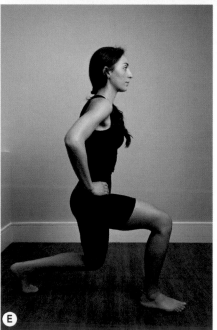

FIGURE 5.6
Progressive hip strength program examples (early stage): (A) double- to single-leg bridge; (B) side-lying hip abduction; (C) quadruped hip extension (short lever); (D) adductor squeeze; (E) split squat.

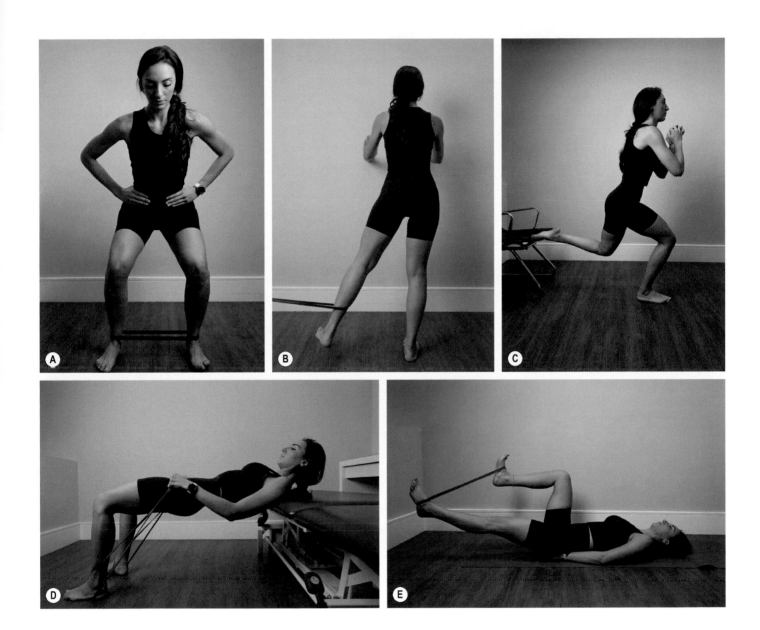

FIGURE 5.7
Progressive hip strength program examples (mid to late stage): (A) ankle lateral band walks; (B) resisted hip adduction;
(C) Bulgarian split squat; (D) banded hip thruster; (E) psoas march.

lunges, hip thruster, step-ups, side to side lateral agilities, forward and backward running with a cord. Exercises such as single-leg squat and dead-lift are beneficial since these create high activity of the gluteus maximus (Distefano et al., 2009). Further, exercises should target the entire kinetic chain and utilize both eccentric and concentric contraction. Additional training with medicine balls, kettle-bells or dumbbells can be added to promote hip strength

(Terrell et al., 2021). When appropriate, plyometric exercises should be introduced and progressed to the level of the activity the patient is returning (Stearns & Powers, 2014).

Trunk and Core Muscles Strengthening

Improving the strength of the trunk muscles in an important target since it has been shown to be reduced in FAI patients following hip arthroscopy (Kemp et al., 2016b). The degree of hip impingement can be affected by the patho-mechanic relationship between the trunk and pelvis (Pierannunzii, 2017). Pelvic position is influenced by trunk mechanics. Therefore, improving trunk muscles strength and stability can improve control around the pelvis, which can alter impingement and reduce pain in FAI patients (Kemp et al., 2020). A pilot randomized controlled trial has shown that addition of trunk stabilization exercises to a typical hip rehabilitation protocol improves clinical outcomes and may augment non-operative rehabilitation in FAIS patients (Aoyama et al., 2018).

There is currently no peer-reviewed evidence on return to play rates with non-operative treatment of FAIS. Athletes may return to sports when they have no pain or tenderness, good muscular strength and appropriate neuromuscular control and demonstrate the ability to attenuate rapid loading of the hip joint (Tranovich et al., 2014). Examples of a progressive trunk and core strength program are outlined in Figure 5.8.

Surgery

If conservative treatment fails despite extended period of rehabilitation, then surgery may be required to address the bony morphology and also to repair/treat the labral lesion and chondral pathology. Historically, this was done through an open procedure. Nowadays, the majority of surgeons are able to offer these interventions through hip arthroscopy. Operative management of FAIS aims to achieve a functional range of motion and restore the femoral head–neck junction offset to a more physiologic state, and relieve stress on nearby muscle groups. This is achieved by resecting cam and pincer lesions and repairing any damage to the labrum using anchors or debridement of degenerative labral tears (Lynch et al., 2020).

Postoperative Rehabilitation

Rehabilitation following hip arthroscopy remains at a preliminary stage, when compared to the growth and technical advancements in hip surgery. Rehabilitation protocols following hip arthroscopy typically consist of four phases (time frames ranging from 12 to 28 weeks), with set goals and progression criteria as outlined in Table 5.6 (Takla et al., 2021).

As there is heterogeneity in patient-specific characteristics and variations in postoperative recommendations by the surgical teams, no determination can be made as to which protocol is most effective and further high-quality comparative studies are needed (Ankem et al., 2020). Readers seeking a more detailed discussion on rehabilitation following hip arthroscopy are encouraged to read work by Domb et al. (2016) and Wilson et al. (2019).

Hip Dysplasia/Hip Instability

Developmental dysplasia of the hip (DDH) is a term that encompasses a spectrum of structural pathology involving the acetabulum and the proximal femur (Gala et al., 2016; Wells et al., 2017). Dysplastic acetabuli can be deficient in shape and/or orientation, often leading to anterior insufficiency but also potentially lateral, posterior, or global deficiency (Gala et al., 2016; Bali et al., 2020). Proximal femoral anomalies can often accompany these acetabular abnormalities, including increased femoral neck anteversion and neck-shaft angle (e.g., coxa valga) (Clohisy et al., 2009). It is well established that severe untreated DDH is a risk factor of early-onset osteoarthritis (Murphy et al., 1995). However, research is also suggesting that mild dysplasia could be linked to the early onset of hip osteoarthritis, in certain individuals (Jacobsen & Sonne-Holm, 2005). Despite this, a lack of awareness and understanding appears to exist among healthcare professionals regarding hip dysplasia. This can obviously create difficulty when trying to provide an effective diagnosis and management of the condition. This section aims to provide a comprehensive outline of hip dysplasia, how to diagnose the condition, and potential management strategies.

Overview of Hip Dysplasia/Hip Instability

The hip is an inherently stable structure with the acetabulum covering approximately 170 degrees of the femoral head, whilst being anteverted 15–20 degrees, with a 45-degree lateral tilt (Kalisvaart & Safran, 2015). The acetabular labrum provides a negative suction and helps to increase both the acetabular volume and surface area by 20–25% (Safran, 2019). The stability of the hip relies upon a combination of factors; bony anatomy within correct physiological parameters, appropriate capsular tension, adequate ligamentous stability, no labral compromise and correct muscle patterning.

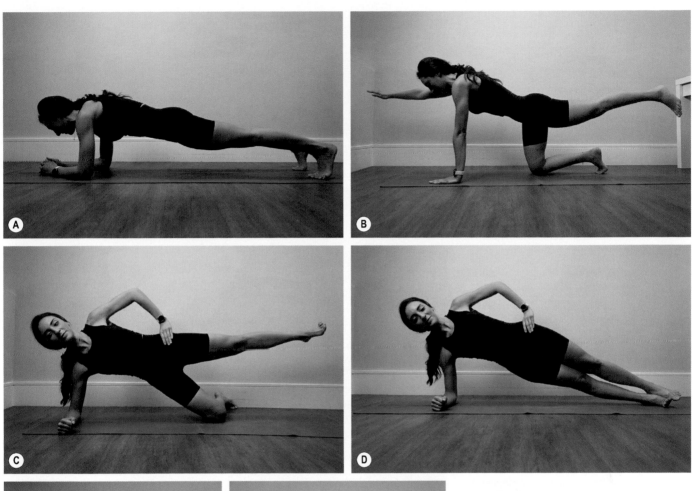

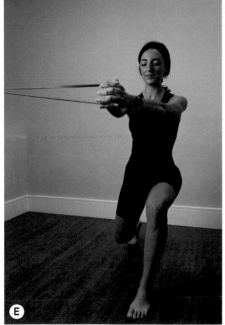

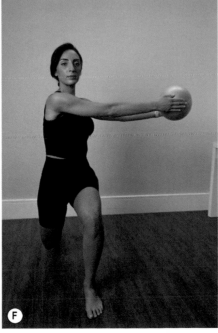

FIGURE 5.8
Progressive trunk and core strength program examples: (A) plank; (B) bird-dog; (C) side-star plank; (D) side plank; (E) split-squat Pallof press; (F) split-squat trunk rotation.

TABLE 5.6 Guidelines for Postoperative Rehabilitation Following Hip Arthroscopy

Stage	Estimate Time (Weeks)	Rehabilitation Goals	Progression Criteria
Immediate postoperative	2–4	Pain control Appropriate gait within weight-bearing status (assistive devices if needed)	90 degrees of asymptomatic flexion 10 degrees of hip extension Tolerate all prescribed exercises
Early impairment	2–4	Symmetrical gait pattern ROM sufficient for ADLs Re-establish neuromuscular control for ADLs	Tolerance of progressive exercise program Establish full weight-bearing status Symmetrical gait pattern ROM >80% of opposite hip in all planes of motion
Late impairment	2–6	ROM symmetrical to non-surgical side Return to low and moderate level ADLs Return to non-labor occupation activities	ROM symmetrical to opposite hip Strength >75% of opposite hip in all planes of motion Maintain single-leg stance × 30s Continuous ambulation >10 min or 1 mile
Functional restoration	2–8	Return to all ADLs Low to moderate fitness activities as aligned with patient goals	Strength >75% of opposite hip in all planes of motion HOS-S >85% for ADL subscale

Note: Time frames are estimated and do not supersede progression criteria

(From Takla et al., 2021.)

If any of these structures are compromised, this can lead to excessive femoral head translation within the acetabulum and thus hip instability. This may lead to abnormal joint contact pressures disrupting the acetabular rim, labrum and articular cartilage, potentially leading to pain (Dangin et al., 2016).

Hip instability can be defined as traumatic or atraumatic, and ranges from subtle micro-instability, to subluxation, to full dislocation of the hip. Patients with instability can be divided into the following six categories: DDH, post-trauma, sports-related micro-trauma, connective tissue disorders, iatrogenic issues, and idiopathic issues (Kalisvaart & Safran, 2015).

Traumatic instability may be as a result of a car accident, or sporting injury, where the mechanisms of injury are usually a posterior dislocation of the hip whilst the hip and knee are flexed, and a posteriorly directed force is transmitted through the knee (Dumont, 2016). Instability can remain post-relocation due to damage to the capsulo-ligamentous structures and the chondrolabral junction.

Other hip disorders: FAI syndrome, hip dysplasia, hip instability

Fractures of the posterior wall can also occur via this mechanism (Safran, 2019). Iatrogenic instability can be induced by arthroscopic surgery. Excessive acetabuloplasty, over-resection of the labrum, division of the capsulo-ligamentous structures, extensive capsulotomy, or psoas tenotomy can all contribute to postoperative instability. There has been much discussion in the literature regarding the requirement for routine closure of the capsulotomy, and it has become more common practice post arthroscopy. Repair of the capsulotomy during arthroscopy surgery is particularly required for patients with connective tissue disorders and those who require extreme physiological hip range of movement for return to optimal function (Dumont, 2016). Abnormal collagen content and formation that is observed in connective tissue disorders such as Ehlers–Danlos syndrome, Down syndrome, Marfan syndrome or generalized hypermobility can predispose patients to develop instability of the hip. These disorders result in decreased capsulo-ligamentous support, which can lead to increased femoral head translation.

Sports such as gymnastics, martial arts, and dancing which require extreme ranges of movement with axial loading and repetitive rotational movement, may induce microtrauma to the ligaments, capsule, or chondrolabral junction. If this is coupled with a background of ligament laxity, then there is a higher risk for increased femoral head translation, micro-instability and pain (Kalisvaart & Safran, 2015).

Idiopathic hip micro-instability is usually seen in patients that may have several very mild associating factors which do not meet clinically significant parameters for diagnosis, such as mild hip dysplasia outside radiographic parameters, or generalized mild ligament laxity, capsular insufficiency, or poor muscular stability (Kalisvaart & Safran, 2015).

Prior to the 1980s, hip dysplasia was more commonly referred to as *congenital dysplasia* of the hip, initially described by Dupuytren in 1832 (Musielak et al., 2015). *Developmental dysplasia of the hip* more appropriately encompasses a dynamic condition capable of worsening or improving as a child develops, or developing in young adulthood. Current notions describe a potential resultant instability of the hip joint thought to lead to chondral degeneration and secondary osteoarthritis (Schmitz et al., 2020).

Prevalence and Etiology

The true prevalence of DDH is difficult to ascertain as the condition can often be asymptomatic, and there are inconsistencies regarding the diagnostic classification in the literature (Schmitz et al., 2020; Jacobsen & Sonne-Holm, 2005). Reports on prevalence range from 1.5% to 20% in the general population (Jacobsen & Sonne-Holm, 2005; Jacobsen et al., 2005; Ortiz-Neira et al., 2012; Tian et al., 2017).

The exact causes of DDH are not known and are likely multifactorial. There are thought to be both mechanical and genetic factors in the etiology of dysplasia. A reduced uterus size reduces fetal leg mobility and is associated with hip dysplasia. This occurs with first-born children and breech presentations. The left hip is more commonly affected, likely due to the left leg being in an adducted position in the uterus against the mother's sacrum. A key external factor in the development of late-presenting DDH is the influence of swaddling (Ishida, 1977; Chaarani et al., 2002).

Rates differ between ethnicity with low rates in African populations and higher rates in Native Americans and Norwegians (Lee et al., 2013). Females are more likely to present for treatment than males (Sankar et al., 2017). A family history of hip disease has also been reported in over a quarter of patients (Sankar et al., 2017).

The psychological impact of hip dysplasia is significant and many patients face an average of 5 years before an accurate diagnosis is made, often seeing multiple medical professionals in that time (Nunley et al., 2011; Gambling & Long, 2019). This delay in diagnosis can lead to psychological effects as patients feel unsupported, stressed and anxious. Early detection of hip dysplasia allows for an increased repertoire of treatment options, including hip preservation surgery which delays the progression to a degenerative joint (Gambling & Long, 2019).

Clinical Evaluation, Presentation, and Diagnosis

The diagnostic criteria for a patient with hip dysplasia lack consensus, particularly in adults with less severe cases. There are three main classifications for defining acetabular dysplasia and structural instability (Table 5.7): anterior, posterior and lateral or global instability (Wilkin et al., 2017).

The traditional measure of DDH is the lateral centre-edge angle (LCEA) of Wiberg radiographically assessed from a

TABLE 5.7 Ottawa Classification for Symptomatic Acetabular Dysplasia

Class	Clinical Findings	Radiographic Findings
Anterior	Anterior hip pain Exacerbated by: • hip extension + external rotation • late stance phase • positive prone apprehension relocation test	Normal LCEA (>25 degrees) Percent anterior coverage <15% Anterior wall index <0.30 Excessive posterior wall coverage
Posterior	Anterior + posterior hip pain ± prior diagnosis of SI joint pathology or piriformis syndrome ± neurologic symptoms in sciatic nerve distribution Exacerbated by: • flexion + internal rotation ± axial load • ascending stairs/slope	Normal LCEA (>25 degrees) Percent posterior coverage <36% Posterior wall index <0.80 Posterior wall sign Ischial spine sign Crossover sign >1 cm from the acetabular roof
Lateral *Anterolateral* *Posterolateral* *Global*	Diffuse activity-related pain Abductor fatigue Symptoms of static overload	LCEA (<20 degrees), or LCEA 20–25 degrees and AI >10 ± features of anterior or posterior under-coverage depending on acetabular version

(Modified from Wilkin et al., 2017.)

weight-bearing AP pelvic view. A value of less than 20 degrees is defined as dysplasia, between 20 and 25 degrees is borderline dysplasia, and 25 to 39 degrees is within normal parameters (Clohisy et al., 2008). The use of the term "borderline" dysplasia has recently been questioned as literature supporting differing classifications grows. As the complex multidirectional nature of DDH has become better understood, the importance of utilizing a combination of radiological and clinical findings is receiving growing recognition (Vaudreuil & McClincy, 2020; Schmitz et al., 2020; Bali et al., 2020).

Diagnosing the dysplastic patient can be challenging, due to the variation in signs and symptoms. Patients commonly exhibit associated conditions such as lumbopelvic pain, greater trochanter pain syndrome (GTPS), and psoas tendinopathy. These can often be the early signs of

hip dysplasia. If these conditions are only diagnosed in isolation, practitioners may miss an underlying hip joint condition. Hip impingement signs can also coexist, both clinically and radiographically.

Unlike FAIS, there is no official diagnostic consensus on hip dysplasia (Griffin et al., 2016). It is important to remember that the physical examination tests for intra-articular hip pathology are sensitive but not specific. Therefore, when a test (such as the Flexion-Adduction-Internal-Rotation test) is positive, this does not confirm FAIS and could potentially be positive for a dysplastic hip.

Patients with hip pain should be screened for DDH risk factors such as: birth history – first born, breech presentation – and any issues identified as a child, family history of dysplasia or hip issues, family history of EDS or hypermobility.

Early commencement of physical therapy may manage some of the associated muscle–tendon pain and address other factors (biomechanics, proprioception, etc.) which therefore aim to reduce shearing forces that may contribute to joint degeneration and pain generation. A detailed assessment of young adult hip pain has been covered in Chapter 12 of this textbook; however, some key points on hip dysplasia tests will be covered.

Clinical Presentation of the Hip Dysplasia Patient

The typical presentation is an insidious onset of hip/groin pain, which is activity-related and eased with rest (Nunley et al., 2011). Eventually, the symptoms may become irritable with prolonged positions such as sitting/standing and daily activities (Dick et al., 2018). Patients may also report symptoms after a period of an unusual increase in activity or post childbirth due to changes in ligamentous stability (Schmitz et al., 2020). Moderate to severe pain on a daily basis has been reported in 77% of patients (Nunley et al., 2011).

The pain location in hip dysplasia is highly variable in adults, with patients complaining of pain in the anterior or lateral hip, groin, anterior aspect of the thigh, or buttock region (Nunley et al., 2011). As with other intra-articular sources such as FAI, patients can demonstrate pain in a C-shaped distribution around the inguinal crease (Schmitz et al., 2020; Dick et al., 2018). Some key differences between FAIS and hip dysplasia clinical presentations are outlined in Table 5.8.

These pain sites may be due to pain directly from the hip joint, or from surrounding musculotendinous structures. Pain in more than one site occurs commonly, with one

TABLE 5.8 Presentation of Hip Dysplasia vs. FAI Syndrome

Characteristics	Hip Dysplasia	FAI Syndrome
Sex	Female (80–90%)	Male and female
Limb dominance	Left hip more likely	No
Range of movement (ROM)	Normal to ↑ Global ROM ↑ Hip rotation in one direction, if associated with version abnormality	↓ Flexion and internal rotation
Generalized ligamentous laxity	Common in up to 50% of patients	Uncommon
Pain triggers	Pain normally with prolonged standing, weight-bearing activities like walking, running	Pain normally when sitting, squatting, flexion-based activities and end-range internal rotation
Apprehension	May be positive	Uncommon
FADIR	+ve with ↑ flexion and IR ROM	+ve with ↓ flexion and IR ROM

Note: These disease characteristics are highly variable with major overlap between FAI and dysplasia.

study reporting a prevalence of 63% of pain in two or more places (Nunley et al., 2011). Common causes of musculo-tendinous pain include the iliopsoas tendon (in approximately half of DDH patients) and gluteus medius/minimus (in approximately one-third of DDH patients) (Jacobsen et al., 2018; Jacobsen et al., 2019).

Iliopsoas tendinopathy is rarely a primary cause, and this should raise a suspicion of dysplasia (Jacobsen et al., 2018). Likewise, pain in the lateral hip can often be diagnosed as greater trochanter pain syndrome (GTPS), but the potential for underlying dysplasia, particularly in a younger patient, should always be considered. Exacerbating activities frequently include: hip flexion and external rotation in weight-bearing, prolonged standing or sitting (Schmitz et al., 2020).

Young and very active patients with severe dysplasia are more likely to be at risk of the joint failing earlier (average age 21) than those patients with mild–moderate dysplasia and mild–moderate activity (average age 28) (Matheney et al., 2016).

Mechanical symptoms such as clicking, catching, popping, locking or giving way are often reported by DDH patients and they may also report feelings of instability (Nunley et al., 2011). This can be due to labral pathology or due to tensor fasciae latae (TFL) tightness, gluteal tendinopathy or psoas tendinopathy. The joint shearing forces

associated with DDH leads to labral hypertrophy and potentially further to labral pathology. This mechanism of labral pathology is likely due to shearing forces, rather than the impingement mechanisms associated with FAIS. Night pain may also be present due to articular damage and labral tears, with a reported prevalence of 59% (Nunley et al., 2011). Limitations in walking distance and associated limping is also often described by patients (Nunley et al., 2011). This can be due to acetabular rim damage, symptomatic labral tears, associated pain inhibition leading to poor muscle patterning and pain on loading of both articular and soft tissue structures.

On physical examination, patients with dysplasia can present with an altered pelvic posture. This can be excessive anterior pelvic tilt to compensate for anterior acetabular deficiency (Fukushima et al., 2018), or swayback position with posterior pelvic tilt (Lewis et al., 2015). An abnormal gait pattern can occur with evidence of Trendelenburg and/or reduced terminal hip extension. This reduces the risk of anterior uncovering during dynamic movement (Kraeutler et al., 2016). The patient should also be evaluated for hypermobility. Beighton test and other specific hip instability tests: anterior apprehension test (AB-HEER test, Figure 5.9), prone instability test (Figure 5.10), hyperextension–external rotation (HEER test, Figure 5.11), dial test, FABER test and FPAW test (foot progression angle walking test) should be performed (Schmitz et al., 2020; Reiman

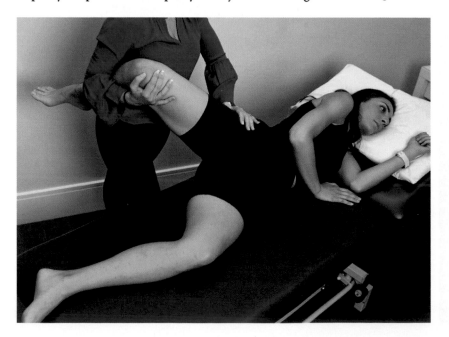

FIGURE 5.9
Abduction–hyperextension–external rotation (AB-HEER) test. Patient is in the side-lying position with the affected side up. The clinician then abducts the hip to 30–45 degrees, hyperextends and externally rotates the hip while providing an anteriorly directed force to the posterior greater trochanter. A positive test is reproduction of the patient's pain or instability sensation over the anterior hip.

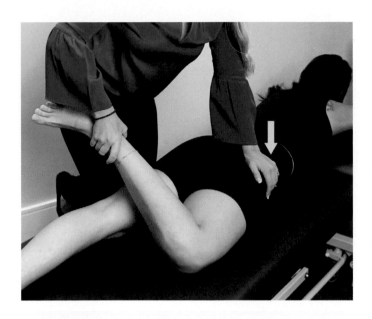

FIGURE 5.10
Prone instability test. Patient is in prone position. The hip is externally rotated, while the clinician applies a downward force on the posterior greater trochanter. A positive test is reproduction of the patient's pain or instability sensation over the anterior hip.

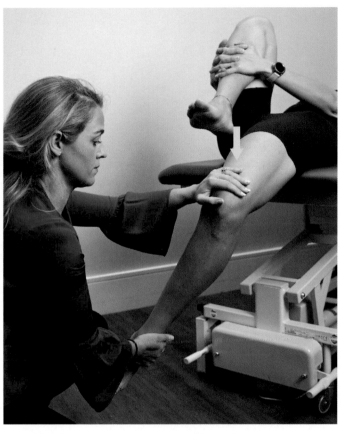

FIGURE 5.11
Hyperextension–external rotation (HEER) test. The patient is lying supine at the end of the bed with their legs hanging over the foot of the bed (Thomas test position). The unaffected hip is flexed up to the chest and held in position, with the affected hip left hanging down. The clinician applies an anteriorly directed force at the hip by performing hyperextension and external rotation of the affected hip. A positive test is reproduction of the patient's pain or instability sensation over the anterior hip.

et al., 2019). Key objective examination tests for hip dysplasia are outlined in Table 5.9. Table 5.10 shows the sensitivity and specificity for common examination tests for hip instability.

Radiographic Parameters

Plain radiographs remain the primary imaging modality in hip dysplasia and are an essential tool in assessment, diagnosis, guiding the treatment plan and also for postoperative review. X-rays provide a clear morphological overview of the entire pelvis; a weightbearing AP pelvis view and false profile view are a fundamental starting point (Tannast et al., 2015; Clohisy et al., 2008). Some important radiographic parameters to look for on a plain AP radiograph include LCEA, acetabular index (AI), posterior wall sign, and crossover sign. Clinicians should review the X-ray themselves, and not solely rely on the radiology report, as often this may only report on the degree of osteoarthritis in the hip. Young adults with hip dysplasia can be missed for this reason, as they may not have yet developed osteoarthritis on X-ray.

MRI and CT are useful for surgical planning and to define the condition of the joint but are not required for primary diagnosis. A 3T MRI is the gold standard to assess for signs of hip instability, such as labral tears, labral hypertrophy, paralabral cysts, and assess for cam morphology which can be concurrent with dysplasia. MRI can also assess joint surfaces, cartilage degradation, bone edema, and muscle bulk around the hip. This all helps in planning the correct operation with the optimal outcome (Hanke et al., 2020).

CT scans provide a three-dimensional picture of the bone anatomy, which shows precisely the location of the deficiency and the shape and orientation of the joint (Hanke et al., 2020).

TABLE 5.9 Key Objective Assessment for Hip Dysplasia

Range of motion	Internal and external rotation in neutral Internal and external rotation at 90 degrees hip flexion	Global ↑ ROM in all directions An increase of rotation in one direction (e.g., internal rotation) combined with a decrease in rotation in another (e.g., external rotation), can be indicative of associated femoral or acetabular anteversion
Apprehension tests	AB-HEER Abduction–hyperextension–external rotation test Prone instability test	When positive, these tests may increase the likelihood of DDH
Beighton's score	A 9-point scale to assess for hypermobility	The presence of hypermobility is an important consideration in the management of DDH
Drehmann sign	Positive or an unavoidable passive external rotation of the hip occurs when performing hip flexion	This may indicate the presence of retroversion. Important to note this can also be present in SCFE, FAI or hip OA

TABLE 5.10 Hip Instability Examination Tests

Test	Sensitivity	Specificity
Anterior apprehension (HEER)	71%	85%
Abduction–hyperextension–external rotation	81%	89%
Prone instability	33%	98%
If all 3 tests mentioned are positive	95% likelihood of micro-instability confirmed at surgery	

(Modified from Safran et al., 2019.)

More recently, cartilage mapping technique such as delayed gadolinium-enhanced magnetic resonance imaging of cartilage (dGEMRIC) has been introduced in the setting of hip dysplasia. This technique helps to quantify cartilage health and defines the degree and area of any degeneration, which can aid in predicting outcomes of surgery in the setting of dysplasia (Beaulé et al., 2020). For example, performing a PAO on a patient with significant cartilage degeneration can contribute to poor outcomes and early conversion to total hip replacement (Larsen et al., 2020). It should be noted that imaging-defined intra-articular hip pathology does not always correlate to pain (Heerey et al., 2018) and is only one component of clinical evaluation.

Femoral Version Abnormalities

Hip dysplasia is multidirectional and the relationship between both the femur and acetabulum will play a part in joint stability. Common variations in proximal femoral morphology include increased anteversion, coxa valga, coxa vara, and a shorter femoral neck. Patients who have versional deformities may present with altered hip rotation and changes in gluteal activation due to lever arm differences.

Increased femoral anteversion may result in increased shearing forces on the anterior acetabular rim, potentially resulting in anterior acetabular labral tears and instability as the anterior aspect of the femoral head may be under-covered (Uding et al., 2019). Those with femoral anteversion often demonstrate an increase in internal rotation and a decrease in external rotation range of movement.

Those with femoral retroversion may demonstrate an increase in external rotation and a decrease in internal rotation (Chadayammuri et al., 2016). Clinically, patients with significant anteversion may walk pigeon-toed and retroverted patients may walk with their feet externally rotated.

Non-surgical Management of Hip Dysplasia

There is limited published resources on managing adult hip dysplasia non-surgically, with no long-term studies investigating these outcomes. Therapists often report a lack of confidence in managing these patients due to the lack of awareness and training in this area. Non-surgical management should be considered when symptoms or deformities are mild, when surgical intervention isn't appropriate, or as a trial prior to surgical intervention. The goals of a comprehensive rehabilitation program (Table 5.11) should be approached for a minimum of 8–12 weeks before consideration of surgical intervention (Hunt et al., 2012; Enseki et al., 2014).

It is important to examine the source of the pain and consider what one can change conservatively. Attempting to identify extra-articular versus intra-articular pathology and whether static or dynamic features are contributing will help to guide the treatment. Aggravating/easing factors and morphological assessment can give insight into potential directional instabilities, which should be considered in rehabilitation. Physical therapy is beneficial in improving muscle patterning and reducing compensatory strategies and provides global strengthening prior to any surgical intervention. Clinically, the authors use symptom modification tests to try to identify one or more methods that reduce their symptoms and/or increase movement and function. Some examples include:

- Distraction of the joint at pain ranges (AP on femoral head at 90 degrees hip flexion). Change in symptoms could indicate articular joint pain/labral pain (Figure 5.12A).

- Compression of the joint at pain ranges. Looking for improved proprioception and therefore reduced pain and irritation on anterior rim (Figure 5.12B).

- Core activation (for example with straight leg raise). Does it change pain? If so, it could be due to anterior shearing overload.

TABLE 5.11 Goals of Treatment	
Educate the patient	An understanding of their hip condition
	An appreciation of factors which could be contributing to their pain
	Guidance on appropriate forms of exercises which are less likely to aggravate their symptoms
	Goal setting: short-term and long-term via a shared decision-making process
Improve physical condition of the hip	Reduce aggravating positions on the hip (through lifestyle modifications)
	(e.g., prolonged sitting, sustained end-range yoga stretches)
	Strengthening muscles and movement which support the hip
	(e.g., gluteus minimus, medius, and deep hip external rotators)
	Reduce load on musculotendinous structures which may be leading to pain and symptoms
	(e.g., iliopsoas and lateral gluteals)
	Proprioceptive training to improve joint stability
Promote general physical wellbeing	Improve cardiovascular health
	(e.g., cross-training, swimming with pool buoy, skip rope)
Improve kinetic chain and reduce hip loads	Lower body strengthening exercises (symmetrical double-leg exercises, reduce depth, e.g., squats and deadlifts)

- Offloading of different muscle groups such as the TFL or rectus femoris (instruct the patient to repeat movement whilst therapist picks up/offloads muscle bulk through the movement).

Conservative management can include physiotherapy, analgesia such as NSAIDS, and intra-articular corticosteroid injections. Physiotherapy should consist of education, lifestyle modifications, load management and strengthening

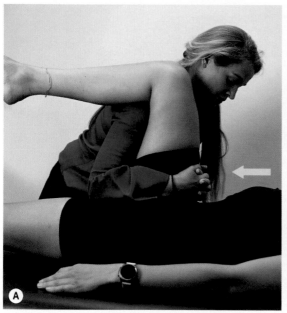
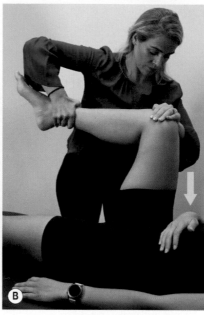

FIGURE 5.12
Symptom modification tests: (A) distraction of the joint at pain ranges (AP on femoral head at 90 degrees hip flexion); (B) compression of the joint at pain ranges.

exercises. Intra-articular injections can be used to create a window of opportunity to reduce pain and inflammation, and to engage with physical therapy, where pain has been a limiting factor. They are also used as a diagnostic tool to confirm that pain is coming from within the joint itself.

The type of dysplasia that a patient has can often correspond to aggravating and easing factors. Understanding the underlying structural abnormalities can be very helpful in advising patients on management. For example, a patient with "anterior dysplasia" will often be symptomatic with hip extension or external rotation movements, e.g., late phase of gait (see Table 5.7). Conversely, a patient with "posterior dysplasia" will often find positions of hip flexion or hip internal rotation irritable, e.g., prolonged sitting. Advice on minimizing or modifying provocative positions and exercises to improve stability during vulnerable tasks should be an important part of management.

Anecdotally, the authors have found proprioceptive rehabilitation to be beneficial as part of the multi-modal management of hip dysplasia (Figure 5.13). Once the fundamentals of posture and pelvic position are understood, then starting rehabilitation on an unstable surface is important in improving the joint position sense and activating the deep stabilizing muscles which have key proprioceptive properties and attachments to the hip capsule. Proprioceptive training has been shown to be beneficial in anterior cruciate ligament rehabilitation (Fitzgerald et al., 2000; Risberg et al., 2007); to the best knowledge of the authors, no published studies have addressed proprioceptive training in the management of labral tears. The labrum has an abundance of free nerve endings which contribute to both pain modulation and proprioception, therefore patients with labral pathology may benefit from proprioceptive training and neuromuscular re-education to improve the joint position sense and dynamic stabilization of the joint under load, with improved recruitment of the deep muscular stabilizers.

Education has been shown to be a key factor in empowering a patient to self-manage and encourage exercise in patients with OA of the hip and knee, and this also applies to the young adult hip population (Gay et al., 2016). Explaining factors contributing to pain, the importance of muscle strength and postural positioning, and the potential onward referral for nutritional advice, weight loss or surgery, are important topics that often need to be discussed. Re-assurance about labral tears should be provided, specifically that whilst they may be painful currently, reducing inflammation and irritation and correcting the shearing forces on the antero-superior rim can reduce pain. Advise that 69–85% of the general population have non-symptomatic labral tears (Register et al., 2012). From the clinical experience of the authors, the language used by

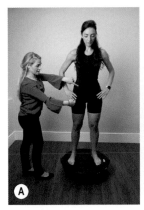 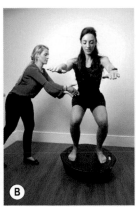 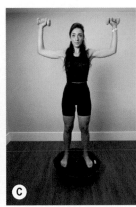 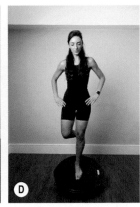 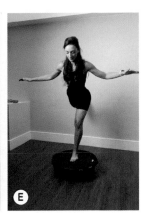

FIGURE 5.13
Proprioception exercises (BOSU Ball Exercises). Exercise program should be progressed on an individual basis. (A) Double leg stance. (B) Squat. (C) Overhead load. (D) Single-leg stance. (E) Single-leg arabesque.

clinicians can define a patient's experience and drive their rehabilitation.

Postural assessment and correction have been shown to improve hip pain in adults with hip dysplasia (Lewis et al., 2015). Many dysplasia patients present in sway back posture with increased posterior tilt of the pelvis, hanging on the front of their hips, where often the bony anatomy is most deficient. This relative hip extension position can increase mechanical stress on the anterior acetabular rim, where often the labral tears are, and also stress the surrounding ligaments, joint capsule and the iliopsoas muscle. Correcting posture by positioning the trunk in line with the pelvis, and correcting hyperextension of the knees may reduce overload on the capsule, ligaments, and muscles and can improve the loading of the femur on the acetabulum into a more neutral range (Figure 5.14).

This can reduce the forces on the anterior rim and therefore reduce labral pain and inflammation. This can then be progressed into dynamic movement during gait, reducing stride length and therefore limiting hip extension moment, potentially reducing the micro-shearing on the anterior rim.

Identification of compensatory movement patterns and poor postures adopted will allow for modification strategies to be implemented. For instance, in a patient getting up from a low chair with labral symptoms of clicking and catching on transitioning from sit to stand, trial changing their pelvic tilt and gluteal activation during the movement and reduce the amount of anterior pelvic tilt causing dynamic impingement as they rise. Sometimes, one can change the mechanical symptoms almost immediately.

Often hip dysplasia patients have increased range of movement in all directions, especially if they are also hypermobile. Identifying specific muscle weakness and addressing this with hip strengthening exercises is crucial. From clinical experience, we often see hypertrophy of TFL with atrophy of gluteus medius. This we find leads to increased reliance on the TFL and iliotibial band (ITB) and results in increased anterior femoral shearing during single-leg stance activities such as walking. Exercises to increase the strength of the gluteus medius whilst disadvantaging TFL (such as sliders in a forward lean position) can be beneficial to reduce this compensatory pattern (Figure 5.15).

We know from the Berlin bed rest study, where patients were placed on bed rest for eight weeks and serial MRIs performed pre and post, that the superficial muscles such as upper gluteus maximus and TFL remain unchanged with unloading, but the deeper muscles such as gluteus medius and minimus and the small lateral rotators are affected significantly by unloading, and atrophy (Belavý et al., 2010). This highlights the importance and requirement for those deep stabilizing muscles (which have articulations with the joint and capsule) to have proprioceptive input. Therefore,

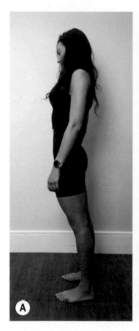

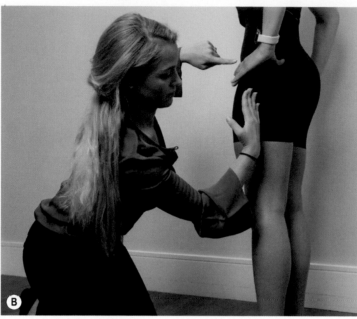

FIGURE 5.14
Postural correction: (A) sway back posture; (B) correction with external cues.

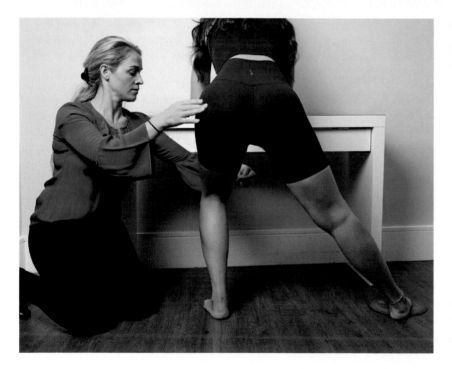

FIGURE 5.15
Hip abduction slider in a supported forward lean position.

closed chain-based exercises which disadvantage the overactive superficial muscles may aid the recruitment of these muscles (Figures 5.16–5.17).

In open-chain hip abduction exercises, patients are more likely to preferentially recruit TFL, rather than the deep stabilizing muscles. Patients with coxa valga often require greater abductor strength and bulk to support body weight, so working into abduction and promoting a wide base of support will help to medialize joint forces. Controlling impact loads and excessive adduction during functional tasks is key. In coxa vara, inner range abduction

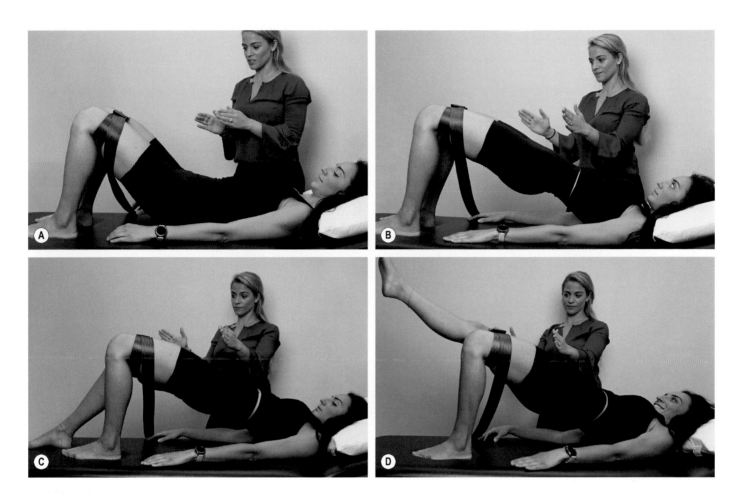

FIGURE 5.16
Closed chain exercises with belt (non-weight-bearing): (A) double-leg bridge (start position); (B) double-leg bridge (end position); (C) off-set bridge; (D) single-leg bridge.

may result in greater trochanter impingement superiorly, so strengthening in positions of external rotation, with a focus on obturator internus should be performed.

Lumbopelvic control and core stability is a vital part of hip dysplasia rehab; intrapelvic stability, peripelvic stability and functional stability all contribute to controlling the forces crossing the hip and pelvis. Optimizing precise joint motion and alignment of the hip joint, avoiding excessive translatory forces is key. By correcting the muscle patterning and improving proprioception, accessory anterior shearing may be reduced (Lewis & Sahrmann, 2006).

Surgery

The surgical treatment of the dysplastic patient aims to improve joint mechanics and usually increase weight-bearing joint contact area. This should reduce static and dynamic overload of the acetabular rim and labrum, and improve muscular lever arms and restore biomechanics. A primary goal of surgery is to delay the development of osteoarthritis and delay the requirement of total hip joint replacement (Salter & Dubos, 1974). There are various osteotomy choices for those with hip dysplasia. The most commonly used osteotomy for young adults with symptomatic hip dysplasia is the Bernese periacetabular osteotomy (PAO), first published

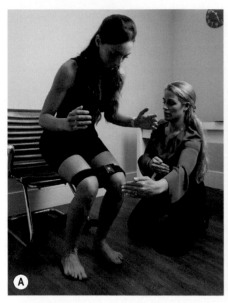
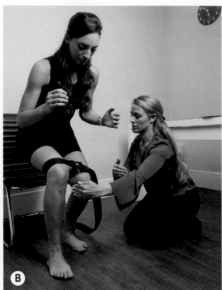
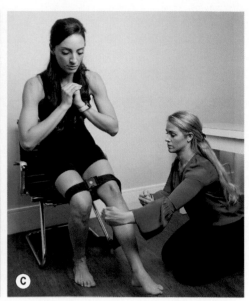

FIGURE 5.17
Closed chain exercises with belt (weight-bearing): (A) sit to stand; (B) staggered sit to stand; (C) single–leg sit to stand.

by Ganz et al. in 1986. Other osteotomy options include the Salter innominate osteotomy, double innominate (e.g., Sutherland), triple innominate (e.g., Steel or Ton105nis), spherical (e.g., Wagner), pericapsular (e.g., Pemberton), and rotational osteotomies (Gillingham et al., 1999). Other salvage operations to improve femoral head coverage include shelf procedures and the Chiari osteotomy.

The PAO is a popular choice as it leaves the posterior column intact, which allows for earlier weight-bearing following surgery. The osteotomy is triplanar which allows for multidirectional corrections of anteversion, retroversion and lateral coverage. This procedure does require careful three-dimensional planning as it is technically more difficult and is shown to have a large learning curve and risk of major complications. Risk factors associated with poor outcomes include high body mass index (BMI), Tonnis grade OA >1, and patient age above 40 years (Sharifi et al., 2008). Complications may include unintended extension of the osteotomy, femoral nerve palsy, excessive bleeding, lateral cutaneous nerve palsy, non-union, osteonecrosis, subluxation of femoral head, heterotrophic ossification, and excessive or insufficient overcorrection (Zaltz et al., 2014).

Postoperative Rehabilitation

There is much debate surrounding the postoperative rehabilitation of the PAO patient and there is very little research. Rehabilitation should consider specifics of the surgical procedure which may vary between surgeons and patients. Ultimately, the therapist must abide by the weight-bearing status set by the operating team, which is usually 20% flat foot toe-touch weight-bearing with aids. A typical postoperative protocol, following PAO, is outlined in Table 5.12.

Conclusion

FAIS and hip dysplasia are leading causes of hip-related pain, physical impairments and impaired quality of life in the active young adult. Awareness and understanding of these pathologies have increased in the last fifteen years. Early and accurate diagnosis is essential for improved outcomes in these patients. A thorough history and comprehensive physical examination, coupled with appropriate diagnostic imaging, can improve the diagnostic accuracy for patients who present with symptoms consistent with FAIS or hip dysplasia. Many patients can be managed

TABLE 5.12 Postoperative Rehabilitation following PAO Surgery	
Phase 1	
Duration	2–6 weeks post-op.
	Orthopedic review varies from 2 to 6 weeks, wound review usually at 11–14 days.
Contraindications	No SLR, weight-bearing status as advised by the surgical team.
Exercise ideas	Core activation, Pilates-based exercises such as single leg lower closed chain, hip twist to regain rotational control, isometric hip abduction and external rotation, hip sliders into flexion, extension, and abduction looking at correct patterning and pelvic control - sliding operated leg, pelvic tilting and awareness.
Cardiovascular and core	Upper body weights.
Other	Potentially start stationary bike from 2 weeks post-op with surgeon clearance.
	Hydrotherapy at chest-height depth when incision site is well-healed (heel raises, mini-squats, walking, side-steps, single-leg balance.
	Alter-G as per hydrotherapy exercises – ensure at 20% body weight.
Goals	Reduction of swelling, optimization of pain management, restoration of joint range of movement, prevention of muscle atrophy within the limits of weight-bearing status, prevention of muscle shortening within limits of weight-bearing status.
Phase 2	
Duration	6–12 weeks.
	Radiographs at 6–8 weeks to confirm bone healing.
Contraindications	Progressing weight-bearing too fast.
Exercise ideas	Gradual progression to 50% body weight and then to full weight-bearing as tolerated. Glute med activation against belt with bridge and sit to stand, single-leg weight transfer, dropdowns, external rotation twisties.
	Symmetrical lower-body exercises. Starting with body weight only initially, and limiting depth: squats (45 degrees), RDL (to knees only), hip thrust or bridge, calf raises.
	Core stability, glutes, hamstrings, quads, gait re-ed, proprioceptive work on BOSU double leg. Short lever pelvic stability such as 4-point kneeling hip extensions with correct pelvic control, progressing to long lever sliders stabilizing on the operative leg sliding the non-op leg into abd or flex/ext in forward lean position to reduce TFL overload.
Goals	Ensure good pelvic awareness, good core stability, prevent overactivity of TFL, ensure good recruitment of all parts of glute med and glute min and good proprioceptive control.

(Continued)

TABLE 5.12 *(Continued)*	
Phase 3	
Duration	12 weeks +.
Contraindications	Nil if bone consolidation present.
Exercise ideas	Asymmetrical and single-leg exercises: lunges, single-leg squats, single-leg hip thrusts. Single-leg proprioceptive work.
	Gradually adding weights. Build up to being able to push body weight double-leg press, progressing to single leg.
	Dynamic loading, commencing with symmetry first, e.g., skipping rope and bounding.
	Core exercises: plank and side planks progressing to on unstable surfaces.
	Return to running and sport-specific rehabilitation.

successfully with conservative measures. Physical therapy should be directed to address muscular weakness, motor patterning, posture, and soft tissue impingement. There is currently no peer-reviewed evidence on return to play rates with non-operative treatment of FAIS or hip dysplasia. When non-surgical treatment is unsuccessful, various surgical approaches addressing hip morphology and addressing the soft tissue damage have been described. Research regarding conservative management of FAIS and hip dysplasia remains in its infancy and additional high-quality studies are needed to establish treatment effectiveness.

References

Agricola R, Bessems JHJM, Ginai AZ, et al. The development of Cam-type deformity in adolescent and young male soccer players. Am J Sports Med. 2012;40:1099–106.

Agricola R, Heijboer MP, Roze RH, et al. Pincer deformity does not lead to osteoarthritis of the hip whereas acetabular dysplasia does: acetabular coverage and development of osteoarthritis in a nationwide prospective cohort study (CHECK). Osteoarthritis Cartilage. 2013;21:1514–21.

Aliprandi A, Di Pietto F, Minafra P, et al. Femoro-acetabular impingement: what the general radiologist should know. Radiol Med. 2014;119:103–12.

Ankem HK, Yelton MJ, Lall AC, et al. Structured physical therapy protocols following hip arthroscopy and their effect on patient-reported outcomes: A systematic review of the literature. J Hip Preservation Surg. 2020;7:357–77.

Aoyama M, Ohnishi Y, Utsunomiya H, et al. A prospective, randomized, controlled trial comparing conservative treatment with trunk stabilization exercise to standard hip muscle exercise for treating femoroacetabular impingement: A pilot study. Clin J Sport Med. 2019;29:267–75.

Audenaert EA, Peeters I, Vigneron L, et al. Hip morphological characteristics and range of internal rotation in femoroacetabular impingement. Am J Sports Med. 2012;40:1329-36.

Austin AB, Souza RB, Meyer JL, et al. Identification of abnormal hip motion associated with acetabular labral pathology. J Orthop Sports Phys Ther. 2008;38:558–65.

Ayeni OR, Farrokhyar F, Crouch S, et al. Pre-operative intra-articular hip injection as a predictor of short-term outcome following arthroscopic management of femoroacetabular impingement. Knee Surg Sports Traumatol Arthrosc. 2014;22:801–5.

Azevedo DC, Paiva EB, Lopes AMA, et al. Pelvic Rotation in femoroacetabular impingement is decreased compared to other symptomatic hip conditions. J Orthop Sports Phys Ther. 2016;46:957–64.

Bagwell JJ, Bauer L, Gradoz M, et al. The reliability of FABER test hip range of motion in measurements. Int J Sports Phys Ther. 2016;11:1101–5.

Bali K, Smit K, Ibrahim M, et al. Ottawa classification for symptomatic acetabular dysplasia assessment of interobserver & intraobserver reliability. Bone J Res. 2020;9:242–9.

Beaulé P, Melkus G, Rakhra K, et al. Quantitative hip cartilage MRI of patients with hip dysplasia. In: Orthopaedic Proceedings. 2020;102(Supp 7):25. The British Editorial Society of Bone & Joint Surgery.

Beck M, Kalhor M, Leunig M, et al. Hip morphology influences the pattern of damage to the acetabular cartilage: femoroacetabular impingement as a cause of early osteoarthritis of the hip. J Bone Joint Surg Br. 2005;87:1012–8.

Belavý DL, Bock O, Börst H, et al. The 2nd Berlin BedRest Study: protocol and implementation. J Musculoskelet Neuronal Interact. 2010;10:207–19.

Byrd JWT. Evaluation of the hip: history and physical examination. N Am J Sports Phys Ther. 2007;2:231–40.

Byrne A, Lodge C, Wallace J. Intrarater test-retest reliability of hip abduction, internal rotation, and external rotation strength measurements in a healthy cohort using a handheld dynamometer and a portable stabilization device: A Pilot Study. Arch Rehabil Res Clinical Translation. 2020;2:100050.

Chadayammuri V, Garabekyan T, Bedi A, et al. Passive hip range of motion predicts femoral torsion and acetabular version. J Bone Joint Surg Am. 2016;98:127–34.

Chaarani MW, Al Mahmeid MS, Salman AM. Developmental dysplasia of the hip before and after increasing community awareness of the harmful effects of swaddling. Qatar Med J. 2002;2002(1):17.

Clohisy JC, Carlisle JC, Beaulé PE, et al. A systematic approach to the plain radiographic evaluation of the young adult hip. J Bone Joint Surg Am. 2008;90(Suppl 4):47.

Clohisy JC, Knaus ER, Hunt DM, et al. Clinical Presentation of patients with symptomatic anterior hip impingement. Clin Orthop Rel Res. 2009;467:638–44.

Clohisy JC, Baca G, Beaulé PE, et al. Descriptive epidemiology of femoroacetabular impingement: a North American cohort of patients undergoing surgery. Am J Sports Med. 2013;41:1348–56.

Dangin A, Tardy N, Wettstein M, et al. Microinstability of the hip: A review. Orthop Traumatol Surg Res. 2016;102:S301–9.

Dick AG, Houghton JM, Bankes MJK. An approach to hip pain in a young adult. BMJ. 2018;361:k1086.

DiSilvestro K, Quinn M, Tabaddor RR. A clinician's guide to femoacetabular impingement in athletes. R I Med J (2013). 2020;103:41–8.

Distefano LJ, Blackburn JT, Marshall SW, et al. Gluteal muscle activation during common therapeutic exercises. J Orthop Sports Phys Ther. 2009;39:532–40.

Domb BG, Sgroi TA, VanDevender JC. Physical therapy protocol after hip arthroscopy: Clinical guidelines supported by 2-year outcomes. Sports Health. 2016;8:347–54.

Dumont GD. Hip instability: current concepts and treatment options. Clin Sports Med. 2016;35(3):435–47.

Egger AC, Frangiamore S, Rosneck J. Femoroacetabular impingement: a review. Sports Med Arthrosc Rev. 2016;24:e53–8.

Emara K, Samir W, Motasem EH, et al. Conservative treatment for mild femoroacetabular impingement. J Orthop Surg. 2011;19:41–5.

Enseki KR, Martin R, Kelly BT. Rehabilitation after arthroscopic decompression for femoroacetabular impingement. Clin Sports Med. 2010;29:247–55

Enseki K, Harris-Hayes M, White DM, et al. Nonarthritic hip joint pain. J Orthop Sports Phys Ther. 2014;44:A1–32.

Fitzgerald GK, Axe MJ, Snyder-Mackler L. The efficacy of perturbation training in nonoperative anterior cruciate ligament rehabilitation programs for physical active individuals. Phys Ther. 2000;80:128–40.

Frank JM, Harris JD, Erickson BJ, et al. Prevalence of femoroacetabular impingement imaging findings in asymptomatic volunteers: a systematic review. Arthroscopy. 2015;31:1199–204.

Freke M, Kemp JL, Svege I, et al. Physical impairments in symptomatic femoroacetabular impingement: a systematic review of the evidence. Br J Sports Med. 2016;50(19):1180.

Fukushima K, Miyagi M, Inoue G, et al. Relationship between spinal sagittal alignment and acetabular coverage: a patient-matched control study. Arch Orthop Trauma Surg. 2018;138:1495–9.

Gala L, Clohisy JC, Beaulé PE. Hip dysplasia in the young adult. J Bone Joint Surg Am. 2016;98(1):63–73.

Gambling TS, Long A. Psycho-social impact of developmental dysplasia of the hip and of differential access to early diagnosis and treatment: A narrative study of young adults. SAGE Open Med. 2019;7:2050312119836010.

Ganz R, Parvizi J, Beck M, et al. Femoroacetabular impingement: a cause for osteoarthritis of the hip. Clin Orthop Relat Res. 2003;41:112–20.

Gay C, Chabaud A, Guilley E, et al. Educating patients about the benefits of physical activity and exercise for their hip and knee osteoarthritis. Systematic literature review. Ann Phys Rehabil Med. 2016;59(3):174–83.

Genovese E, Spiga S, Vinci V, et al. Femoroacetabular impingement: role of imaging. Musculoskelet Surg. 2013;97:S117–126.

Gillingham BL, Sanchez AA, Wenger DR. Pelvic osteotomies for the treatment of hip dysplasia in children and young adults. J Am Acad Orthop Surg. 1999;7:325–37

Griffin DR, Dickenson EJ, O'Donnell J, et al. The Warwick Agreement on femoroacetabular impingement syndrome (FAI syndrome): an international consensus statement. Br J Sports Med. 2016;50:1169–76.

Griffin DR, Dickenson EJ, Wall PD, et al. Hip arthroscopy versus best conservative care for the treatment of femoroacetabular impingement syndrome (UK FASHIoN): a multicentre randomised controlled trial. Lancet. 2018;391(10136):2225–35.

Hack K, Di Primio G, Rakhra K et al. Prevalence of cam-type femoroacetabular impingement morphology in asymptomatic volunteers. J Bone Joint Surg Am. 2010;92:2436–44.

Hadeed MM, Cancienne JM, Gwathmey FW. Pincer impingement. Clin Sports Med. 2016;35:405–18.

Hale RF, Melugin HP, Zhou J, et al. Incidence of femoroacetabular impingement and surgical management trends over time. Am J Sports Med. 2021;49:35–41.

Halim A, Badrinath R, Carter CW. The importance of sex of patient in the management of femoroacetabular impingement. Am J Orthop. 2015;44:172–5.

Hanke MS, Schmaranzer F, Steppacher SD, et al. Hip preservation. EFORT Open Reviews. 2020;5:630–40.

Harris-Hayes M, Czuppon S, Van Dillen LR, et al. Movement-pattern training to improve function in people with chronic hip joint pain: A Feasibility Randomized Clinical Trial. J Orthop Sports Phys Ther. 2016;46:452–61.

Heerey J, Risberg MA, Magnus J, et al. Impairment-based rehabilitation following hip arthroscopy: postoperative protocol for the HIP arthroscopy international randomized controlled trial. J Orthop Sports Phys Ther. 2018;48:336–42.

Heerey JJ, Kemp JL, Mosler AB, et al. What is the prevalence of imaging-defined intra-articular hip pathologies in people with and without pain? A systematic review and meta-analysis. Br J Sports Med. 2018;52:581–93.

Hernigou P. Smith-Petersen and early development of hip arthroplasty. Int Orthop. 2014;38:193–8.

Hoit G, Whelan DB, Dwyer T, et al. Physiotherapy as an initial treatment option for femoroacetabular impingement: A systematic review of the literature and meta-analysis of 5 randomized controlled trials. Am J Sports Med. 2020;48:2042–50.

Hu H, Zhan S, Cai Z. Biomechanics of hip joints. In: Zhang C, editor. Hip Surgery: A Practical Guide [Internet]. Singapore: Springer; 2021:17–23.

Hunt D, Prather H, Harris Hayes M, et al. Clinical outcomes analysis of conservative and surgical treatment of patients with clinical indications of prearthritic, intra-articular hip disorders. PM R. 2012;4:479–87.

Ishida K. Prevention of the development of the typical dislocation of the hip. Clin Orthop Relat Res. 1977;126:167–9.

Jacobsen JS, Bolvig L, Hölmich P, et al. Muscle-tendon-related abnormalities detected by ultrasonography are common in symptomatic hip dysplasia. Arch Orthop Trauma Surg. 2018;138:1059–67.

Jacobsen JS, Søballe K, Thorborg K, et al. Patient-reported outcome and muscle-tendon pain after periacetabular osteotomy are related: 1-year follow-up in 82 patients with hip dysplasia. Acta Orthop. 2019;90:40–5.

Jacobsen S, Sonne-Holm S. Hip dysplasia: a significant risk factor for the development of hip osteoarthritis. A cross-sectional survey. Rheumatology. 2005;44:211–8.

Jacobsen S, Sonne-Holm S, Søballe K, et al. Hip dysplasia and osteoarthrosis: a survey of 4151 subjects from the Osteoarthrosis Substudy of the Copenhagen City Heart Study. Acta Orthop. 2005;76:149–58.

Jauregui JJ, Salmons HI, Meredith SJ, et al. Prevalence of femoro-acetabular impingement in non-arthritic patients with hip pain: a meta-analysis. Int Orthop. 2020;44:2559–66.

Kahlenberg CA, Han B, Patel RM, et al. Time and cost of diagnosis for symptomatic femoroacetabular impingement. Orthop J Sports Med. 2014;2:2325967114523916.

Kalisvaart MM, Safran MR. Microinstability of the hip: it does exist: etiology, diagnosis and treatment. J Hip Preserv Surg. 2015;2:123–35.

Kemp JL, Makdissi M, Schache AG, et al. Is quality of life following hip arthroscopy in patients with chondrolabral pathology associated with impairments in hip strength or range of motion? Knee Surg Sports Traumatol Arthrosc. 2016a;24:3955–61.

Kemp JL, Risberg MA, Schache AG, et al. Patients with chondrolabral pathology have bilateral functional impairments 12 to 24 months after unilateral hip arthroscopy: a cross-sectional study. J Orthop Sports Phys Ther. 2016b;46:947–56.

Kemp JL, King MG, Barton C, et al. Is exercise therapy for femoroacetabular impingement in or out of FASHIoN? We need to talk about current best practice for the non-surgical management of FAI syndrome. Br J Sports Med. 2019;53(19):1204–5.

Kemp JL, Mosler AB, Hart H, et al. Improving function in people with hip-related pain:

a systematic review and meta-analysis of physiotherapist-led interventions for hip-related pain. Br J Sports Med. 2020;54:1382–94.

Keogh MJ, Batt ME. A review of femoroacetabular impingement in athletes. Sports Med. 2008;38:863–78.

Khan W, Khan M, Alradwan H, et al. Utility of intra-articular hip injections for femoroacetabular impingement: A Systematic Review. Orthop J Sports Med. 2015;3:2325967115601030.

Kivlan BR, Martin RL, Sekiya JK. Response to diagnostic injection in patients with femoroacetabular impingement, labral tears, chondral lesions, and extra-articular pathology. Arthroscopy. 2011;27:619–27.

Knapik DM, Salata MJ. Hip injuries in the contact athlete. Oper Tech Sports Med. 2019;27:145–51.

Kolber MJ, Cheatham SW, Hanney WJ, et al. Training considerations for individuals with femoral acetabular impingement. Strength Conditioning J. 2015;37:35–47.

Kraeutler MJ, Garabekyan T, Pascual-Garrido C, et al. Hip instability: a review of hip dysplasia and other contributing factors. Muscles Ligaments Tendons J. 2016;6:343–53.

Kubiak-Langer M, Tannast M, Murphy SB, et al. Range of motion in anterior femoroacetabular impingement. Clin Orthop Relat Res. 2007;458:117–24.

Larsen JB, Mechlenburg I, Jakobsen SS, et al. 14-year hip survivorship after periacetabular osteotomy: a follow-up study on 1,385 hips. Acta Orthop. 2020;91:299–305.

Larson CM, Pierce BR, Giveans MR. Treatment of athletes with symptomatic intra-articular hip pathology and athletic pubalgia/sports hernia: a case series. Arthroscopy. 2011;27:768–75.

LeBeau RT, Nho SJ. The use of manual therapy post-hip arthroscopy when an exercise-based therapy approach has failed: a case report. J Orthop Sports Phys Ther. 2014;44:712–21.

Lee CB, Mata-Fink A, Millis MB, Kim Y-J. Demographic differences in adolescent-diagnosed and adult-diagnosed acetabular dysplasia compared with infantile developmental dysplasia of the hip. J Pediatr Orthop. 2013;33:107–11.

Lewis CL, Sahrmann SA. Acetabular labral tears. Phys Ther. 2006;86:110–21.

Lewis CL, Khuu A, Marinko L. Postural correction reduces hip pain in adult with acetabular dysplasia: a case report. Man Ther. 2015;20:508–12.

Lim S-J, Park Y-S. Plain radiography of the hip: A review of radiographic techniques and image features. Hip Pelvis. 2015;27:125–34.

Lynch TS, Minkara A, Aoki SK, et al. Best practice guidelines for hip arthroscopy in femoroacetabular impingement: results of a Delphi Process. Orthop J Sports Med. 2020;28(2):81–9.

Maffiuletti NA, Bizzini M, Sutter R, et al. Hip muscle strength asymmetries and their associations with hip morphology and symptoms are sex-specific in patients with femoroacetabular impingement syndrome. Phys Ther Sport. 2020;42:131–8.

Mascarenhas VV, Castro MO, Rego PA, et al. The Lisbon agreement on femoroacetabular impingement imaging-part 1: overview. Eur Radiol. 2020;30:5281–97.

Matheney T, Zaltz I, Kim Y-J, et al. Activity level and severity of dysplasia predict age at Bernese periacetabular osteotomy for symptomatic hip dysplasia. J Bone Joint Surg Am. 2016;98:665–71.

Matsumoto K, Ganz R, Khanduja V. The history of femoroacetabular impingement. Bone Joint Res. 2020;9:572–7.

McGovern RP, Martin RL, Kivlan BR, et al. Non-operative management of individuals with non-arthritic hip pain: A literature review. Int J Sports Phys Ther. 2019;14:135–47.

Melugin HP, Hale RF, Zhou J, et al. Risk factors for long-term hip osteoarthritis in patients with femoroacetabular impingement without surgical intervention. Am J Sports Med. 2020;48:2881–6.

Murphy SB, Ganz R, Müller ME. The prognosis in untreated dysplasia of the hip. A study of radiographic factors that predict the outcome. J Bone Joint Surg Am. 1995;77:985–9.

Musielak B, Idzior M, Jóźwiak M. Evolution of the term and definition of dysplasia of the hip: A review of the literature. Arch Med Sci. 2015;11:1052–7.

Nakano N, Khanduja V. Femoroacetabular impingement: the past, current controversies and future perspectives. Phys Sportsmed. 2018;46:270–2.

Nawabi DH, Bedi A, Tibor LM, et al. The demographic characteristics of high-level and recreational athletes undergoing hip arthroscopy for femoroacetabular impingement: A sports-specific analysis. Arthroscopy 2014;30:398–405.

Nunley M, Prather H, Hunt D, et al. Clinical presentation of symptomatic acetabular dysplasia in skeletally mature patients. J Bone Joint Surg Am. 2011;93:17–21.

Ortiz-Neira CL, Paolucci EO, Donnon T. A meta-analysis of common risk factors associated with the diagnosis of developmental dysplasia of the hip in newborns. Eur J Radiol. 2012;81:e344-51.

Padaki AS, Lynch TS, Larson CM, et al. Femoroacetabular impingement and core muscle injury in athletes: Diagnosis and algorithms for success. Sports Med Arthrosc Rev. 2021;29:9–14.

Palmer AJ, Gupta VA, Fernquest S, et al. Arthroscopic hip surgery compared with physiotherapy and activity modification for the treatment of symptomatic femoroacetabular impingement: multicentre randomised controlled trial. BMJ. 2019;364:l185.

Patel RV, Han S, Lenherr C, et al. Pelvic tilt and range of motion in hips with femoroacetabular impingement syndrome. J Am Acad Orthop Surg. 2020;28:e427–32.

Philippon MJ, Maxwell R, Johnston TL, et al. Clinical presentation of femoroacetabular impingement. Knee Surg Sports Traumatol Arthrosc. 2007;15:1041–7.

Pierannunzii L. Pelvic posture and kinematics in femoroacetabular impingement: a systematic review. J Orthop Traumatol. 2017;18:187–96.

Register B, Pennock AT, Ho CP, et al. Prevalence of abnormal hip findings in asymptomatic participants: a prospective, blinded study. Am J Sports Med. 2012;40:2720–4.

Reiman MP, Matheson JW. Restricted hip mobility: clinical suggestions for self-mobilization and muscle re-education. Int J Sports Phys Ther. 2013;8:729–40.

Reiman MP, Décary S, Mathew B, et al. Accuracy of clinical and imaging tests for the diagnosis of hip dysplasia and instability: a systematic review. J Orthop Sports Phys Ther. 2019;49:87–97.

Reiman MP, Agricola R, Kemp JL, et al. Consensus recommendations on the classification, definition and diagnostic criteria of hip-related pain in young and middle-aged active adults from the International Hip-related Pain Research Network, Zurich 2018. Br J Sports Med. 2020;54:631–41.

Retchford TH, Crossley KM, Grimaldi A, et al. Can local muscles augment stability in the hip? A narrative literature review. J Musculoskelet Neuronal Interact. 2013;13:1–12.

Reynolds D, Lucas J, Klaue K. Retroversion of the acetabulum. A cause of hip pain. J Bone Joint Surg Br. 1999;81:281–8.

Riley GM, McWalter EJ, Stevens KJ, et al. Magnetic resonance imaging of the hip for the evaluation of femoroacetabular impingement; past, present, and future. J Magn Reson Imaging. 2015;41:558–72.

Risberg MA, Holm I, Myklebust G, Engebretsen L. Neuromuscular training versus strength training during first 6 months after anterior cruciate ligament reconstruction: a randomized clinical trial. Phys Ther. 2007;87:737–50.

Roach KE, Miles TP. Normal hip and knee active range of motion: the relationship to age. Phys Ther. 1991; 71:656–65.

Ross JR, Nepple JJ, Philippon MJ, et al. Effect of changes in pelvic tilt on range of motion to impingement and radiographic parameters of acetabular morphologic characteristics. Am J Sports Med. 2014;42:2402–9.

Ross JR, Stone RM, Larson CM. Core muscle injury/sports hernia/athletic pubalgia, and femoroacetabular impingement. Sports Med Arthrosc Rev. 2015;23:213–20.

Safran MR. Microinstability of the hip-gaining acceptance. J Am Acad Orthop Surg. 2019;27:12-22.

Salter RB, Dubos JP. The first fifteen year's personal experience with innominate osteotomy in the treatment of congenital dislocation and subluxation of the hip. Clin Orthop Relat Res. 1974;98:72103.

Samora JB, Ng VY, Ellis TJ. Femoroacetabular impingement: a common cause of hip pain in young adults. Clin J Sport Med. 2011;21:51–6.

Sankar WN, Duncan ST, Baca GR, et al. Descriptive epidemiology of acetabular dysplasia: The Academic Network of Conservational Hip Outcomes Research (ANCHOR) Periacetabular Osteotomy. J Am Acad Orthop Surg. 2017;25:150–9.

Satpathy J, Kannan A, Owen JR, et al. Hip contact stress and femoral neck retroversion: a biomechanical study to evaluate implication of femoroacetabular impingement. J Hip Preserv Surg. 2015;2:287–94.

Schmitz MR, Murtha AS, Clohisy JC, ANCHOR Study Group. Developmental dysplasia of the hip in adolescents and young adults. J Am Acad Orthop Surg. 2020;28:91–101.

Sharifi E, Sharifi H, Morshed S, et al. Cost-effectiveness analysis of periacetabular osteotomy. J Bone Joint Surg Am. 2008;90:1447–56.

Short SM, MacDonald CW, Strack D. Hip and groin injury prevention in elite athletes and team sport – current challenges and opportunities. Int J Sports Phys Ther. 2021;16(1):270.

Siebenrock KA, Ferner F, Noble PC, et al. The cam-type deformity of the proximal femur arises in childhood in response to vigorous sporting activity. Clin Orthop Relat Res. 2011;469:3229–40.

Stearns KM, Powers CM. Improvements in hip muscle performance result in increased use of the hip extensors and abductors during a landing task. Am J Sports Med. 2014;42:602–9.

Strosberg DS, Ellis TJ, Renton DB. The role of femoroacetabular impingement in core muscle injury/athletic pubalgia: diagnosis and management. Front Surg. 2016;3:6.

Takla A, O'Donnell J, Voight M, et al. The 2019 International Society of Hip Preservation (ISHA) physiotherapy agreement on assessment and treatment of femoroacetabular impingement syndrome (FAIS): an international consensus statement. J Hip Preserv Surg. 2021;7(4):631–42.

Tannast M, Siebenrock KA, Anderson SE. Femoroacetabular impingement: radiographic diagnosis – what the radiologist should know. Am J Roentgenol. 2007;188:1540–52.

Tannast M, Hanke MS, Zheng G, et al. What are the radiographic reference values for acetabular under- and overcoverage? Clin Orthop Relat Res. 2015;473:1234–46.

Terrell SL, Olson GE, Lynch J. Therapeutic exercise approaches to nonoperative and postoperative management of femoroacetabular impingement syndrome. J Athl Train. 2021;56(1):31–45.

Thorborg K, Bandholm T, Schick M, et al. Hip strength assessment using handheld dynamometry is subject to intertester bias when testers are of different sex and strength. Scand J Med Sci Sports. 2013;23:487–93.

Tian F-D, Zhao D-W, Wang W, et al. Prevalence of developmental dysplasia of the hip in Chinese adults: a cross-sectional survey. Chin Med J. 2017;130:1261–8.

Tijssen M, Cingel REH van, de Visser E, et al. Hip joint pathology: relationship between patient history, physical tests, and arthroscopy findings in clinical practice. Scand J Med Sci Sports. 2017;27:342–50.

Tranovich MJ, Salzler MJ, Enseki KR, et al. A review of femoroacetabular impingement and hip arthroscopy in the athlete. Phys Sportsmed. 2014;42:75–87.

Trindade CAC, Briggs KK, Fagotti L, et al. Positive FABER distance test is associated with higher alpha angle in symptomatic patients. Knee Surg Sports Traumatol Arthrosc. 2019;27:3158–61.

Uding A, Bloom NJ, Commean PK, et al. Clinical tests to determine femoral version category in people with chronic hip joint pain and asymptomatic controls. Musculoskelet Sci Pract. 2019;39:115–22.

van Klij P, Reiman MP, Waarsing JH, et al. Classifying cam morphology by the alpha angle: A systematic review on threshold values. Orthop J Sports Med. 2020;8:2325967120938312.

Vaudreuil NJ, McClincy MP. Evaluation and treatment of borderline dysplasia: moving beyond the lateral center edge angle. Curr Rev Musculoskelet Med. 2020;13:28–37.

Wall PDH, Fernandez M, Griffin DR, et al. Nonoperative treatment for femoroacetabular impingement: a systematic review of the literature. PM R. 2013;5:418–26.

Ward SR, Winters TM, Blemker SS. The architectural design of the gluteal muscle group:

implications for movement and rehabilitation. J Orthop Sports Phys Ther. 2010;40:95–102.

Wells J, Nepple JJ, Crook K, et al. Femoral morphology in the dysplastic hip: three-dimensional characterizations with CT. Clin Orthop Relat Res. 2017;475:1045–54.

Wilson KW, Kannan AS, Kopacko M, et al. Rehabilitation and return to sport after hip arthroscopy. Operative Techn Orthopaedics. 2019;29:100739.

Wilkin GP, Ibrahim MM, Smit KM. A contemporary definition of hip dysplasia and structural instability: toward a comprehensive classification for acetabular dysplasia. The Journal of arthroplasty. 2017;32(9):S20–7.

Wright AA, Tarara DT, Gisselman AS, et al. Do currently prescribed exercises reflect

contributing pathomechanics associated with femoroacetabular impingement syndrome? A scoping review. Phys Ther Sport. 2021;47:127-33.

Wylie JD, Kim Y-J. The natural history of femoroacetabular impingement. J Pediatr Orthop. 2019;39:S28–32.

Zaltz I, Baca G, Kim Y-J, et al. Complications associated with the periacetabular osteotomy: a prospective multicenter study. J Bone Joint Surg Am. 2014;96:1967–74.

Zhou J, Melugin HP, Hale RF, et al. The prevalence of radiographic findings of structural hip deformities for femoroacetabular impingement in patients with hip pain. Am J Sports Med. 2020;48:647–53.

Muscle and tendon injuries of the hip and knee: quadriceps, hamstrings, adductors, gluteals

John J. Mischke, Richard W. Willy, Craig Purdam

6

Introduction

Muscular and tendinous injuries of the hip and knee result in considerable time lost from sports participation. Muscle injuries represent 31% of all injuries sustained by professional soccer players, resulting in 27% of the total injury absence (Ekstrand et al., 2011). Additionally, patellar tendon injuries are also experienced by 25.2% of Australian football players throughout a season (Docking et al., 2018). Proper diagnosis and management of musculotendinous injuries of the hip and knee are imperative to minimize loss of function and time away from sport.

Progressive loading is the cornerstone of contemporary management of hip and knee muscle and tendon injuries. Passive interventions (e.g., manual therapy, modalities, dry needling, or extra-corporeal shockwave therapy) should also be part of a multimodal therapy program, but it is critical that progressive loading is the mainstay of rehabilitation programs. Although specific management programs are presented in this chapter, patient outcomes will be maximized using a treatment approach tailored to each patient, aiming for a durable return to play or activity.

To streamline the clinician's approach to muscle and tendon disorders of the hip and knee, the chapter divides pathology into several body regions: anterior thigh and knee, buttock and posterior thigh, medial thigh and groin, and lateral hip. This chapter discusses the relevant anatomy, epidemiology, risk factors, presentation, differential diagnosis, and management of several muscle and tendon injuries in the hip and knee regions.

Anterior Thigh and Knee

Quadriceps Muscle Strain

Background

The rectus femoris, vastus lateralis, vastus intermedius, and vastus medius make up the quadriceps musculature. The two-joint nature of the rectus femoris allows the muscle to serve as both a hip flexor and as a knee extender which may predispose it to injury; rectus femoris is the most commonly strained muscle of the quadriceps (Cross et al., 2004). Quadriceps injury rates occur in 1.07/10,000 athletic exposures in collegiate athletes, but vary widely per sport (Eckard et al., 2017a). The highest overall quadriceps strain rates occur in men's and women's soccer, women's indoor track, and women's softball (Eckard et al., 2017a). Quadriceps muscle strains result in an average 17 days' absence from sport and have a 17% re-injury rate (Ekstrand et al., 2011).

Risk Factors

A non-statistically significant trend toward increased risk of quadriceps strain exists in shorter, heavier players (Fousekis et al., 2011). Consensus on modifiable risk factors for quadriceps strains is currently lacking. However, one study found a non-significant trend toward increased risk in soccer players with quadriceps flexibility or eccentric quadriceps strength asymmetries (Fousekis et al., 2011).

Prevention

Injury prevention efforts that include a standardized warm-up consisting of balance exercises, plyometrics, strengthening, and running, i.e., the FIFA 11+ program (RR: 0.73, 95%CI 0.48 to 1.12), reduce risk of quadriceps injuries (low quality evidence) (Ishoi et al., 2020).

Differential Diagnosis

The differential diagnosis for proximal thigh symptoms includes, but is not limited to: rectus femoris avulsion, quadriceps contusion, iliopsoas-related groin pain, hip-related groin pain, lumbar spine referral, femoral neck stress fracture, abdominal viscera referral, and genitourinary pathology. The differential diagnosis for distal thigh symptoms includes, but is not limited to: quadriceps tendinopathy, anterior knee pain, quadriceps contusion, stress fractures of the anterior femoral shaft, lumbar spine referral, and femoral nerve irritation.

Clinical Presentation

Patients with an acute quadriceps muscle strain recall a memorable event resulting in sudden onset of anterior thigh pain. The mechanism of injury may be reported as a forceful eccentric contraction, as seen in sprint deceleration, change

TABLE 6.1 Clinical Grading System of Muscle Strains

Grade	Pain	Strength	Physical Examination
1	Minimal and highly localized pain with palpation. Pain aggravated by movement	No or minimal strength loss	Minor disability but absent gait disturbances, no obvious muscle defect, and minimal to absent ecchymosis
2	Substantial pain with palpation that is poorly localized. Pain is aggravated by movement	Moderate strength loss	Moderate disability and greatly disturbed gait; moderate swelling that develops within 12–24 hours, ecchymosis, localized tenderness; stretching and tearing of fibers, without complete disruption with a small muscle defect
3	Severe and intractable pain to palpation and with attempts to contract muscle. Pain is diffuse in nature	Severe/complete strength loss	Severe disability, cannot weight bear, severe swelling that develops rapidly within an hour, ecchymosis, hematoma, palpable muscle defect and loss of muscle function

(Adapted from Grassi et al., 2016.)

of direction, jumping, or in the backswing of kicking. The presence of edema and ecchymosis are commonly present in Grade II and III injuries, but are not typical of Grade I quadriceps strains (Table 6.1) (Grassi et al., 2016).

Pain with palpation, resisted hip flexion, resisted knee extension, passive hip extension, or passive knee flexion are the most common clinical tests for a quadriceps strain. Presence (LR+ 11.20, 95%CI 4.85 to 25.86) or absence (LR– 0.0) of pain with palpation of the rectus femoris muscle, and resisted knee extension in the modified Thomas test position as a negative test (LR+ 4.17, 95%CI 2.54 to 6.82; LR– =0.0), are the most effective clinical diagnostic tests (Ishoi et al., 2020). Diagnostic imaging can be helpful with grading the injury and determining the exact tissue involved.

Management

Initial treatment of an acute quadriceps strain should begin immediately after the injury (first 72 hours) and should entail a combination of protection, optimal loading, cryotherapy, compression, and elevation (Bleakley et al., 2012). Optimal loading in the acute phase will depend on the injury extent and may include activity modification as well as initiating sub-maximal isometric exercises in a shortened quadriceps position. Grade II and III injuries often require crutches to

protect the injured musculature (Kary, 2010). Aggressive stretching is not appropriate in the acute phase and rarely appropriate throughout the rehabilitation program.

Following the acute phase, management includes progressive strengthening, balance training, a graded return to sprinting (Table 6.2 provides an example program), and finally, sport-specific activities. Progressive muscular strengthening is introduced first at shorter lengths using isometric contractions, progressing to concentric contractions, then finally, eccentric contractions which appear critical to reducing the risk of re-injury in other muscle strains (Kary, 2010; Askling et al., 2013). Eccentric exercises in this phase of rehabilitation may include reverse lunges, hip flexion against external resistance, and the Reverse Nordic exercise (Figure 6.1) The addition of energy storage and release exercises, i.e., plyometrics, decelerations, and kicking, are integral to bridging the gap between controlled strengthening exercises and return to sport exercises. Chapter 19 shows other exercises for the quadriceps musculature.

Return to sport decision-making should assess the patient's readiness for the sport-specific demands, including functional field or court tests, while also implementing a shared decision-making approach (Ardern et al., 2016). Specific criteria for return to sport clearance after a quadriceps strain are not established. The application of generalized return

TABLE 6.2 Intensity and Distance of the 9-Stage Progressive Sprinting Protocol

Stage	Acceleration Phase	Hold Phase	Deceleration Phase
1	Walk 20 meters	Jog 10 meters	Walk 20 meters
2	Walk 15 meters	Jog 20 meters	Walk 15 meters
3	Walk 10 meters	Jog 30 meters	Walk 10 meters
4	Jog 20 meters	Run 10 meters	Jog 20 meters
5	Jog 15 meters	Run 20 meters	Jog 15 meters
6	Jog 10 meters	Run 30 meters	Jog 10 meters
7	Run 20 meters	Sprint 10 meters	Run 20 meters
8	Run 15 meters	Sprint 20 meters	Run 15 meters
9	Run 10 meters	Sprint 30 meters	Run 10 meters

Walk is defined as regular gait, jog as less than 50% of perceived maximal running speed, run as less than 70% of perceived maximal running speed, and sprint as greater than 90% of perceived maximal running speed.

(Adapted from Hickey et al., 2020.)

to sport criteria for muscle strains may guide clinical decision-making (Table 6.3) (Hickey et al., 2020).

Surgical intervention is rare, but may be considered for patients with severe Grade II and Grade III quadriceps tears, displaced avulsion injuries, or in patients with recalcitrant symptoms who have previously failed conservative management.

Patellar Tendinopathy

Background

Patellar tendinopathy, often referred to as "jumper's knee," is a common overuse injury in athletes participating in sports loading the knee extensors. The overall prevalence of patellar tendinopathy among elite athletes has been reported at 14% and is most prevalent in volleyball and basketball athletes (Lian et al., 2005).

Risk Factors

Patellar tendinopathy is more common in males (OR 2.0, 95%CI 1.1 to 3.5) (de Vries et al., 2015) in their 20s and 30s. Greater activity volume, greater counter-movement jump height, decreased ankle dorsiflexion range of motion, decreased posterior thigh and quadriceps flexibility, and greater volume of jump training have been shown to be potentially modifiable risk factors for patellar tendinopathy (Sprague et al., 2018).

CHAPTER SIX

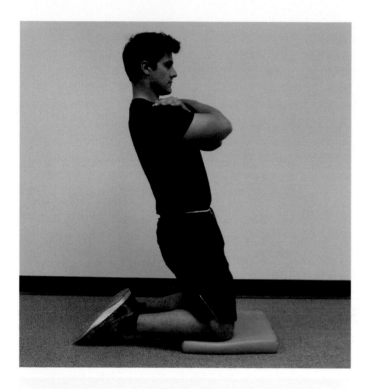

FIGURE 6.1
Reverse Nordic exercise. The patient starts in the tall kneeling position, then slowly lowers their upper body posteriorly toward the ground while maintaining a rigid spine and hip position.

TABLE 6.3 Return to Play Clearance Criteria
• No pain on palpation of injured muscle
• No pain during active knee extension or passive straight leg raise test, with range of motion at 90% or greater of that of the uninjured leg
• No pain during maximal-effort isometric knee flexor contraction at 0/0 degrees and 90/90 degrees of hip/knee flexion
• No pain or apprehension during sprinting at 100% of perceived maximal running intensity
(Adapted from Hickey et al., 2020.)

Clinical Presentation

Patellar tendinopathy commonly presents as load-dependent, localized pain at the inferior pole of the patella with an insidious onset, generally after a recent spike in jump-landing loads or decelerations. Initial symptom onset is typically preceded by an alteration in loading (e.g., an excessive increase in loading over a short period).

Jumping and landing on the affected leg, stair descent, single-leg squatting, resisted knee extension and passive knee flexion often reproduce symptoms. Symptom severity and functional limitations can be assessed with the Victorian Institute of Sport Assessment – Patella (VISA-P) questionnaire. More about the psychometric data of VISA-P can be found in Chapter 9 of this textbook. The single-leg decline squat (+LR: 4.5; –LR: 0.4) has also been shown to be a valid test for patellar tendon pain provocation (Purdam et al., 2003, Mendonca et al., 2016). However, this test loads several anterior knee structures (e.g., patellofemoral joint, Hoffa's fat pad, quadriceps tendon) and results should be interpreted with caution. Patellar tendon palpation is commonly used in the diagnosis of PT (+LR: 2.18; –LR: 0.76) (Cook et al., 2001); however, caution should be used when interpreting the presence/absence of a tender patellar tendon and the tendon may be symptomatic to palpation in alternative diagnoses. Overall, a combined approach of patient history coupled with pain provocation in the decline squat test seems advisable.

Pathological tendon findings on imaging may be considered a risk factor for symptom development (Comin et al., 2013), although imaging abnormalities are also seen in the patellar tendons of asymptomatic basketball players (Cook et al., 2000). Imaging should be used in combination with examination findings and may be most helpful when ruling out competing diagnoses.

Differential Diagnosis

The differential diagnosis of anterior knee pain should include conditions at the knee as well as remote conditions that can refer to the knee. Anterior knee pain differential diagnostic considerations are depicted in Table 6.4.

Management

Malliaris et al. (2015) described a 4-stage approach to treating patellar tendinopathy: (1) isometric loading; (2) heavy,

TABLE 6.4 Differential Diagnosis of Anterior Knee Pain

Common	Less Common	Important (Not to Miss)
• Patellar tendinopathy	• Patellar subluxation	• Sinister pathology (cancer, infection)
• Patellofemoral pain	• Medial plica irritation	• Patella fracture
• Lumbar spine referral	• Quadriceps tendinopathy	• Acute patella dislocation
• Hip joint referral	• Femoral nerve irritation	• Femoral stress fracture
• Hoffa's fat pad irritation	• Saphenous nerve irritation	• Slipped capital femoral epiphysis (pediatric patients)
• Meniscus injury	• Articular cartilage lesion	• Osgood–Schlatter disease (pediatric patients)
• Intra-articular ligament injury (i.e., anterior cruciate ligament)		• Sinding–Larsen–Johansson disease (pediatric patients)

slow resistance training; (3) plyometrics; and (4) return to sport. Minimal pain (1–3/10 on a numeric pain rating scale) during loading exercises is permitted; however, avoidance of exacerbation of pain in the 24 hours after a loading bout is a better metric to monitor the appropriateness of rehabilitation loads. Chapter 19 of this textbook discusses those proposals for exercise progressions in individuals with patellar tendinopathy.

Isometric loading serves as a way to load the tendon without an increase in irritability in the early stages of rehabilitation. Rio et al. (2015) suggested that isometric exercise in individuals with patellar tendinopathy may induce analgesia due to central neurophysiologic mechanisms. Mid-range isometric loading can be performed via a knee extension machine to isolate the quadriceps, or via Spanish squats (Figure 6.2). Initial suggested dosage may include 5 sets of 45 seconds at 70% 1-RM (Malliaras et al., 2015). The heavy, slow resistance training phase should initially include 3–4 sets at 15-RM progressing to 6-RM every other day performing single-leg exercises (knee extensions, leg press, split squats) that stress the patellar tendon and quadriceps.

Plyometrics can be initiated when progress appears to plateau with heavy, slow resistance training, or when the patient meets a strength metric (i.e., single leg press 1.5x body weight). Plyometric exercises begin with double-leg exercises while monitoring for symptom response and progressing to single leg as symptoms allow.

The final stage, return to sport, should progressively replicate the demand of the patient's sport on the patellar

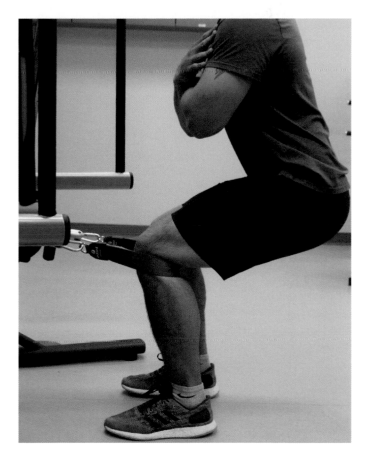

FIGURE 6.2
Spanish squat performed at 70–90 degrees of knee flexion with the lower legs remaining perpendicular to the floor and rigid straps below the knees.

tendon and other body regions. This progression should include most, if not all, of the sport demands to ensure there are no novel loads as the patient fully returns to sport. Sport technique and kinetic chain energy sharing are also addressed in the return to sport phase in an attempt to decrease injury risk and enhance performance.

Quadriceps Tendon Rupture

Background

The vasti and rectus femoris converge distally at the junction of the quadriceps tendon. Isolated quadriceps tendon ruptures make up approximately 3% of all tendon ruptures (Kannus & Józsa, 1991) with an incidence of 2.82/100,000 patients per year (Reito et al., 2019).

Risk Factors

Quadriceps tendon rupture has far greater prevalence in males than females (male:female ratio 4.2:1, mean age: 51.1 years) (Clayton & Court-Brown, 2008) with an elevated risk with increasing age (Shah, 2002). The risk of quadriceps tendon rupture increases with diabetes mellitus, parathyroidism, chronic renal failure, obesity, systemic lupus erythematosus, and gout (Shah, 2002).

Clinical Presentation

In the athletic population, the mechanism of injury typically entails a forceful eccentric contraction of the quadriceps with the knee flexed and foot planted. The mechanism of injury for non-athletic individuals may include a fall or spontaneous rupture in those with multiple comorbidities. The patient may feel or hear a "pop," often accompanied by a tearing sensation. Acute quadriceps tendon ruptures present with gait disturbances, anterior knee pain, difficulty or inability to extend the knee, diffuse swelling, and a palpable defect.

Differential Diagnosis

Quadriceps ruptures are readily diagnosed clinically, whereas partial tears are commonly missed (Perfitt et al., 2014). Ultrasound (US) imaging is highly sensitive (sens: 1.00) and positive findings should be confirmed by the gold standard, magnetic resonance imaging (MRI)

(Perfitt et al., 2014). The differential diagnosis should include quadriceps contusion, quadriceps strain, patellar tendon rupture, lumbar spine referral, femoral fracture, patella fracture, femoral nerve pathology, and patellofemoral pain.

Management

Conservative management is preferred for patients with a partially torn quadriceps tendon who can extend the leg. Conservative management commonly involves a period of immobilization in full knee extension followed by a gradual introduction of knee flexion range of motion, progressive quadriceps strengthening, and return to activity.

Patients with a complete tendon rupture or partially torn tendon combined with the inability to actively extend the leg undergo surgical repair of the quadriceps tendon. The repair is protected via immobilization in full knee extension for an average of 6 weeks, although some rehabilitation guidelines include the use of early mobilization. Early mobilization rehabilitation programs are associated with double the risk for adverse events compared with delayed mobilization programs (Serino et al., 2017). Often, patients are allowed to perform weight-bearing as tolerated in the locked brace within the first two weeks after surgery.

Acute postoperative precautions avoid closed kinetic chain knee flexion and open kinetic chain knee extension for the first 6 weeks. Patients then undergo a graded strengthening program for the quadriceps and other lower extremity musculature. Postoperative rehabilitation may also include proprioception training, neuromuscular electric stimulation, and functional strengthening. Re-rupture rates for quadriceps tendon repair are low (~2%), and outcomes are typically good to excellent (Ciriello et al., 2012). Poorer outcomes are associated with delayed surgery (>3 weeks) following rupture and increasing age (Ciriello et al., 2012). Postoperative average return to activity has been reported at 18.1 weeks (O'Shea et al., 2002). However, this is dependent on many factors including the patient's prior level of function.

Patellar Tendon Rupture

Background

The patellar tendon comprises a superficial and a deep layer; the superficial layer runs as a continuation of the central fibers of the rectus femoris tendon and the deep layer traveling from its origin on the apex of the patella to the attachment at the tibial tubercle (Basso et al., 2001; Andrikoula et al., 2006). Though relatively rare, with an incidence of 0.68/100,000 (Clayton & Court-Brown, 2008), traumatic injuries to the patellar tendon cause immediate disability due to disruption of the knee extensor mechanism. The injury is more common in males (Clayton & Court-Brown, 2008) in the 3rd and 4th decades of life (Ramseier et al., 2006), and typically occurs at the proximal portion of the tendon (Lobenhoffer & Thermann, 2000).

Risk Factors

The mechanism of injury can be either high velocity (e.g., high falls, motor vehicle accidents, basketball) or indirect, low velocity (e.g., falls, slips) due to a hyperflexion injury (Kasten et al., 2001). Contrary to the risk factors for quadriceps tendon rupture, systemic diseases and other comorbidities are not known risk factors for patellar tendon rupture.

Clinical Presentation

Patellar tendon rupture may present similarly to quadriceps tendon rupture with diffuse edema, ecchymosis, pain, quadriceps weakness, and potential inability to actively extend the knee. In a complete tear, the patient will likely present with patella alta. Depending on the extent of the tear, patients may be unable to perform routine functional activities including ambulation, transfers, and other activities of daily living.

Differential Diagnosis

Similar to quadriceps tendon rupture, early diagnosis is essential to proper management in those with patellar tendon rupture. The differential diagnosis for patellar tendon rupture is consistent with quadriceps tendon rupture (above).

Management

Small partial tendon ruptures may be treated conservatively if the knee extensor mechanism remains intact. Conservative management entails initial immobilization (commonly 6 weeks) followed by graded loading, strengthening, and return to function.

Complete patellar tendon ruptures and partial tendon ruptures with a loss of the knee extensor mechanism require surgical fixation. Several techniques exist for patellar tendon rupture repair and technique choice depends on several factors, including tissue quality, patient comorbidities, time since injury, and surgeon preference (Gilmore et al., 2015).

Conflicting evidence exists regarding the most appropriate immobilization period following surgery (early mobilization versus 6 weeks of immobilization). This decision will likely be made on an individual basis and clinicians must consider a variety of factors when making this decision. Patients will gradually return to ambulation, strengthening, proprioceptive activities, and graded quadriceps loading within the parameters of the postoperative rehabilitation guidelines.

Post-surgical functional outcomes in patients treated early after injury tend to be good to excellent with low failure rates (Huleatt et al., 2019).

Buttock and Posterior Thigh

Hamstring Strain

Background

Hamstring injuries (HSI) are the most common lower limb muscle injury, representing 12% of all injuries and 37% of all muscle injuries among professional soccer players. In professional soccer players (Ekstrand et al., 2011), the prevalence of HSI increased by 4% annually between 2001 and 2014, which is concerning due to the considerable burden (19.7 days/1000 hours of exposure) of this injury. Nearly 12%–25% of people who sustain a first-time HSI will experience recurrence of this injury (Wing & Bishop, 2020).

Risk Factors

The semimembranosus, semitendinosus, and the long head of the biceps femoris are biarticular in nature, and function to extend the hip and flex the knee, with a secondary function of stabilizing the lumbopelvic region. Sprinting/high-velocity running is the most cited mechanism of HSI across sports, while kicking-related HSI often result in the most lost time (Wing & Bishop, 2020). During sprinting, the hamstrings forcefully contract eccentrically to decelerate the simultaneously flexing hip and extending knee during terminal swing (Opar et al., 2012). During this phase of sprinting, the biceps femoris undergoes the greatest stretch of the hamstring muscles and is the most implicated muscle in HSI (Ekstrand et al., 2012). Overstretch injuries are a unique HSI subset, occurring commonly during the follow-through motion of kicking or during stretching exercises in dance, and are managed differently than other HSI (Askling et al., 2008).

Prevention of HSI is an area of intense interest among clinicians and coaching staff due to the high incidence, the associated burden, and the high rate of recurrence among sprinters and field athletes. Non-modifiable risk factors for HSI include older age, the prior occurrence of HSI or calf strains, and previous anterior cruciate ligament injury. Prevention efforts target the modifiable risk factors associated with HSI, including insufficient warm-up, eccentric hamstring strength deficits (Wing & Bishop, 2020), short fascicle length of the long head of the biceps femoris, and excessive progression of high-speed running training loads (Duhig et al., 2016). Nordic hamstring exercises (Figure 6.3) are perhaps the most popular intervention to reduce the risk of HSI, with a recent meta-analysis suggesting a 51% reduction in HSI injuries among athletes who regularly perform this exercise (van Dyk et al., 2019). The FIFA 11+ warm-up program, which includes the Nordic hamstring exercise, results in a number needed to treat of 3.31 for biceps femoris injuries and a number needed to treat of 10.7 to prevent recurrent HSI (Nouni-Garcia et al., 2018). The addition of Nordic hamstring exercises to an athlete's conditioning program appears to result in greater eccentric hamstring strength, hamstring hypertrophy, and greater fascicle length of the biceps femoris (van Dyk et al., 2019); together, these training effects address several modifiable risk factors associated with HSI. Other exercises focusing on HIS can be found in Chapter 19.

Clinical Presentation

Prognosis is determined by HSI grade and mechanism of injury, underscoring the importance of a full subjective assessment and a thorough examination. In soccer players, Grade I HSI averaged 17 ± 10 days, Grade II HSI averaged 22 ± 11 days, and Grade III HSI averaged 73 ± 60 days to return to play (Ekstrand et al., 2012). HSI that occurs

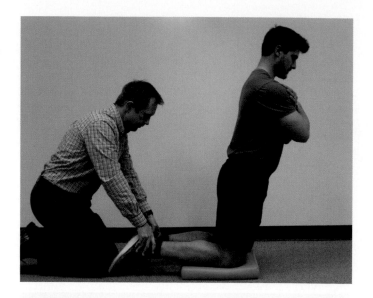

FIGURE 6.3
Nordic hamstring exercise. The patient starts in the tall kneeling position while the partner holds the patient's feet in contact with the floor. The patient slowly lowers their upper body toward the ground while maintaining a rigid spine and hip position. Hands and arms are used to break the descent and push the patient back up to the starting position.

during sprinting most often involves the intramuscular tendon of the biceps femoris (Type I HSI), whereas HSI sustained during kicking or dance (overstretch mechanism of injury) most often involves the proximal free tendon of the semimembranosus (Type II HSI) (Askling et al., 2007). Type I and Type II HSI average 16 weeks (range 6–50 weeks) and 50 weeks (range 30–76 weeks), respectively, to return to pre-injury performance levels (Askling et al., 2006).

Athletes with HSI describe a memorable event, characterized by sudden onset of posterior thigh pain during sprinting or activities that involve high eccentric forces in an elongated muscle, such as kicking or dancing. While edema, ecchymosis, loss of hamstring strength, and gait disruption are common with Grade II and Grade III HSI, these clinical signs are rarely present with Grade I HSI (Heiderscheit et al., 2010). Palpation is a critical assessment tool as more proximal sites of hamstring pain (likely indicating a Type II HSI), require longer to return to pre-injury performance levels (Askling et al., 2007). Passive straight leg raise and active knee extension (with hip positioned in 90 degrees of hip flexion) are key initial range of motion measurements with this injury. Isometric dynamometry to isolate the hip extension and knee flexion actions of the hamstrings should be included in the initial assessment, as well as regularly throughout rehabilitation to track progress. Hip adductor strains, particularly involving the adductor magnus, should be ruled out. Sciatic nerve irritation, assessed via forward slump test, should be suspected when posterior thigh pain is present without a memorable event (Heiderscheit et al., 2010). Imaging can be useful to rule out other competing diagnoses, such as avulsion fracture of the ischial tuberosity.

Management

Athletes who begin rehabilitation, which should include hamstring mobilization, 2 days post-injury, can be expected to miss 25.3% fewer days than those who wait until 9 days post-injury to begin rehabilitation (early mobilization: 62.5 days, interquartile range, 48.8 to 77.8 vs. delayed mobilization: 83.0 days, interquartile range, 64.5 to 97.3) (Bayer et al., 2017).

In a moderate quality trial, progressive, end-range, eccentric loading of the hamstrings resulted in a return to sport of 28 days (range 8–58 days) post-HSI, compared with 51 days (range 12–94 days) for return to sport for a program of hamstring stretching and mid-range hamstring strengthening (Askling et al., 2013) (Figure 6.4 shows the eccentric loading program used in this study). Eccentric hamstring strengthening should be performed in ranges of motion and with loads that elicit up to 4/10 pain on a 0–10 numeric pain rating scale since greater hamstring strength gains and greater fascicle lengths can be achieved compared with pain-avoidance rehabilitation loads (Hickey et al., 2020). Once athletes can walk with a non-antalgic gait, a progressive return to sprinting program is commenced (see Table 6.2 for a sample program).

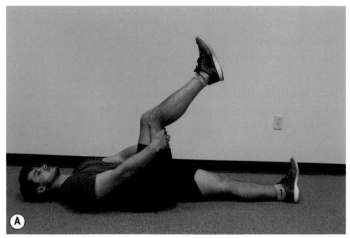

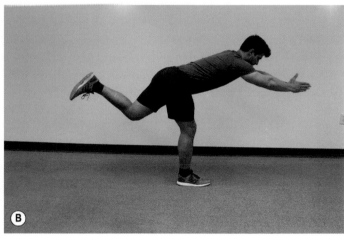

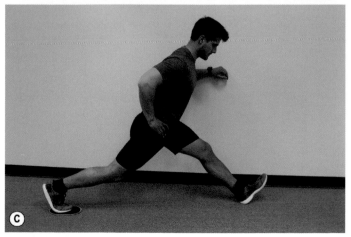

FIGURE 6.4
(A) The Extender. The thigh is stabilized in 90 degrees of hip flexion while the knee is actively extended just prior to the point of pain. (B) The Diver. From an upright trunk position, simultaneously stretching the arms forward as the standing hip is flexed. The standing knee position is maintained at 10–20 degrees throughout. (C) The Glider. From a starting position with upright trunk, the motion is started by gliding backward with one leg and stopped prior to pain onset.

(Adapted from Askling et al., 2013.)

Return to play criteria for athletes recovering from HSI are described in Table 6.3. Other tests to determine return to play readiness following HSI may include isokinetic strength testing and the Askling H-test (Askling et al., 2013; Hickey et al., 2017); Only 1.3%–3.6% of athletes recovering from HSI who pass the Askling H-test experienced re-injury (Askling et al., 2013, 2014). Straight leg raise range of motion and isometric hamstring strength deficits tend to resolve 40–50 days post-injury; however, concentric and eccentric strength deficits persist even after return to play (Maniar et al., 2016). Long-term eccentric hamstring deficits increase the risk of re-injury (Timmins et al., 2016), strongly supporting eccentric hamstring strengthening protocols in those with past HSI.

Proximal Hamstring Tendinopathy

Background

Hamstring tendinopathy affects athletes and non-athletes, and is a difficult condition to understand and manage. Proximal hamstring tendinopathy (PHT) forms the majority of presentations and will be addressed. Pain is generally localized to the ischial region and provoked on loaded trunk/hip flexion or on compression in sitting. In the athletic population it is present in many football players, although not a great cause of time lost from training or playing. PHT is frequently encountered in distance runners, both at high and recreational levels, as well as in disciplines such as hurdling or race-walking. Diagnosis is often confounded by sciatic neuritis; hip, lumbar or sacroiliac issues; or nearby muscle–tendon involvement.

Risk Factors

The anatomy of the hamstring origin is well described. The long head of biceps femoris and semitendinosus arise from the medial facet of the ischial tuberosity, whereas the semimembranosus arises more laterally and anterior (Sato et al., 2012; Feucht et al., 2015). Each tendon may be subjected to increased compression loads, although the biceps femoris/semitendinosus common tendon more with anterior pelvic tilt (Goom et al., 2016). Similarly, the semimembranosus tendon may be subjected to increased compression when there is poor frontal plane pelvic control. Recognizing and understanding these factors is crucial to successful management.

The pathology of hamstring tendinopathy is well described by Lempainen et al. (2009) who suggested involvement predominantly of semimembranosus whereas Benazzo et al. (2013) found it more distributed across all tendons. The histological changes parallel that of other tensile tendinopathies, notably cellular proliferation, proteoglycan and collagenous matrix changes and variable neurovascular ingrowth. Additionally, bone edema may be seen at the enthesis on MRI (De Smet et al., 2012).

Clinical Presentation

In athletes, the onset is generally after a period of increased load into hip/trunk flexion, often following a period of reduced loading (Drew et al., 2016). Pain is localized to the medial or anterolateral ischial tuberosity. The sciatic nerve lies in close proximity to the ischial tuberosity and may be involved in PHT and complicate the diagnostic picture. Pain on sitting is a common presenting symptom in PHT which is shared with sciatic neuritis. Tendinopathy pain should be provoked with a combination of high tendon tensile and compressive loading such as bent knee and hip hamstring bridging (Figure 6.5), lunges or arabesques (Chapter 19). Cacchio et al. (2012) devised a suite of 3 tests with good sensitivity and specificity. The Modified Bent-Knee Stretch Test can be seen in Figure 6.6.

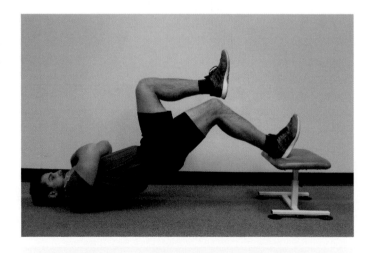

FIGURE 6.5
single-leg bent-knee bridge. A low load clinical test in which the patient presses through the heel and extends the hip.

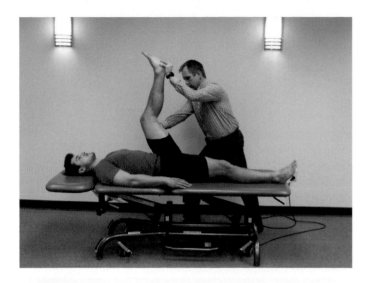

FIGURE 6.6
Modified bent-knee stretch test (end position). The patient lies supine with knees extended. The examiner maximally flexes the hip and knee, then rapidly extends the knee.

Pain is usually increased with the speed of running, or with increasing hip flexion in activities such as lunges or Romanian deadlifts (RDLs). It is not uncommon for the patient to present with ipsilateral hip or lumbar joint impairments which may contribute to the development of PHT.

Hamstring and gluteus maximus (de Jesus et al., 2015) weakness is often present in those with a long history of PHT. In non-athletes, periods of prolonged sitting on hard chairs or an overemphasis of hamstring stretching may precede symptom onset.

Differential Diagnosis

Principal differential diagnostic considerations are depicted in Table 6.5. In acute injury, partial tears of the semimembranosus tendon secondary to overstretch have been described (Askling et al., 2008). Bony avulsion in the adolescent or soft tissue avulsion in the older person should also be considered (Lempainen et al., 2009, 2015). All three conditions, semimembranosus tendon partial tear, bony avulsion, and soft tissue avulsion, are managed quite specifically. Whilst acute care and timeframes may differ, the progression of reloading is similar to that undertaken for isolated tendinopathy.

In insidious onset of ischial pain, the more common differentials include sciatic neuritis, proximal adductor magnus (Obey et al., 2016) or deep gluteal muscle myotendinous strains. Less usual presentations are ischial bursitis, ischiofemoral impingement (Gomez-Hoyos et al., 2016) or stress fractures (most commonly seen in distance runners). Less localized or referred pain may emanate from the lumbar spine, sacroiliac joint, sacrotuberous ligament, and/or posterior hip joint.

Imaging may be used when the diagnosis is unclear. However, asymptomatic tendon signal changes may be seen on MRI (De Smet et al., 2012) and imaging findings should correspond to clinical findings.

TABLE 6.5 Differential Diagnosis of Proximal Hamstring Pain

Common	Less Common	Important (Not to Miss)
• PHT	• Ischiofemoral impingement	• Proximal hamstring avulsion
• Sciatic nerve irritation/DGS	• Posterior femoral cutaneous nerve irritation	• Stress fracture (ischial or pubic ramus)
• Lumbar spine referral	• Pudendal/inferior cluneal nerve irritation	• Seronegative disorders (e.g., ankylosing spondylitis)
• SIJ pathology	• Sacro-tuberous ligament irritation	
• Hip-related ischial pain	• Deep gluteal muscle strain including piriformis	
• Ischiogluteal bursitis		
• Adductor magnus strain		

PHT: proximal hamstring tendinopathy; DGS: deep gluteal syndrome; SIJ: sacroiliac joint.

Specialized physical tests are available to detect sciatic neuritis (Martin et al., 2014, 2015). These tests include the Seated Piriformis test (adducting the internally rotated leg with the knee in extension and palpating the piriformis region) as well as the Active Piriformis test in side-lying. Piriformis entrapment is not the sole mechanism for sciatic neuritis, and a number of other entrapment sites exist, including adventitious fibrous bands deep to gluteus maximus (Hernando et al., 2015; Carro et al., 2016). MRI or US may sometimes identify these bands, but false negatives are not uncommon. Surgery may be required in recalcitrant cases.

Ischiofemoral impingement is rare, but well described. Specific tests adducting and extending the ipsilateral hip and walking with exaggerated long strides may reproduce the symptoms (Gomez-Hoyos et al., 2016). MRI may be used to confirm the suspected diagnosis.

In many long-standing presentations, cases may involve multiple comorbidities, not uncommonly being a combination of spinal/hip/sacroiliac joint, peripheral neural and myotendinous components, requiring the integration of other interventions beyond simple rehabilitation of the hamstring tendon.

Management

Primary PHT management principles include: (1) provocative load reduction; (2) non-provocative, controlled tensile loading; (3) tensile re-loading; (4) hypertrophy-biased interventions; (5) reintroduction of previously symptomatic hip flexion range; and (6) return to running and sport-specific activities.

Initially, provocative loads should be reduced, especially those involving compression combined with tension. Examples include reduction in deep or fast lunging, change of direction, deep squatting, or RDLs. Sitting on hard chairs should also be avoided or modified by off-loading the affected region with towels or other padding to reduce direct or prolonged compression of the ischial region.

Next, controlled tensile load avoiding direct provocation of the region is introduced. This may be in hip neutral or extended positions, and as semimembranosus is the most affected tendon, avoiding adduction of the thigh in hip flexed positions. Where long head biceps femoris is the issue, care with exaggeration of anterior pelvic rotation as the hamstring is loaded is also important (Goom et al., 2016). This may be the result of technical faults in running or lunging.

The tensile re-loading phase may take the form of graduated isometric loading in a hip neutral and slightly abducted position (Rio et al., 2016). This may also be supplemented by range-protected slow isotonic or eccentric exercises, gradually increasing range over time.

Alongside tendon tensile loading, hypertrophy-biased programs may be instituted to address not only associated hamstring weakness, but also to capture any deficits in the synergists (e.g., gluteus maximus and medius/minimus, the external rotators, and other regions). Further, other issues such as lumbar, sacroiliac or hip joint dysfunction (Gerhardt, 2019) should be addressed at this time.

Once PHT pain is controlled on provocative tests and muscle strength is close to normalized, a gradual reintroduction of working into the previously symptomatic hip flexion range may recommence at low speeds. Monitoring of the next-day response (Goom et al., 2016) is a key element to determine if loads and ranges are within the optimal window. Further progression of weight first, then range, then speed, must be completed to successfully progress to full function. Highly provocative activities, such as lunges or step-ups, are closely monitored and undertaken twice weekly.

The final phase of PHT management includes return to running and sport activities. Return to running, again initially twice weekly, is progressed in speed, then expanded to include change of direction drills, graduating from structured to unstructured sessions whilst monitoring workloads in metrics specific to the hamstring tendon (e.g., accelerations, decelerations, deep lunges, squats, kicking).

Medial Thigh and Groin Pain
Adductor-related Groin Pain
Background

Groin injuries are typically seen in team sports associated with kicking, cutting and/or change of direction. The adductors are the second most frequently injured muscle group in professional soccer players (Ekstrand et al., 2011) and the most commonly injured muscle group in those presenting with acute groin injury (Serner et al., 2015).

Adductor muscle injuries are also commonly seen in ice hockey players and account for approximately 10% of all hockey injuries (Lorentzon et al., 1988). Adductor muscle group groin injuries can be difficult to assess, diagnose, and manage due to a myriad of factors. The inherent complexity and diagnostic terminology variation in groin injuries has led to expert recommendations for uniform diagnostic terminology of "adductor-related groin pain" (Weir et al., 2015). Although adductor-related groin injuries are relatively common, they are difficult to appropriately manage, are associated with considerable lost-time, and have a high recurrence rate (16%–30% in collegiate ice hockey) (Eckard et al., 2017b).

Risk Factors

Diagnostic terminology inconsistencies in research are a main limitation for identifying risk factors for adductor-related groin pain and more high-quality research using consistent terminology is warranted.

Risk factors for groin injury include higher level of play, lower levels of sport-specific training, previous groin injury, and reduced hip adductor strength (Whittaker et al., 2015). Harøy et al. (2019) have found a 41% decrease in the prevalence of soccer-related groin injuries in athletes performing a progressive adductor strengthening program throughout preseason and competitive season.

Total hip range of motion may also be related to groin injuries; however, these range differences may be too small to consistently detect on physical examination (Tak et al., 2017). Hip abductor weakness and knee flexor weakness may also be seen in those prior to a sports-related groin injury (Kloskowska et al., 2016).

Differential Diagnosis

A comprehensive differential diagnosis list and a thorough clinical reasoning process are paramount for accurate diagnosis of adductor-related groin pain. A list of differential diagnoses for groin pain can be seen in Table 6.6.

Presentation

Adductor longus is the most commonly injured adductor muscle followed, in descending order, by adductor brevis, pectineus, obturator externus, gracilis, and adductor magnus (Serner et al., 2018). Adductor longus is the most commonly injured muscle during kicking-related mechanisms of injury (Serner et al., 2015). The most common mechanism of injury for adductor-related groin pain in footballers (soccer players) is change of direction followed by kicking, then reaching (Serner et al., 2019).

Symptom location may assist the clinician in properly diagnosing the specific muscle involved in adductor-related groin pain; however, it may not be definitive due to radiating and/or vague symptom location.

Physical examination should include testing to rule out the lumbar spine, sacroiliac joints, and hip joint as potential referral sources. Lumbar spine screening may include repeated motion testing, quadrant testing, and passive accessory mobility assessment. In order to rule out the sacroiliac joints, the provider can use a cluster of provocation tests as described in Chapter 13 (Laslett et al., 2005). Hip joint screening can be performed using tests with higher reported sensitivities including the Flexion Adduction Internal Rotation (FADDIR) and Flexion-Internal Rotation tests (Reiman et al., 2015).

TABLE 6.6 Differential Diagnosis of Groin Pain

Common	Less Common	Important (Not to Miss)
• Adductor-related groin pain	• Iliopsoas-related groin pain	• Visceral referral (i.e., urinary, genital, etc.)
• Hip-related groin pain	• Inguinal-related groin pain	• Sinister pathology (cancer, infection)
• Femoroacetabular impingement	• Pubic-related groin pain	• Pelvic stress fracture
• Lumbar spine referral	• Femoral nerve irritation	• Femoral stress fracture
• Sacroiliac joint pathology	• Obturator nerve irritation	• Slipped capital femoral epiphysis (pediatric patients)
		• Legg–Calvé–Perthes disease (pediatric patients)

Patients with adductor-related groin pain experience symptom reproduction with adductor muscle palpation, movements that elongate the adductors (passive abduction, passive combined abduction/external rotation/extension), and resisted adduction. The Adductor Squeeze Test may also assist in diagnosing adductor-related groin pain and has been described in both 0 degrees and 45 degrees of hip flexion (Chapter 19). A comprehensive examination should also include examination of related impairments, functional, and performance testing.

Medical imaging, including US or MRI, may be considered in the event of recalcitrant adductor-related groin pain, or if adductor avulsion, bone stress or non-musculo-skeletal injury is suspected.

Management

Adductor-related groin injury management can be challenging, especially for the in-season athlete. Proper management is crucial as recurrent injuries are oftentimes more severe than the initial injury resulting in longer absence from sport (Ekstrand et al., 2020).

Several paradigms exist regarding management of adductor-related groin pain, including impairment-based, criteria-based, and rehabilitation targeting intersegmental control. Successful management of adductor-related groin pain will likely require a combination of approaches using an individualized plan of care for the patient.

Lumbopelvic control and muscle strength exercises, with an emphasis on the adductors, have been shown to provide favorable outcomes (Holmich et al., 1999; Weir et al., 2011; Yousefzadeh et al., 2018). The Holmich and Modified Holmich protocols are two such programs emphasizing abdominal recruitment and strengthening in addition to progressive adductor strengthening (Holmich et al., 1999; Yousefzadeh et al., 2018). Rehabilitation targeting intersegmental control with an emphasis on technique and progressive loading has also shown promising results (King et al., 2018). The progression in this study started with intersegmental control and strengthening, progressing to linear mechanics and running load, then to multidirectional mechanics and sprinting, and finally to return to play (King et al., 2018).

Exercises as a part of a criteria-based rehabilitation program have been described in patients with acute adductor injuries and demonstrate moderate return to sport rates (grades 0–2: median = 18 days, grade 3: median = 78 days) (Serner et al., 2020). The 4 phases in the groin exercise portion of the program include: (1) active flexibility; (2) early resistance; (3) load progression; and (4) high load, high speed. Figure 6.7 shows the Copenhagen adduction exercise from the high load, high speed phase of the program. More data on adductor exercises are provided in Chapter 19.

Adductor-related groin pain return to sport should be made within an interdisciplinary healthcare team. Factors influencing return to sport include injury severity, impairment-based measures (strength, range of motion, pain), functional and performance testing, ability to perform symptom-free sports-related activities, and functional outcome measure scores.

Surgical intervention may be warranted in those with adductor avulsion or refractory cases of adductor-related groin pain. Selective partial adductor release for chronic adductor-related groin pain has been shown to have promising results (Schilders et al., 2013); however, this should be used as a last resort due to complication risk and the potential for ensuing adductor muscle weakness.

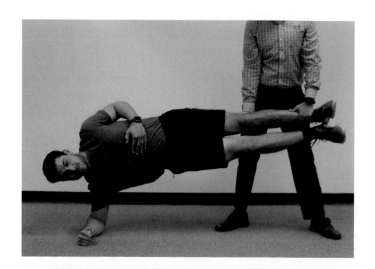

FIGURE 6.7
Copenhagen Adduction Exercise (End Position). The partner holds the patient's top leg while the patient lifts their pelvis and lower leg into a plank position. The patient slowly lowers their pelvis and lower leg back to the ground.

Lateral Hip Pain

Greater Trochanteric Pain Syndrome/Gluteal Tendinopathy

Background

Greater trochanteric pain syndrome (GTPS) is a common condition affecting 17.6% of community-based adults 50 to 79 years old (Segal et al., 2007). GTPS is an umbrella-like diagnosis encompassing several pathologies in the greater trochanteric region including the most common, gluteal tendinopathy (Grimaldi & Fearon, 2015). In a Dutch-based study, GTPS was found to have the highest incidence (3.29 per 1000 person-years) and prevalence (4.22 per 1000 person-years) of all lower limb tendinopathies (Albers et al., 2016). GTPS is difficult to diagnose due to the region's relationship to the lumbar spine, the referral patterns of intra-articular hip pathology, and the vague symptom location. Previously thought to be trochanteric bursitis; however, minimal bursal inflammation is present upon imaging in those presenting with GTPS (Silva et al., 2008; Long et al., 2013).

Risk Factors

Gluteal tendinopathy is most common in individuals over the age of 40, affecting women 2.4–4 to 1 more than men (Grimaldi and Fearon, 2015). MRI shows gluteus medius and minimus pathology is also correlated to advancing age (Chi et al., 2015).

Higher body mass index, altered gait parameters, and lower hip abduction muscle strength are commonly found in those with GTPS, although causation cannot be established (Plinsinga et al., 2019). GTPS is also associated with iliotibial band syndrome (Segal et al., 2007), knee osteoarthritis (Segal et al., 2007) and low back pain (Tortolani et al., 2002; Segal et al., 2007; Tan et al., 2018).

Clinical Presentation

GTPS presents as lateral hip pain near the greater trochanter. Pain may radiate down the lateral thigh and mimic lumbar referral or radiculopathy. Symptoms are often reported with activities or positions that compress the lateral hip/gluteal tendon, such as side-lying, sitting cross-legged, or "hip hanging" (standing with weight shifted predominantly toward the involved limb) which can be seen in Figure 6.8.

Performing functional activities that load a single limb (stair ambulation, single-leg stance while dressing) may also be problematic. Although a specific mechanism of injury is possible, most patients report a gradual insidious symptom onset preceded by increased activity.

Patients may demonstrate symptom reproduction with greater trochanter and/or surrounding area palpation. Palpation should be used with caution due to the presence of centrally mediated factors such as hyperalgesia and allodynia that may affect symptom response (French et al., 2019; Ferrer-Peña et al., 2019). Patients also commonly have symptoms with resisted hip abduction and/or rotation.

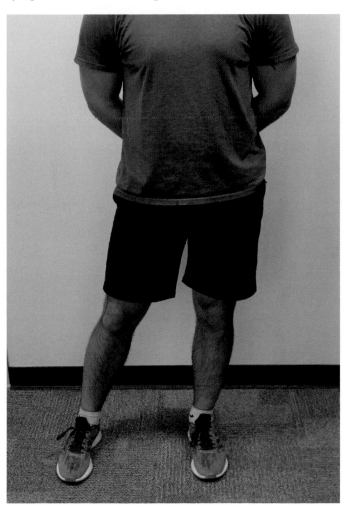

FIGURE 6.8
"Hip hanging" – standing with weight shifted predominantly toward the involved limb.

Special tests used to aid the diagnosis of GTPS include resisted isometric abduction with the limb in adduction (+LR 5.7; –LR: 0.66), resisted FADER (+LR 6.6; –LR: 0.60), and 30-second single-leg stance test (+LR 12.2; –LR: 0.62) (Grimaldi et al., 2017). The FABER test (+LR 2.1; –LR: 0.73) can be helpful in differentiating between hip osteoarthritis and sacroiliac dysfunction and GTPS. Due to the moderate –LRs of these aforementioned tests, clinicians should conduct a thorough examination to rule out competing diagnoses, as described in Chapter 13.

Differential Diagnosis

Non-musculoskeletal diagnoses such as bony metastasis (consider if presence of unrelenting pain that may be worse at night) and rheumatoid diseases (presence of warmth and symmetrical presentation) should be ruled out. Musculoskeletal diagnoses including femoral neck fracture (recent fall, presence of osteoporosis), hip joint pathology (pain in groin, medial knee, deep buttock), and lumbar spine referral should also be considered. GTPS and hip osteoarthritis are common differential diagnoses in lateral hip pain (Grimaldi & Fearon, 2015). Reported pain with donning/doffing shoes may assist in differentiating GTPS from hip osteoarthritis – absence of pain with shoe/sock manipulation implicates GTPS (Fearon et al., 2013). Additional features differentiating GTPS, hip osteoarthritis, and lumbar spine referral can be seen in Table 6.7.

Radiography and scintigraphy are considered to rule out competing diagnoses, whereas MRI and US are more helpful in the diagnosis of GTPS. US has shown a higher positive predictive value (PPV: .95–1.00) and sensitivity (sens: .79–1.00) (Westacott et al., 2011).

Management

Proper management of GTPS includes a combination of activity modification, load management, and loading exercise. Early management consists of patient education

---

TABLE 6.7 Diagnostic Features of GTPS, Hip OA, and Lumbar Spine Referral

	GTPS	Hip OA	Lumbar Spine Referral
History	• Pain with activities compressing gluteal tendon (i.e., hip hanging, side-lying) • Night pain if reactive • Location of symptoms at or near greater trochanter	• Morning stiffness ≤60 minutes • Groin/buttock pain • Difficulty in donning shoes/socks • Night pain in advanced OA	• Low back pain • Vague report of symptom location in the lower extremity • Paresthesia • Pain with lumbar loading (i.e., lumbar flexion)
Physical Examination	• Pain with SLS ≤30 secs • Pain with resisted hip abduction in pre-positioned adduction • Pain with resisted external derotation test • Negative hip joint provocation tests	• Positive hip joint provocation tests (i.e., FADDIR, Scour) • Absent gluteal tendon tenderness • Decreased hip ROM in two directions (i.e., IR, flexion) • Pain with passive ROM hip IR	• Pain with lumbar loading (i.e., lumbar flexion, repeated movements) • Negative hip and GTPS testing • Positive lumbar PAIVMs • Positive neurodynamic tests (radicular) • Diminished or absent deep tendon reflexes (radicular)

GTPS: greater trochanteric pain syndrome; OA: osteoarthritis; SLS: single-leg stance; FADDIR: Flexion Adduction Internal Rotation; IR: internal rotation; PAIVMs: passive accessory intervertebral movements.

and modifying activities to reduce tendon and lateral hip compressive loads including avoiding hip adduction stretches.

Loading exercise can be initiated isometrically in non-compressive positions, i.e., hip in neutral flexion, abducted slightly, and in neutral rotation, to decrease pain and initiate tendon loading. Isometric parameters and exercise progressions (intensity, length of holds, number of repetitions, and permissible pain during repetitions) should optimize progressive tendon loading, while avoiding symptom exacerbation after each loading bout (Grimaldi & Fearon, 2015).

In the next phase, isotonic weight-bearing and non-weight-bearing exercises are added to progressively load the tendon. At first, patients and clinicians should limit tendon compression in the early stages of rehabilitation, with gradual reintroduction of compressive loads as the patient recovers. Finally, functional loading and return to sport activities should be employed to replicate the demands of sport/everyday activities.

Proper management should also address contributing factors in the lumbar spine and lower extremity. Manual therapy and modalities may also be employed; however, literature supporting their use in GTPS is scarce.

Historically, corticosteroid injections have been used in the treatment of GTPS despite its known deleterious effects on tendon structure. A high-quality trial found greater short-term and long-term outcomes in those with GTPS who received patient education and exercise compared with corticosteroids (Mellor et al., 2018).

Return to Play Considerations

Rehabilitation programs should progressively expose the athlete to loads that ensure that novel loads are not experienced once return to play commences. Thus, it is imperative to perform a systematic, graded loading approach to return to running/sprinting, plyometrics, and sport-specific activities prior to the athlete being cleared for full participation. Utilizing a progressive framework that initially emphasizes progressive resistance training (emphasizes heavy loads applied in a controlled manner), progressing to plyometrics (builds energy storage and release capacity), and eventual gradual reintroduction to sport-specific loads via sport-specific exercises (builds tolerance to cumulative and unpredictable loads) ensures the athlete is physically prepared for return to sport (Breda et al., 2021).

Objective criteria should determine when the athlete is ready to return to sport. Return to competition should involve shared decision-making involving the athlete, coaching staff, and the medical team (Ardern et al., 2016). Return to play decisions can be challenging, especially when external pressure exists for the athlete to make their return. Fear of re-injury often affects an athlete's ability to return to full participation; thus, considering psychological readiness is key in return to sport decisions. The Injury Psychological Readiness to Return to Sport scale (Glazer, 2009) may provide the athlete and clinical team with important insights into the athlete's confidence in returning to sport.

Conclusions

Hip and knee muscle and tendon injuries include some of the most common, yet challenging-to-manage diagnoses in the sporting population. These injuries can result in significant disability and time away from sport/everyday activities. As was discussed throughout the chapter, proper diagnosis and management are crucial to effective injury management that decreases time away from sport and activities of daily living. In all cases, a multimodal approach may be warranted; however, the cornerstone to hip and knee muscle and tendon injury management should include a progressive loading component. Return to play considerations should be multifactorial and include shared decision-making that includes the athlete and rest of the healthcare team. This chapter serves as a concise overview of several key diagnoses and we recommend the astute clinician turn to the literature regarding updates on evaluating and managing patients with these diagnoses.

Conflict of Interest

Dr. Mischke offers continuing education courses. Dr. Willy offers continuing education courses and provides professional consulting services to professional sports teams and athletes. The authors have no other conflicts of interest to report.

CHAPTER SIX

References

Albers IS, Zwerver J, Diercks RL, et al. Incidence and prevalence of lower extremity tendinopathy in a Dutch general practice population: a cross sectional study. BMC Musculoskelet Disord. 2016;17:16.

Andrikoula S, Tokis A, Vasiliadis HS, Georgoulis A. The extensor mechanism of the knee joint: an anatomical study. Knee Surg Sports Traumatol Arthrosc. 2006;14:214–20.

Ardern CL, Glasgow P, Schneiders A, et al. Consensus statement on return to sport from the First World Congress in Sports Physical Therapy, Bern. Br J Sports Med. 2016;50:853–64.

Askling C, Saartok T, Thorstensson A. Type of acute hamstring strain affects flexibility, strength, and time to return to pre-injury level. Br J Sports Med. 2006;40:40–4.

Askling CM, Tengvar M, Saartok T, Thorstensson A. Acute first-time hamstring strains during high-speed running: a longitudinal study including clinical and magnetic resonance imaging findings. Am J Sports Med. 2007;35:197-206.

Askling CM, Tengvar M, Saartok T, Thorstensson A. Proximal hamstring strains of stretching type in different sports: injury situations, clinical and magnetic resonance imaging characteristics, and return to sport. Am J Sports Med. 2008;36:1799-804.

Askling CM, Tengvar M, Thorstensson A. Acute hamstring injuries in Swedish elite football: a prospective randomised controlled clinical trial comparing two rehabilitation protocols. Br J Sports Med. 2013;47:953–9.

Askling CM, Tengvar M, Tarassova O, Thorstensson A. Acute hamstring injuries in Swedish elite sprinters and jumpers: a prospective randomised controlled clinical trial comparing two rehabilitation protocols. Br J Sports Med. 2014;48(7):532–9.

Basso O, Johnson DP, Amis AA. The anatomy of the patellar tendon. Knee Surg Sports Traumatol Arthrosc. 2001;9:2–5.

Bayer ML, Magnusson SP, Kjaer M, Tendon Research Group Bispebjerg. Early versus delayed rehabilitation after acute muscle injury. N Engl J Med. 2017;377:1300–1.

Benazzo F, Marullo M, Zanon G, et al. Surgical management of chronic proximal hamstring tendinopathy in athletes: a 2 to 11 years of follow-up. J Orthop Traumatol. 2013;14:83–9.

Bleakley CM, Glasgow P, MacAuley DC. PRICE needs updating, should we call the POLICE? Br J Sports Med. 2012;46:220–1.

Breda SJ, Oei EHG, Zwerver J, et al. Effectiveness of progressive tendon-loading exercise therapy in patients with patellar tendinopathy: a randomised clinical trial. Br J Sports Med. 2021;55:501–9.

Cacchio A, Borra F, Severini G et al. Reliability and validity of three pain provocation tests used for the diagnosis of chronic proximal hamstring tendinopathy. Br J Sports Med. 2012;46:883–7.

Carro LP, Hernando MF, Cerezal L, et al. Deep gluteal space problems: piriformis syndrome, ischiofemoral impingement and sciatic nerve release. Muscles Ligaments Tendons J. 2016;6:384–96.

Chi AS, Long SS, Zoga AC et al. Prevalence and pattern of gluteus medius and minimus tendon pathology and muscle atrophy in older individuals using MRI. Skeletal Radiol. 2015;44:1727–33.

Ciriello V, Gudipati S, Tosounidis T, et al. Clinical outcomes after repair of quadriceps tendon rupture: a systematic review. Injury. 2012;43:1931–8.

Clayton RA, Court-Brown CM. The epidemiology of musculoskeletal tendinous and ligamentous injuries. Injury. 2008;39:1338–44.

Comin J, Cook J, Malliaras P, et al. The prevalence and clinical significance of sonographic tendon abnormalities in asymptomatic ballet dancers: a 24-month longitudinal study. Br J Sports Med. 2013;47:89–92.

Cook JL, Khan KM, Kiss ZS, Griffiths L. Patellar tendinopathy in junior basketball players: a controlled clinical and ultrasonographic study of 268 patellar tendons in players aged 14–18 years. Scand J Med Sci Sports. 2000;10:216–20.

Cook JL, Khan KM, Kiss ZS, et al. Reproducibility and clinical utility of tendon palpation to detect patellar tendinopathy in young basketball players. Victorian Institute of Sport tendon study group. Br J Sports Med. 2001;35:65–9.

Cross TM, Gibbs N, Houang MT, Cameron M. Acute quadriceps muscle strains: magnetic resonance imaging features and prognosis. Am J Sports Med. 2004;32:710–9.

de Jesus J, Bryk F, Moreira V, et al. Gluteus maximus inhibition in proximal hamstring tendinopathy. Medical Express. 2015;2:1.

De Smet AA, Blankenbaker DG, Alsheik NH, Lindstrom MJ. MRI appearance of the proximal hamstring tendons in patients with and without symptomatic proximal hamstring tendinopathy. AJR Am J Roentgenol. 2012;198:418–22.

de Vries AJ, van der Worp H, Diercks RL, et al. Risk factors for patellar tendinopathy in volleyball and basketball players: A survey-based prospective cohort study. Scand J Med Sci Sports. 2015;25:678–84.

Docking SI, Rio E, Cook J, et al. The prevalence of Achilles and patellar tendon injuries in Australian football players beyond a time-loss definition. Scand J Med Sci Sports. 2018;28:2016-22.

Drew MK, Cook J, Finch CF. Sports-related workload and injury risk: simply knowing the risks will not prevent injuries: Narrative review. Br J Sports Med. 2016;50:1306–8.

Duhig S, Shield AJ, Opar D, et al. Effect of high-speed running on hamstring strain injury risk. Br J Sports Med. 2016;50:1536–40.

Eckard TG, Kerr ZY, Padua DA, et al. Epidemiology of quadriceps strains in National Collegiate Athletic Association Athletes, 2009-2010 Through 2014-2015. J Athl Train. 2017a;52:474–81.

Eckard TG, Padua DA, Dompier TP, et al. Epidemiology of hip flexor and hip adductor strains in National Collegiate Athletic Association Athletes, 2009/2010-2014/2015. Am J Sports Med. 2017b;45:2713–22.

Ekstrand J, Hägglund M, Waldén M. Epidemiology of muscle injuries in professional football (soccer). Am J Sports Med. 2011;39:1226-32.

Ekstrand J, Healy JC, Walden M, et al. Hamstring muscle injuries in professional football: the correlation of MRI findings with return to play. Br J Sports Med. 2012;46:112–7.

Ekstrand J, Krutsch W, Spreco A et al. Time before return to play for the most common injuries in professional football: a 16-year follow-up of the UEFA Elite Club Injury Study. Br J Sports Med. 2020;54:421–6.

Fearon AM, Scarvell JM, Neeman T, et al. Greater trochanteric pain syndrome: defining the clinical syndrome. Br J Sports Med. 2013;47:649-53.

Ferrer-Peña R, Muñoz-García D, Calvo-Lobo C, Fernández-Carnero J. Pain expansion and severity reflect central sensitization in primary care patients with greater trochanteric pain syndrome. Pain Med. 2019;20:961–70.

Feucht MJ, Plath JE, Seppel G, et al. Gross anatomical and dimensional characteristics of the proximal hamstring origin. Knee Surg Sports Traumatol Arthrosc. 2015;23:2576–82.

Fousekis K, Tsepis E, Poulmedis P, et al. Intrinsic risk factors of non-contact quadriceps and hamstring strains in soccer: a prospective study of 100 professional players. Br J Sports Med. 2011;45:709–14.

French HP, Jong CC, McCallan M. Do features of central sensitisation exist in Greater Trochanteric Pain Syndrome (GTPS)? A case control study. Musculoskelet Sci Pract. 2019;43:6–11.

Gerhardt M. Editorial Commentary: Proximal Hamstring Injuries-Is the Hip to Blame? Arthroscopy. 2019;35:1403–5.

Gilmore JH, Clayton-Smith ZJ, Aguilar M, et al. Reconstruction techniques and clinical results of patellar tendon ruptures: Evidence today. Knee. 2015;22:148–55.

Glazer DD. Development and preliminary validation of the Injury-Psychological Readiness to Return to Sport (I-PRRS) scale. J Athl Train. 2009;44:185–9.

Gomez-Hoyos J, Martin RL, Schroder R, et al. Accuracy of 2 clinical tests for ischiofemoral impingement in patients with posterior hip pain and endoscopically confirmed diagnosis. Arthroscopy. 2016;32:1279–84.

Goom TS, Malliaras P, Reiman MP, Purdam CR. Proximal hamstring tendinopathy: Clinical aspects of assessment and management. J Orthop Sports Phys Ther. 2016;46:483–93.

Grassi A, Quaglia A, Canata GL, Zaffagnini S. An update on the grading of muscle injuries: a narrative review from clinical to comprehensive systems. Joints. 2016;4:39–46.

Grimaldi A, Fearon A. Gluteal Tendinopathy: Integrating pathomechanics and clinical features in its management. J Orthop Sports Phys Ther. 2015;45:910–22.

Grimaldi A, Mellor R, Nicolson P, et al. Utility of clinical tests to diagnose MRI-confirmed gluteal tendinopathy in patients presenting with lateral hip pain. Br J Sports Med. 2017;51:519–24.

Harøy J, Clarsen B, Wiger EG, et al. The Adductor Strengthening Programme prevents groin problems among male football players: a cluster-randomised controlled trial. Br J Sports Med. 2019;53:150–7.

Heiderscheit BC, Sherry MA, Silder A, Chumanov ES, Thelen DG. Hamstring strain injuries: recommendations for diagnosis, rehabilitation, and injury prevention. J Orthop Sports Phys Ther. 2010;40: 67-81.

Hernando MF, Cerezal L, Perez-Carro L, et al. Deep gluteal syndrome: anatomy, imaging, and management of sciatic nerve entrapments in the subgluteal space. Skeletal Radiol. 2015;44:919–34.

Hickey JT, Timmins RG, Maniar N, et al. Criteria for progressing rehabilitation and determining return-to-play clearance following hamstring strain injury: a systematic review. Sports Med. 2017;47(7):1375–87.

Hickey JT, Timmins RG, Maniar N, et al. Pain-free versus pain-threshold rehabilitation following acute hamstring strain injury: A Randomized Controlled Trial. J Orthop Sports Phys Ther. 2020;50:91–103.

Holmich P, Uhrskou P, Ulnits L, et al. Effectiveness of active physical training as treatment for long-standing adductor-related groin pain in athletes: randomised trial. Lancet. 1999;353:439–43.

Huleatt JB, Gebrelul A, Premkumar A, Xerogeanes J. Suture anchor repair of quadriceps tendon and patellar tendon ruptures. Techniques in Orthopaedics. 2019;34:134–9.

Ishoi L, Krommes K, Husted RS, et al. Diagnosis, prevention and treatment of common lower extremity muscle injuries in sport - grading the evidence: a statement paper commissioned by the Danish Society of Sports Physical Therapy (DSSF). Br J Sports Med. 2020;54:528–37.

Kannus P, Józsa L. Histopathological changes preceding spontaneous rupture of a tendon. A controlled study of 891 patients. J Bone Joint Surg Am. 1991;73:1507–25.

Kary JM. Diagnosis and management of quadriceps strains and contusions. Curr Rev Musculoskelet Med. 2010;3:26–31.

Kasten P, Schewe B, Maurer F, et al. Rupture of the patellar tendon: a review of 68 cases and a retrospective study of 29 ruptures comparing two methods of augmentation. Arch Orthop Trauma Surg. 2001;121:578–82.

King E, Franklyn-Miller A, Richter C, et al. Clinical and biomechanical outcomes of rehabilitation targeting intersegmental control in athletic groin pain: prospective cohort of 205 patients. Br J Sports Med. 2018;52:1054–62.

Kloskowska P, Morrissey D, Small C, et al. Movement patterns and muscular function before and after onset of sports-related groin pain: A Systematic Review with Meta-analysis. Sports Med. 2016;46:1847–67.

Laslett M, Aprill CN, McDonald B, Young SB. Diagnosis of sacroiliac joint pain: validity of individual provocation tests and composites of tests. Man Ther. 2005;10:207–18.

Lempainen L, Johansson K, Banke IJ, et al. Expert opinion: diagnosis and treatment of proximal hamstring tendinopathy. Muscles Ligaments Tendons J. 2015;5:23–8.

Lempainen L, Sarimo J, Mattila K, et al. Proximal hamstring tendinopathy: results of surgical management and histopathologic findings. Am J Sports Med. 2009;37:727–34.

Lian OB, Engebretson L, Bahr R. Prevalence of jumper's knee among elite athletes from different sports: a cross-sectional study. Am J Sports Med. 2005;33:561–7.

Lobenhoffer P, Thermann H. [Quadriceps and patellar tendon ruptures]. Orthopade. 2000;29:228–34.

Long SS, Surrey DE, Nazarian LN. Sonography of greater trochanteric pain syndrome and the rarity of primary bursitis. AJR Am J Roentgenol. 2013;201:1083–6.

Lorentzon R, Wedrèn H, Pietilä T. Incidence, nature, and causes of ice hockey injuries. A three-year prospective study of a Swedish elite ice hockey team. Am J Sports Med. 1988;16:392–6.

Malliaras P, Cook J, Purdam C, Rio E. Patellar Tendinopathy: Clinical diagnosis, load management, and advice for challenging case presentations. J Orthop Sports Phys Ther. 2015;45:887–98.

Maniar N, Shield AJ, Williams MD, et al. Hamstring strength and flexibility after hamstring strain injury: a systematic review and meta-analysis. Br J Sports Med. 2016;50:909–20.

Martin HD, Kivlan BR, Palmer IJ, Martin RL. Diagnostic accuracy of clinical tests for sciatic nerve entrapment in the gluteal region. Knee Surg Sports Traumatol Arthrosc. 2014;22:882–8.

Martin HD, Reddy M, Gómez-Hoyos J. Deep gluteal syndrome. J Hip Preserv Surg. 2015;2:99-107.

Mellor R, Bennell K, Grimaldi A P, et al. Education plus exercise versus corticosteroid injection use versus a wait and see approach on global outcome and pain from gluteal tendinopathy: prospective, single blinded, randomised clinical trial. Br J Sports Med. 2018;52:1464–72.

Mendonca LdM, Ocarino JM, Bittencourt NF, et al. The accuracy of the VISA-P questionnaire, single-leg decline squat, and tendon pain history to identify patellar tendon abnormalities in adult athletes. J Orthop Sports Phys Ther. 2016;46:673-80.

Nouni-Garcia R, Carratala-Munuera C, Orozco-Beltran D, et al. Clinical benefit of the FIFA 11 programme for the prevention of hamstring and lateral ankle ligament injuries among amateur soccer players. Inj Prev. 2018;24:149–54.

Obey MR, Broski SM, Spinner RJ, et al. Anatomy of the adductor magnus origin: implications for proximal hamstring injuries. Orthop J Sports Med. 2016;4:2325967115625055.

Opar DA, Williams MD, Shield AJ. Hamstring strain injuries: factors that lead to injury and re-injury. Sports Med. 2012;42:209–26.

O'Shea K, Kenny P, Donovan J, et al. Outcomes following quadriceps tendon ruptures. Injury. 2002;33:257–60.

Perfitt JS, Petrie MJ, Blundell CM, Davies MB. Acute quadriceps tendon rupture: a pragmatic approach to diagnostic imaging. Eur J Orthop Surg Traumatol. 2014;24:1237–41.

Plinsinga ML, Ross MH, Coombes BK, Vicenzino B. Physical findings differ between individuals with greater trochanteric pain syndrome and healthy controls: A systematic review with meta-analysis. Musculoskelet Sci Pract. 2019;43:83–90.

Purdam CR, Cook JL, Hopper DM, et al. Discriminative ability of functional loading tests for adolescent jumper's knee. Phys Ther Sport. 2003;4:3–9.

Ramseier LE, Werner CM, Heinzelmann M. Quadriceps and patellar tendon rupture. Injury. 2006;37:516–9.

Reiman MP, Goode AP, Cook CE, et al. Diagnostic accuracy of clinical tests for the diagnosis of hip femoroacetabular impingement/labral tear: a systematic review with meta-analysis. Br J Sports Med. 2015;49:811.

Reito A, Paloneva J, Mattila VM, Launonen AP. The increasing incidence of surgically treated quadriceps tendon ruptures. Knee Surg Sports Traumatol Arthrosc. 2019;27:3644–9.

Rio E, Kidgell D, Purdam C, et al. Isometric exercise induces analgesia and reduces inhibition in patellar tendinopathy. Br J Sports Med. 2015;49:1277–83.

Rio E, Kidgell D, Moseley GL, et al. Tendon neuroplastic training: changing the way we think about tendon rehabilitation: a narrative review. Br J Sports Med. 2016;50:209–15.

Sato K, Nimura A, Yamaguchi K, Akita K. Anatomical study of the proximal origin of hamstring muscles. J Orthop Sci. 2012;17:614–8.

Schilders E, Dimitrakopoulou A, Cooke M, et al. Effectiveness of a selective partial adductor release for chronic adductor-related groin pain in professional athletes. Am J Sports Med. 2013;41:603–7.

Segal NA, Felson DT, Torner JC, et al. Greater trochanteric pain syndrome: epidemiology and associated factors. Arch Phys Med Rehabil. 2007;88:988–92.

Serino J, Mohamadi A, Orman S, et al. Comparison of adverse events and postoperative mobilization following knee extensor mechanism rupture repair: A systematic review and network meta-analysis. Injury. 2017;48:2793–9.

Serner A, Mosler AB, Tol JL, et al. Mechanisms of acute adductor longus injuries in male football players: a systematic visual video analysis. Br J Sports Med. 2019;53:158–64.

Serner A, Tol JL, Jomaah N K, et al. Diagnosis of acute groin injuries: A prospective study of 110 athletes. Am J Sports Med. 2015;43:1857–64.

Serner A, Weir A, Tol JL, et al. Return to sport after criteria-based rehabilitation of acute adductor injuries in male athletes: A prospective cohort study. Orthop J Sports Med. 2020;8:2325967119897247.

Serner A, Weir A, Tol JL, et al. Characteristics of acute groin injuries in the adductor muscles: A detailed MRI study in athletes. Scand J Med Sci Sports. 2018;2:667–76.

Shah MK. Simultaneous bilateral rupture of quadriceps tendons: analysis of risk factors and associations. South Med J. 2002;95:860–6.

Silva F, Adams T, Feinstein J, Arroyo RA. Trochanteric bursitis: refuting the myth of inflammation. J Clin Rheumatol. 2008;14:82–6.

Sprague AL, Smith AH, Knox P, et al. Modifiable risk factors for patellar tendinopathy in athletes: a systematic review and meta-analysis. Br J Sports Med. 2018;52:1575–85.

Tak I, Engelaar L, Gouttebarge V, et al. Is lower hip range of motion a risk factor for groin pain in athletes? A systematic review with clinical applications. Br J Sports Med. 2017;51:1611–21.

Tan LA, Benkli B, Tuchman A, et al. High prevalence of greater trochanteric pain syndrome among patients presenting to spine clinic for evaluation of degenerative lumbar pathologies. J Clin Neurosci. 2018;53:89–91.

Timmins RG, Bourne MN, Shield AJ, et al. Short biceps femoris fascicles and eccentric knee flexor weakness increase the risk of hamstring injury in elite football (soccer): a prospective cohort study. Br J Sports Med. 2016;50:1524–35.

Tortolani PJ, Carbone JJ, Quartararo LG. Greater trochanteric pain syndrome in patients referred to orthopedic spine specialists. Spine J. 2002;2:251–4.

van Dyk N, Behan FP, Whiteley R. Including the Nordic hamstring exercise in injury prevention programmes halves the rate of hamstring injuries: a systematic review and meta-analysis of 8459 athletes. Br J Sports Med. 2019;53:1362-70.

Weir A, Brukner P, Delahunt E et al. Doha agreement meeting on terminology and definitions in groin pain in athletes. Br J Sports Med. 2015;49:768–74.

Weir A, Jansen JA, van de Port IG, et al. Manual or exercise therapy for long-standing adductor-related groin pain: a randomised controlled clinical trial. Man Ther. 2011;16:148–54.

Westacott DJ, Minns JI, Foguet P. The diagnostic accuracy of magnetic resonance imaging and ultrasonography in gluteal tendon tears--a systematic review. Hip Int. 2011;21:637–45.

Whittaker JL, Small C, Maffey L, Emery CA. Risk factors for groin injury in sport: an updated systematic review. Br J Sports Med. 2015;49:803-9.

Wing C, Bishop C. Hamstring Strain Injuries: Incidence, mechanisms, risk factors, and training recommendations. Strength Conditioning J. 2020;42:40–57.

Yousefzadeh A, Shadmehr A, Olyaei GR, et al. The effect of therapeutic exercise on long-standing adductor-related groin pain in athletes: Modified Hölmich Protocol. Rehabil Res Pract. 2018;2018:8146819.

Knee disorders: ligament and meniscus postoperative rehabilitation

Benjamin Geletka, Allison Toole, Carol A. Courtney

Introduction

Knee injury is common and experienced in people of all ages. Ligamentous and meniscal injuries occur regularly during sport and with trauma. Surgical management is routinely required in these cases. Physical therapist management plays an integral role in this process by helping control pain and inflammation, restoring joint range of motion (ROM) and muscular strength, as well as establishing appropriate control and mechanics with returning to higher level movement and sport. In this chapter, common ligamentous and meniscal injuries will be discussed, as well as surgical interventions, and postoperative rehabilitation. Readers are referred to the figure and to anatomical textbooks for the precise anatomy of the knee (Figure 7.1).

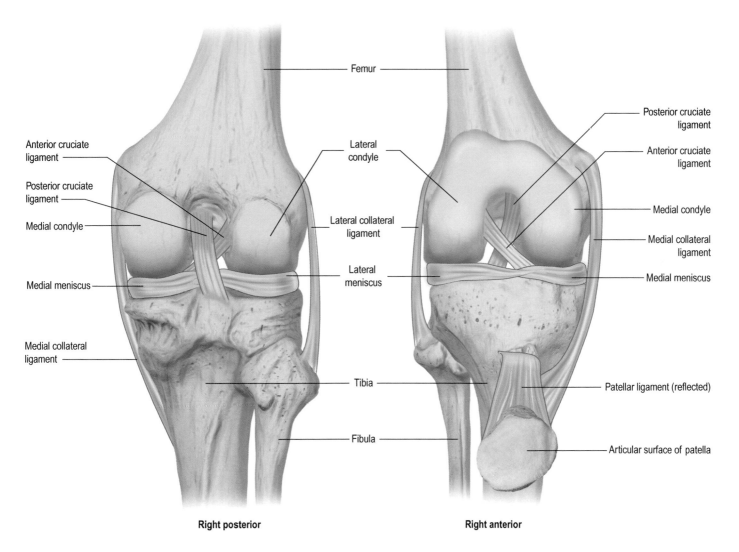

Right posterior

Right anterior

FIGURE 7.1
Bone and ligamentous anatomy of the knee.

Anterior Cruciate Ligament

The anterior cruciate ligament (ACL) is one of the most important ligaments for maintaining knee stability. It serves as a primary restraint to anterior tibial translation relative to the femur as well as limiting internal rotation of the tibia (Butler et al., 1980). The ultimate tensile force of the ACL varies between 600 newtons (N) and 2300 N and strain of about 20% before failing. Older ACLs fail under lower loads than younger ACLs, and forces placed on an intact ACL range from about 100 N during passive knee extension to about 400 N with walking and 1700 N with cutting, acceleration and deceleration activities (Marieswaran et al., 2018).

The ACL is made up of many small strands and is organized into an anteromedial bundle and posterolateral bundle. It originates at the medial area of the lateral femoral condyle in the intercondylar notch and inserts onto the anterior intercondylar surface of the tibial plateau, where it partially blends with the lateral meniscus (Domnick et al., 2016). The blood supply to the ACL is largely supplied from the middle and inferior geniculate branches of the popliteal artery, while the posterior articular nerve (a branch of the posterior tibial nerve) provides innervation.

Injury to the ACL is devastating, especially for young or professional athletes. An estimated 100,000–250,000 ACL injuries occur each year and females have a 2- to 8-fold greater ACL injury rate compared to their male counterparts (Hewett et al., 1999). The differences in anatomy, hormones, neuromuscular control, and biomechanics likely contribute to ACL injury rate disparity between males and females (Arendt & Dick, 1995; Hewett et al., 1999). The majority (approximately 70%) of ACL injuries are noncontact in nature and typically occur with a quick change in direction, cutting, or landing from a jump that involves a quick combination of anterior tibial translation, internal rotation and abduction of the tibia on a planted foot and semi-extended knee. Contact injuries make up about 30% of ACL injuries and are described as an injury that occurs as the result of a direct blow to the knee (McNair et al., 1990; Myklebust et al., 2003). At the time of ACL injury, other structures in the knee can be damaged as well. Due to the magnitude of the injury, this often includes chondral damage in the form of a tibial–femoral bone bruise, medial collateral ligament (MCL) injury, and up to 70% can have a torn meniscus as well (Krüger-Franke et al., 1995; Marks et al., 1992).

Examination

When evaluating a patient with a potential ACL injury, it is important to determine whether the ACL tear is isolated or in combination with injury to other structures. Patient history, physical examination, and imaging techniques are utilized in confirming a proper diagnosis. The patient typically will report hearing or feeling a "pop" in the knee, and about 80% of patients will report a rapid onset of swelling after the injury (Alford & Fadale, 2003). The swelling is a result of a hemarthrosis from rupture of the ACL, which is highly vascular and bleeds into the joint when it is torn. Patients may also report instability in the knee or inability to bear weight on the injured limb directly following an injury. Upon physical examination, the examiner may notice swelling, bruising, and point tenderness around the knee, which could also indicate injury or involvement of other structures (Alford & Fadale 2003). For example, focal joint-line tenderness to palpation and discomfort with rotation–compression techniques of the knee may indicate possible meniscus tear. Involvement of the collateral ligaments needs to be considered as well following traumatic injury. The physical examination primarily consists of maneuvers that attempt to test the stability of the knee, and these special tests can be referenced in Table 7.1. When considering special tests, it is important to note that they do not serve as a stand-alone in final diagnosis and should rather help guide the diagnostic process in combination with history, examination findings, and imaging. Plain film radiography should be the primary imaging study ordered when there is a suspected ACL injury. An avulsion of the insertion of the ACL within the intercondylar eminence may be seen, as well as a possible Segond fracture. A Segond fracture results from an avulsion of the lateral capsule from the tibia at a location posterior to Gerdy's tubercle and superior/anterior to the fibular head. In addition to plain film radiographs, magnetic resonance imaging (MRI) is also recommended when evaluating damage to the ACL in addition to other structures including meniscus, bone bruising, chondral injuries, and complex ligamentous injuries.

Treatment

The treatment options for ACL injury include both surgical and non-surgical management. Non-operative treatment of the ACL deficient knee may be indicated in older, sedentary people. However, ACL reconstruction is commonly chosen by people who wish to undergo surgical intervention with

TABLE 7.1 Special Tests for the Knee

Special Test (Structure Tested)	Description	Accuracy
Lachman Test (ACL)	The patient's involved limb is placed in 20–30 degrees knee flexion and slightly externally rotated. The femur is firmly stabilized by the examiner's out hand; an anteriorly directed force is applied to the proximal tibia. The examiner estimates displacement in millimeters in comparison to the contralateral limb and assess for presence or absence of an end point. Laxity is measured as a comparison to the contralateral side.	Sensitivity: 0.86 Specificity: 0.91 LR +: 9.56 LR −: 0.15
Anterior Drawer Test (ACL)	The patient lies supine on a plinth with their hips flexed to 45 degrees, knees flexed to 90 degrees and feet flat on the plinth. The examiner sits on the toes of the tested extremity to help stabilize it. The examiner grasps the proximal lower leg, just below the tibial plateau or tibiofemoral joint line, and attempts to translate the lower leg anteriorly. The test is considered positive if there is a lack of end feel or excessive anterior translation relative to the contralateral side.	Sensitivity: 0.62 Specificity: 0.88 LR +: 5.17 LR −: 0.43
Pivot Shift Test (ACL)	The patient lies supine with legs relaxed. The examiner grasps the heel of the involved leg with examiner's opposite hand placed laterally on the proximal tibia just distal to the knee. The examiner then applies a valgus stress and an axial load while internally rotating the tibia as the knee is moved into flexion from a fully extended position. A positive test is indicated by subluxation of the tibia while the femur rotates externally followed by a reduction of the tibia at 30–40 degrees of flexion.	Sensitivity: 0.32 Specificity: 0.98 LR +: 16.5 LR −: 0.68
Posterior Sag Sign (PCL)	The patient is in a supine position. Have the patient's involved limb in a position of 45 degrees hip flexion and 90 degrees knee flexion. Look for the tibia to "sag" compared to the position of the femur.	Sensitivity: .79 Specificity: 1.0 +LR: 79 −LR: .21
Quadriceps Active Test (PCL)	The patient is in the supine position. Have the patient's involved limb in a position of 45 degrees hip flexion and 90 degrees knee flexion. The patient gently contracts their quadriceps muscle without extending the knee. Look for relocation/reduction of the proximal tibia from a "sagged" position	Sensitivity: 0.54 Specificity: 0.97 +LR: 18 −LR: 0.47
Posterior Drawer Test (PCL)	This is performed with the patient supine. Have the patient's involved limb in a position of 45 degrees hip flexion, 90 degrees knee flexion, and foot in a neutral position. The examiner sits on the patient's foot, with fingers behind the proximal tibia and thumbs on the tibial plateau. A posterior force is applied to the proximal tibia, assessing for increased posterior displacement and an "end point."	Sensitivity: 0.90 Specificity: 0.99 +LR: 90 −LR: 0.10

(Continued)

TABLE 7.1 *(Continued)*

Special Test (Structure Tested)	Description	Accuracy
McMurray's Maneuver (Meniscus)	With the knee maximally flexed, internal rotation, as well as a valgus force, is applied to the foot and ankle. The knee is then brought from full flexion to approximately 90 degrees. This technique is then repeated with external rotation and a varus force.	Sensitivity: 29 Specificity: 96 LR+: 7.3 LR–: .74
Apley's Maneuver (Meniscus)	With patient in prone, the examiner half kneels, placing their knee on the hamstring of the patient, and flexes the patient's knee to 90 degrees. The examiner grasps the patient's foot with both hands, distracts the tibia, and rotates the tibia and assesses for pain. A positive test is indicated by worse pain with rotation and is indicative of a soft tissue sprain. The examiner then leans on the patient's foot, providing a compressive force to the tibia and again rotates the tibia. A positive test for a meniscus tear is indicated by more pain in compression than with distraction.	Sensitivity: 13 Specificity: 90 LR+: 1.3 LR–: 0.97
Thessaly's Maneuver (Meniscus)	Patient standing flat footed on the affected limb with the knee in 20 degrees of flexion. With the examiner holding the patient's hands, the patient rotates the knee and body 3 times in each direction while keeping the knee flexed. Test is performed on the unaffected limb initially for comparison. Test is positive if there is medial or lateral joint line discomfort or has a sense of locking or catching.	Sensitivity: 75 Specificity: 87 LR+: 5.6 LR–: 0.28
Valgus Stress Test (MCL/PCL)	The patient is supine with the hip slightly abducted and extended so the thigh is resting on the table. The knee is flexed 30 degrees over the side of the table and the examiner places one hand over the lateral aspect of the knee while the other hand grasps the ankle. A lateral to medial force is applied gently to the knee. The test is repeated in full extension. A positive test is excessive medial opening and pain when compared to the uninvolved knee. If the test is positive at 30 degrees, the MCL is implicated. If the test is positive at 0 degrees, then the MCL and PCL are implicated.	Sensitivity: 56–100 Specificity: 91 LR+: 6.4 LR–: 0.5
Varus Stress Test (LCL, PLC)	The femur is stabilized to the examination table with one hand, which is also used to assess the amount of lateral compartment gapping, while the other hand is used to hold the patient's foot or ankle and apply a varus force. Lateral compartment gapping in comparison to the contralateral side, with the knee flexed to 30 degrees, indicates an injury to the LCL and potentially to the secondary stabilizers of the PLC. If stability is restored when tested in full extension, an isolated injury to the LCL is presumed. However, if the varus instability persists in full extension, a combined LCL, PLC and cruciate ligament injury is assumed.	Sensitivity: 25 Specificity: NT LR+: NA LR–: NA
Reverse Pivot Shift (PLC)	The patient lies supine with the knee flexed to near 90 degrees. The joint line is palpated, a valgus load is applied through the knee, and external rotation force is applied to the tibia and the knee is slowly extended. If the previously subluxated lateral tibial plateau reduces at approximately 35–40 degrees of flexion, this is a positive test.	Sensitivity: 26 Specificity: 95 LR+: 5.2 LR–: 0.78

(Continued)

TABLE 7.1 *(Continued)*

Special Test (Structure Tested)	Description	Accuracy
Dial Test (PLC/PCL)	With the patient in the prone or supine position and the knee flexed to 30 degrees, the femur is fixed with one hand while the ankle and foot are externally rotated. An increase of more than 10 degrees of external rotation compared with the contralateral side suggests an injury to the PLC. The knee is then flexed to 90 degrees. Because of its role as an important secondary stabilizer, a knee with an intact PCL will see a decrease in external rotation. If, at 90 degrees, there is an increase in external rotation, as compared with 30 degrees, a combined PLC and PCL injury is presumed.	Sensitivity: NT Specificity: NT LR+: NA LR–: NA
Posterolateral Drawer Test (PLC)	Patient lies supine with the hip flexed at 45 degrees and the knee flexed to 90 degrees. The posterior drawer test is performed in neutral, external, and internal tibial rotation of 15 degrees. A positive test is indicated by a relative posterior appearance of the lateral tibial condyle during the push phase of the drawer test when compared with the medial tibial condyle.	Sensitivity: NT Specificity: NT LR+: NA LR–: NA
External Rotation Recurvatum Test (PLC)	The patient lies supine with the examiner holding the heel of the leg in 30 degrees of knee flexion. The examiner gradually extends the knee from 30 degrees of flexion while the opposite hand gently grasps the posterolateral aspect of the knee joint. A positive test is the relative hyperextension and external rotation felt by examiner compared to the opposite knee.	Sensitivity: 3 Specificity: 99 LR+: 3.0 LR–: 0.98
Patellar Apprehension Test (patellofemoral instability)	Patient is positioned supine with a relaxed knee passively flexed to 30 degrees over the side of the table with foot resting on examiner. The examiner presses both thumbs on the medial aspect of the patella to exert a lateral force. A positive test occurs when the patient shows signs of apprehension or pain is reproduced.	Sensitivity: 32 Specificity: 86 LR+: 2.3 LR–: 0.79
Positive J Sign (patellofemoral instability)	Demonstrated when the patient sits on the edge of the examination table and moves their knee from a position of flexion to extension; in patients with a tight lateral retinaculum, the patella may appear to shift laterally as the knee extends	Sensitivity: NT Specificity: NT LR+: NT LR–: NT

(From: Benjaminse et al., 2006; Buchanan et al., 2016; Chahla et al., 2016; Cook and Hegedus, 2008; Dean & LaPrade, 2020; Kastelein et al., 2008; Lowery et al., 2006; Prins, 2006; Rosinski et al., 2019; Rubinstein et al., 1994; Sheehan et al., 2010; Smith et al., 2015.)

CHAPTER SEVEN

the goal of regaining knee stability and returning to a high level of function. The choice of graft can vary depending on the surgeon's preference with a given procedure as well as the activity level or sport of the patient. When making the decision on the type of graft, there is also a consideration for the person's age, goals, line of work, and lifestyle. Natural grafts can be classified as autografts or allografts. Autografts are grafts that are harvested from the patient's own tendon, while allografts are obtained from human cadavers. A summary of graft types, and their advantages and disadvantages, can be seen in Table 7.2.

Preoperative Considerations

Prior to undergoing ACL reconstruction, many studies have shown both short-term and long-term advantages to

TABLE 7.2 Anterior Cruciate Ligament (ACL) Graft Types

Type of Graft	Advantages	Disadvantages	Rehab Considerations
Allograft	• Reduced surgery time • Reduced donor site morbidity • More appropriate for older, lower functioning individuals	• Higher infection rate • Higher risk of rejection of graft • Higher graft failure rate	• Slower revascularization, so crutches and brace may be utilized longer • Care with progression of higher-level activity secondary to increase failure rate
Bone Patellar Tendon Bone Autograft	• Stronger fixation because of bone plugs • Lower re-tear rates	• Anterior knee pain • Donor site morbidity • Extensor mechanism dysfunction	• Patellar tendon pain common • Consider patellar taping or strap to reduce pain • Gradual progression with exercises that may irritate anterior knee pain
Hamstring Tendon Autograft	• No anterior knee pain associated with patellar tendon or quad tendon graft	• Donor site morbidity • Loss of hamstring strength • Higher incidence of re-tear	• No isolated resisted hamstring strengthening for 8 weeks
Quadriceps Tendon Autograft	• Less anterior knee pain with kneeling • Less graft site pain • Less sensation loss • Similar anterior knee stability as patellar tendon autograft • Good option for skeletally immature patients	• Donor site morbidity • Extensor mechanism dysfunction	• Achieving full knee extension early postoperatively is vital to avoid arthrofibrosis

(From: Gifstad et al., 2014; Kim et al., 2009; Lund et al., 2014; Marieswaran et al., 2018; Maletis et al., 2016; Papalia et al., 2015; Persson et al., 2014.)

participating in preoperative rehabilitation. Quadriceps weakness is a frequently observed barrier to effective rehabilitation following ACL injury and reconstruction. It may lead to further problems including extension deficit, gait abnormality, quadriceps atrophy, poor function, dynamic instability, persistent knee pain and early osteoarthritis (Sonnery-Cottet et al., 2019). Properly preparing for surgery and resolving deficits in muscle mass, strength, ROM, quality of gait, and swelling can enhance postoperative function. Most "pre-rehabilitation" programs focus on initial impairment resolution, including little to no swelling or pain, full ROM, progressive strengthening, restoration of normal gait pattern, and neuromuscular training. The available research indicates that participation in rehabilitation prior to surgery results in superior knee functional outcomes postoperatively compared to those who did not participate (Failla et al., 2016; Grindem et al., 2015; Shaarani et al., 2013). In fact, a preoperative Quads Index (QI) <66% has been associated with a greater risk of unsuccessful return to sport (Kitaguchi et al., 2020).

Posterior Cruciate Ligament

The posterior cruciate ligament (PCL) is the largest and strongest ligament of the knee joint and is made up of two independent bundles including the larger anterolateral bundle and smaller posterior-medial bundle (Pache et al., 2018). The primary function of the PCL is to limit posterior tibial translation relative to the femur and biomechanical studies show a codominant relationship between the anterolateral bundle and posteromedial bundle in restricting this translation (Ahmad et al., 2003). As the knee goes through flexion and extension, there are changes in the orientation of each bundle that prevent either from possessing complete dominance in the restraint of posterior tibial translation. The PCL has also been identified as a secondary restraint to rotation, particularly between 90 and 120 degrees of flexion (Kennedy et al., 2014).

The synovium surrounding the PCL is significantly stronger than the ACL and provides an increased blood supply that allows for a strong intrinsic healing capability for low-grade tears. The blood supply of the PCL comes from the middle geniculate artery, and branches of the tibial nerve innervate the complex (Lynch et al., 2021).

PCL injuries often present as part of a multi-ligamentous knee injury, with isolated PCL injuries being rare. Isolated

PCL tears are typically produced by external trauma such as the classic "dashboard injury," resulting from a posteriorly directed force on the anterior aspect of the proximal tibia with the knee flexed (Pache et al., 2018). In athletics, the typical mechanism of injury for isolated PCL tears is a direct blow to the anterior tibia or a fall onto the knee with the foot in a plantarflexed position (Fanelli & Edson, 1995). Football, rugby, soccer and skiing are among the sports with the highest incidence of PCL tears (Pache et al., 2018). Non-contact mechanisms, such as hyperflexion or hyperextension, are less common.

Examination

When evaluating a patient with a potential PCL injury, it is important to determine whether the PCL tear is isolated or combined with other injuries because it determines the long-term results of the treatment. Patient history, physical examination and correct imaging techniques are used in confirming a proper diagnosis. Isolated PCL injuries may have more subtle symptoms including stiffness, swelling, and pain localized to the posterior knee or pain with deep knee flexion (Bedi et al., 2016; Wind et al., 2004). The majority of the physical examination includes attempts to demonstrate posterior instability and subluxation of the knee. The most frequently used special tests can be seen in Table 7.1. Due to the presence of the neurovascular bundle in the posterior aspect of the knee, a neurovascular examination is essential and should include checking pulses (dorsalis pedis, posterior tibial), as well as motor/sensory examination findings (Wind et al., 2004). Any concern regarding the vascular status of the limb should be evaluated with an arteriogram. Imaging techniques including plain film radiographs, stress radiographs, and MRI are recommended in further confirming injury to the PCL, with MRI being the preferred imaging technique (Bedi et al., 2016; Wind et al., 2004).

Treatment

In recent years, a better understanding of the anatomy and biomechanics of the PCL has emerged, thus leading to an improved understanding of treatment and rehabilitation. However, controversy still exists regarding the decisions for non-operative vs. operative treatment, optimal surgical technique, and rehabilitation. Historically, isolated PCL injury has been initially managed with a trial of conservative treatment, regardless of the severity (Wind et al., 2004).

In general, non-surgical treatment has been advocated for patients with isolated grade I or II tears, or those with grade III injuries but have mild symptoms or only participate in low-demand activities (Bedi et al., 2016). The clinical outcomes after non-operative treatment of isolated PCL injuries have demonstrated good long-term subjective outcomes, a high return to sport rate, and evidence of successful healing on MRI (Wang et al., 2018). Dynamic PCL braces can help keep the tibia reduced during healing by avoiding posterior tibial translation and have been suggested in the treatment of non-operative management for the first three months (Jacobi et al., 2010; LaPrade et al., 2015).

Operative treatment of PCL injuries is typically recommended to patients with complete tears displaying inadequate functional improvement in response to non-operative treatment (Winkler et al., 2021). A side-to-side difference in posterior tibial translation greater than 8 to 10 mm indicates a complete PCL tear and presents as an indication for operative treatment for symptomatic patients. Because of the complex anatomy and nature of the PCL, there is currently no consensus for a specific operative technique when considering PCL reconstruction (PCL). Many biomechanical and research efforts have allowed the development of techniques focusing on anatomic restoration of native knee kinematics, though there is no consistent agreement on which operative technique is best (Devitt et al., 2018; Owesen et al., 2017; Spiridonov et al., 2011).

Medial Collateral Ligament

The MCL is one of the most commonly injured ligaments of the knee (Motamedi et al., 2017), with injury occurring primarily in physically active individuals (Roach et al., 2014). The injury incidence has been reported to be 0.24 per 1000 people in the United States in any given year and to be twice as high in males (0.36) compared to females (0.18) (Laprade & Wijdicks, 2012). The MCL consists of a superficial and deep layer. The superficial layer originates from the posterior aspect of the medial epicondyle of the femur and has a proximal insertion, primarily to soft tissue, approximately 1 cm distal to the medial joint line, and a distal insertion at the tibia approximately 6 cm distal to the joint line (Andrews et al., 2017). The deep layer is a thickening of the joint capsule and has two components (meniscofemoral and meniscotibial) that have attachments on the medial meniscus (Laprade & Wijdicks, 2012). Most MCL injuries occur due to a valgus force directly applied to the knee with the foot planted, particularly in stance position. The main role of the MCL is to provide medial knee stability and prohibit valgus stress; however, the superficial layer of the MCL provides both valgus and external rotational stability (Robinson et al., 2006), limiting these motions. While external rotational laxity is often attributed to a posterolateral corner injury, consideration of the patient with a traumatic knee injury should include assessment for medial structural insult. Due to the attachment of the deep layer with the medial meniscus, trauma to the MCL should prompt a meniscal examination. With more severe injuries, the anterior cruciate ligament may be implicated due to a shared role in limiting valgus stress. A popping sensation or audible pop may accompany an injury to this ligament that results in immediate pain. Familiar pain is reproduced with palpation along the MCL (Reider, 1996).

The integrity of the MCL is determined with a valgus stress test applied at 30 degrees of knee flexion (Table 7.1). Diagnosis of MCL injury is best determined by combining information from the subjective examination (e.g., mechanism of injury) with pain and laxity during valgus stress testing (Kastelein et al., 2008). The reference standard (gold standard) for the diagnosis of MCL tear is MRI (Kurzweil & Kelley, 2006).

The MCL has a good blood supply allowing for healing post-injury. With appropriate rehabilitation, an isolated MCL injury can typically be managed non-operatively with a return to activity within 2–5 weeks (Motamedi et al., 2017; Roach et al., 2014). Surgical intervention may be considered when patients do not respond to the initial non-operative measures or demonstrate residual valgus instability. In a 2017 systematic review, Varelas et al. (2017) found only 275 patients who underwent MCL reconstruction in the past 11 years, illustrating the fact that MCL reconstructions are extremely uncommon. In patients sustaining a Grade 3 MCL injury, nearly 78% of patients had an injury to another associated structure, with 95% involving the ACL (Grant et al., 2012). These individuals often elect to surgically repair their knees. Some will delay ACL reconstruction by 5–6 weeks to allow healing of the MCL (Laprade & Wijdicks, 2012). Concomitant reconstruction of the MCL and ACL is associated with an increased prevalence of postoperative arthrofibrosis (Varelas et al., 2017).

Lateral Collateral Ligament

The lateral collateral ligament (LCL) is an extracapsular ligament at the lateral knee that extends from the posterior and superior aspect of the femoral lateral epicondylar ridge to the fibular head (LaPrade et al., 2004). The LCL courses deep to the superficial layer of the iliotibial band and is cord-like, unlike the broad, flattened structure of the MCL. The LCL serves as the primary restraint to varus stress on the knee, but also acts as a secondary restraint to tibial external rotation and posterior displacement. Isolated injury to the LCL is rare (Bushnell et al., 2010), with an incidence of 7.9% (Swenson et al., 2013). Posterolateral corner (PLC) structures such as the ITB, biceps femoris tendon, lateral gastrocnemius tendon, posterior cruciate ligament, popliteofibular ligament, popliteus muscle, arcuate ligament complex, and joint capsule of the tibiofemoral joint may be injured in conjunction with the LCL. It has been reported that 25%–30% of traumatic lateral knee injuries are sports-related, while 52% are from motor vehicle collisions (Krukhaug et al., 1998).

Acute LCL sprain is typically from a blow to the anteromedial knee or some varus force to the knee near full knee extension. This will most commonly occur in sports such as gymnastics, football, soccer, or skiing (Quarles & Hosey, 2004). Patients will typically complain of lateral knee pain, swelling or instability, perhaps associated with a pop.

Injury to the LCL will be accompanied by swelling and ecchymosis around the lateral knee that will correlate with the extent of the injury. Palpation will be painful and the varus stress test (Table 7.1), performed in approximately 30 degrees of knee flexion, will demonstrate laxity and loss of firm end feel. Whenever an LCL injury is suspected, the posterolateral corner should be examined. MRI is considered the imaging modality of choice for LCL injury detection (Grawe et al., 2018).

Posterior Lateral Corner Injury

The PLC of the knee serves to resist varus and external rotation forces at the tibia. The three main stabilizing structures are the LCL, the popliteus tendon, and the popliteofibular ligament (Kennedy et al., 2019). Figure 7.2 visualizes the structures of the posterior lateral corner of the knee.

Injury to the PLC of the knee occurs typically with trauma from athletics, motor vehicle accidents, or with falls

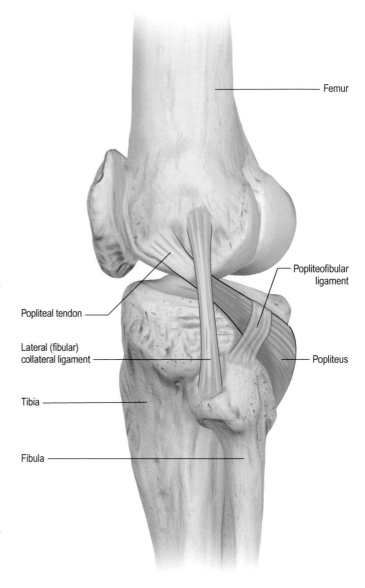

Femur

Popliteofibular ligament

Popliteal tendon

Lateral (fibular) collateral ligament

Popliteus

Tibia

Fibula

FIGURE 7.2
Structures of the posterior lateral corner of the knee.

(Lunden et al., 2010). Commonly this happens with a blow to the anteromedial aspect of the knee in extension, hyperextension injury, or with valgus contact force with the knee in a flexed position. PLC injury frequently occurs with ACL or PCL tears, with only 28% of all PLC injuries occurring in isolation (Chahla et al., 2016). This can be a devastating injury with significant structural damage, dislocation, and neurovascular compromise (Chahla et al., 2019; The STaR Trial Investigators et al., 2017). In this type of injury, failure to recognize vascular compromise can lead to catastrophic limb dysfunction and potential amputation. A medical assessment is typically necessary to investigate a popliteal artery injury, as a palpable pulse may be present distal to the injury secondary to collateral blood flow. When signs of ischemia are present (cool limb, pulseless, color changes), immediate vascular surgery consultation is warranted (Fanelli et al., 2010). Following injury, patients present with complaints of pain over the posterolateral aspect of the knee, instability, and difficulty with ambulation over uneven ground. Ecchymosis, swelling, and foot drop may be present (Dean & LaPrade, 2020). When a related peroneal nerve injury occurs, early placement in an ankle–foot orthosis is important to prevent equinus deformity (Fanelli et al., 2010).

The physical examination of a possible PLC injury can be detailed, given the incidence of other ligamentous injuries that can occur in conjunction. Common special tests (Table 7.1) include the Lachman test, pivot shift, reverse pivot shift, dial test, posterolateral drawer test, varus stress test, and external recurvatum test (Dean & LaPrade, 2020). MRI is advocated for the assessment of suspected acute PLC injury (Chahla et al., 2019), as well as bilateral varus stress radiographs to determine side-to-side differences in lateral gapping (Dean & LaPrade, 2020).

PLC injuries are graded as I, II, or III. Grades I and II are considered partial tears and defined as mild or moderate varus instability, respectively, with an intact PCL. These are typically treated non-operatively as they lack chronic ligament insufficiency, positive return to activity levels, and little to no radiographic evidence of posttraumatic OA. Alternatively, grade III injuries demonstrate severe varus translation, PCL rupture, and have been found to display persistent instability that does not heal when treated non-operatively, and therefore surgical management is recommended (Kennedy et al., 2019; Shon et al., 2017). Acute grade III cases are typically addressed surgically within 2–3 weeks following injury (Chahla et al., 2019).

Surgical management consists of repair, reconstruction, or potentially both. Reconstruction is typically associated with lower failure rates and this seems to be the preferred procedure in most cases (Kennedy et al., 2019). Postoperative complications are seen in 20% of cases, usually including arthrofibrosis, infection, or neurovascular injury. PLC repairs or reconstructions failed in ~10% of cases (Maheshwer et al., 2021).

Meniscus

The medial and lateral menisci are crescent-shaped fibrocartilaginous wedges (Figure 7.3) that are situated between the femoral condyles and tibial plateaus (Bronstein & Schaffer, 2017; Chirichella et al., 2019). They function to stabilize the knee joint, distribute load with weight-bearing, and maintain the health of the articular cartilage (Bronstein & Schaffer, 2017; Markes et al., 2020; Wolf & Gulbrandsen, 2020).

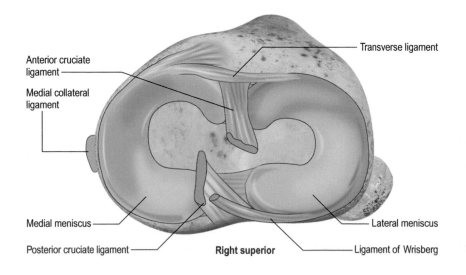

FIGURE 7.3
Anatomy of menisci: superior view of right knee.

Anterior cruciate ligament

Medial collateral ligament

Transverse ligament

Medial meniscus

Posterior cruciate ligament

Right superior

Lateral meniscus

Ligament of Wrisberg

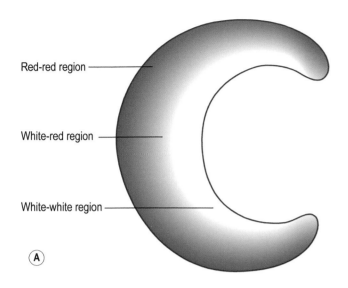

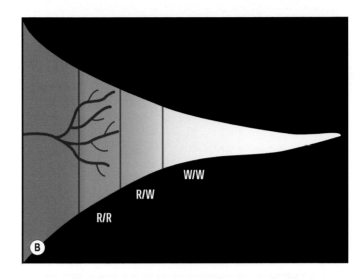

Red-red region

White-red region

White-white region

W/W

R/W

R/R

FIGURE 7.4
Regions of vascularity in the meniscus (A) demonstrating the red–red region, red–white region, and white–white region, and (B) a cross-section of the meniscus demonstrating the regions.

They are primarily made up of type I collagen, which in the deep and peripheral regions is arranged circumferentially, and in the medial and superficial regions radially. This arrangement allows for appropriate transmission of force between the femur and the tibia. Vascular supply is via genicular vessels, which mainly supply the periphery of the menisci (Figure 7.4), with the remainder of the meniscus receiving nourishment from the synovial fluid (Chirichella et al., 2019).

Meniscal injuries are the second most common to the knee, with a prevalence of 12%–14% and incidence of 61/100,000 persons (Abram et al., 2020; Logerstedt et al., 2018; Twomey-Kozak & Jayasuriya, 2020). They can occur in isolation, though they are commonly associated with ACL tears and tibial plateau fractures (Gee et al., 2020). Traditionally, meniscal tears are classified as traumatic (typically occurring in athletes) or degenerative (common in older adults, Figure 7.5) (Chang & Brophy, 2020). When injured, the medial meniscus is 2 to 3 times more likely to be implicated (Gee et al., 2020). A pediatric exception to this is the discoid lateral meniscus, which is a congenital variant that involves abnormal morphology and potential instability of the lateral meniscus (Kocher et al., 2017).

Short-term ramifications after injury include disability with daily life, loss of time at work, and inability to return to sport. Knee osteoarthritis is a potential long-term concern following meniscal tears (Snoeker et al., 2015).

Examination

Detection of meniscal injury in primary care can be challenging (Snoeker et al., 2015). It must be completed via a thorough subjective history, objective examination, and potential imaging studies. Acute/traumatic meniscal tears present typically with a twisting knee injury, commonly during sport. This is usually associated with a snap or a pop and a tearing sensation, followed by a sharp pain localized to the medial or lateral joint line (Chirichella et al., 2019; Logerstedt et al., 2018; Wolf & Gulbrandsen, 2020). Delayed swelling is common, and mechanical symptoms (clicking, catching, locking, "give way") can be reported (Bhan, 2020). There is also strong evidence that delay in ACL reconstruction >12 months after injury is a risk factor for medial meniscus tears (Snoeker et al., 2013).

In the case of degenerative tears, the patient will complain of knee pain and intermittent swelling along with mechanical symptoms. Degenerative tears present more often in males, those greater than 60 years of age, and with work-related kneeling, squatting, or climbing (Chirichella et al., 2019; Snoeker et al., 2015; Snoeker et al., 2013).

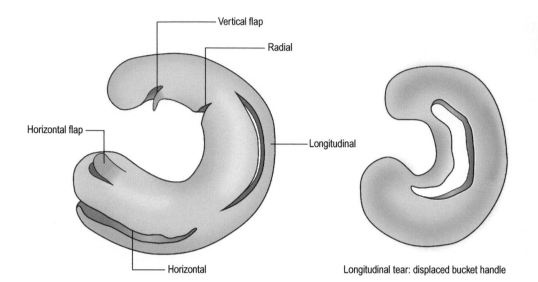

Vertical flap

Radial

Horizontal flap

Longitudinal

Horizontal

Longitudinal tear: displaced bucket handle

FIGURE 7.5
Illustration of various meniscal tear types.

Risk Factors

Modifiable risk factors for meniscal injury consist of higher Body Mass Index (BMI) and activity level. Regarding body mass, individuals with greater than 25 kg/m² BMI have an increased probability of having meniscus surgery, and odds are 15 times greater when BMI is greater than 40 kg/m² (Laberge et al., 2012; Snoeker et al., 2013). Increased activity is a recognized risk factor for meniscal tears and has been well studied in athletes (Ackerman et al., 2017; Mitchell et al., 2016; Snoeker et al., 2013) and in the military (Jones et al., 2012). Sports most commonly identified as high risk for meniscal injury are football, rugby, soccer, basketball, and wrestling (Kilcoyne et al., 2012; Mitchell et al., 2016; Stanley et al., 2016).

Other non-modifiable risk factors that present themselves are anatomically related. These include posterior tibial slope and medial meniscal slope angles, biconcave medial tibial plateau, and knee malalignment (Gee et al., 2020). Discoid meniscus is a risk factor in children (Gee et al., 2020; Kocher et al., 2017; Lee et al., 2019a).

During the physical examination, common findings are pain with forced hyperextension, pain with maximum passive knee flexion, joint-line tenderness, and positive findings with special tests (Logerstedt et al., 2018). Tests such as McMurray's, Apley's, and Thessaly's (Table 7.1) have been historically recommended to diagnose meniscal tears, though the diagnostic accuracy of these tests remains in question (Bhan, 2020; Smith et al., 2015; Snoeker et al., 2015).

A Meniscal Pathology Composite Score (Table 7.3) has been recommended to detect meniscal tears (Lowery et al., 2006) with increased specificity with increased positive findings.

Diagnostic imaging, specifically MRI, demonstrates sensitivity and specificity for diagnosing meniscus tears as high as 93% and 88%, respectively (Bhan, 2020; Snoeker et al., 2015).

TABLE 7.3 Meniscus Pathology Composite Score	
1. History of catching or locking	>5 positive findings Sn 11.2%, Sp 99%
2. Pain with forced hyperextension	≥4 positive findings Sn 16.86%, SP 96.1%
3. Pain with maximum passive knee flexion	≥3 positive findings Sn 30.8%, Sp 90.2%
4. Joint line tenderness	≥2 positive findings Sn 51.4%, Sp 71.6%
5. Pain or audible click with McMurray's Maneuver	≥1 positive finding Sn 76.6%, Sp 43.1%
	0 positive findings Sn 23.4%, Sp 56.9%
Sn = Sensitivity, Sp = Specificity.	
(From Lowery et al., 2006.)	

Other studies have demonstrated clinical examination performed by well-trained clinicians being as accurate as MRI in diagnosing meniscal tears. Cost is also a prohibitive factor. It is therefore proposed the MRI should be reserved for more complicated and confusing cases, and more so in preoperative planning and prognosis (Kocabey et al., 2004; Logerstedt et al., 2018; Madhusudhan et al., 2008).

Abstinence, Meniscectomy, and Repair

Historically, the meniscus was underestimated in its importance and was the victim of regular open total meniscectomy (Beaufils & Pujol, 2017a; Bhan, 2020; Englund et al., 2008; Papalia et al., 2011; Smillie, 1967). Advances in technology gave rise to the less invasive arthroscopic partial meniscectomy (APM), with the first procedure being performed in 1962 (DeMaio, 2013). With time and research, the risk of progression to osteoarthritis following meniscectomy became well known, and was even reported as early as 1948 (Fairbank, 1948). Osteoarthritis is common following meniscectomy, and more so when associated with an ACL tear (Beaufils & Pujol, 2017b). Despite this knowledge, the APM continues to be one of the most routine surgical procedures performed (Beaufils & Pujol, 2017b; Chirichella et al., 2019). Randomized controlled trials comparing APM versus non-operative management by a physical therapist after meniscal tear both resulted in significant functional improvement and decreased pain, though studies have not been able to demonstrate APM superiority over non-operative treatment (Beaufils & Pujol, 2017b; Chirichella et al., 2019; Katz et al., 2013; Kise et al., 2016; Noorduyn et al., 2020; Sharma, 2021; Thorlund et al., 2015). Given this, an effort to preserve the meniscus via repair or abstention from surgical intervention has been advocated, as a meniscal lesion does not necessarily require repair (Beaufils & Pujol, 2017b). Not all tears are symptomatic (Gee et al., 2020). Incidental meniscal findings on MRI of the knee are common and increase with age. One MRI study noted 61% of subjects who had meniscal tears were without pain, aching, or stiffness (Englund et al., 2008).

Conservative management recommendations consist of modification of risk factors, diet, exercise, and self-management programs (Sharma, 2021). Patients that present after injury without severe restriction of ROM, locking, or instability should be managed non-operatively (Chirichella et al., 2019).

Medial Patellofemoral Ligament

Lateral patellar dislocations account for around 3% of all knee injuries and typically occur in younger females (Koh & Stewart, 2014). These injuries are commonly associated with a traumatic event caused by a twisting knee injury or a direct blow to the medial aspect of the patella. The medial patellofemoral ligament (MPFL) is the primary passive stabilizer preventing lateral displacement of the patella, and complete dislocation is always accompanied by MPFL injury (Matuszewski et al., 2018). Individuals prone to patellofemoral instability can display both primary (trochlear dysplasia, excessive tibial tubercle–trochlear groove distance, patella alta) and secondary (excessive femoral anteversion or lateral tibial torsion, recurvatum, genu valgum) risk factors (Chouteau, 2016). MPFL repair or reconstruction are common surgical management techniques after injury. MPFL repair consists of the utilization of sutures and anchors to reestablish the stability of the MPFL. Reconstruction aims to rebuild the primary medial restraint to lateral patellar translation with a graft with higher stiffness and load to failure than the native tissue (Koh & Stewart, 2014). Grafts can be autografts or allografts and can be harvested from multiple donor sites. A variety of surgical techniques have been described, though it is critical to reproduce the anatomy and isometry of the native ligament (Matzkin, 2019). Correct tunnel positioning and graft tensioning restore normal joint kinematics and articular cartilage contact (Stephen et al., 2016). Reconstruction appears to be more reliable than repair, as it is associated with improved outcomes and decreased recurrence rates (Puzzitiello et al., 2019; Strickland, 2019). Bony procedures, such as trochleoplasty or tibial tubercle osteotomy, may also be utilized in the case of recurrent dislocations (Hodax et al., 2019).

Upon presentation after dislocation, the patient can present with pain and swelling of the knee, difficulty with knee ROM, and may show a positive patellar apprehension test, a positive J sign (Table 7.1), and more than two quadrants of lateral patellar translation (Rosinski et al., 2019). In the case of routine first-time dislocations, and in the absence of cartilaginous lesions or symptomatic loose bodies, non-operative management is recommended (Askenberger et al., 2018). After a second dislocation, recurrent dislocations become more likely, and surgery is often required.

Non-operative rehabilitation often includes a brief period of immobilization (~1 week), as well as pain and swelling management. This is followed by progressive ROM and strengthening. On average, patients tend to obtain full knee ROM by six weeks after injury. Return to sport can vary from 6 weeks to 3 months (Vellios et al., 2020).

General Principles of Rehabilitation

General Considerations

Though there is variation with surgical interventions, precautions, and protocols following ligamentous and meniscal procedures, there is overlap in postoperative management, especially noted in the later stages and with return to sport (RTS). Most nuances are noted in the early phase of rehabilitation to protect the involved structures. The plan of care following any joint injury should include consideration of the biological healing properties of musculoskeletal tissues and the stage of healing. Management should follow the EdUReP principle, which stands for Educate the patient, Unload the injured tissues, Reload these structures, and Prevent re-injury (Davenport et al., 2005). The main components of rehabilitation that should be considered include control of inflammation, muscle performance including quadriceps reactivation and strengthening of hip and core musculature, motor control and endurance, recovery of active and passive ROM at the knee, modulation of pain, promotion of static and dynamic balance, return to function and activity participation including cardiovascular conditioning and prevention of re-injury.

Early rehabilitation should focus on control of inflammation and quadriceps reactivation. Uncontrolled joint inflammation facilitates mechanisms of pain and may cause arthrogenic muscle inhibition (AMI) of the quadriceps muscle (Rice & McNair, 2010), leading to muscle weakness, giving way and movement dysfunction. A major error in the management of knee ligament injury by some clinicians is poor control of inflammation and over-aggressive rehabilitation with no regard for joint effusion.

Manual therapy approaches may be valuable in regaining ROM not only at the tibiofemoral and patellofemoral joints, but also at other lower extremity joints that may also be limited and contributing to movement dysfunction. The initiation of early motion in flexion (Figure 7.6) and extension (Figure 7.7) may result in greater tensile strength of the healing ligament. In addition, mechanistic studies in persons with chronic knee pain have demonstrated a

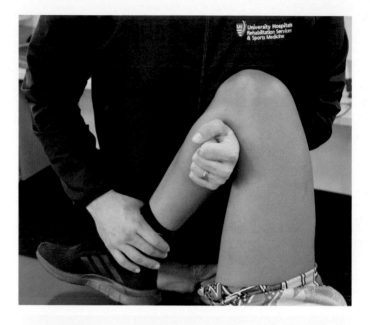

FIGURE 7.6
Knee flexion mobilization with wedge. Used to decrease stiffness in the anterior knee and control flexion when patient is painful into greater degrees of knee flexion.

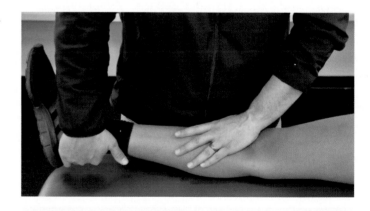

FIGURE 7.7
Knee extension mobilization technique. Used to gain knee extension and decrease stiffness in the posterior knee.

down-modulation of nociceptive pathways following the application of manual therapy (Courtney et al., 2011, 2016).

Weight-Bearing

If the patient's injury was managed surgically, consultation with the surgeon and review of the surgical procedure would aid in developing an appropriate plan of rehab care. Post-operative protocols vary depending on surgical technique, structures involved, as well as surgeon preference. Bracing and crutches are typically issued following knee surgery, and weight-bearing precautions may be implemented. As appropriate, the patient is able to wean off of crutches to full weight-bearing once they are able to ambulate without antalgia or asymmetry. Bracing is removed once the patient is able to demonstrate appropriate quad control. This is assessed via repetitions of a straight leg raise exercise without lag during performance, and without complaints of weakness or instability with ambulation in the postoperative knee brace. A step-up test has also been recommended to assess for appropriate strength prior to discontinuation of the brace (The STaR Trial Investigators et al., 2017).

Rehabilitation after Anterior Cruciate Ligament Reconstruction

Immediate Postoperative Phase

Most protocols combine both time-based and criteria-based guidelines following ACL reconstruction. Despite time-based factors, the patient should not be progressed to subsequent stages unless specific criteria milestones are met. Immediate postoperative considerations and focus should be on reducing pain and swelling, combatting quadriceps inhibition, and regaining adequate ROM. The Stroke Test (Table 7.4, Figures 7.8 and 7.9) is a reliable method of rating knee effusion in an outpatient setting (Sturgill et al., 2009).

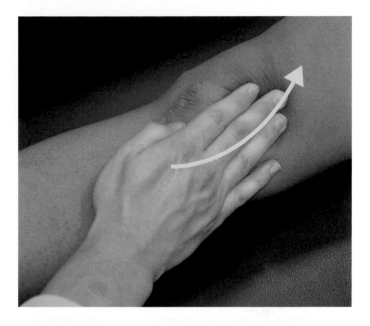

FIGURE 7.8
Stroke test to assess effusion. First step: examiner strokes upwards from the medial joint line towards the suprapatellar pouch.

TABLE 7.4 Modified Stroke Test	
Grade	**Result**
Zero	No wave produced on downstroke
Trace	Small wave on medial side with downstroke
1+	Larger bulge on medial side with downstroke
2+	Effusion spontaneously returns to medial side after upstroke (no downstroke necessary)
3+	So much fluid that it is not possible to move effusion out of the medial aspect of knee
(From Sturgill et al., 2009.)	

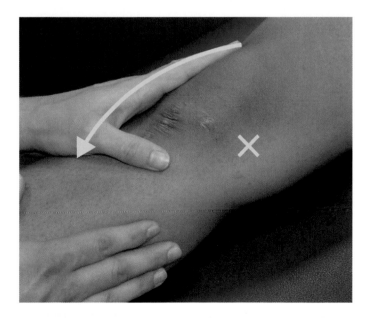

FIGURE 7.9
Stroke test to assess effusion. Second step: a downward stroke on the distal lateral thigh from the suprapatellar pouch towards the lateral joint line is performed; a wave of fluid is observed at the medial knee (X indicates region to assess effusion with downstroke).

Early observation of the surgical site should be monitored for signs of infection or deep vein thrombosis (DVT) as well. The Well's criteria checklist is a reliable clinical tool to assess the risk of DVT (Modi et al., 2016). The milestones for this phase include active/passive ROM equal to 0 degrees to 90 degrees and the performance of an active quadriceps contraction (Adams et al., 2012). Postoperative restrictions may limit ROM and weight-bearing status initially depending on other soft tissue procedures, such as meniscal repair. Gaining extension ROM back early is critical given that even small losses of knee extension (3 to 5 degrees) can adversely affect subjective and objective outcomes following ACL reconstruction (Shelbourne & Gray, 2009). The early accomplishment of full knee extension also decreases the risk of postoperative complications such as arthrofibrosis (Graf et al., 1994). Techniques to help achieve knee extension ROM include low-load long-duration stretching, patellar mobilizations, and joint mobilizations. Although deficits in quadriceps strength following ACL reconstruction can persist for months or years, neuromuscular electrical stimulation (NMES, Figure 7.10) has been used in addition to quadriceps strengthening exercises and has been shown to improve outcomes (Adams et al., 2012). After surgery AMI affects the quadriceps muscles and limits volitional contraction; however, NMES directly recruits the motor neurons to produce better quadriceps strength gains than voluntary exercises alone. Another treatment that can be utilized in the immediate postoperative phase to help improve quadriceps strength and combat the negative effects of AMI is blood flow restriction (BFR), which is demonstrated in Figure 7.11 (Lu et al., 2020). This is a newer area of research; however, current data and utilization looks promising.

Early Postoperative Phase

If the patient is able to meet the criteria from the first phase, then they may progress to the next, which typically begins around week 2. The milestones of this phase include knee flexion ROM to 110 degrees, restoring normal gait pattern without the use of crutches, reciprocal stair climbing, and straight leg raise without an extension lag (Adams et al., 2012). The treatment in this phase consists of weight-bearing activities (closed chain exercises, Figure 7.12) such as wall squats and pain-free step-ups as well non-weight-bearing exercises (open chain exercises). Research has shown that

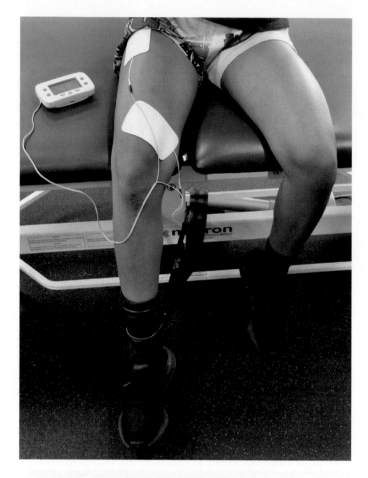

FIGURE 7.10
Neuromuscular electric stimulation for quadriceps strength. Isometric long arc quad performed with parameters as follows: 3" × 5" electrodes placed (1) proximally ~2" from the AIIS and (2) distally over the VMO diagonally. 50–80pps; 2 second ramp; 12 seconds on, 50 seconds rest; intensity of maximum tolerance (at least 50% maximal volitional isometric contraction); 10–15 contractions/session with the involved limb at 60–75 degrees of knee flexion (Adams et al., 2012). Recommended frequency 3×/week in clinic, or if able to perform at home 1–2×/day.

early utilization of open chain knee extension exercises in a restricted ROM (90–45 degrees) and progressing to full knee extension by week 12 has led to higher quadriceps strength gains without causing increased laxity in the ACL graft (Fukuda et al., 2013; Mikkelsen et al., 2000).

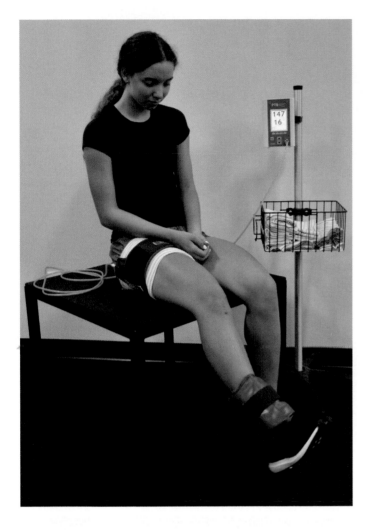

FIGURE 7.11
Blood flow restriction rehabilitation with performance of a long arc quad exercise. Blood flow restriction has been shown to improve strength and hypertrophy in muscle when combined with lower resistance loads. It also may preserve bone density and protect against bone loss following ACL reconstruction (Hughes et al., 2017; Lambert et al., 2019).

Intermediate Postoperative Phase

Milestones of this phase include achieving knee flexion ROM to within 10 degrees of the uninvolved side and demonstrating quadriceps strength to at least 60% of the uninvolved side (Adams et al., 2012). Quadriceps strength symmetry helps to guide clinical decision-making regarding

progressing the patient appropriately through rehabilitation. The gold standard for measuring the maximal volitional isometric contraction of the quadriceps is performed using an isokinetic dynamometer and can be implemented at 12 weeks postoperative. However, use of a handheld isometric dynamometer with the knee maintained at 85–90 degrees of knee flexion or a 1 repetition maximum on an open chain knee extension machine from 90–45 degrees of knee flexion have also been shown to be reliable alternatives for assessing quadriceps strength (Sinacore et al., 2017). Caution is given with these two alternative methods, though, as they can often overestimate knee strength when compared to actual results on the isokinetic dynamometer. This phase is featured by continued focus and attention on regaining quadriceps strength and nearing full knee ROM. Patients in this phase will also begin balance and neuromuscular re-education exercises. Neuromuscular alterations (example: muscle inhibition or impaired sensorimotor function) around the ACL reconstruction knee may contribute to clinical impairments such as strength loss, atrophy, and altered function (Ingersoll et al., 2008). Optimizing neuromuscular function is considered a key aspect in both prevention and rehabilitation following ACL injury. Several publications have investigated neuroplastic changes that may occur after ACL injury and compensations in neuromuscular control (Gokeler et al., 2019; Kapreli et al., 2009; Needle et al., 2017; Roy et al., 2017). Grooms et al. (2017) have suggested that people after ACL reconstruction may be more reliant upon a visual-motor strategy (the patient becomes much more visually dependent) as opposed to a sensory-motor strategy to engage in knee movement. Strategies to address these include principles of motor learning to assist in the restoration of neuromuscular control (Gokeler et al., 2019; Grooms et al., 2017) as can be seen in Figure 7.13. Traditionally, when teaching a patient how to perform novel motor skills, instructions have been delivered in a manner that directs the patient's attention to their own movements (internal focus of attention). However, directing a patient's attention to the effects of the movements on the environment (an external focus of attention) results in more effective and efficient movement (Gokeler et al., 2019; Wulf et al., 2010). It has been shown that the use of external focus of attention has resulted in improved jump-landing motor control as well as postural stability when compared to the use of internal focus of

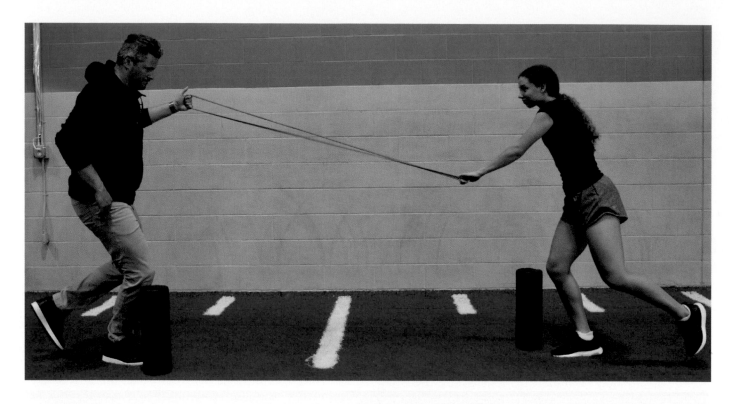

FIGURE 7.12
Balance battles. The patient and therapist provide perturbations to attempt to force their opponent off of single-leg stance. External cue is used for appropriate motor control and positioning.

attention (Gokeler et al., 2015). Some examples of different exercises with external focus are seen in Figures 7.14–7.16. Internal versus external focus examples can be seen in Table 7.5. Utilizing this information in rehabilitation has been hypothesized to be important for the reduction of secondary injury.

Late Postoperative Phase

The milestones of the late postoperative phase include quadriceps strength to at least 80% of the uninvolved side, normal gait pattern, full knee ROM compared to the uninvolved side and knee effusion of trace or less. The quadriceps index of 80% represents a minimal deficit in strength and has been previously used to distinguish between poor and good quadriceps strength (Adams et al., 2012; Lewek et al., 2002; Nyland et al., 2003). With the continued focus on improving quadriceps strength, exercises will start to transition from double leg (Figure 7.17) to single leg and

will increase in terms of difficulty to the patient to ensure they are progressing towards their milestones (Figures 7.18 and 7.19).

Transitional Phase

Once a patient has met the milestones of the previous phase and has clearance from their physician, a running progression may begin (Rambaud et al., 2018). The benefits of a running progression include unilateral strengthening and increased force generation from the nature of running. The running progression begins as a two-part activity, with a balance between jogging and walking. The ratio of jogging to walking is gradually increased (Adams et al., 2012). Progression to the next level is based off completion of the current level without increased effusion or pain. It is also important during this phase that the patient continues to focus on unilateral lower extremity strengthening and neuromuscular control to

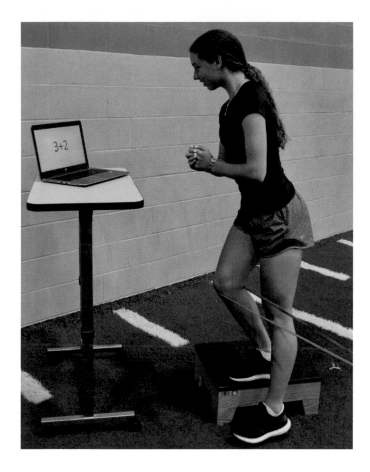

FIGURE 7.13
Lateral step down with knee valgus resistance with cognitive dual task. The patient performs step-down task while viewing a slideshow with math problems where they move up or down based on odd or even answers.

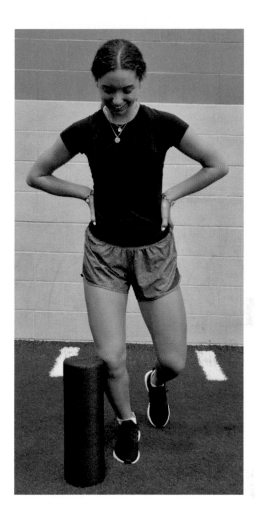

FIGURE 7.14
Single-leg squat with external focus.

work towards improving limb symmetry. The patient is also progressed towards sport-specific activity/movement patterns, agility exercises and functional testing during this phase.

Return to Sport

Return to the pre-injury level of sport is the main goal for patients after ACL reconstruction (Lynch et al., 2015). Current studies show that patient expectations of returning to pre-injury level of sport are high both preoperatively (94%) and postoperatively (88%) (Feucht et al., 2016; Webster & Feller, 2019). Research indicates that there is a discrepancy between the reality of return to sport (RTS) rates after ACL

injury and patients' expectations. Professional athletes tend to return to the pre-injury level at about 78% to 98% around two years after ACL reconstruction (Busfield et al., 2009; Erickson et al., 2014; Harris et al., 2013). Unfortunately, for amateur athletes only 65% of the patients return to their pre-injury level of sport two years after ACL reconstruction (Ardern et al., 2014). The risk for sustaining a secondary ACL injury for athletes has been reported to be as high as 23% for those athletes who are 25 years or younger, combined with the return to high-level sport (Wiggins et al., 2016). Due to the high rate of secondary injury following return to sport (RTS) after ACL reconstruction, it is critical to assess a patient's readiness and ultimately clearance for RTS. Several factors contribute to clearance for RTS after

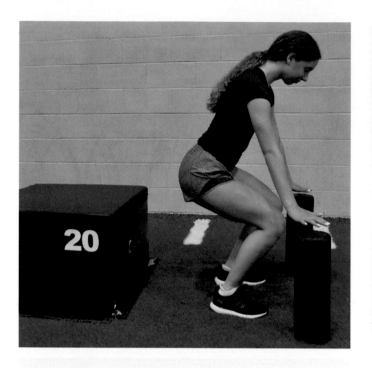

FIGURE 7.15
Drop vertical jump with external focus. The patient drops off of box and is cued to "reach towards the targets" to encourage hip and knee flexion.

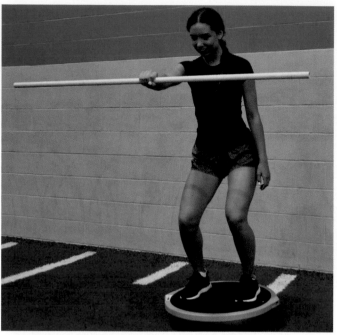

FIGURE 7.16
Stability exercise with external focus. The patient balances on the BOSU while keeping the base and the bar horizontal.

TABLE 7.5 Instructions with Internal Focus versus External Focus

Exercise	Internal Focus of Attention	External Focus of Attention	Technology Use
Short Arc Quad	"Squeeze your quad muscle and lift your heel off the table"	"Press your thigh down into the table and pull your toes toward your knee while following tempo"	Metronome, biofeedback device
Supine Bridge	"Squeeze your glutes and lift your hips off the table"	"Drive your heels down into the table, then lift up your hips"	Metronome
Single-leg Squat	"Try to keep your knee aligned over your second toe"	"Try to keep your knee pointed towards the foam roller"	Foam roller, cone, laser pointer on knee
Postural Stability on BOSU ball	"Try to minimize movements of your feet"	"Try to keep the bar horizontal while holding it out in front of you"	Dowel rod

(From Faltus et al., 2020; Gokeler et al., 2019.)

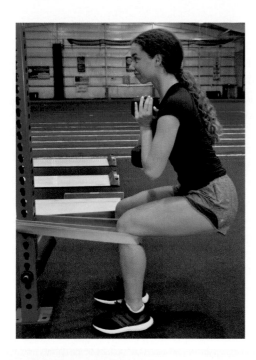

FIGURE 7.17
Spanish squat.

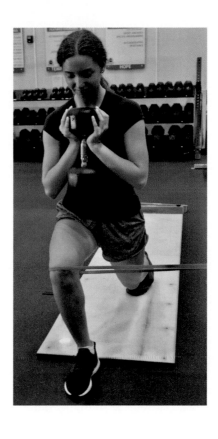

FIGURE 7.19
Reverse slide
board lunge
with valgus
resistance.

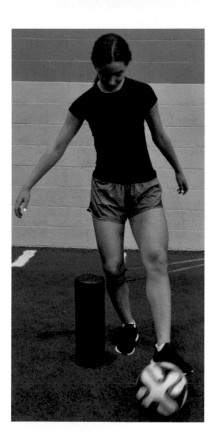

FIGURE 7.18
Passing drill with
resisting valgus
and external
cue. The patient
resists a valgus
force at the knee
while in single-leg
stance, keeping
knee towards
the target while
passing and
receiving the ball.

ACL reconstruction, including time from surgery, greater muscle strength, higher scores on functional tests, quality of movement assessment, psychological readiness, and patient-reported outcome measures.

Traditionally, RTS is recommended after six months; however, this timeframe has been questioned in the literature since the risk of sustaining a secondary ACL injury is the highest during the early period of RTS (6–12 months) (Ardern et al., 2014; Dingenen & Gokeler 2017; Gokeler et al., 2017). To reduce the risk of re-injury, it has been recommended to delay RTS to at least nine months after ACL reconstruction (Grindem et al., 2016; Kyritsis et al., 2016). The current recommendations on muscle strength include obtaining at least 90% symmetry on quadriceps and hamstring strength testing via isokinetic dynamometer, although most of the research literature recommendations are closer to 95%–100% limb symmetry. The functional tests that are most commonly used and referred to in the literature include four functional hop tests: single-leg hop for distance, triple hop, cross-over hop, and 6-meter timed hop. The goal on these tests is again achieving at least 90% symmetry and these hop tests have been found to show good inter- and intra-rater reliability (Ross et al., 2002). However, motor control should also be monitored and assessed during these hop tests, as it is quite common for patients to achieve symmetrical hop performance yet still display motor control or strength deficits. Research has shown that those who achieve higher quadriceps and hamstring strength, as well as more symmetrical hop testing, demonstrate a higher likelihood for RTS and higher knee-related function (Grindem et al., 2016; Kyritsis et al., 2016; Welling et al., 2020). Other functional tests that are often utilized and also further assess movement quality include the Y-balance test, tuck jump assessment and the landing error scoring system (LESS). While the gold standard for assessing movement quality involves the use of a 3-D biomechanical technology, the use of a 2-D system on a tablet or smartphone can be clinically useful in determining proper movement patterns during this phase.

Psychological readiness has also been shown to affect a patient's recovery. Fear of re-injury is a common reason cited by athletes who do not RTS after ACL reconstruction (Kvist et al., 2005). The Tampa Scale of Kinesiophobia (TSK-11) assesses pain-related fear of movement or re-injury and has been used to assess fear of movement/re-injury in patients who have undergone ACL reconstruction (Chmielewski et al., 2008; George et al., 2012). Research has shown that patients with greater fear on the TSK-11 with a score of 17 or greater were four times more likely to report lower levels of activity, seven times more likely to have a hop limb symmetry lower than 95% and six times more likely to have quadriceps strength symmetry lower than 90%. Further, patients with a TSK-11 score of 19 or greater at the time of RTS were 13 times more likely to suffer a second ACL tear within 24 months after RTS (Paterno et al., 2018). The Anterior Cruciate Ligament – Return to Sport after Injury (ACL-RSI) scale was developed to assess psychological readiness in relation to RTS (Webster et al., 2008). The current recommended cut-off score on the ACL-RSI is 77 or greater. A recent study showed that younger patients who experienced a second ACL injury had lower psychological readiness measured at 12 months after ACL reconstruction. Patients who scored below 77 on the ACL-RSI scale indicate they are at higher risk of a second ACL injury (McPherson et al., 2019).

Other patient-reported outcome measures that assess overall knee function are also recommended in RTS decision-making after ACL reconstruction. The International Knee Documentation Committee (IKDC) subjective knee form is a commonly used measure of self-reported knee function. Multiple studies have shown that individuals who returned to pre-injury level of sport after ACL reconstruction had a higher IKDC score than those who did not, with the current recommendation score being 90 or better (Czuppon et al., 2014; Lentz et al., 2012). Another commonly used self-reported knee function outcome measure is the Knee Injury and Osteoarthritis Outcome Score (KOOS), which is made up of 5 subscales evaluating different areas of knee-related function including pain, other symptoms, function in daily living, function in sport and recreation, and knee-related quality of life. Similar to the IKDC, the recommended score on the KOOS is a 90 or better (Grindem et al., 2016; Roos et al., 1998; Roos & Lohmander 2003; Salavati et al., 2011).

Despite current recommendations for return to sport, there is still a need for continued research on what the best criteria are when determining return to sport readiness after ACL reconstruction. Current literature shows very low percentage of patients meeting all recommended criteria prior to being released for return to sport. Due to the longevity of rehabilitation and high secondary injury rates, the return to sport decision continues to be evolving and one that should be made by the patient, clinicians, and surgeon providing care to the patient.

Rehabilitation after Posterior Cruciate Ligament Reconstruction

Although different rehabilitation programs exist, there are key elements that should lay the foundation for any protocol. These include progressive weight-bearing, prevention of posterior tibial subluxation, safe restoration of ROM, and early quadriceps activation (Senese et al., 2018). Unfortunately, there is much variability in the literature to date and the recommendations for specific components of rehabilitation following PCL reconstruction. There are currently no studies that directly compare the outcomes of the various aspects of rehabilitation protocols and current rehabilitation recommendations are based on low-level evidence.

Postoperatively, the surgeon is often concerned about recurrent laxity and therefore often discourages accelerated rehabilitation that does not protect the healing PCL beyond patellar mobilization and quadriceps strength. Early in rehabilitation, the focus is on slow progression of ROM, highlighting avoidance of hyperextension and caution with flexion. The graft is typically tensioned between 70 degrees and 90 degrees of flexion, and since greater flexion angles directly stretch the graft, flexion is limited beyond that range for 2–4 weeks. Regarding the progression of ROM, the majority of studies found that 90 degrees of flexion was allowed at 4–8 weeks postoperatively and 120 degrees flexion at 6–12 weeks (Senese et al., 2018). Range of motion is typically performed in the prone position so that during the flexion action, gravity imparts an anterior force on the tibia, rather than a typical 90-degree hip and knee flexion activity (supine wall slides), in which gravity exerts a posterior force on the tibia. In addressing weight-bearing, the majority of the studies showed full weight-bearing was delayed until 6 weeks postoperatively (Senese et al., 2018). The recommendations on wearing a protective brace to prevent posterior tibial subluxation varied, and the majority of the studies recommended wearing a brace for 6–8 weeks locked in extension; however, some recommended its use until 12 weeks postoperatively (Senese et al., 2018). Regarding strengthening, isometric quadriceps strengthening and straight leg raise training were initially started and followed by open kinetic chain exercise in the majority of studies. Stress on the PCL can occur during midrange knee extension, with studies showing lower stress force from 60 degrees to 0 degrees; therefore, knee extension is recommended to be performed in this range initially. The starting point of closed kinetic chain exercises varied from immediate postoperatively to 6 weeks, and one study notes delay until 12 weeks. The majority of all studies delayed active hamstring exercise for at least 12 weeks or more (Senese et al., 2018). Initial implementation of knee flexion exercises should be performed from 0 degrees to 90 degrees in prone or standing rather than seated to minimize the posterior force of gravity. Resisted knee flexion exercises should be approached with caution until adequate healing of the PCL occurs (at least four months after PCL reconstruction) because of the high PCL loads with hamstring contraction. With regards to return to sport, most studies recommend a combination of timeframe, strength and functional performance to reduce the risk of re-injury upon return to sport (Senese et al., 2018).

As is typical in the early stages, pain control and edema management are prioritized. A knee immobilizer is utilized, and the patient is non-weight-bearing for six weeks (Serra Cruz et al., 2016; Shon et al., 2017). Passive ROM can be limited initially to 0–90 degrees for the first two weeks, then progressed as tolerated (Chahla et al., 2016). Early mobilization is implemented to avoid arthrofibrosis (Chahla et al., 2019). An exception to this is in the multiligament-injured knee reconstruction, where knee extension can be maintained for 2–3 weeks prior to beginning knee ROM (Alentorn-Geli et al., 2019; Levy et al., 2010). Other studies have noted early mobility was not associated with increased joint instability in acutely managed patients, and those that were immobilized in the early postoperative stages demonstrated more severe ROM deficits (Mook et al., 2009). Aggressive stretching and mobilization is not advocated in the first 4–6 weeks, especially with extension, which is limited to neutral (avoiding hyperextension). After six weeks the patient will begin to progress weight-bearing and wean off crutches. Once they are full weight-bearing, they can progressively start a strengthening program. Isolated hamstring strengthening is often limited for 4 months to avoid stress to the reconstruction. Running usually occurs ~6 months post-surgery. Return to sport is recommended after 9 months and based on objective functional testing, and often is impacted by other associated concurrent ligamentous procedures (Chahla et al., 2016, 2019).

Rehabilitation Considerations for Collateral Ligament Injuries

MCL injuries are commonly associated with meniscal damage so rehabilitation protocols must take into consideration activities that may affect meniscal healing. With LCL injury, clinicians should consider the potential of proximal tibiofibular joint dysfunction secondary to its attachment to the fibula. Reports also show that approximately 35% of PLC injuries may have an associated peroneal nerve palsy. This comorbidity is likely due to the proximity of the peroneal nerve to the LCL. Both MCL and LCL injury may be associated with rotary instability so caution must be taken to avoid rehabilitation interventions that may promote transverse plane laxity. Considering the rotation that occurs at both end-range knee flexion and extension, impulsive end-range knee extension/varus loading that sometimes occurs in individuals following ACL injury may result in pain and inflammation (Ismail et al., 2019) and ultimately promote laxity at the joint. Depending on the patient and their sport or activity, the use of a hinged brace may be used early in the rehabilitative process, and sometimes with a return to competition. While the evidence for the use of braces following collateral ligament injury is equivocal, their use may be indicated in some instances.

Guidelines for appropriate ROM following MCL surgical intervention should be communicated by the surgeon to the physical therapist to ensure safe knee ROM. A hinged knee brace set from 0 to 90 degrees of knee flexion is often used to prevent stress to the healing ligament. Depending on the location of the repair, range of motion recommendations will vary. Distal repairs need to be cautious with knee flexion ROM to allow healing and prevent long-term valgus laxity. Therefore, flexion is limited to 90 degrees for the first four weeks, and then afterwards progressed as tolerated. Proximal or mid-substance repairs are followed by more accelerated/aggressive knee flexion ROM to prevent arthrofibrosis and loss of functional ROM (Laprade & Wijdicks, 2012). Early weight-bearing is encouraged, with patients increasing their weight-bearing as tolerated. Early rehabilitation often includes isometric exercise which promotes muscle activation, particularly of the quadriceps muscle. Recent studies in chronic knee conditions suggest that low load, long duration isometric exercise may be valuable down-modulating nociplastic pain if present (Rio et al., 2015). Progressive strengthening of quadriceps, hamstrings, and gastrocnemius musculature is indicated; however, the clinician should also consider muscle performance in the entire lower quarter. Hip abduction weakness during dynamic activities can place a valgus stress across the knee, excessively loading the reconstructed complex. Furthermore, core stability training has also been demonstrated to significantly reduce strength asymmetries during functional assessment such as hop testing (Logan et al., 2016).

For LCL reconstruction, protection of the lateral repair is critical early in rehabilitation. For the first two to six weeks, it is important to avoid placing stresses on the repair, so bracing or immobilization is recommended with the knee in 30 degrees of flexion to place the collateral ligaments on slack. Bracing may be utilized, and most rehabilitation protocols involve a period of immobilization to protect the repair from unwanted stresses. Rehabilitation

following LCL and MCL repair is based on biological healing time frames, where early ROM is critical in the recovery process in addition to restoring quadriceps strength (Wilk et al., 1996).

Meniscus: Conservative Management, Meniscectomy, and Repair

The focus of conservative rehabilitation initially should entail pain management, control of knee effusion, ROM, and joint mobility. Offloading has been advocated for comfort, though full weight-bearing can be established when tolerated (Chirichella et al., 2019). Manual therapy interventions have been advocated in the literature for knee osteoarthritis and meniscal injury (Deyle et al. 2016; Jansen et al., 2011; Safran-Norton et al., 2019; Sullivan et al., 2018). In a systematic review by Jansen et al. (2011) it was noted that exercise combined with manual mobilization showed a moderate effect size on pain compared to the small effect sizes for strength training or exercise therapy alone. Examples of manual interventions aimed towards the meniscus can be seen in Figures 7.20–7.24. Therapeutic interventions consisting of strengthening of the gluteus, quadriceps, and

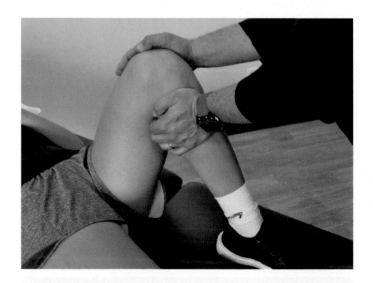

FIGURE 7.20
Tibial internal rotation in end-range flexion. Utilized to improve accessory motion in knee flexion and decrease stiffness. Proximal hand maintains flexion and stabilizes while the distal hand provides an internal rotation force at the anterior medial tibia.

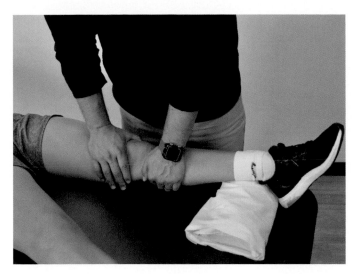

FIGURE 7.21
Tibial external rotation in end-range extension. Utilized to improve accessory motion in knee extension and decrease stiffness. Proximal hand maintains extension while the distal hand provides an external rotation force at the posterior medial tibia.

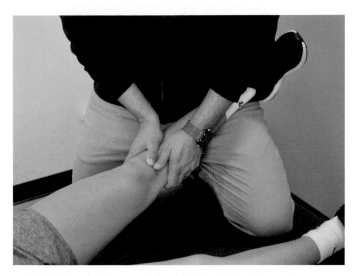

FIGURE 7.23
Knee extension and valgus mobilization. Used to increase extension and to decrease stiffness in the posterior medial knee. Hip is internally rotated and hands work in coordinated effort to impart extension/valgus mobilization at the knee.

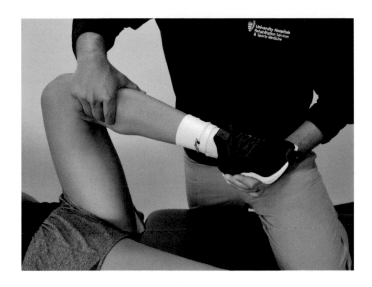

FIGURE 7.22
Internal tibiofemoral rotation mobilization. Used to increase accessory mobility into flexion and to decrease stiffness when further knee flexion is not tolerated. Knee is taken to tolerated amount of flexion and both hands work in a coordinated effort to internally rotate the tibia into resistance.

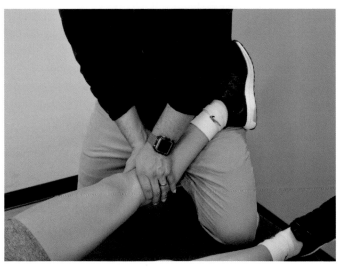

FIGURE 7.24
Knee extension and varus mobilization. Used to increase extension and to decrease stiffness in the posterior lateral knee. Hip is externally rotated and hands work in a coordinated effort to impart extension/varus mobilization at the knee.

hamstring muscles, proprioceptive training, and conditioning exercises such as stationary cycling and aquatic exercise can be utilized (see Chapter 19 of this textbook). Sport-specific activity can be completed once pain, swelling, ROM, and strength are adequate.

Rehabilitation following APM is similar, with an initial focus on pain control, effusion management, joint mobilization, and ROM without restriction (Koch et al., 2020). Resolution of quadriceps strength after arthroscopy is of particular concern, and this is initiated immediately and progressed per patient tolerance with multiple approaches, including exercise, NMES, and BFR. Weaning off of bracing and crutches is as described previously. Once pain and swelling are well controlled and ROM has normalized, progressive strengthening and motor control training can take place. RTS following APM, on average, is reported to be around 2 months (Agarwalla et al., 2019; Lee et al., 2019b).

Rehabilitation protocols following meniscal repair vary widely in the literature. A close working relationship with the surgeon is advocated as meniscal tear type and repair may impact the postoperative plan of care (Harput et al., 2020). Typical recommendations have the patient non-weight-bearing and with restricted ROM for the first 4–6 weeks following repair (Dean et al., 2020; Harput et al., 2020; Koch et al., 2020; Lin et al., 2013; Mueller et al., 2016), as there is concern for failure with increased stress through the repair with early weight-bearing and with higher degrees of knee flexion. These restrictions might be advocated more so with certain procedures such as meniscal root repairs (Dean et al., 2020). Contrary to these concerns, research indicates that clinical success rates following restricted postoperative protocols are comparable to accelerated programs, where early weight-bearing and unrestricted ROM is implemented (Harput et al., 2020; Koch et al., 2020; Lin et al., 2013; O'Donnell et al., 2017; VanderHave et al., 2015). Manual interventions can be implemented following repair, though the judicious selection of technique is important to avoid increased stress through the repaired tissue. Rotational techniques (Figures 7.25 and 7.26) might be best reserved for once appropriate tissue healing has taken place, or avoidance of posterior to anterior techniques when combined with ACL reconstruction. Return to sport after isolated meniscal repair on average is ~6 months versus ~12 months when accompanied by concurrent ACL reconstruction (Lee et al., 2019b; Spang et al., 2018).

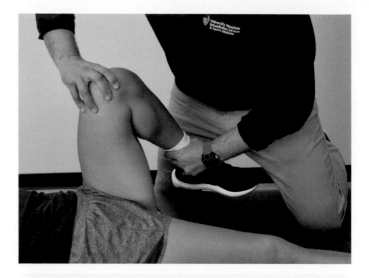

FIGURE 7.25
Knee flexion combined with abduction and internal rotation. Used to improve accessory mobility into flexion and decrease stiffness. One hand stabilizes the femur while the other hand imparts motion into knee flexion while internally rotating and abducting the tibia.

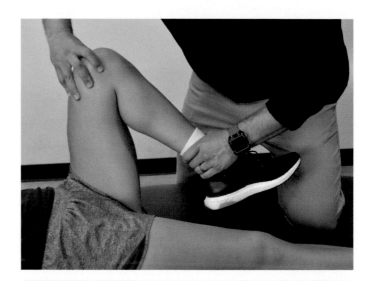

FIGURE 7.26
Knee flexion combined with adduction and external rotation. Used to improve accessory mobility into flexion and decrease stiffness. One hand stabilizes the femur while the other hand imparts motion into knee flexion while externally rotating and adducting the tibia.

Rehabilitation Considerations Following MPFL Repair and Reconstruction

Regarding protocols, there is substantial variability in the content and timing of the phases of rehabilitation (Lieber et al., 2019). Common complications after surgical reconstruction are stiffness, patellar fracture, quadriceps atrophy, pain in the femur and along the graft, and recurrence of dislocation (Chouteau, 2016). Early controlled mobilization is advised to increase ROM, reduce pain, and limit adverse changes to soft tissue structures (McGee et al., 2017). Knee flexion is initiated progressively and early, though limitations may be implemented per surgeon preference. Patellar mobilization is also utilized early to restore normal movement in all planes. Readers are referred to Chapter 16 for visualizing manual interventions of the patella.

Mobilization has been advocated in all directions in the immediate postoperative phase without restriction after reconstruction (Fithian et al., 2010; Manske & Prohaska, 2017) as the strength of the graft far exceeds that of the previous native tissue and, with appropriate fixation, concern with stress to the reconstructed tissue is not warranted. Others note that patellar mobilization may stress the surgical site and should be avoided or only completed in a very low grade (Manske & Prohaska 2017; McGee et al., 2017). Typically weight-bearing can begin immediately with crutches, and a brace may be used until full limb control can be demonstrated (Fithian et al., 2010). Early muscular activity with exercise and NMES is implemented for quadriceps facilitation. Weight-bearing and ROM restrictions can vary per physician preference (Zaman et al., 2018). Intermediate stages of rehabilitation focus on progress to full ROM, maintaining and protecting the surgery, and initiating progressive functional activity. Emphasis is shifted to control rotational forces of the lower extremity and work on neutral alignment, which is important for avoidance of re-injury. This should be reinforced with all exercise, and particular attention should be given to deficits noted from the ipsilateral hip and the foot. Any impairments noted should be addressed to allow for increased dynamic control of the knee.

Regarding RTS guidelines, most studies report use of time-based criteria for returning to sport, with the majority suggesting six months as ideal. A minority of studies used objective or subjective patient-centric criteria (Zaman et al., 2018). Those that utilized a criteria-based system were poorly defined and inconsistent with the agreement in recommendations. Further investigation to determine safe and effective guidelines for RTS after MPFL reconstruction and repair has been recommended (Chatterji et al., 2020; Lieber et al., 2019; Zaman et al., 2018).

Conclusion

Despite the routine frequency of ligamentous and meniscal injury, researchers continue to seek the best methods for appropriate management and progression throughout the stages of rehabilitation. Injury prevention and avoidance of re-injury continues to challenge us, especially with returning to sport. And though the patient is typically focused on the finale of rehab and to return to pre-injury functional levels or return to play, clinicians cannot overlook the importance of appropriate progression through each stage of rehabilitation, utilizing time and criteria-based strategies to help them meet their goals. The guidelines outlined in this chapter are based on current evidence-based practice and desire to bring attention to the facilitation of healing, increasing joint mobility, increasing muscular strength, and progressive increase in endurance and motor control to assist the patient in reaching their final outcome. A patient-centered approach and a strong working relationship with the surgeon, the athletic trainer, the coaches, and the family will foster these ideals and help to optimize the patient's journey.

CHAPTER SEVEN

References

Abram SGF, Hopewell S, Monk AP, et al. Arthroscopic partial meniscectomy for meniscal tears of the knee: a systematic review and meta-analysis. Br J Sports Med. 2020;54:652–63.

Ackerman IN, Kemp JL, Crossley KM, et al. Hip and knee osteoarthritis affects younger people, too. J Orthop Sports Phys Ther. 2017;47:67–79.

Adams D, Logerstedt D, Hunter-Giordano A, et al. Current concepts for anterior cruciate ligament reconstruction: A criterion-based rehabilitation progression. J Orthop Sports Phys Ther. 2012;42:601–14.

Agarwalla A, Gowd AK, Liu JN, et al. Predictive factors and duration to return to sport after isolated meniscectomy. Orthop J Sports Med. 2019;7:2325967119837940.

Ahmad CS, Cohen ZA, Levine WN, et al. Codominance of the individual posterior cruciate ligament bundles. An analysis of bundle lengths and orientation. Am J Sports Med. 2003;31:221–5.

Alentorn-Geli E, Lazarides AL, Utturkar GM, et al. Factors predictive of poorer outcomes in the surgical repair of multiligament knee injuries. Knee Surg Sports Traumatol Arthrosc. 2019;27:445–59.

Alford JW, Fadale PD. Evaluation of postoperative bupivacaine infusion for pain management after anterior cruciate ligament reconstruction. Arthroscopy. 2003;19:855–61.

Andrews K, Lu A, Mckean L, Ebraheim N. Review: Medial collateral ligament injuries. J Orthop. 2017;14:550–4.

Ardern CL, Taylor NF, Feller JA, Webster KE. Fifty-five per cent return to competitive sport following anterior cruciate ligament reconstruction surgery: an updated systematic review and meta-analysis including aspects of physical functioning and contextual factors. Br J Sports Med. 2014;48:1543–52.

Arendt E, Dick R. Knee injury patterns among men and women in collegiate basketball and soccer. NCAA data and review of literature. Am J Sports Med. 1995;23:694–701.

Askenberger M, Bengtsson Moström E, et al. Operative repair of medial patellofemoral ligament injury versus knee brace in children with an acute first-time traumatic patellar dislocation: a randomized controlled trial. Am J Sports Med. 2018;46:2328–40.

Beaufils P, Pujol N. Does anyone still need meniscectomy? Joint Bone Spine. 2017a;84:389–92.

Beaufils P, Pujol N. Management of traumatic meniscal tear and degenerative meniscal lesions. Save the meniscus. Orthop Traumatol Surg Res. 2017b;103:S237–44.

Bedi A, Musahl V, Cowan JB. Management of posterior cruciate ligament injuries: An evidence-based review. J Am Acad Orthop Surg. 2016;24:277–89.

Benjaminse A, Gokeler A, van der Schans CP. Clinical diagnosis of an anterior cruciate ligament rupture: a meta-analysis. J Orthop Sports Phys Ther. 2006;36:267–88.

Bhan K. Meniscal Tears: Current Understanding, Diagnosis, and Management. Cureus [Internet]. 2020 Jun 13; Available from: https://www.cureus.com/articles/34300-meniscal-tears-current-understanding-diagnosis-and-management

Bronstein RD, Schaffer JC. Physical examination of the knee: meniscus, cartilage, and patellofemoral conditions. J Am Acad Orthop Surg. 2017;25:365–74.

Buchanan G, Torres L, Czarkowski B, Giangarra CE. Current concepts in the treatment of gross patellofemoral instability. Int J Sports Phys Ther. 2016;11:867–76.

Busfield BT, Kharrazi FD, Starkey C, et al. Performance outcomes of anterior cruciate ligament reconstruction in the National Basketball Association. Knee Surg Sports Traumatol Arthrosc. 2009;25:825–30.

Bushnell BD, Bitting SS, Crain JM, et al. Treatment of Magnetic Resonance Imaging-documented isolated grade iii lateral collateral ligament injuries in National Football League Athletes. Am J Sports Med. 2010;38:86–91.

Butler DL, Noyes FR, Grood ES. Ligamentous restraints to anterior drawer in the human knee: a biomechanical study. J Bone Joint Surg Am. 1980;62:259–70.

Chahla J, Moatshe G, Dean CS, LaPrade RF. Posterolateral corner of the knee: Current concepts. Arch Bone Jt Surg. 2016;4:97–103.

Chahla J, Murray IR, Robinson J, et al. Posterolateral corner of the knee: an expert consensus statement on diagnosis, classification, treatment, and rehabilitation. Knee Surg Sports Traumatol Arthros. 2019;27:2520–9.

Chang PS, Brophy RH. As goes the meniscus goes the knee. Clin Sports Med. 2020;39:29–36.

Chatterji R, White AE, Hadley CJ, et al. Return-to-play guidelines after patellar instability surgery requiring bony realignment: A systematic review. Orthop J Sports Med. 2020;8:232596712096613.

Chirichella PS, Jow S, Iacono S, et al. Treatment of knee meniscus pathology: rehabilitation, surgery, and orthobiologics. PM&R. 2019;11:292-308.

Chmielewski TL, Jones D, Day T, et al. The association of pain and fear of movement/reinjury with function during anterior cruciate ligament reconstruction rehabilitation. J Orthop Sports Phys Ther. 2008;38:746–53.

Chouteau J. Surgical reconstruction of the medial patellofemoral ligament. Orthop Traumatol Surg Res. 2016;102:S189–94.

Cook C, Hegedus EJ. Orthopedic physical examination tests: an evidence-based approach. Upper Saddle River, NJ: Pearson Prentice Hall; 2008.

Courtney CA, Durr RK, Emerson-Kavchak AJ, et al. Heightened flexor withdrawal responses following ACL rupture are enhanced by passive tibial translation. Clin Neurophysiol. 2011;122:1005–10.

Courtney CA, Steffen AD, Fernández-de-las-Peñas C, et al. Joint mobilization enhances mechanisms of conditioned pain modulation in individuals with osteoarthritis of the knee. J Orthop Sports Phys Ther. 2016;46:168–76.

Czuppon S, Racette BA, Klein SE, Harris-Hayes M. Variables associated with return to sport following anterior cruciate ligament reconstruction: a systematic review. Br J Sports Med. 2014;48:356–64.

Davenport TE, Kulig K, Matharu Y, Blanco CE. The EdUReP model for nonsurgical management of tendinopathy. Phys Ther. 2005;85:1093–103.

Dean RS, LaPrade RF. ACL and posterolateral corner injuries. Curr Rev Musculoskelet Med. 2020;13:123–32.

Dean RS, DePhillipo NN, Monson JK, LaPrade RF. Peripheral stabilization suture to address meniscal extrusion in a revision meniscal root repair: surgical technique and rehabilitation protocol. Arthrosc. Tech 2020;9:e1211–8.

DeMaio M. Giants of Orthopaedic Surgery: Masaki Watanabe MD. Clin Orthop. 2013;471:2443–8.

Devitt BM, Dissanayake R, Clair J, et al. Isolated posterior cruciate reconstruction results in improved functional outcome but low rates of return to preinjury level of sport: A systematic review and meta-analysis. Orthop J Sports Med. 2018;6:2325967118804478.

Deyle GD, Gill NW, Rhon DI, et al. A multicentre randomised, 1-year comparative effectiveness, parallel-group trial protocol of a physical therapy approach compared to corticosteroid injections. BMJ Open. 2016;6:e010528.

Dingenen B, Gokeler A. Optimization of the return-to-sport paradigm after anterior cruciate ligament reconstruction: A critical step back to move forward. Sports Med Auckl NZ. 2017;47:1487–500.

Domnick C, Raschke M, Herbort M. Biomechanics of the anterior cruciate ligament: Physiology, rupture and reconstruction techniques. World J Orthop. 2016;7:82–93.

Englund M, Guermazi A, Gale D, et al. Incidental meniscal findings on knee MRI in middle-aged and elderly persons. N Engl J Med. 2008;359:1108–15.

Erickson BJ, Harris JD, Cole BJ, et al. Performance and return to sport after anterior cruciate ligament reconstruction in National Hockey League Players. Orthop J Sports Med. 2014;2:2325967114548831.

Failla MJ, Logerstedt DS, Grindem H, et al. Does extended preoperative rehabilitation influence outcomes 2 years after ACL reconstruction? A comparative effectiveness study between the MOON and Delaware-Oslo ACL Cohorts. Am J Sports Med. 2016;44:2608–14.

Fairbank TJ. Knee joint changes after meniscectomy. J Bone Joint Surg Br. 1948;30B:664–70.

Faltus J, Criss CR, Grooms DR. Shifting focus: A clinician's guide to understanding neuroplasticity for anterior cruciate ligament rehabilitation. Curr Sports Med Rep. 2020;19:76-83.

Fanelli GC, Edson CJ. Posterior cruciate ligament injuries in trauma patients: Part II. Arthroscopy. 1995;11:526–9.

Fanelli GC, Stannard JP, Stuart MJ, et al. Management of complex knee ligament injuries. J Bone Joint Surg Am. 2010;92:2235–46.

Feucht MJ, Cotic M, Saier T, et al. Patient expectations of primary and revision anterior cruciate ligament reconstruction. Knee Surg Sports Traumatol Arthrosc. 2016;24:201–7.

Fithian DC, Powers CM, Khan N. Rehabilitation of the knee after medial patellofemoral ligament reconstruction. Clin Sports Med. 2010;29:283-90.

Fukuda TY, Fingerhut D, Moreira VC, et al. Open kinetic chain exercises in a restricted range of motion after anterior cruciate ligament reconstruction: a randomized controlled clinical trial. Am J Sports Med. 2013;41:788–94.

Gee SM, Tennent DJ, Cameron KL, Posner MA. The burden of meniscus injury in young and physically active populations. Clin Sports Med. 2020;39:13–27.

George SZ, Lentz TA, Zeppieri G, et al. Analysis of shortened versions of the tampa scale for kinesiophobia and pain catastrophizing scale for patients after anterior cruciate ligament reconstruction. Clin J Pain. 2012;28:73–80.

Gifstad T, Foss OA, Engebretsen L, et al. Lower risk of revision with patellar tendon autografts compared with hamstring autografts: a registry study based on 45,998 primary ACL reconstructions in Scandinavia. Am J Sports Med. 2014;42:2319–28.

Gokeler A, Benjaminse A, Welling W, et al. The effects of attentional focus on jump performance and knee joint kinematics in patients after ACL reconstruction. Phys Ther Sport. 2015;16:114–20.

Gokeler A, Welling W, Zaffagnini S, et al. Development of a test battery to enhance safe return to sports after anterior cruciate ligament reconstruction. Knee Surg Sports Traumatol Arthrosc. 2017;25:192–9.

Gokeler A, Neuhaus D, Benjaminse A, et al. Principles of motor learning to support neuroplasticity after ACL Injury: Implications for optimizing performance and reducing risk of second ACL Injury. Sports Med Auckl NZ. 2019;49:853–65.

Graf BK, Ott JW, Lange RH, Keene JS. Risk factors for restricted motion after anterior cruciate reconstruction. Orthopedics 1994; 17: 909–12.

Grant JA, Tannenbaum E, Miller BS, Bedi A. Treatment of combined complete tears of the anterior cruciate and medial collateral ligaments. Arthrosc J Arthrosc Relat Surg. 2012;28:110–22.

Grawe B, Schroeder AJ, Kakazu R, Messer MS. Lateral collateral ligament injury about the knee: Anatomy, evaluation, and management. J Am Acad Orthop Surg. 2018;26:e120–7.

Grindem H, Granan LP, Risberg MA, et al. How does a combined preoperative and postoperative rehabilitation programme influence the outcome of ACL reconstruction 2 years after surgery? A comparison between patients in the Delaware-Oslo ACL Cohort and the Norwegian National Knee Ligament Registry. Br J Sports Med. 2015;49:385–9.

Grindem H, Snyder-Mackler L, Moksnes H, et al. Simple decision rules can reduce reinjury risk by 84% after ACL reconstruction: the Delaware-Oslo ACL cohort study. Br J Sports Med. 2016;50:804–8.

Grooms DR, Page SJ, Nichols-Larsen DS, et al. Neuroplasticity associated with anterior cruciate ligament reconstruction. J Orthop Sports Phys Ther. 2017;47:180–9.

Harput G, Guney-Deniz H, Nyland J, Kocabey Y. Postoperative rehabilitation and outcomes following arthroscopic isolated meniscus repairs: A systematic review. Phys Ther Sport. 2020;45:76–85.

Harris JD, Erickson BJ, Bach BR, et al. Return-to-sport and performance after anterior cruciate ligament reconstruction in National Basketball Association Players. Sports Health. 2013;5:62–8.

Hewett T, Lindenfeld T, Riccobene J, Noyes F. The effect of neuromuscular training on the incidence of knee injury in female athletes: A prospective study. Am J Sports Med. 1999;27:699–706.

Hodax JD, Leathers MP, Ding D, et al. Tibial tubercle osteotomy and medial patellofemoral ligament imbrication for patellar instability due to trochlear dysplasia. Orthop J Sports Med. 2019;7:232596711986517.

Hughes L, Paton B, Rosenblatt B, et al. Blood flow restriction training in clinical musculoskeletal rehabilitation: a systematic review and meta-analysis. Br J Sports Med. 2017;51:1003–11.

Ingersoll CD, Grindstaff TL, Pietrosimone BG, Hart JM. Neuromuscular consequences of anterior cruciate ligament injury. Clin Sports Med. 2008;27:383–404.

Ismail SA, Simic M, Salmon LJ, et al. Side-to-side differences in varus thrust and knee abduction moment in high-functioning individuals with chronic anterior cruciate ligament deficiency. Am J Sports Med. 2019;47:590–7.

Jacobi M, Reischl N, Wahl P, et al. Acute isolated injury of the posterior cruciate ligament treated by a dynamic anterior drawer brace: a preliminary report. J Bone Joint Surg Br. 2010;92:1381–4.

Jansen MJ, Viechtbauer W, Lenssen AF, et al. Strength training alone, exercise therapy alone, and exercise therapy with passive manual mobilisation each reduce pain and disability in people with knee osteoarthritis: a systematic review. J Physiother. 2011;57:11–20.

Jones JC, Burks R, Owens BD, Sturdivant RX. Incidence and risk factors associated with meniscal injuries among active-duty US Military Service Members. J Athl Train. 2012;47:7.

Kapreli E, Athanasopoulos S, Gliatis J, et al. Anterior cruciate ligament deficiency causes brain plasticity: a functional MRI study. Am J Sports Med. 2009;37:2419–26.

Kastelein M, Wagemakers HPA, Luijsterburg PAJ, et al. Assessing medial collateral ligament knee lesions in general practice. Am J Med. 2008;121:982–8.

Katz JN, Brophy RH, Chaisson CE, et al. Surgery versus physical therapy for a meniscal tear and osteoarthritis. N Engl J Med. 2013;368:1675–84.

Kennedy MI, Bernhardson A, Moatshe G, et al. Fibular collateral ligament/ posterolateral corner injury. Clin Sports Med. 2019;38:261–74.

Kennedy NI, LaPrade RF, Goldsmith MT, et al. Posterior cruciate ligament graft fixation angles, part 1: biomechanical evaluation for anatomic single-bundle reconstruction. Am J Sports Med. 2014;42:2338–45.

Kilcoyne KG, Dickens JF, Haniuk E, et al. Epidemiology of meniscal injury associated with ACL Tears in young athletes. Orthopedics. 2012;35:208–12.

Kim SJ, Kumar P, Oh KS. Anterior cruciate ligament reconstruction: autogenous quadriceps tendon-bone compared with bone-patellar tendon-bone grafts at 2-year follow-up. Arthrosc J Arthrosc Relat Surg. 2009;25:137–44.

Kise NJ, Risberg MA, Stensrud S, et al. Exercise therapy versus arthroscopic partial meniscectomy for degenerative meniscal tear in middle aged patients: randomised controlled trial with two year follow-up. BMJ. 2016;50:1473-80.

Kitaguchi T, Tanaka Y, Takeshita S. Preoperative quadriceps strength as a predictor of return to sports after anterior cruciate ligament reconstruction in competitive athletes. Phys Ther Sport. 2020;45:7–13.

Kocabey Y, Tetik O, Isbell W, et al. The value of clinical examination versus magnetic resonance imaging in the diagnosis of meniscal tears and anterior cruciate ligament rupture. Arthrosc J Arthrosc Relat Surg. 2004;20:696–700.

Koch M, Memmel C, Zeman F, et al. Early functional rehabilitation after meniscus surgery: Are currently used orthopedic rehabilitation standards up to date? Rehabil Res Pract. 2020;2020:1–8.

Kocher MS, Logan CA, Kramer DE. Discoid lateral meniscus in children: Diagnosis, management, and outcomes. J Am Acad Orthop Surg. 2017;25:736–43.

Koh JL, Stewart C. Patellar instability. Clin Sports Med. 2014;33:461–76.

Krüger-Franke M, Reinmuth S, Kugler A, Rosemeyer B. [Concomitant injuries with anterior cruciate ligament rupture. A retrospective study]. Unfallchirurg. 1995;98:328-32.

Krukhaug Y, Mølster A, Rodt A, Strand T. Lateral ligament injuries of the knee. Knee Surg Sports Traumatol Arthrosc. 1998;6:21–5.

Kurzweil PR, Kelley ST. Physical examination and imaging of the medial collateral ligament and posteromedial corner of the knee. Sports Med Arthrosc Rev. 2006;14:67–73.

Kvist J, Ek A, Sporrstedt K, Good L. Fear of re-injury: a hindrance for returning to sports after anterior cruciate ligament reconstruction. Knee Surg Sports Traumatol Arthrosc. 2005;13:393–7.

Kyritsis P, Bahr R, Landreau P, et al. Likelihood of ACL graft rupture: not meeting six clinical discharge criteria before return to sport is associated with a four times greater risk of rupture. Br J Sports Med. 2016;50:946–51.

Laberge MA, Baum T, Virayavanich W, et al. Obesity increases the prevalence and severity of focal knee abnormalities diagnosed using 3T MRI in middle-aged subjects—data from the Osteoarthritis Initiative. Skeletal Radiol. 2012;41:633–41.

Lambert B, Hedt CA, Jack RA, et al. Blood flow restriction therapy preserves whole limb bone and muscle following ACL reconstruction. Orthop J Sports Med. 2019;7:2325967119S0019.

LaPrade CM, Civitarese DM, Rasmussen MT, LaPrade RF. Emerging updates on the Posterior Cruciate Ligament: A review of the current literature. Am J Sports Med. 2015;43:3077–92.

LaPrade RF, Tso A, Wentorf FA. Force measurements on the fibular collateral ligament, popliteofibular ligament, and popliteus tendon to applied loads. Am J Sports Med. 2004;32:1695-701.

Laprade RF, Wijdicks CA. The management of injuries to the medial side of the knee. J Orthop Sports Phys Ther. 2012;42:221–33.

Lee DH, D'Lima DD, Lee SH. Clinical and radiographic results of partial versus total meniscectomy in patients with symptomatic discoid lateral meniscus: A systematic review and meta-analysis. Orthop Traumatol Surg Res. 2019a;105:669–75.

Lee YS, Lee O-S, Lee SH. Return to sports after athletes undergo meniscal surgery: A systematic review. Clin J Sport Med. 2019b;29:29–36.

Lentz TA, Zeppieri G, Tillman SM, et al. Return to preinjury sports participation following anterior cruciate ligament reconstruction: contributions of demographic, knee impairment, and self-report measures. J Orthop Sports Phys Ther. 2012;42:893–901.

Levy BA, Dajani KA, Morgan JA, Shah JP, Dahm DL, Stuart MJ. Repair versus reconstruction of the fibular collateral ligament and posterolateral corner in the multiligament-injured knee. Am J Sports Med 2010; 38: 804–9.

Lewek M, Rudolph K, Axe M, Snyder-Mackler L. The effect of insufficient quadriceps strength on gait after anterior cruciate ligament reconstruction. Clin Biomech. 2002;17:56–63.

Lieber AC, Steinhaus ME, Liu JN, et al. Quality and variability of online available physical therapy protocols from academic orthopaedic surgery programs for medial patellofemoral ligament reconstruction. Orthop J Sports Med. 2019;7:232596711985599.

Lin DL, Ruh SS, Jones HL, et al. Does high knee flexion cause separation of meniscal repairs? Am J Sports Med. 2013;41:2143–50.

Logan CA, O'Brien LT, LaPrade RF. Post-operative rehabilitation of grade iii medial collateral ligament injuries: evidence-based rehabilitation and return to play. Int J Sports Phys Ther. 2016;11:1177–90.

Logerstedt DS, Scalzitti DA, Bennell KL, et al. Knee Pain and Mobility Impairments: Meniscal and Articular Cartilage Lesions Revision 2018: Clinical Practice Guidelines Linked to the International Classification of Functioning, Disability and Health From the Orthopaedic Section of the American Physical Therapy Association. J Orthop Sports Phys Ther. 2018;48:A1–50.

Lowery DJ, Farley TD, Wing DW, et al. A clinical composite score accurately detects meniscal pathology. Arthroscopy. 2006;22:1174–9.

Lu Y, Patel BH, Kym C, et al. Perioperative blood flow restriction rehabilitation in patients undergoing ACL reconstruction: a systematic review. Orthop J Sports Med. 2020;8:2325967120906822.

Lund B, Nielsen T, Faunø P, et al. Is quadriceps tendon a better graft choice than patellar tendon? a prospective randomized study. Arthroscopy. 2014;30:593–8.

Lunden JB, Bzdusek PJ, Monson JK, et al. Current concepts in the recognition and treatment of posterolateral corner injuries of the knee. J Orthop Sports Phys Ther. 2010;40:502–16.

Lynch AD, Logerstedt DS, Grindem H, et al. Consensus criteria for defining "successful outcome" after ACL injury and reconstruction: a Delaware-Oslo ACL cohort investigation. Br J Sports Med. 2015;49:335–42.

Lynch TB, Chahla J, Nuelle CW. Anatomy and biomechanics of the posterior cruciate ligament. J Knee Surg. 2021;34:499–508.

Madhusudhan T, Kumar T, Bastawrous S, Sinha A. Clinical examination, MRI and arthroscopy in meniscal and ligamentous knee Injuries: a prospective study. J Orthop Surg. 2008;3:19.

Maheshwer B, Drager J, John NS, et al. Incidence of intraoperative and postoperative complications after posterolateral corner reconstruction or repair: A systematic review of the current literature. Am J Sports Med. 2021;036354652098169.

Maletis GB, Chen J, Inacio MCS, Funahashi TT. Age-related risk factors for revision anterior cruciate ligament reconstruction: A cohort study of 21,304 patients from the kaiser permanent anterior cruciate ligament registry. Am J Sports Med. 2016;44:331–6.

Manske RC, Prohaska D. Rehabilitation following medial patellofemoral ligament reconstruction for patellar instability. Int J Sports Phys Ther. 2017;12:494–511.

Marieswaran M, Jain I, Garg B, Sharma V, Kalyanasundaram D. A review on biomechanics of anterior cruciate ligament and materials for reconstruction. Appl Bionics Biomech. 2018;2018:4657824.

Markes AR, Hodax JD, Ma CB. Meniscus form and function. Clin Sports Med. 2020;39:1–12.

Marks PH, Goldenberg JA, Vezina WC, et al. Subchondral bone infractions in acute ligamentous knee injuries demonstrated on bone scintigraphy and magnetic resonance imaging. J Nucl Med. 1992;33:516–20.

Matuszewski Ł, Tramś M, Ciszewski A, et al. Medial patellofemoral ligament reconstruction in children: A comparative randomized short-term study of fascia lata allograft and gracilis tendon autograft reconstruction. Medicine. 2018;97:e13605.

Matzkin E. Medial patellofemoral ligament reconstruction: indications, technique, and outcomes. Arthroscopy. 2019;35:2970–2.

McGee TG, Cosgarea AJ, McLaughlin K, et al. Rehabilitation after medial patellofemoral ligament reconstruction. Sports Med Arthrosc Rev. 2017;25:105–13.

McNair PJ, Marshall RN, Matheson JA. Important features associated with acute anterior cruciate ligament injury. N Z Med J. 1990;103:537–9.

McPherson AL, Feller JA, Hewett TE, Webster KE. Psychological readiness to return to sport is associated with second anterior cruciate ligament injuries. Am J Sports Med. 2019;47:857–62.

Mikkelsen C, Werner S, Eriksson E. Closed kinetic chain alone compared to combined open and closed kinetic chain exercises for quadriceps strengthening after anterior cruciate ligament reconstruction with respect to return to sports: a prospective matched follow-up study. Knee Surg Sports Traumatol Arthrosc. 2000;8:337–42.

Mitchell J, Graham W, Best TM, et al. Epidemiology of meniscal injuries in US high school athletes between 2007 and 2013. Knee Surg Sports Traumatol Arthrosc. 2016;24:715–22

Modi S, Deisler R, Gozel K, et al.Wells criteria for DVT is a reliable clinical tool to assess the risk of deep venous thrombosis in trauma patients. World J Emerg Surg. 2016;11:24.

Mook WR, Miller MD, Diduch DR, et al. Multiple-ligament knee injuries: A systematic review of the timing of operative intervention and postoperative rehabilitation: J Bone Joint Surg Am. 2009;91:2946–57.

Motamedi AR, Gowd AK, Nazemi AK, et al. Incidence, positional distribution, severity, and time missed in medial collateral ligament injuries of the knee in NCAA Division I Football Athletes. JAAOS Glob Res Rev. 2017;1:e019.

Mueller BT, Moulton SG, O'Brien L, LaPrade RF. Rehabilitation following meniscal root repair: a clinical commentary. J Orthop Sports Phys Ther. 2016;46:104–13.

Myklebust G, Engebretsen L, Braekken IH, et al. Prevention of anterior cruciate ligament injuries in female team handball players: a prospective intervention study over three seasons. Clin J Sport Med. 2003;13:71–8.

Needle AR, Lepley AS, Grooms DR. Central nervous system adaptation after ligamentous injury: A summary of theories, evidence, and clinical interpretation. Sports Med Auckl NZ. 2017;47:1271–88.

Noorduyn JCA, Glastra van Loon T, van de Graaf VA, et al. Functional outcomes of arthroscopic partial meniscectomy versus physical therapy for degenerative meniscal tears using a patient-specific score: A Randomized Controlled Trial. Orthop J Sports Med. 2020;8:232596712095439.

Nyland J, Cook C, Keen J, Caborn DNM. Lower extremity neuromuscular recovery following anterior cruciate ligament reconstruction; a 2-week case study. Electromyogr Clin Neurophysiol. 2003;43:41–9.

O'Donnell K, Freedman KB, Tjoumakaris FP. Rehabilitation protocols after isolated meniscal repair: a systematic review. Am J Sports Med. 2017;45:1687–97.

Owesen C, Sandven-Thrane S, Lind M, et al. Epidemiology of surgically treated posterior cruciate ligament injuries in Scandinavia. Knee Surg Sports Traumatol Arthrosc. 2017;25:2384-91.

Pache S, Aman ZS, Kennedy M, et al. Posterior cruciate ligament: Current concepts review. Arch Bone Jt Surg. 2018;6:8–18.

Papalia R, Del Buono A, Osti L, et al. Meniscectomy as a risk factor for knee osteoarthritis: a systematic review. Br Med Bull. 2011;99:89–106.

Papalia R, Franceschi F, D'Adamio S, et al. Hamstring tendon regeneration after harvest for anterior cruciate ligament reconstruction: A systematic review. Arthrosc J Arthrosc Relat Surg. 2015;31:1169–83.

Paterno MV, Flynn K, Thomas S, Schmitt LC. Self-reported fear predicts functional performance and second ACL injury after ACL reconstruction and return to sport: a pilot study. Sports Health. 2018;103:228–33.

Persson A, Fjeldsgaard K, Gjertsen JE, et al. Increased risk of revision with hamstring tendon grafts compared with patellar tendon grafts after anterior cruciate ligament reconstruction: a study of 12,643 patients from the Norwegian Cruciate Ligament Registry, 2004-2012. Am J Sports Med. 2014;42:285–91.

Prins M. The Lachman test is the most sensitive and the pivot shift the most specific test for the diagnosis of ACL rupture. Aust J Physiother. 2006;52:66.

Puzzitiello RN, Waterman B, Agarwalla A, et al. Primary medial patellofemoral ligament repair versus reconstruction: rates and risk factors for instability recurrence in a young, active patient population. Arthrosc J Arthrosc Relat Surg. 2019;35:2909–15.

Quarles JD, Hosey RG. Medial and lateral collateral injuries: prognosis and treatment. Prim Care. 2004;31:957–75.

Rambaud AJM, Ardern CL, Thoreux P, et al. Criteria for return to running after anterior cruciate ligament reconstruction: a scoping review. Br J Sports Med. 2018;52:1437–44.

Reider B. Medial collateral ligament injuries in athletes. Sports Med. 1996;21:147–56.

Rice DA, McNair PJ. Quadriceps arthrogenic muscle inhibition: Neural Mechanisms and Treatment Perspectives. Semin Arthritis Rheum. 2010;40:250–66.

Rio E, Kidgell D, Purdam C, et al. Isometric exercise induces analgesia and reduces inhibition in patellar tendinopathy. Br J Sports Med. 2015;49:1277–83.

Roach CJ, Haley CA, Cameron KL, et al. The epidemiology of medial collateral ligament sprains in young athletes. Am J Sports Med. 2014;42:1103–9.

Robinson JR, Bull AMJ, Dew Thomas RR, Amis AA. The role of the medial collateral ligament and posteromedial capsule in controlling knee laxity. Am J Sports Med. 2006;34:1815–23.

Roos EM, Lohmander LS. The Knee injury and Osteoarthritis Outcome Score (KOOS): from joint injury to osteoarthritis. Health Qual Life Outcomes. 2003;1:64.

Roos EM, Roos HP, Lohmander LS, et al. Knee Injury and Osteoarthritis Outcome Score (KOOS): Development of a self-administered outcome measure. J Orthop Sports Phys Ther. 1998;28:88–96.

Rosinski A, Chakrabarti M, Gwosdz J, et al. Double-bundle medial patellofemoral ligament reconstruction with allograft. Arthrosc Tech. 2019;8:e513–20.

Ross MD, Langford B, Whelan PJ. Test-retest reliability of 4 single-leg horizontal hop tests. J Strength Cond Res. 2002;16:617–22.

Roy JS, Bouyer LJ, Langevin P, Mercier C. Beyond the joint: The role of central nervous system reorganizations in chronic musculoskeletal disorders. J Orthop Sports Phys Ther. 2017;47:817–21.

Rubinstein RA, Shelbourne KD, McCarroll JR, et al. The accuracy of the clinical examination in the setting of posterior cruciate ligament injuries. Am J Sports Med. 1994;22:550–7.

Safran-Norton CE, Sullivan JK, Irrgang JJ, et al. A consensus-based process identifying physical therapy and exercise treatments for patients with degenerative meniscal tears and knee OA: The TeMPO physical therapy interventions and home exercise program. BMC Musculoskelet Disord. 2019;20:514.

Salavati M, Akhbari B, Mohammadi F, et al. Knee injury and Osteoarthritis Outcome Score (KOOS); reliability and validity in competitive athletes after anterior cruciate ligament reconstruction. Osteoarthritis Cartilage. 2011;19:406–10.

Senese M, Greenberg E, Todd Lawrence J, Ganley T. Rehabilitation following isolated posterior cruciate ligament reconstruction: a literature review of published protocols. Int J Sports Phys Ther. 2018;13:737–51.

Serra Cruz R, Mitchell JJ, Dean CS, et al. Anatomic posterolateral corner reconstruction. Arthrosc Tech. 2016;5:e563–72.

Shaarani SR, O'Hare C, Quinn A, et al. Effect of prehabilitation on the outcome of anterior cruciate ligament reconstruction. Am J Sports Med. 2013;41:2117–27.

Sharma L. Osteoarthritis of the knee. Engl J Med. 2021;384:51–9.

Sheehan FT, Derasari A, Fine KM, et al. Q-angle and J-sign: Indicative of maltracking subgroups in patellofemoral pain. Clin Orthop. 2010;468:266–75.

Shelbourne KD, Gray T. Minimum 10-year results after anterior cruciate ligament reconstruction: how the loss of normal knee motion compounds other factors related to the development of osteoarthritis after surgery. Am J Sports Med. 2009;37:471–80.

Shon OJ, Park JW, Kim BJ. Current concepts of posterolateral corner injuries of the knee. Knee Surg Relat Res. 2017;29:256–68.

Sinacore JA, Evans AM, Lynch BN, et al. Diagnostic accuracy of handheld dynamometry and 1-repetition-maximum tests for identifying meaningful quadriceps strength asymmetries. J Orthop Sports Phys Ther. 2017;47:97–107.

Smillie IS. The current pattern of internal derangements of the knee joint relative to the menisci. Clin Orthop. 1967;51:117–22.

Smith BE, Thacker D, Crewesmith A, Hall M. Special tests for assessing meniscal tears within the knee: a systematic review and meta-analysis. Evid Based Med. 2015;20:88–97.

Snoeker BAM, Bakker EWP, Kegel CAT, Lucas C. Risk factors for meniscal tears: a systematic review including meta-analysis. J Orthop Sports Phys Ther. 2013;43:352–67.

Snoeker BAM, Lindeboom R, Zwinderman AH, et al. Detecting meniscal tears in primary care: Reproducibility and accuracy of 2 weight-bearing tests and 1 non–weight-bearing test. J Orthop Sports Phys Ther. 2015;45:693–702.

Sonnery-Cottet B, Saithna A, Quelard B, et al. Arthrogenic muscle inhibition after ACL reconstruction: a scoping review of the efficacy of interventions. Br J Sports Med. 2019;53:289–98.

Spang III RC, Nasr MC, Mohamadi A, et al. Rehabilitation following meniscal repair: a systematic review. BMJ Open Sport Exerc Med. 2018;4:e000212.

Spiridonov SI, Slinkard NJ, LaPrade RF. Isolated and combined grade-III posterior cruciate ligament tears treated with double-bundle reconstruction with use of endoscopically placed femoral tunnels and grafts: operative technique and clinical outcomes. J Bone Joint Surg Am. 2011;93:1773–80.

Stanley LE, Kerr ZY, Dompier TP, Padua DA. Sex differences in the incidence of anterior cruciate ligament, medial collateral ligament, and meniscal injuries in collegiate and high school sports: 2009-2010 through 2013-2014. Am J Sports Med. 2016;44:1565–72.

Stephen JM, Kittl C, Williams A, et al. Effect of medial patellofemoral ligament reconstruction method on patellofemoral contact pressures and kinematics. Am J Sports Med. 2016;44:1186–94.

Strickland SM. Medial patellofemoral ligament repair versus reconstruction: still a question or a clear winner? Arthrosc J Arthrosc Relat Surg. 2019;35:2916–7.

Sturgill LP, Snyder-Mackler L, Manal TJ, Axe MJ. Interrater reliability of a clinical scale to assess knee joint effusion. J Orthop Sports Phys Ther. 2009;39:845–9.

Sullivan JK, Irrgang JJ, Losina E, et al. The TeMPO trial (treatment of meniscal tears in osteoarthritis): rationale and design features for a four arm randomized controlled clinical trial. BMC Musculoskelet Disord. 2018;19:429.

Swenson DM, Collins CL, Best TM, et al. Epidemiology of Knee Injuries among U.S. High School Athletes, 2005/2006–2010/2011. Med Sci Sports Exerc. 2013;45:462–9.

The STaR Trial Investigators, Lynch AD, Chmielewski T, Bailey L, et al. Current concepts and controversies in rehabilitation after surgery for multiple ligament knee injury. Curr Rev Musculoskelet Med. 2017;10:328–45.

Thorlund JB, Juhl CB, Roos EM, Lohmander L. Arthroscopic surgery for degenerative knee: systematic review and meta-analysis of benefits and harms. Br J Sports Med. 2015;49:1229–35.

Twomey-Kozak J, Jayasuriya CT. Meniscus repair and regeneration. Clin Sports Med. 2020;39:125-63.

VanderHave KL, Perkins C, Le M. Weightbearing versus non-weight bearing after meniscus repair. Sports Health Multidiscip Approach. 2015;7:399-402.

Varelas AN, Erickson BJ, Cvetanovich GL, Bach BR. Medial collateral ligament reconstruction in patients with medial knee instability: a systematic review. Orthop J Sports Med. 2017;5:232596711770392.

Vellios EE, Trivellas M, Arshi A, Beck JJ. Recurrent patellofemoral instability in the pediatric patient: management and pitfalls. Curr Rev Musculoskelet Med. 2020;13:58–68.

Wang D, Graziano J, Williams RJ, Jones KJ. Nonoperative treatment of pcl injuries: goals of rehabilitation and the natural history of conservative care. Curr Rev Musculoskelet Med. 2018;11:290–7.

Webster KE, Feller JA. Expectations for return to preinjury sport before and after anterior cruciate ligament reconstruction. Am J Sports Med. 2019;47:578–83.

Webster KE, Feller JA, Lambros C. Development and preliminary validation of a scale to measure the psychological impact of returning to sport following anterior cruciate ligament reconstruction surgery. Phys Ther Sport. 2008;9:9–15.

Welling W, Benjaminse A, Lemmink K, Gokeler A. Passing return to sports tests after ACL reconstruction is associated with greater likelihood for return to sport but fail to identify second injury risk. Knee. 2020;27:949–57.

Wiggins AJ, Grandhi RK, Schneider DK, et al. Risk of secondary injury in younger athletes after anterior cruciate ligament reconstruction. Am J Sports Med. 2016;44:1861–76.

Wilk KE, Andrews JR, Clancy WG. Nonoperative and postoperative rehabilitation of the collateral ligaments of the knee. Oper Tech Sports Med. 1996;4:192–201.

Wind WM, Bergfeld JA, Parker RD. Evaluation and treatment of posterior cruciate ligament injuries: revisited. Am J Sports Med. 2004;321:765–75.

Winkler PW, Zsidai B, Wagala NN, et al. Evolving evidence in the treatment of primary and recurrent posterior cruciate ligament injuries, Part 2: surgical techniques, outcomes and rehabilitation. Knee Surg Sports Traumatol Arthrosc. 2021;29:682–93.

Wolf BR, Gulbrandsen TR. Degenerative meniscus tear in older athletes. Clin Sports Med. 2020;39:197–209.

Wulf G, Shea C, Lewthwaite R. Motor skill learning and performance: a review of influential factors. Med Educ. 2010;44:75–84.

Zaman S, White A, Shi WJ, et al. Return-to-play guidelines after medial patellofemoral ligament surgery for recurrent patellar instability: a systematic review. Am J Sports Med. 2018;46:2530–9.

Clinical examination of hip and knee pain disorders

Megan Burrowbridge Donaldson, Alicia Emerson

Purpose of the Interview

Introduction

The clinical interview is one of the most useful diagnostic and therapeutic tools for a healthcare practitioner, albeit also one of the most challenging skills to master. It should blend the art and style of good communication with evidence-based questions that guide the practitioner's decisions. This type of communication with the patient is intentional. It should blend purposeful questioning for diagnostic reasoning and interpersonal skills to establish rapport with the patient and facilitate conversation. The interview determines the accuracy of the diagnostic/prognostic assessment, management decisions, and the quality of the practitioner–patient relationship, thereby affecting the entire diagnostic–therapeutic process. In essence, excellent communication results in better diagnosis and treatment for the patients.

This chapter outlines the factors for consideration when interviewing, a communication style and approach, specific knowledge base and interview skill set, and verbal/non-verbal behaviors relevant to effective communication during the clinical interview. This chapter does not intend to present a critical review of the literature on communication methods and interviewing strategies in healthcare, nor is it an in-depth discussion of the knowledge base and skills to be learned. Instead, it guides practitioners on foundational communication and medical interviewing strategies to apply with patients seeking healthcare.

Why should clinicians or educators be interested in communication, interviewing, and effective history-taking for patients with lower extremity syndromes? Effective communication in clinical settings increases the likelihood that: (1) the information gathered from patients is accurate and reliable to improve hypothesis generation for further testing or diagnostic assessment; (2) patients recognize the practitioner is genuinely interested in them, their health, and their care; (3) a common ground is developed to form a patient–practitioner therapeutic relationship; and (4) patients develop an active role in their own decisions and outcomes. Additionally, engaged communication strategies can minimize risk for implicitly biased management, improve patient outcomes, and can increase overall satisfaction for patients and clinicians.

Patient-centered Care

The biopsychosocial model is both a philosophy of clinical care and a practical clinical guide for centering care around a patient. At the practical level, it is a way of understanding the patient's subjective experience as an essential contributor to accurate diagnosis, health outcomes, and humane care. Critically, it is now generally accepted that illness and health result from an interaction between biological, psychological, and social factors. Wade and Halligan (2017) identified a need to increase the proportion of healthcare resources devoted to chronic disorders, and the accompanying need to improve patient outcomes requires action; better understanding and employment of the biopsychosocial model by those charged with healthcare funding could help improve healthcare outcomes while also controlling costs. Clinicians should consider utilizing tools, scales, or outcome measures to gain insight into the interplay of the injury and/or disease and its impact on the patient beyond the biological or physiological factors (see Chapter 9 of this textbook). Embracing non-physical factors related to the treatment of the patient's whole system provides an opportunity for improved trust between the patient and clinician, better adherence to medical care, and ultimately better outcomes. Social and contextual factors may be gleaned from tools developed by Ware (1993), such as the 36-Item Short Form Survey (SF-36) or the tool created by Zimet et al. (1988), the Multidimensional Scale of Perceived Social Support (MSPSS). Chapter 9 of this textbook discusses the outcomes for patients with hip and knee problems.

Lakke and Meerman (2016) found that clinicians who can develop a therapeutic relationship or alliance with the patient have been shown to positively affect patient outcomes, patient satisfaction, and reduction of communication barriers. Pinto et al. (2012) identify that the communication factors, including interaction styles and verbal or non-verbal behaviors, appear to be associated with constructs of the therapeutic alliance. This alliance is a collaboration, agreement, or trust bond developed between health practitioners and patients. Babatunde et al. (2017) suggest that patient-centered interaction styles related to providing emotional support and allowing patient involvement in the consultation process enhance the therapeutic alliance.

Patient-centered Interviewing

There are various history-taking or interview approaches described in the literature. Dwamena et al. (2012) found that a patient-centered or collaborative interview is a style of interviewing that has led to better interventions and improved patient outcomes. Centering the care around the patient encourages: (1) shared control of the consultation, decisions about interventions or management of the health problems with the patient, and/or (2) a focus in the consultation on the patient as a whole person who has individual preferences situated within social contexts. Beck et al. (2002) identify that centering the interview around the patient can be a challenge for every clinician. Although patient-centered interviewing is learned during entry-level education, it is not adequate to learn these skills without significant practice. Clinicians are reminded that strategies and questions should be reflective and tailored to the individual. Some patients may be athletes and require a different set of questions from those of an elderly patient to clearly understand the impact of the condition on the patient's quality of life. Walter et al. (2005) and Asnani (2009) provide evidence clearly illustrating the fundamental relationships between effective communication and the quality of working relationships, the degree of patient safety, and the satisfaction levels of both the patient and the clinicians.

Facilitators and Barriers to Communication

The clinician that adopts engaging communication strategies can improve their chances of achieving a congruent interview. Babatunde et al. (2017) found that purposeful communication skills allow for an enhanced therapeutic alliance to be established and improve the accuracy of information gathered. An interview that can build an alliance with the patient may also decrease the risk of chronic musculoskeletal pain development. In the social communication model of pain, healthcare practitioners' verbal and non-verbal communication styles may influence patients' pain experiences. As such, clinicians understanding the patient and validating their concerns appear to offer the opportunity to optimize patient outcomes, in part, by mitigating the stress of not being heard during the interview.

Facilitators to engage in communication include a variety of verbal and non-verbal behaviors. Non-verbal communication behaviors such as body language can be used to demonstrate that a healthcare practitioner is interested, paying attention, and caring. Examples of engaged and supportive non-verbal behaviors include maintaining eye contact, appropriately nodding, and using facial expressions to convey concern or empathy. Lee et al. (2016) identify that patient outcomes were positively associated with healthcare practitioners who demonstrated empathy and attentiveness. Patients may have preferences on gender, physical appearance, and/or attire of their practitioner, which could influence perceived patient comfort and competence assessment. Identifying factors that encourage conversation may facilitate patient trust and communication to enable practitioners to anticipate challenges in a clinical encounter to optimize communication. Additionally, Douglas et al. (2017) encourage healthcare practitioners to be aware of when patients demonstrate non-verbal communication behaviors that indicate a lack of engagement in the interview and thoughtfully consider how to check-in with the patient and/or adjust their communication style. This skill can be considered similar to the metacognitive strategies expert clinicians use when managing the interview.

Verbal communication behaviors use spoken language to convey a message. Interviewing styles will be covered in more detail later in the chapter. Facilitators to verbal communication include asking straightforward open-ended questions, not interrupting the patient, and deploying active listening strategies during follow-up communication. Active listening strategies include restating back to the patient what the patient said and asking close-ended clarifying questions. Another good strategy a clinician can use during the interview is to summarize what the patient stated. Summarizing offers the opportunity for the patient to confirm or better clarify so that the healthcare practitioner gathers a complete picture.

FitzGerald and Hurst (2017) conducted a systematic review recognizing the challenges on both sides of the practitioner–patient relationship, such as implicit biases, incongruent pain judgments, or unmet patient expectations during the interview and impact outcomes. When practitioners address these challenges directly, a positive therapeutic alliance and improved patient outcomes can occur. However, they can also be barriers when steps are not taken to mitigate them. Therefore, thoughtful consideration when approaching the interview is warranted. Careful history-taking requires practitioners to recognize and overcome their implicit biases related to race, ethnicity, gender, patients' educational level, and religious identity. Patient-perceived stigma and misinformation regarding diagnosis or treatment may limit patient disclosure of clinical history during the interview. Specific to physical therapy, Jones and Forhan (2019) reported a perceived stigma related to obesity and their chronic pain. Ross and Setchelle (2019) recognized that within the communities of lesbian, gay, bisexual, transgender, intersex, queer, or related identities (LGBTIQA+), taking time during the clinical conversation to avoid unintentional stigmatizing behaviors may help to minimize implicit healthcare biases that may impact care adversely.

The Art of Communication: Style and Approach

Although there are many purposes to taking a good history, the style and approach to which the clinical interview or history-taking is conducted appear to impact the patient's clinical outcome based on the systematic review and meta-analysis by Henry et al. (2012). The interview is a process of clinician seeking information, reflective listening, and exploring various related medical conditions based on the patient's clinical presentation/symptoms. The Calgary-Cambridge guides provide suggestive models for conducting the interview used widely throughout Europe and North America for teaching and assessment by Silverman et al. (2011). These guides have been presented and substantiated within the literature and should be considered for educational training of clinicians and use in clinical practice. These interview guides by Kurtz and Silverman (1996) provide structure and emphasize relationship building with the patient simultaneously. The basic process includes: (1) initiating the session; (2) gathering information; (3) performing the physical examination; (4) explanation and planning; and (5) closing the session. Continuous awareness to provide structure to the interview and building a relationship must be maintained through this framework.

This communication guide identifies the role that the patient's perception may have regarding their medical condition. The open conversation regarding the patient's fears and motivation, and commitment level to participating in care allows the clinician to explore barriers to care. Rollnick et al. (2008) found that adapting a style of inquisitiveness and curiosity for collaborative conversation, such

as motivational interviewing, provides a patient-centered approach that acknowledges the patient's expertise in his/her own problems and empowers the patient. It is essential to encourage patients in solving problems, making decisions, overcoming barriers and setbacks within a supportive relationship with their clinician. This appears to be essential for patients that have recurrent issues or difficulty following through with treatment plans. VanBuskirk and Wetherell (2013) conducted a systematic review and meta-analysis on motivational interviewing identifying that only one session may enhance readiness to change and action directed toward reaching health behavior-change goals.

Additionally, a large body of literature supports the systematic review by VanBuskirk and Wetherell (2013) suggesting that involvement of the patient in the interview may improve adherence with prescription and treatment. Nijs et al. (2020) recently developed a practical guide to integrate the concepts of pain education and motivational interviewing. Motivational interviewing allows clinicians to explore concepts such as pain knowledge/beliefs, awareness, willingness to explore psychological factors that are potentially associated with pain; this includes musculoskeletal-related or complex pain syndromes.

The spirit of motivational interviewing uses inquiry and communication skills to facilitate a patient-centered approach to clinical encounters. These communication strategies or skills include open-ended questioning, non-verbal communication skills such as purposeful silence or non-verbal encouragement, attentive listening, and summarizing or paraphrasing. Effective patient–practitioner communication and shared decision-making require the incorporation of these techniques into everyday practice. Table 8.1 provides five-staged interviews that embody a blend of the models and styles to facilitate a patient-centered interaction.

Interview Content

Within the USA, all states, the District of Columbia, and the US Virgin Islands allow physical therapists to evaluate patients without a referral from another healthcare professional. The majority of those states further improve accessibility by allowing physical therapists to evaluate and treat, under certain conditions, patients without a referral. Patients with lower extremity syndromes may present

TABLE 8.1 Five-Staged Interview

Stage	Description	Actions to facilitate patient-centered interaction
1	**Preparation:** Set the stage for the patient-centered medical interview	• Provide screening tools, surveys, or outcome measures to explore constructs from the biopsychosocial model • Welcome patient, ask for the patient's preferred name, clinician introduction of him/herself, ask permission to assist the patient if necessary • Ensure patient readiness and privacy • Identify SDoH screen to reduce communication, language, or literacy barriers • Establish patient comfort, allow the patient to position themself for comfort (sit, stand, lie down) if in pain (for the interview)
2	**Explore:** Identify the chief complaint and what brings the patient to seeking care	• Explore patient goals and desired outcomes • Obtain the list of issues the patient wants to discuss and preferences for care • Summarize/finalize agenda, prioritize items for current encounter versus future encounter
3	**Gather:** Open-ended questions for an understanding of present illness (non-focused)	• Ask open-ended questions and attentive listening • Use active listening, which includes verbal and non-verbal encouragement • Summarize or paraphrase subjective findings or concerns • Inform patient that style of questioning will now change ("I'm now going to ask you several specific medical questions about your symptoms") to use a funnel strategy to create more specific yes/no questions for differential diagnosis
4	**Perform:** Patient-centered medical interview and history of present illness (focused)	• Use focused, but open-ended, questions to obtain a description of physical symptoms during the physical examination (provoking, relieving, familiar symptoms, etc.) • Explore patient description of symptoms, emotional or social context of symptoms associated with physical movements or physical examination methods
5	**Explain and Plan:** Ensure strategies for patient–practitioner ongoing therapeutic relationship	• Summarize conversation, findings, and confirm the accuracy of information. Blend the subjective with the objective • Discuss the plan (treat, treat and refer, or refer) • Develop tailored and patient-centered goals within the domains associated with the International Classification of Functioning (ICF) Model • Communicate the plan for the next session

with a myriad of clinical presentations for physical therapy to differentiate; some may be well-defined, and some very complex. In many instances, physical therapists are involved in primary care settings which require an advanced skill set of screening, differential diagnosis, and clinical decision-making to treat this population appropriately. The interview suggested by Jarvik and Deyo (2002) is part of the examination process with three interrelated components: (1) screening/patient history; (2) systems review/differential diagnosis inquiry; and (3) tests and measures. Often, a clinical pattern emerges from the interview that guides the tests and measures.

The value of the interview has been significant in primary care, with physicians reporting that the history alone was sufficient to make a diagnosis in around 75% of patients, physical examination in around 10%, and lab or imaging investigation in a further 10% (Goodman and Snyder, 2009). The diagnostic value of the subjective clinical report remains widely understudied throughout the literature within types of study designs for diagnostic accuracy studies. However, based on the best evidence that exists to date, some questions or content items are contained within the interview that should help the clinician differentiate between lower extremity pain syndromes from other conditions.

There are various clinical presentations in many lower extremity pain syndromes; therefore, it is suggested to take a systems approach within the content items in the interview. The systems approach should be screened as an initial process to aid in a differential diagnosis and ruling out other systems as potential pain generators. Woolf (2003) suggests three goals at the end of the interview: (1) understanding the patient's problem and potential causes; (2) identify the effect of the problem on the patient's lifestyle; and (3) plan the objective examination.

Screening from Patient History

The interview is a critical component of an examination for decision-making, screening, and differential diagnosis. Edwards et al. (2004) suggested that a thorough examination uses a well-constructed interview as the foundation to develop a plan for the physical examination that will provide diagnostic value for both the clinician and the patient. The use of intake forms to gain information regarding demographics and clinical history may save significant time when completed outside of the interview (Goodman & Snyder, 2009). Integrating the findings from the patient intake form, self-reported outcome forms, initial referral (if one exists), and observing the patient in the waiting room can evoke a wide range of clinical hypotheses for consideration. These forms should help initiate the conversation and allow the therapist to generate clarifying and/or additional questions to assist in the decision-making process. Higgs (1992) suggested that initial hypotheses are derived from

the clinician's knowledge base and clinical experience, and differences exist between novice and expert clinicians.

Many lower extremity syndromes and conditions, including significant healthcare burdens such as low back pain (LBP) and osteoarthritis (OA) of the hip, knee, and ankle, are recurrent, progressive, and lead to a significant decrease in quality of life. Harris-Hayes et al. (2013) proposed alignment with the biopsychosocial model framework to use self-reported outcome measures to capture the information contained within the domains of pain, disability, function, quality of life, job satisfaction, fear, and/or psychosocial concerns which are essential for the complexity of lower extremity syndromes. The practitioner should consider the physical diagnostic possibilities contributing to the problem and explore the full range of factors that may contribute to the patient's health. This includes understanding the impact of the condition on the patient's life; capturing information from more than one domain may be helpful in understanding and managing the patient with lower extremity pain syndromes. Table 8.2 provides a list of questionnaires or tools that may provide insight into the patient lower extremity condition. Readers are referred to Chapter 9 for more data about specific outcome for patients with hip and knee conditions.

Systems Review and Differential Diagnosis Inquiry

Red Flags

Boissonnault (2011) proposed that the goal of the screening process is to recognize the need for a physician referral, speeding up the diagnosis of systemic and other pathologic processes. The purpose is to identify symptoms unusual for neuro-musculoskeletal conditions, which may have been overlooked during the investigation of the patient's chief presenting complaints, which is a primary purpose for the screen. Koes et al. (2006) found considerable commonalities between disease and neuro-musculoskeletal condition complaints. The history should aim to specify potential sources. Table 8.3 provides a planned list of general health status indicators to be used at the initial physical therapy visit during intake, which may indicate a more in-depth systems review during the history or physical examination.

The presence of any of the "red flags" should be noted at the initial assessment. This step is critical in determining

TABLE 8.2 Self-reported Outcome Measures for Patients with Lower Extremity Pain Syndromes

Name of Outcome Measure	Description
Fear-Avoidance Belief Questionnaire	The FABQ assesses patient beliefs about the effect of physical activity and works on their low back pain. It consists of 16 items and patients rate their agreement with each statement on a 7-point Likert scale. A higher score indicates more strongly held fear-avoidance beliefs. Two subscales are contained: 7-item work subscale and 4-item physical activity scale.
	Previous studies have found the FABQ work subscale to be associated with current and future disability and work loss in patients with chronic and acute low back pain (Waddell et al., 1993; Williamson, 2006).
Functional Rating Index (FRI)	This FRI measure is specifically designed to quantitatively measure the subjective perception of function and pain of the spinal musculoskeletal system in a clinical environment. The measure appears to have good reliability and validity (Feise & Menke, 2001).
Knee Outcome Survey	There is an indication to use this knee outcome survey tool with patients with a nonspecific knee injury. It has reliability and validity. It is responsive to functional limits for a variety of impairments (Irrgang et al., 1998).
Lower Extremity Functional Scale (LEFS)	Indications for the use of the LEFS includes all lower extremity conditions; reliability and validity: strong for hip and knee total arthroplasty; useful with patients following arthroplasty. In a 1999 study, this scale was administered with the SF-36, the acute version. In the conclusion of the study, they found that the retest reliability of the LEFS scores was excellent. They found that the minimal detectable clinical change within the score was at least 9 scale points and recommended this scale over the SF-36 (Binkley et al., 1999; Stratford et al., 1999).
Multidimensional Scale of Perceived Social Support	The Multidimensional Scale of Perceived Social Support (MSPSS) is a brief questionnaire designed to measure perceptions of support from 3 sources: Family, Friends, and a Significant Other. The scale consists of a total of 12 items, with 4 items for each subscale. Due to linguistic and cultural differences, there is a need to test the psychometrics of the adapted versions. MSPSS yielded a three-factor structure, high internal consistency ($\alpha = 0.88$), stability (yielded $\alpha = 0.85$ after 3 months from first administration) and moderate construct validity as the SS scores were negatively correlated to anxiety ($r = -0.18$; $p < 0.01$) and depression scores ($r = -24$; $p < 0.01$) (Dambi et al., 2018).
Oswestry Low Back Disability Questionnaire (OLBDQ)	This tool quantifies a patient's functional status and assesses pain-related disability in persons with LBP. This measure has been studied and is a reliable and valid tool (Fairbank et al., 1980).
Pain Self-Efficacy Questionnaire	The Pain Self-Efficacy Questionnaire (PSEQ) is a 10-item questionnaire, developed to assess the confidence people with ongoing pain have in performing activities while in pain. The PSEQ is applicable to all persisting pain presentation. It covers a range of functions, including household chores, socializing, work, as well as coping with pain without medication. Internal consistency is high (0.92 Cronbach's alpha) and test–retest reliability is high of a 3-month period (Nicholas, 2007).

(Continued)

TABLE 8.2 *(Continued)*	
Name of Outcome Measure	**Description**
Patient-Specific Functional Scale (PSFS)	This useful questionnaire can be used to quantify activity limitation and measure functional outcome for patients with any orthopedic condition (Stratford et al., 1995). It is a self-report outcome measure of function that could be used in patients with varying levels of independence. Investigates functional status by asking patients to nominate activities that are difficult to perform based on their condition and rate the level of limitation with each activity. It is a valid, reliable, responsive and efficient outcome measure applicable to a large number of lower extremity syndromes and clinical presentations.
Roland–Morris Disability Questionnaire	This is a health status measure, designed by Roland & Morris (1986) to assess physical disability due to low back pain.
Short Form-36	SF-36 is a valid and reliable tool to measure health at the individual level in clinical practice and research and at the population level for health policy evaluations, and general population surveys (Ware et al., 2000). Scores for the different domains are converted and pooled using a scoring key, for a total score indicating a range of low to high QOL. Two component scores can also be tallied; a physical component summary and a mental component summary. Similarly, research also suggests that the SF-36 cannot be used as a single index of overall health-related QOL because it measures two dimensions (physical and mental).
WOMAC (Western Ontario and McMaster University Osteoarthritis Index)	This tool, created by Bellamy et al. (1998), measures symptoms and physical disability, originally developed for people with OA of the hip and knee. It has been studied with reliability and validity for OA.

who is and is not a candidate for physical therapy. This step requires recognizing and ruling out the presence of red flags. Sizer et al. (2007) defined red flags as signs and symptoms that may tie a disorder to a severe pathology but may mimic a musculoskeletal condition. Boissonnault (2011) recommends that clinicians recognize red flags from a patient's clinical history and physical examination. Fritz and Flynn (2005) recommended several regional screening tools to help recognize potential severe disorders (red or yellow flags) that aid in the differential diagnosis of musculoskeletal conditions commonly encountered by physical therapists and require questions during the interview.

Cook et al. (2011) identify that LBP, buttock pain, and/or pain in the lower extremity may be related to spinal malignancy. Although the incidence of spinal cancer is low, clinicians need to conduct a thorough red flag screening as low back movements may reproduce mechanical pain in patients with or without cancer. A systematic review by Henschke et al. (2013) found that previous history of cancer meaningfully increases the likelihood of cancer with a high positive likelihood ratio. Furthermore, it was identified that other red flags have high false-positive rates leading to unnecessary and potentially harmful investigations, such as radiation. Currently, there is a lack of evidence and studies that have sufficient statistical power to produce precise estimates of sensitivity and specificity of "red flags." However, despite their inclusion in the guidelines, the usefulness of screening for "red flags" for malignancy in patients with LBP continues to be debated, and there remains very little information on their diagnostic accuracy and how best to use them in clinical practice. Furthermore, Henschke et al. (2013) recommended that clinicians ask more than one red flag question as presented in Table 8.4.

Fractures are also a typical red flag and can produce LBP and spine-related leg pain or symptoms. Vertebral compression fractures are the most common osteoporosis-related

TABLE 8.3 General Systems Review Questions

Vasculogenic screen including pulmonary system questions	Visercogenic system questions
Dyspnea	Swallowing difficulties
Cough	Indigestion, heartburn
Palpitations	Food intolerance
Syncope	Bowel dysfunction
Sweats	Color of stool
Cold distal extremities	Shape, caliber of stool
Skin discoloration	Constipation
Open wounds/ulcers	Diarrhea
Clubbing of the nails	Difficulty initiating
Wheezing, stridor	Incontinence

Genitourinary system questions	Reproductive system questions
Urinary changes	Male gender
Color	Urethral discharge
Flow	Sexual dysfunction
Reduced caliber or force of urine stream	Pain during intercourse
	Female gender
Incontinence	Vaginal discharge
	Pain with intercourse
	Menstruation changes
	Menopause

(Adapted from Boissonnault, 2011.)

TABLE 8.4 Red Flags to Screen for Malignancy in Patients with Low Back Pain

Clinical History Questions	Post-test Probability
Do you have a previous history of cancer?	4.6%
Have you experienced any unexplained weight loss?	1.2%
Have your symptoms improved after one month (if not)?	0.9%
Age >50 years?	0.8%
Have you had symptoms (this episode) >1 month?	0.8%
Do you have severe pain?	0.5%
Have you tried bed rest with no relief?	0.6%

(From Henschke et al., 2013.)

(Downie et al., 2013). The authors reported that many red flags in current guidelines provide virtually no change in fracture probability or have untested diagnostic accuracy.

Vasculogenic Screen

Cardiovascular systems can refer pain and/or symptoms (including edema) into the lower extremity and require a differential diagnosis. Boissonnault (2011) provided some considerations for the clinician to rule out related reasons for peripheral edema, including venous insufficiency, congestive heart failure, pulmonary hypertension, and deep venous thrombosis associated with unilateral edema. Siracuse et al. (2012) recognized that occlusive arterial disease is a common problem in the elderly and smokers and may present in a similar manner to claudication. Like other lower extremity syndromes, it may present as pain, edema, and/or a cramping sensation in buttocks, thighs, or calves. However, claudication

spinal fractures presenting with clinical signs and symptoms of back pain, posture changes, loss of height, functional impairment, disability, and diminished quality of life. A systematic review identified three red flags that would be useful to detect fracture in a primary care setting, including significant trauma, older age, and corticosteroid use pain is typically associated with increased physical activity and is relieved by rest. de Virgilio and Chan (2010) identified that aortic aneurysms are potentially dangerous conditions and demonstrate symptomatic behaviors manifested by a deep, diffuse, throbbing, or aching mid-back, chest, left shoulder, or abdominal pain. If symptom onset is related to recent surgical events or a lower level of activity, screening for deep vein thrombosis may be required. The Wells Clinical Prediction Rule is a reliable and valid tool for a clinical assessment for predicting the risk of deep venous thrombosis in the lower extremity (Wells et al., 1997).

Viscerogenic Screen

In the gastrointestinal system, the viscera can refer pain and/or symptoms into the lower extremity and should be ruled out as a pain generator with patients presenting with lower extremity pain syndromes. Intake questions regarding changes in bowel habits should be a part of an initial screen. However, Goodman and Snyder (2009) recommend that additional questions regarding blood in stools or black stools should be screened for colon cancer. Additionally, the behavior of symptoms from visceral organs varies depending on the function of the organ. The report of fluctuation of the symptoms may be related to eating habits or bowel or bladder function. Certain foods may precipitate the onset of symptoms or may affect the intensity of symptoms. Other disorders may be associated with bladder fullness or constipation, urination, or defecation. It is essential to question the patient regarding the total area of pain or related symptoms to ultimately determine all contributing pain if changes within this system are reported.

Neurogenic Screen

Neurological symptoms associated with leg paresthesias, numbness, and weakness as progressive neurologic symptoms may involve a peripheral nerve entrapment or spinal nerve root lesion and require further inquiry. Additionally, any unusual descriptions of altered sensation, bilateral extremity deficits, difficulty urinating, or change in frequency require further investigation of this system. Concerns regarding bilateral symptoms and urination are derived from a medical diagnosis of cauda equina. Deyo et al. (1992) identify that medical questions regarding symptoms of urinary retention have a sensitivity of 90% and specificity of 95% for cauda equina. Additionally, cauda equina presents

with unilateral or bilateral leg pain, numbness, and weakness, which are common in over 80% of medical cases.

Spondylogenic or Non-mechanical Pathologies: Differential Diagnosis

Koes et al. (2006) suggested that non-mechanical pathologies should be considered in lower extremity syndrome differential diagnosis and screening. Many of these conditions can worsen at night, although presenting as common lower extremity pain syndromes and behaving similarly with mechanical pain presentations. Seronegative spondyloarthropathies need to be considered when a young patient with progressive back pain presents with inflammatory symptom behaviors, including morning stiffness and improvement with exercise. Atlas and Deyo (2001) suggest various conditions for screening, including the following: ankylosing spondylitis, Reiter's syndrome, psoriatic arthritis, and arthritis of inflammatory bowel disease, which require additional medical testing for diagnosis. Ankylosing spondylitis (AS) may be identified with the following questions: a slow onset, age population <40, long-term discomfort (>3 months), and inflammatory behaviors of morning stiffness and improvement of discomfort with exercise. The diagnostic accuracy associated with these questions includes a sensitivity of 23% and a specificity of 82% and helps rule in AS.

Psychogenic Screen and Biopsychosocial Factors

Psychosocial factors may also manifest in musculoskeletal pain and be associated with regional or widespread pain in the presentation. A systematic review identified baseline predictors of persistent disabling LBP including maladaptive pain coping behavior, functional impairment, low general health status, and the presence of anxiety and depressive comorbidities (Chou & Shekelle, 2010). An umbrella review also found psychological stress to increase the odds of having low back pain and sciatica (Parreira et al., 2018). Consistent evidence found that various psychological factors impact prognosis (Nicholas et al., 2011; Grovle et al., 2013). However, the literature is less consistent as to which factors are the most prognostic variables. A recent systematic review noted that patients with lower levels of depression or fear of movement were more likely to return to work (Oosterhuis et al., 2019). Given the entirety of these findings, it remains crucial to screen for biopsychosocial factors during the interview.

Persistent Pain Screening

Courtney et al. (2011) suggested that conditions in the lower extremity require clinicians to consider the entire lower quadrant as persistent low back pain can refer to the leg and be considered spinal-related leg pain. In the absence of sinister pathology, Lesnak and Sluka (2019) propose that persistent pain that continues outside of typical, expected healing time frames requires further investigation into possible contributing factors, including peripheral and central sensitization. Central sensitization is operationally defined as an amplification of neural signaling within the central nervous system that elicits pain hypersensitivity. Woolf (2011) operationally defined peripheral sensitization as increased responsiveness and reduced threshold of nociceptors to stimulation of their receptive fields, including nociceptive pain, which refers to pain conditions predominantly driven by the activation of peripheral nociceptive sensory fibers. Clinical examination of the predominant sensitization mechanisms, peripheral and/or central, could lead to a clinical hypothesis for treatment.

Social Determinants of Health (SDoH)

Emerging evidence from Healthy People (2020) identified the importance of screening for SDoH, health behaviors, and other biopsychosocial factors. Screening for these factors better informs diagnosis, prognosis and health outcomes, particularly for socioeconomically vulnerable populations. Therefore, a well-structured interview involving screening and/or inquiry into the critical information about the patient's general health status, lifestyle, and well-being is needed. This is particularly salient as SDoH can be associated with an increased risk for chronic musculoskeletal pain development.

Health People (2020) organizes the SDoH around five key domains: (1) economy (e.g., financial stability); (2) education (i.e., access and quality); (3) access to the health system and healthcare; (4) neighborhood and built environment; and (5) social and community context. Therefore, screening for risk factors can help healthcare practitioners foster interdisciplinary care when patients present with lower extremity syndromes and have increased risk factors. Yet within the USA, the appropriate role for the healthcare practitioners in addressing SDoH remains poorly defined. Additionally, Gottlieb et al. (2017) suggest using tools for effectively collecting the information to assess SDoH.

However, the impact of these unmet needs in clinical settings is currently not well understood. Physical therapists have a role in SDoH screening in ambulatory or primary care settings. Improved knowledge and skills could improve healthcare teams' ability to understand the factors impacting their patients' health and ability to act on healthcare strategies or recommendations.

Additionally, the screening and understanding of the SDoH may guide the therapeutic alliance to better inform clinical care decisions, and identify patients in need of referral to community resources to address identified needs. Manchanda and Gottlieb (2015) suggest there are readily available tools online, such as a free portable document format (PDF) that provides validated SDoH items to be used as a screening tool before the interview. Access to these tools allows clinicians to have improved knowledge of the SDoH and its possible impact on the patient who seeks healthcare.

Health Behaviors

Healthy People (2020) initiatives are broadly categorized into over a dozen different types of health behaviors. Those relevant to this book chapter include health communication, sleep, nutrition, and healthy eating, and physical activity. Intake forms that can incorporate validated measures related to health literacy, sleep quality, food insecurity, and physical activity can help shape the interviewing questions. When healthcare practitioners screen/identify low health literacy, they can then seek ways to improve the patient's understanding of their condition and management. Other health behaviors can inform a more accurate diagnosis/prognosis. For example, Nijs et al. (2018) found that poor sleep quality is both a result of and can be predictive of persistent musculoskeletal pain.

Symptom Investigation and Referral Pattern

Regardless of the content-specific questions, the interview should be planned carefully and should utilize a good intake form/strategy that includes many critical questions about the patient's condition. Table 8.5 presents a suggested guide to developing an intake form. The clinician seeking to become an expert should consider using a body diagram to foster clinical decision-making. The body diagram is a visual illustration of all of the symptoms the patient may be experiencing. Pattern recognition can help to inform and drive the interview. Early in the interview, it is important to help the patient identify the primary reason for seeking care. Some of the initial symptom investigations can be completed on the clinical history intake form to streamline the interview.

During intake and/or during the interview identifying specific movement patterns that alter the patient's

symptoms better and/or worse are imperative. Understanding what worsens or improves symptoms helps the clinician with the hypothesis generation and informs the physical examination. Some authors refer to this as the concordant sign and are distinguished from other symptoms produced during the physical assessment. Maitland (2001) described a concordant sign that needs to be identified during the interview to allow both the patient and the clinician to identify the critical complaint. Laslett et al. (2003) suggest

TABLE 8.5 Suggested Intake Information for Patients with Lower Extremity Pain Syndromes

Intake Questions Related to:	Purpose of the Content
Patient Profile and Demographics	• Relates to the epidemiology with prevalence and incidence of related conditions based on age, gender, and ethnicity • Outcome measures to evaluate the biopsychosocial aspects to care • Social Determinants of Health
Description of the Problem	• Characterize the problem and determine cause (if one exists), determine chief complaint, and other related concerns • Concordant/familiar/comparable – movement associated with the pain in which the patient is seeking care • Patient's perspective of the condition (concerns, expectations, feelings, beliefs)
Nature and Behavior of the Condition	• *Severity:* intensity of the patient's symptoms as they relate to a functional activity or time of day • *Irritability:* how quickly a stable condition degenerates in the presence of pain-causing inputs • *Nature:* represents the structures at fault, or involved in the syndrome. May also inquire as to the aggravating factors or relieving factors. May also inquire as to presentation: constant, intermittent, and/or episodic • *Stage of pathology:* assessment of the stage of healing in which the condition is presenting • *Stability:* symptom progression over time (better, worse, staying the same)
Pertinent Medical History	• Use intake forms to minimize questions for screening • Review of systems for differential diagnosis of viscerogenic, vasculogenic, spondylogenic, neurogenic, and/or psychogenic pain generators • Determine if potential related medical components may be related to clinical presentation • Baseline for current medication use, general wellness, activity level, current medical conditions and/or medical test for present condition
Patient Goals and Barriers to Care	• Commonly used to identify motivation to improving current health status • Related to adherence to plan of care and self-efficacy which are prognostic variables to successful outcomes • Treatment alternatives in accordance with patient-centered care

that lower extremity syndromes may also present with one or more discordant signs and may be described as painful or abnormal but not related to concordant signs.

Severity, Nature, and Behavior of the Symptoms

The severity, nature, and behavior of the condition help frame questions regarding the severity, nature, irritability, stage of pathology, and stability of the symptoms. Again, as with many other history-taking components, many of these concepts are not well described or studied within the literature. The severity of the symptoms relates to the intensity of the patient's symptoms related to a functional activity or time of day. Farrar et al. (2001) suggested that the Numeric Pain Rating Scale be used to provide a baseline for comparison and it should be captured with various movements during the physical examination to promote clinical decision-making. The nature of the patient's symptoms refers to the pain presentation as being constant, intermittent, and/or episodic in behavior. The nature of symptoms can be descriptive (i.e., sharp, dull) or can identify symptom location (i.e., deep or superficial) or other quality (i.e., stiffness, burning, tingling) that may need further investigation. Chimenti et al. (2018) suggest that the nature of symptoms can also guide clinicians' decisions regarding nociceptive processing and indicate a more effective influence on the patient's pain experience.

The behavior of symptoms should include inquiry as to the aggravating factors or relieving factors for the patient. Questions regarding symptom behavior during the day are associated with neuro-musculoskeletal impairments or movement disorders. These conditions typically fluctuate as mechanical loads on the body increase or decrease with time of day, onset or cessation of specific activities, and adoption or avoidance of certain postures. Irritability is another pain behavior concept that appears to be unique and relates to how quickly a condition may flare in the presence of pain-causing inputs. Based on the studies examining this concept of irritability, three questions prove helpful:

1. What does the patient have to do to set this condition off?

2. How long do the symptoms last, and how severe are the symptoms?

3. How long and what does the patient have to do to calm the symptoms down?

The narrative from Chimenti et al. (2018) further advances how our understanding of pain science can help to conceptualize the irritability of the patient's condition. Patients who only have pain with specific movements and the pain resolves immediately upon cessation indicate a more mechanical or nociceptive presentation. This presentation is considered low irritability. Patients with high pain severity whose pain continues to persist after ceasing the activity indicate higher levels of irritability. Higher irritability is commonly associated with central nocioplasticity and may be categorized as neuropathic or non-neuropathic. Zusman (1998) suggested that in patients with higher irritability of symptoms or pain, clinicians require to be cautious of aggressive treatment because they worsen with selected activities.

History of Current Condition

The patient needs to understand the cause if one exists of their lower extremity condition. History questions can distinguish onset related to trauma versus acute-on-chronic flares when prioritizing tests and follow-up measures. The stage of the pathology or condition relates specifically to the stage of healing for the injury or symptom presentation. In contrast, the stability of the symptom presentation refers to the symptom progression over time as improving, worsening, or staying the same. Additionally, understanding contributing factors such as patient demographics and the mechanism of injury can assist with pattern recognition. Upon a complete interview and the subsequent tests and measures, the patient should present a consistent symptom pattern to a musculoskeletal condition. Suppose the symptoms are not present during an examination, or the patient cannot express any activities. In that case, a further medical workup may be warranted, and the therapist should refer to the appropriate provider.

History-taking Questions Specific to Lower Extremity Pain Syndromes

The following sections regarding history-taking present subjective history questions studied for their diagnostic values and may assist the clinician with hypothesis generation and decision-making. Cook et al. (2007) suggest clinicians should be mindful of diagnostic odds ratios (DOR), sensitivity (the ability of the test to positively identify an individual who has the problem according to the reference test), specificity (the ability of the test to positively exclude an individual who does not have the problem according to the reference test), likelihood ratios (+LR or –LR), will be reported with the characterization statements, subjective history questions, and/or self-report questionnaire items affiliated with a specific condition.

Specific Low Back-associated Musculoskeletal Pain Syndromes

There are various low back or spinal conditions that should be considered when addressing a patient with lower extremity pain syndromes. Many studies have suggested various questions that can be used to identify a specified lower quarter condition. Specifically, within the lumbar spine, several studies have examined the diagnostic accuracy of history-taking items for persistent pain (spinal-related leg pain), lumbar spinal stenosis, lumbar sacral nerve root compression/radiculopathy, lumbar disc herniation, and clinical lumbar instability.

Persistent Pain (Spinal-related Leg Pain)

Leg pain is a frequent accompaniment to low back pain but can often be present in the absence of low back pain. Schafer et al. (2009) suggest the structures often involved with leg pain (with or without low back pain) for this chapter will be presented and classified as (1) central sensitization; (2) peripheral nerve sensitization (with or without denervation); and (3) musculoskeletal pain from non-neural structures. Each of the various structures involved can present a distinct pattern of signs and symptoms that the patient may describe during the interview or intake form. However, more research in the pain sciences identifies a significant crossover. Smart et al. (2012a, 2012b) suggest that patients experiencing pain disproportionate to injury, disproportionate aggravating/easing factors, and other psychosocial symptoms were very likely to be diagnosed with central sensitization, now refer as nociplasticity (DOR: 15.19, 30.69, and 7.65, respectively). Individuals complaining of localized or intermittent pain are more likely to be diagnosed with nociceptive low back pain (DOR: 69.79 and 4.25, respectively).

Lumbar Spinal Stenosis (LSS)

There are a variety of personal history questions/self-report items studied for the diagnosis of LSS. All of the following self-report items presented met the criteria for at least a small increase in the probability of a diagnosis of LSS. The most diagnostic combination included a cluster of (1) bilateral symptoms, (2) leg pain more than back pain, (3) pain during walking/standing, (4) pain relief upon sitting, and (5) age >48 years. Failure to meet the condition of any one of five positive examination findings demonstrated high sensitivity (SN: 0.96) and a low LR– (0.19). Cook et al. (2011) found that meeting the condition of four of five examination findings yielded an LR+ 4.6 and a post-test probability of 76%. Other studies found that increasing the patient's age above 48 increased the LR+ of having the condition (Konno et al., 2007; Katz et al., 1995; Sugioka et al., 2008). The following questions appear to be helpful: does the patient have severe leg pain (LR+ of 2.00); no pain when seated (LR+ of 6.60); symptoms that improve when seated (LR+ of 3.10); leg numbness (LR+ of 2.62)? Additional questions include worse pain when walking but relieved by taking a rest (DOR: 70.77), worse when standing (DOR: 11.38), and numbness around the buttocks (DOR: 77.0). For patients with LSS, asking if the patient's pain was reported for more than six months (DOR: 2.17), or if they have reports of walking more slowly than usual (DOR: 2.28), and sitting down because of lower extremity pain (DOR: 2.01), and if the patient needed to wake up to urinate at night (DOR: 2.34), slightly to moderately altered the probability of having LSS.

Nerve Root Compression/Radiculopathy

The most significant history component for nerve root compression is the location of pain and/or if the symptoms present in a dermatomal distribution, and if symptom radiation was the most significant history complaint (DOR: 24.29) (Smart et al., 2012a; 2012b). The patient experiencing more pain with coughing, sneezing, or straining (DOR: 3.20), self-noticed muscle weakness (DOR: 2.20), self-noticed sensory loss (DOR: 2.10), and self-reports of disturbed urinary passage (DOR: 2.3) have been associated with the diagnosis of lumbar sacral nerve root compression/radiculopathy. Additionally, Vroomen et al. (2002) identify an age relationship, as age 51–81 years alters the probability of this patient having this condition (DOR: 2.2).

Lumbar Disc Herniation

For the diagnosis of lumbar disc herniation, only a few studies have compared findings to a gold standard, and some have a significant risk of bias. Vucetic et al. (1997) identify the key history items elicited from the interview; any previous non-spinal surgery (DOR: 3.52), a low education level (DOR: 3.22), and progressive sciatic pain (DOR: 2.77) yielded some benefit in screening for lumbar disc herniation.

Lower Extremity-associated Musculoskeletal Pain Syndromes

Hip Osteoarthritis

Recent systematic review conducted by Wright et al. (2021) explored the diagnostic accuracy of patient history in the diagnosis of hip-related pain. For the diagnosis of hip osteoarthritis, some of the key history items suggested for diagnosis screening include: for hip osteoarthritis, a family history of OA (+LR 2.13), history of knee OA (+LR 2.06), report of groin or anterior thigh pain (+LR 2.51–3.86), self-reported limitation in range of motion of one or both hips (+LR 2.87), constant low back pain/buttock pain (+LR 6.50), and groin pain on the same side (+LR 3.63), and a screening questionnaire (+LR 3.87–13.29). The review by Metcalfe et al. (2019) found that the most useful findings for identifying a patient with hip OA included squat causing posterior pain (+LR 6.1), groin pain on passive abduction/adduction (+LR 5.7), abductor weakness (+LR 4.5), and decreased passive hip adduction (+LR 4.2) or internal rotation (+LR 3.2).

Other Hip Pathologies

Still, much more research is needed in the realm of diagnostic accuracy of intra-articular hip pathology from both the patient's subjective or self-reported history and objective clinical examination standpoint. Burgess et al. (2011) examined the diagnostic accuracy of the subjective statements associated with labral pathology. Studies identified that patients with labral pathology present with anterior groin pain sensitivity of 100% and a specificity of 40%, reports of clicking ranged with sensitivity from 57% to 100%. Tijssen et al. (2012) conducted a systematic review where the authors grouped the mechanical symptoms of clicking, locking, popping, or giving way together from three of their included studies and found that reports of mechanical symptoms yielded a range of sensitivity from 53% to 100%. Little is known about the diagnostic value of the clinical history-taking on femoroacetabular impingement (FAI). In a systematic review by Wright et al. (2021) of intra-articular hip pathology, crepitus

(+LR 3.56) was the most significant finding. This condition has been increasingly recognized as a causative factor of many intra-articular hip lesions and labral pathology. Some studies have described the clinical characteristics and symptoms. However, no studies have examined the diagnostic accuracy of these history questions for FAI.

Knee Osteoarthritis (OA)

The knee is a significant target of this degenerative disease. Morvan et al. (2009) found three questions during the interview identified a small shift in the probability of having this knee OA. Pain for at least 4 weeks yielded a sensitivity of 0.95, the specificity of 0.46, LR+ of 1.77, and LR– of 0.10; pain while climbing stairs or walking down slopes: sensitivity of 0.81, specificity of 0.63, LR+ of 2.19, and LR– of 0.30; and having swelling in one or both knees yielded a sensitivity of 0.47 of 0.84, LR+ of 3.10 and LR– of 0.62.

Patellofemoral Pain (PFP)

A recent clinical practice guideline on patellofemoral pain was published by Willy et al. (2019) including the examination methods. Specific to the diagnostic value of the self-reported symptoms, Cook et al. (2012) conducted a systematic review that identified some questions that may help identify patients with PFP. Their included studies identified that self-reported pain during squatting presents with a range of low LR+ ranging from 1.3–1.8 and LR– between 0.9 and 0.1 from three studies reported in a systematic review. Additionally, self-reports of pain during kneeling also have a low LR+ of 1.7 and LR– of 0.3. During prolonged sitting or flexion of the knee, self-reported pain was captured in three studies and ranged from low to moderate shift in probabilities from LR+ of 1.7–7.4 and LR– of 0.3–0.5. Pain reports during stair climbing had a wider range of LR+ from 1.3 to 11.6 and LR– from 0.6–0.1 from three studies that captured this item. The wide ranges of differential diagnosis identified by the systematic review authors may be due to the reference standard for diagnosis. The definition of PFP is highly variable amongst the studies on this topic.

Knee Meniscal Injury

Two history-taking items have been reported for identifying knee meniscal injuries. One study included the self-reported sensation of giving way and locking had an accuracy of 49.2% and 60.9% compared to MRI and yielded a specificity of 0.84 and 0.96, respectively (Yan et al., 2011). Wagemakers et al. (2008) identified a question cluster of being older (age over 40 years), the continuation of activity being impossible, and reports of a weight-bearing trauma to yield a small shift in probability LR+ of 2.0 for meniscal injury. Thorlund et al. (2019) further report that mechanical symptoms such as self-reported catching or locking of the knee or inability to straighten the knee are equally prevalent in patients with and without a meniscal tear.

Knee Ligamentous Injury

More diagnostic accuracy studies have examined anterior cruciate ligament (ACL) injury than the other types of ligamentous injuries. This study further examined history-taking clusters for both partial and complete ACL lesions. The history-taking items reported: swelling/effusion LR+ of 1.6, LR– of 0.8 for partial tears, and LR+ of 2.0 and LR– of 0.6 for identifying complete tears. The reports of a popping sensation yielded LR+ of 2.3, LR– of 0.5 for partial tears, and LR+ of 2.1, and LR– of 0.5 for complete tears. The self-reported sensation of giving way yielded a small shift with LR+ of 1.6, LR– of 0.6 for partial tears, and LR+ of 1.7, and LR– of 0.6 for complete tears. When combined in a cluster, the history findings yielded a specificity of 0.99, a sensitivity of 0.18 and a LR+ of 17.7 for partial tears when compared

to MRI. Wagemakers et al. (2012) identified that complete ACL tears yielded a large, albeit slightly smaller, shift than partial tears, with a LR+ of 9.8 and LR– of 0.8 and similar specificity (0.98) and sensitivity (0.18) for the history test cluster.

Conclusions

As evidence-based clinicians, physical therapists need to utilize the best evidence to develop a biopsychosocial model-based, patient-centered interview. The history-taking approach, interview style and content questions are both understudied within the current literature in physical therapy. However, several tools, outcome measures, and screening questions that may aid in decision-making have been presented based on structures often involved with lower extremity syndromes. In clinical practice, the history and clinical examination are not isolated. History questions form within the interview, and their contributing value for decision-making remains understudied in the literature compared to the physical examination test studies. We may not know the actual value of the history regarding diagnostic accuracy to specific conditions. However, using the patient's narrative and understanding their condition and its impact on their quality of life does improve patient satisfaction with care and patient outcomes with many musculoskeletal conditions.

References

Alqarni AM, Schneiders AG, Hendrick PA. Clinical tests to diagnose lumbar segmental instability: A systematic review. J Orthop Sports Phys Ther. 2011;41:130–140.

Anstiss T. Motivational interviewing in primary care. J Clin Psychol Med Settings. 2009;16:87–93.

Asnani MR. Patient-physician communication. West Indian Med. 2009;58:357–61.

Atlas SJ, Deyo RA. Evaluating and managing acute low back pain in the primary care setting. J General Int Med. 2001;16:120–131.

Babatunde F, MacDermid J, MacIntyre N. Characteristics of therapeutic alliance in musculoskeletal physiotherapy and occupational therapy practice: a scoping review of the literature. BMC Health Services Research. 2017;17:375.

Beck RS, Daughtridge R. Sloane PD. Physician-patient communication in the primary care

office: a systematic review. J Am Board Fam Pract. 2002;15:25–38.

Bellamy N, Buchanan WW, Goldsmith CH, et al. Validation study of WOMAC: a health status instrument for measuring clinically important patient-relevant outcomes following total hip or knee arthroplasty in osteoarthritis. J Orthop Rheumatol. 1998;1:95–108

Benjaminse A, Gokeler A, van der Schans CP. Clinical diagnosis of an anterior cruciate ligament rupture: a meta-analysis. J Orthop Sports Phys Ther. 2006;36:267–88.

Binkley JM, Stratford PW, Lott SA, et al. The Lower Extremity Functional Scale (LEFS): scale development, measurement properties, and clinical application: North American Orthopaedic Rehabilitation Research Network. Phys Ther. 1999;79:371–383.

Boissonnault WG. Primary care for the physical therapist: Examination and triage. St Louis, MO: Elsevier Saunders; 2011.

Burgess RM, Rushton A, Wright C, et al. The validity and accuracy of clinical diagnostic tests used to detect labral pathology of the hip: A systematic review. Man Ther. 2011;16:318–26.

Chimenti RL, Frey-Law LA, Sluka KA. A mechanism-based approach to physical therapist management of pain. Phys Ther. 2018;98(5):302–14.

Chou R, Shekelle P. Will this patient develop persistent disabling low back pain? J Am Med Assoc. 2010;303:1295–302.

Cole C, Seto C, Gazewood J. Plantar fasciitis: evidence-based review of diagnosis and therapy. Am Fam Physician. 2005;72:2237–42.

Cook CE, Brismee JM, Sizer PS. Subjective and objective descriptors of clinical lumbar spine instability: A Delphi Study. Man Ther. 2006;11:11–21.

Cook C, Cleland J, Huijbregts P. Creation and critique of studies of diagnostic accuracy: Use of the STARD and QUADAS Methodological

Quality Assessment Tools. J Man Manip Ther. 2007;14:93–100.

Cook C, Ross MD, Isaacs R, et al. Investigation of non-mechanical findings during spinal movement screening for identifying and/or ruling out metastatic cancer. Pain Practice. 2011;12:426–33.

Cook C, Mabry L, Reiman MP, et al. Best test/clinical findings for screening and diagnosis of patellofemoral pain syndrome: a systematic review. Physiother. 2012;98:93–100.

Courtney CA, Clark JD, Duncombe AM, et al. Clinical presentation and manual therapy for lower quadrant musculoskeletal conditions. J Man Manip Ther. 2011;19:212–22.

de Virgilio C, Chan T. Assessment of vascular patients and indications for therapy. Periph Endovascular Interv. 2010;6:37–44.

Dambi JM, Corten L, Chiwaridzo M. A systematic review of the psychometric properties of the cross-cultural translations and adaptations of the Multidimensional Perceived Social Support Scale (MSPSS). Health Qual Life Outcomes. 2018;16:80.

Deyo RA. Nonsurgical care of low back pain. Neurosurg Clin N Am. 1991;2:851–62.

Deyo RA, Rainville J, Kent DL. What can the history and physical examination tell us about low back pain? J Am Med Assoc. 1992;268:760–5.

Douglas SL, De Souza LR, Yudin MH. Identification of patient-perceived barriers to communication between patients and physicians. Fam Med Med Sci Res. 2017;6:214.

Downie A, Williams CM, Henschke N, et al. Red flags to screen for malignancy and fracture in patients with low back pain: systematic review. BMJ. 2013;347:f7095.

Dwamena F, Holmes-Rovner M, Gaulden CM, et al. Interventions for providers to promote a patient-centered approach in clinical consultations. Cochrane Database Syst Rev. 2012;12:CD003267.

Edwards I, Jones M, Carr J, et al. Clinical reasoning strategies in physical therapy. Phys Ther. 2004;84:312–30.

Fairbank J, Couper J, Davies J, et al. The Oswestry Low Back Pain Questionnaire. Physiother. 1980;66:271–3.

Farrar JT, Young JP, LaMoreaux L, et al. Clinical importance of changes in chronic pain intensity measured on an 11-point numerical pain rating scale. Pain. 2001;94:149–58.

Feise RJ, Menke J. Functional Rating Index: A new valid and reliable instrument to measure the magnitude of clinical change in spinal conditions. Spine. 2001;26:78–86.

FitzGerald C, Hurst S. Implicit bias in healthcare professionals: a systematic review. BMC Med Ethics. 2017;18:19.

Fritz J, Flynn TW. Autonomy in physical therapy: less is more. J Orthop Sports Phys Ther. 2005;35:696–8.

Goodman CC, Snyder TE. Differential diagnosis in physical therapy, 3rd edn. Philadelphia: WB Saunders; 2009.

Gottlieb LM, Wing H, Adler NE. A systematic review of interventions on patients' social and economic needs. Am J Prev Med. 2017;53:719–29.

Grovle L, Haugen AJ, Keller A, et al. Prognostic factors for return to with in patients with sciatica. Spine. 2013;13:1849–57.

Harris-Hayes M, McDonough CM, Leunig M. Clinical outcomes assessment in clinical trials to assess treatment of femoroacetabular impingement: use of patient-reported outcome measures. J Am Acad Orthop Surg. 2013;21:S39–46.

Healthy People. Social Determinants of Health. Office of Disease Prevention and Health Promotion. 2020. Available at: https://www.healthypeople.gov/2020/topics-objectives/topic/social-determinants-of-health.

Henschke N, Maher CG, Ostelo RW et al. Red flags to screen for malignancy in patients with low-back pain. Cochrane Database Syst Rev.2013;2:CD008686.

Henry SG, Fuhrel-Forbis A, Rogers M, et al. Association between nonverbal communication during clinical interactions and outcomes: a systematic review and meta-analysis. Patient Educ Couns. 2012;86:297–315.

Higgs J. Developing knowledge: A process of construction, mapping and review. New Zealand J Physiother. 1992;20:23–30.

Irrgang JJ, Snyder-Mackler L, Wainner RS, et al. Development of a patient-reported measure of function of the knee. J Bone Joint Surg. 1998;80:1132–45.

Jarvik JG, Deyo RA. Diagnostic evaluation of low back pain with emphasis on imaging. Ann Intern Med. 2002;137:586–97.

Jones AC, Forhan M. Addressing weight bias and stigma of obesity amongst physiotherapists. Physiother Theor Pract. 2019;1–9.

Katz JN, Dalgas M, Stucki G et al. Degenerative lumbar spinal stenosis: Diagnostic value of the history and physical examination. Arthritis Rheum. 1995;38:1236–41.

Koes BW, van Tulder MW, Thomas S. Diagnosis and treatment of low back pain. Br Med J. 2006;332:1430–4.

Konno SI, Kikuchi SI, Tanaka Y, et al. A diagnostic support tool for lumbar spinal stenosis: a self-administered, self-reported history questionnaire. BMC Musculoskeletal Dis. 2007;8:102.

Kurtz SM, Silverman JD. The Calgary-Cambridge observation guides: an aid to defining the curriculum and organizing the teaching in communication training programmes. Med Educ. 1996;30:83–9.

Lakke SE, Meerman S. Does working alliance have an influence on pain and physical functioning in patients with chronic musculoskeletal pain; a systematic review. J Compassionate Health Care. 2016;3:1.

Laslett M, Young S, April C, et al. Diagnosing painful sacroiliac joints: A validity study of a McKenzie evaluation and sacroiliac provocation tests. Aust J Physiother. 2003;49:89–97.

Lee H, Mansell G, McAuley JH, et al. Causal mechanisms in the clinical course and treatment of back pain. Best Pract Res Clin Rheumatol. 2016;30:1074–83.

Lesnak J, Sluka KA. Chronic non-inflammatory muscle pain: central and peripheral mediators. Curr Opin Physiol. 2019;11:67–74.

Maitland GD. Maitland's vertebral manipulation. 6th ed. London: Butterworth-Heinemann; 2001.

Manchanda R., Gottlieb L. Upstream risks screening tool & guide V2.6. 2015. Available at: https://www.aamc.org/download/442878/data/chahandout1.pdf.

McPoil TG, Martin RL, Cornwall MW, et al. Heel Pain-Plantar Fasciitis: Clinical Practice Guidelines Linked to the International Classification of Function, Disability, and Health from the Orthopaedic Section of the American Physical Therapy Association. J Orthop Sports Phys Ther. 2008;38:A1–18.

Metcalfe D, Perry DC, Claireaux HA, et al. Does this patient have hip osteoarthritis? The rational clinical examination systematic review. JAMA. 2019;322:2323–33.

Morvan J, Roux CH, Fautrel B, et al. A case-control study to assess sensitivity and specificity of a questionnaire for the detection of hip and knee osteoarthritis. Arthritis Rheum. 2009;61(1):92–9.

Nicholas MK. The pain self-efficacy questionnaire: Taking pain into account. Eur J Pain. 2007;11:153–63.

Nicholas MK, Linton SJ, Watson PJ, et al. Early identification and management of psychological risk factors ("Yellow Flag") in patients with low back pain: a reappraisal. Phys Ther. 2011;91:737-53.

Nijs J, Mairesse O, Neu D, et al. Sleep disturbances in chronic pain: neurobiology, assessment, and treatment in physical therapist practice. Phys Ther. 2018;98:325–35.

Nijs J, Wijma AJ, Willaert W, et al. Integrating motivational interviewing in pain neuroscience education for people with chronic pain: a practical guide for clinicians. Phys Ther. 2020;100:846–59.

Oosterhuis T, Smaardijk VR, Kuijer PPF, et al. Systematic review of prognostic factors for work participation in patients with sciatica. Occup Environ Med. 2019;76:772–9.

Parreira P, Maher CG, Steffens D, et al. Risk factors for low back pain and sciatica: an umbrella review. Spine. 2018;18:1715–21.

Pinto RZ, Ferreira ML, Oliveira VC, et al. Patient-centered communication is associated with positive therapeutic alliance: a systematic review. J Physiother. 2012;58:77–87.

Roland M, Morris R. A Study of the natural history of back pain, part I: The development of a reliable and sensitive measure of disability of low back pain. Spine. 1986;8:141–4.

Roland M, Fairbank J. The Roland-Morris Disability Questionnaire and the Oswestry Disability Questionnaire. Spine. 2000;25:3115-22.

Rollnick S, Miller WR, Butler CC. Motivational interviewing in health care. New York: Guilford Press; 2008.

Ross MH, Setchell J. People who identify as LGBTIQ+ can experience assumptions, discomfort, some discrimination, and a lack of knowledge while attending physiotherapy: a survey. J Physiother. 2019;65:99–105.

Schafer A, Hall T, Briffa K. Classification of low back-related leg pain: A proposed patho-mechanism-based approach. Man Ther. 2009;14:222–30.

Silverman J, Archer J, Gillard S. Initial evaluation of epscale, a rating scale that assesses the process of explanation and planning in the medical interview. Patient Educ Couns. 2011;82:89–93.

Siracuse JJ, Giles KA, Pomposelli FB. Results for primary bypass versus primary angioplasty/stent for intermittent claudication due to superficial femoral artery occlusive disease. J Vascular Surg. 2012;55:1001–7.

Sizer P, Brismee JM, Cook C. Medical screening for red flags in the diagnosis and management of musculoskeletal spine pain. Pain Pract. 2007;7:53–71.

Smart KM, Blake C, Staines A, et al. Mechanisms-based classifications of musculoskeletal pain: Part 1 of 3: Symptoms and signs of central sensitization in patients with low back (±leg) pain. Man Ther. 2012a;17:336–44.

Smart KM, Blake C, Staines A, et al. Mechanisms-based classifications of musculoskeletal pain: Part 3 of 3: Symptoms and signs of nociceptive pain in patients with low back (±leg) pain. Man Ther. 2012b;17:352–7.

Stratford P, Gill C, Westway M, et al. Assessing disability and change on individual patients: A report of a patient specific measure. Physiother Can. 1995;47:258–63.

Stratford P, Binkley J, Lott S, et al. The Lower Extremity Functional Scale (LEFS): Scale Development, Measurement Properties, and Clinical Application. J Am Phys Ther Assoc. 1999;79:371–83.

Sugioka T, Hayashino Y, Konno S, et al. Predictive value of self-reported patient information for the identification of lumbar spinal stenosis. Family Practice. 2008;25:237–44.

Thorlund JB, Pihl K, Nissen N, et al. Conundrum of mechanical knee symptoms: signifying feature of a meniscal tear? Br J Sports Med. 2019;53(5):299–303.

Tijssen M, van Cingel R, Willemsen L, de Vissre Enrico. Diagnostics of femoroacetabular impingement and labral pathology of the hip: A systematic review of the accuracy and validity of physical tests. J Arthroscopic Rela Surg. 2012;28:860–71.

VanBuskirk KA, Wetherell JL. Motivational interviewing with primary care populations: a systematic review and meta-analysis. J Behav Med. 2013;2:11.

Vucetic N, Bri ED, Svensson O. Clinical history in lumbar disc herniation: a prospective study in 160 patients. Acta Orthopaedica. 1997;68:116–20.

Vroomen PC, de Krom MC, Wilmink JT, et al. Diagnostic value of history and physical examination in patients suspected of lumbosacral nerve root compression. J Neurol Neurosurg Psych. 2002;72:630–4.

Waddell G, Newton M, Henderson I. A Fear Avoidance Beliefs Questionnaire (FABQ) and the role of fear-avoidance beliefs in chronic low back pain and disability. Pain. 1993;52:157–68.

Wade DT, Halligan PW. The biopsychosocial model of illness: a model whose time has come. Clin Rehabil. 2017;31:995–1004.

Wagemakers HP, Heintjes EM, Boks SS, et al. Diagnostic value of history-taking and physical examination for assessing meniscal tears of the knee in general practice. Clin J Sport Med. 2008;18:24–30.

Wagemakers HP, Luijsterburg PA, Boks SS, et al. Diagnostic accuracy of history taking and physical examination for assessing anterior cruciate ligament lesions of the knee in primary care. Arch Phys Med Rehabil. 2012;91:1452–9.

Walter A, Bundy C, Dornan T. How should trainees be taught to open a clinical interview? Med Educ. 2005;39:492–6.

Ware JE, Snow KK, Kolinsky M, et al. SF-36 Health Survey: Manual and Interpretation Guide. Boston: The Health Institute; 1993.

Ware J. SF-36 Health Survey Update. Spine. 2000;24:3130–9.

Wells PS, Anderson DR, Bormanis J, et al. Value of assessment of pretest probability of deep-vein thrombosis in clinical management. Lancet. 1997;350:1795–8.

Williamson E. Fear Avoidance Beliefs Questionnaire (FABQ). Austr J Physiother. 2006;52:149.

Willy RW, Hoglund LT, Barton CJ, et al. Patellofemoral Pain. Clinical Practice Guidelines Linked to the International Classification of Functioning, Disability, and Health from the Academy of Orthopaedic Physical Therapy of the American Physical Therapy Association. J Orthop Sports Phys Ther. 2019;49(9):CPG1–CPG95.

Woolf AD. How to assess musculoskeletal conditions: History and physical examination. Best Practice Res Clin Rheumatol. 2003;17:381-402.

Woolf CJ. Central sensitization: implications for the diagnosis and treatment of pain. Pain. 2011;152:S2–15.

Wright AA, Ness BM, Donaldson M. Diagnostic accuracy of patient history in the diagnosis of hip-related pain: a systematic review. Arch Phys Med Rehabil. 2021. Online ahead of print.

Yan R, Wang H, Yang Z, et al. Predicted probability of meniscus tears: comparing history and physical examination with MRI. Swiss Med Wkly. 2011;141:13314.

Zimet GD, Dahlem NW, Zimet SG, Farley GK. The Multidimensional Scale of Perceived Social Support. J Personality Assessment. 1998;52:30-41.

Zusman M. Irritability. Man Ther. 1998;3(4):195-202.

Hip and knee outcome measures: are they valid for clinical settings?

9

Alessandra N. Garcia, Chad Cook, Bradley J. Myers, Joshua Cleland

Introduction

Clinical measures are an essential component of the patient examination process in any practice setting (Jewell, 2014). Clinical measures are more commonly used to quantify and/or describe patients' impairments in body functions and structures (Jewell, 2014). These measures may also assist healthcare providers in distinguishing among different levels of severity of a problem and in having a better understanding of how patients' impairments impact patients' activity limitations and participation restrictions (Jewell, 2014). Results obtained from clinical measures serve as a foundation for developing a plan of care and indications of patients' progress during the treatment. Patient-reported outcome measures (PROMs) are one of many other clinical measures widely used in clinical practice.

In the past few decades, there has been an increasing focus on the importance of using PROMs in the healthcare system (Sorensen et al., 2019). PROMs have been increasingly incorporated into clinical practice to describe patients' impairments, support shared decision-making and patient-centered care, and inform efforts to improve the quality and safety of the healthcare system (Williams et al., 2016). This chapter focuses on the use of PROMs for individuals with hip and knee disorders. We discuss the concept of PROMs, how to select PROMs in clinical practice, and how to determine if a PROM is valid in a clinical setting. In addition, we provide a few examples of the most common PROMs recommended for individuals with hip and knee disorders, and we conclude by indicating the clinical application of the use of PROMs.

Patient-reported Outcome Measures (PROMs)

Patient-reported outcomes (PROs) pertain to the patient's symptoms, health-related quality of life, or functional status reported by the patient without interference or interpretation of the patient's response by a healthcare professional (Weldring et al., 2013). Patient-reported outcome measures (PROMs) are self-reporting instruments, mostly used in a questionnaire fashion to capture PROs (Marshall et al., 2006; Williams et al., 2016). Analysis of PROMs usually focuses on the change in scores between initial examination and post-intervention (Williams et al., 2016). PROMs were initially developed for use in research and were gradually adopted by individual clinicians and hospitals to enhance individual patients' clinical management (Black, 2013).

At present, PROMs are used to assess patients' outcomes, support clinical decision-making, health policies and reimbursement processes. These instruments are also used to assess the healthcare effectiveness at different levels of the health system to inform efforts to improve healthcare quality and safety (Black, 2013; Impellizzeri et al., 2020; Williams et al., 2016). England, the United States, the Netherlands, and Sweden have been recognized as the most advanced countries in implementing PROMs at a national level (Williams et al., 2016). Figure 9.1 displays a few examples of the usefulness of PROMs from the perspectives of patients, healthcare providers, healthcare organizations and health system policymakers (Wilson et al., 2019).

PROMs can be either general in nature (generic) or disease-specific (Black, 2013; Weldring & Smith, 2013). Generic PROMs measure single or multiple aspects of health (e.g., pain, self-care, mobility, quality of life) (Black, 2013; Williams et al., 2016). These measures also allow comparison of outcomes across conditions. Examples of generic PROMs include the Short Form-36 (SF-36), SF-12, Nottingham Health Profile, Sickness Impact Profile, and WHOQOL-Brief (Williams et al., 2016). Disease-specific PROMs include clinical and physiological measures and outcome-related indicators to assess a particular population. These measures provide more detailed information about a patient's perceptions of symptoms across the trajectory of treatment and recovery for the disorder (Williams et al., 2016). Examples of disease-specific PROMs include the Oxford Hip Score and the self-reported Kessler-10 Psychological Distress Scale (Black, 2013; Williams et al., 2016). When used together, both types of PROMs can provide complementary information and contribute to shared clinical decision-making (Williams et al., 2016).

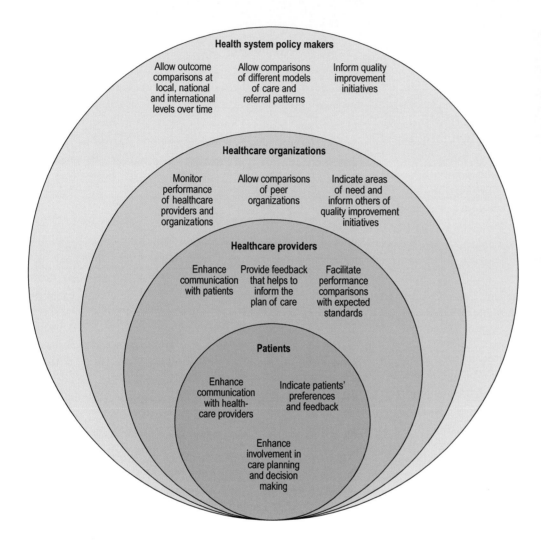

FIGURE 9.1
Usefulness of PROMs from different perspectives.

Within the figure:

Health system policy makers
- Allow outcome comparisons at local, national and international levels over time
- Allow comparisons of different models of care and referral patterns
- Inform quality improvement initiatives

Healthcare organizations
- Monitor performance of healthcare providers and organizations
- Allow comparisons of peer organizations
- Indicate areas of need and inform others of quality improvement initiatives

Healthcare providers
- Enhance communication with patients
- Provide feedback that helps to inform the plan of care
- Facilitate performance comparisons with expected standards

Patients
- Enhance communication with health-care providers
- Indicate patients' preferences and feedback
- Enhance involvement in care planning and decision making

Selection of PROMs in Clinical Practice

PROMs are increasingly being introduced to clinical practice routines across a range of health services. Before selecting a PROM, a healthcare provider needs to determine the outcome of interest (e.g., function, mobility), the population of interest (e.g., age, sex, diagnostic, duration of symptoms), and whether the focus is on generic or disease-specific measures (Chiarotto, 2019; Prinsen et al., 2018). Biomedical databases and PROM-specific databases (e.g., *Rehabilitation Measures Database* – www.sralab.org/rehabilitation-measures) can be systematically searched for identifying potential PROMs. Given that PROMs are frequently used to support clinical decision-making and health policies, the valid interpretation of data obtained using PROMs is of paramount importance (Hawkins et al.,

2018; Impellizzeri et al., 2020). Thus, the next step – after determining the outcome and population of interest and identification of potential PROMs to be used – consists of assessing the quality of these PROMs. The availability and quality of a PROM (i.e., sufficient measurement properties) are pre-conditions to its use and a vital component of the validity of the inferences drawn from its data in its development context (Hawkins et al., 2018; Jewell, 2014; Prinsen et al., 2018).

The COnsensus-based Standards for the selection of health Measurement INstruments (COSMIN) initiative developed a taxonomy of measurement properties relevant for evaluating PROMs, as well as several methodologies and practical tools for assessing the quality of PROMs in terms of measurement properties and feasibility (Chiarotto, 2019;

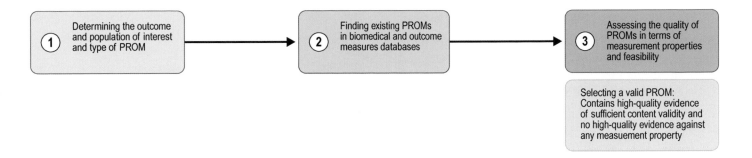

FIGURE 9.2
Selection of a valid PROMs to be used in clinical practice.

Impellizzeri et al., 2020; Mokkink et al., 2018; Prinsen et al., 2018; Terwee et al., 2018). The COSMIN guidelines can be used by researchers and clinicians to select the most appropriate PROM (Impellizzeri et al., 2020). In assessing the quality of a PROM, COSMIN distinguishes three domains: reliability, validity, and responsiveness. The domain reliability refers to the "degree to which the measurement is free from measurement error" (Jewell, 2014). This domain contains three measurement properties: internal consistency, reliability, and measurement error. A PROM that has demonstrated sufficient reliability produces stable results over time (Jewell, 2014). The domain of validity indicates "the degree to which a PROM measures the construct(s) it purports to measure." It contains three measurement properties: content validity (including face validity), structural validity, hypothesis testing for construct validity, cross-cultural validity, and criterion validity. The domain responsiveness refers to the ability of a PROM to detect change over time in the construct to be measured and contains only one measurement property, which is also called responsiveness. A PROM that has demonstrated sufficient validity is said to correctly capture what is supposed to be measured, whereas a responsive PROM has demonstrated the ability to detect change in the phenomenon of interest (Jewell, 2014).

Among these measurement properties, content validity (i.e., qualitative approach with patients) and structural validity (i.e., quantitative psychometric approach) are the measurement properties that require priority in PROM assessment. Sufficient content validity indicates that a PROM includes aspects that are relevant, comprehensive, and comprehensible for the targeted outcome and population (Chiarotto, 2019; Terwee et al., 2018). A PROM with sufficient structural validity would be expected to determine whether the dimensionality of a PROM is aligned with that of the domain (Chiarotto, 2019). The other measurement properties should be assessed when a PROM meets these first two criteria (Chiarotto, 2019). The feasibility of a PROM is also an important aspect to consider. It includes interpretability, ease of administration, length, completion time, ease of standardization, costs, copyright, and ease of score calculation (Chiarotto, 2019). Selecting an appropriate PROM in clinical practice involves finding an instrument with (at least) high-quality evidence of sufficient content validity and no high-quality evidence against any other property (Chiarotto, 2019). Based on measurement properties' results and feasibility characteristics, one can select the best available PROM for a given outcome and population (Chiarotto, 2019) (Figure 9.2).

PROMs for Hip and Knee Pain Conditions

There exists a plethora of commonly utilized PROMs for collecting self-reported health status in individuals with hip and knee pain, and providing a commentary on all of them is beyond the scope of this chapter. In this section, we will selectively describe many of the recommended and commonly utilized outcome measures for individuals with non-arthritic knee and hip joint pain and arthritic knee and hip joint pain, in addition to their related measurement properties. However, it is the responsibility of the clinician to select the most appropriate PROM based on measurement properties for the population they are likely to implement it with and its intended use.

PROMs for Hip Disorders (Table 9.1)

A number of PROMs have been recommended for individuals with non-arthritic hip pain in clinical practice guidelines, including the Hip Outcome Score, the Copenhagen Hip and Groin Outcome Score, and the International Hip Outcome Tool (iHOT-33) (Enseki et al., 2014). The Hip Outcome Score (HOS) is a self-report measurement tool that includes both an activity of daily living and a sports subscale. There is a total of 26 items with 17 in the ADL subscale; they include activities such as getting in and out of a car, going up and down stairs, walking, squatting, work duties, and recreational activities. The sports subscale contains 9 items such as fast walking, jumping, landing, running, cutting, and the ability to participate in sport.

TABLE 9.1 Summary of Patient-reported Outcome Measures (PROMs) for Hip Disorders

PROM	Hip disorder	Domains	Score/interpretation	Examples of measurement properties investigated*
Hip Outcome Score (HOS)	Non-arthritic hip pain	Activity of daily living and a sport	26 items (0–100) Higher scores indicate higher function in both scales	Sufficient reliability and construct validity
The Copenhagen Hip and Groin Outcome Score (HAGOS)	Non-arthritic hip pain (young to middle-aged, physically active patients with hip and/or groin pain)	Symptoms, pain, function in daily living, function in sport and recreation (sports/rec), participation in physical activities and hip and/or groin-related quality of life	Six scores (0–100). Higher scores indicate no symptoms	Sufficient reliability
International Hip Outcome Tool (iHOT-33)	Non-arthritic hip pain (health-related quality of life in young, active patients with hip disorders)	Symptoms and functional limitations; sports and recreational activities; job-related concerns; and social, emotional, and lifestyle concerns	33 items (0–100). Higher scores indicate a higher quality-of-life score	Sufficient reliability and construct validity
Lower Extremity Functional Scale (LEFS)	Hip osteoarthritis	Standing, squatting, walking, lifting, getting in and out of the car and performing usual activities	20 items (0–80). Higher scores indicate greater levels of function	Sufficient reliability

(Continued)

TABLE 9.1 *(Continued)*

PROM	Hip disorder	Domains	Score/interpretation	Examples of measurement properties investigated*
Hip disability and Osteoarthritis Outcome Score (HOOS)	Hip osteoarthritis	Pain, other symptoms, function in activities of daily living, function in sport/recreation, and hip-related quality of life	45 items (0–100). Higher scores indicate extreme problems	Sufficient reliability
Western Ontario and McMaster Universities Osteoarthritis Index (WOMAC)	Hip osteoarthritis	Pain, stiffness, and physical function	24 items (the scores for each subscale are summed up, with a possible score range of 0–20 for pain, 0–8 for stiffness, and 0–68 for physical function. Higher scores indicate worse outcomes	Sufficient reliability and construct validity

* Interpretation according to the original reports.

Each item is scored from 4 to 0, with 4 being "no difficulty" and 0 being "unable to do." There is a "nonapplicable" option that is not counted in scoring. The total number of items with a response is multiplied by 4 to get the highest potential score (Enseki et al., 2014; Martin et al., 2006; Martin et al., 2007). A person's score is divided by the highest potential score, then multiplied by 100 to get a percentage. Higher scores are indicative of higher function in both the ADL and sports subscales.

Martin and Philippon (2008) examined the reliability and responsiveness of the HOS in 126 subjects who had undergone hip arthroscopy for either a labral repair, chondral defect, osteoplasty, or capsular tightening. Test–retest reliability for both the ADL subscale and the sport subscale were found to be excellent (ICC 0.98, 0.92 respectively). At the time of the follow-up, the authors classified patients as either "changed" if the individual reported they were "much improved" or "somewhat improved" and having a "normal" or "nearly normal" level of functioning or "stable" if the patient's condition remained unchanged. Similarly, Kemp et al. (2013) found a test–retest reliability of ICC 0.95 (0.92–0.97) for the ADL subscale and 0.96 (0.92–0.98) for the sport subscale. The calculated minimal detectable change (MDC) has been found to be 13 for the ADL subscale and 16 for the sports subscale (Kemp et al., 2013). The minimal clinically important difference for the function subscale was found to be 9 points while it was 6 points in the sports subscale (Martin & Philippon, 2008). Furthermore, the ADL and sports subscales exhibited construct validity when compared to the Medical Outcomes Study 36-Item Short-Form Health Survey physical function and physical component scores. The ADL subscale demonstrated a correlation of 0.74 and 0.76, while the correlation with the sports subscale was 0.72 and 0.68, respectively (Martin & Philippon, 2008).

The Copenhagen Hip and Groin Outcome Score (HAGOS) has been recommended as a PROM for assessing disability in young to middle-aged, physically active patients with hip and/or groin pain (Enseki et al., 2014). The HAGOS is a self-report questionnaire with 6 dimensions: Symptoms, Pain, Function in Daily Living (ADL), Function in Sport and Recreation (Sports/Rec), Participation in Physical Activities (PA) and hip and/or groin-related Quality of Life (QOL). Each item is scored on a Likert scale ranging from 0 to 4, where 0 indicates no difficulties (Thorborg et al., 2011). Each subscale is scored separately, with a score of 100 indicating no symptoms.

In a sample of physically active patients, Thorborg et al. (2011) found the test–retest reliability to be excellent, ranging from an ICC of 0.82 to 0.91. Of the reliability values, the lowest bound confidence interval on any of the scales was found to be 0.68. Kemp et al. (2013) found the reliability to be excellent, also with an ICC between 0.92 and 0.97. Similarly, and more recently, in a Dutch population, Giezen et al. (2017) found the HAGOS subscales exhibited test-reliability values between 0.80 and 0.95. The MDC for the six HAGOS individual subscales in the Kemp study (Kemp et al., 2013) ranged from 8 to 19 and in the Giezen study 18.3 to 34.1, which brings into question whether the HAGOS is the best tool for monitoring physical function over time (Giezen et al., 2017).

The International Hip Outcome Tool (iHOT-33) was developed as a self-administered evaluative tool to measure health-related quality of life in young, active patients with hip disorders (Mohtadi et al., 2012). The iHOT-33 is a disease-specific self-report questionnaire with questions related to four domains. The 33 questions were distributed within the four domains, including: symptoms and functional limitations (16 questions), sports and recreational activities (6 questions), job-related concerns (4 questions), and social, emotional, and lifestyle concerns (7 questions). Each question is scored on a 100-mm visual analog scale. The test–retest reliability was identified in the original validation study as an ICC of 0.78. Furthermore, Mohtadi et al. (2012) reported good construct validity as correlation with the Non-Arthritic Hip was 0.81. The measurement properties of the iHOT-33 were evaluated in a population of adults undergoing hip arthroscopy as well (Kemp et al., 2013). The test–retest reliability was excellent with an ICC of 0.93 (0.87–0.96) with an MDC of 16. Griffin et al. (2012) shortened the original iHOT33 down to 12 questions referred to as the iHOT-12. Test–retest reliability ranged from 0.59 to 0.93 for the individual items. The smallest detectable change ranged from 17.1 to 44.9.

Clinical Practice Guidelines have recommended the use of a variety of PROMs, including the Lower Extremity Functional Scale (LEFS), the Hip disability and Osteoarthritis Outcome Score (HOOS), and the Western Ontario and McMaster Universities Osteoarthritis Index (WOMAC) as PROMs for use in individuals with osteoarthritis (OA). The LEFS was originally developed by Binkley et al. (1999) and is a scale consisting of 20 items addressing numerous functional activities, including standing, squatting, walking, lifting, getting in and out of the car and performing usual activities. Each item is scored on a 5-point Likert scale ranging from 0 to 4 where "0" is extreme difficulty and "4" is no difficulty. The scores for each item are summed, with the highest possible score being an 80 (Binkley et al., 1999). Higher scores indicate greater levels of function.

A systematic review reported the LEFS is reliable, valid and responsive (Mehta et al., 2016). However, the review combined pathologies of the lower extremity (hip, knee, foot/ankle). In a patient population with hip OA, Pua et al. (2009) found the LEFS exhibits excellent test reliability with an ICC of 0.92 (95%CI 0.85–0.96). In a sample of Dutch patients with hip OA the ICC was found to be 0.78. The authors also identified the standard error of measure of 3.6 points (upper bound estimate of CI was 4.6 points) and an MDC of 9.9 points (upper bound estimate of CI was 12.5 points) while Hoogeboom et al. (2012) found the ICC to be 12 points. Therefore, it could be suggested that the LEFS is an appropriate and reasonable outcome measure of physical functioning in patients with hip OA.

Probably the most commonly used outcome measure in both clinical practice and research is the WOMAC, which has been recommended for individuals with hip OA. The WOMAC consists of three subscales: pain (5 items), stiffness (2 items), and physical function (17 items). Users answer the 24 condition-specific questions on a numeric rating scale ranging from 0 (no symptoms) to 10 (extreme symptoms), or alternatively on a Likert-type scale from 0 to 4. Scores from each subscale are summed, with higher scores indicating more pain, stiffness, and disability in individuals with hip or knee OA and have been widely studied in the literature. Pua et al. (2009) found the WOMAC exhibited test–retest reliability of ICC 0.90 (95%CI 0.81–0.94) and an MDC of 9.1 (11.6) in patients with hip OA. A systematic review reporting on the measurement properties of the WOMAC (Gandek, 2015) found that the test–retest reliability was excellent for pain (0.86, 95%CI 0.77–0.91), stiffness (0.82, 95%CI 0.77, 0.86), and function (0.92, 95%CI 0.90–0.94). The authors also identified 15 studies that examined the correlations between the WOMAC pain and function subscales and reported a median correlation of r = 0.76 (range 0.64–0.86), which suggests that the pain and functional scales may have considerable overlap (Ryser et al., 1999). Therefore, it is plausible that both subscales may be providing similar information regarding patient status or that the pain scale might be measuring pain during functional activities rather than the construct of pain in isolation (Gandek, 2015).

The Hip Disability and Osteoarthritis Outcome Score (HOOS) is an additional PROM recommended for use in adults with arthritic hip pain and has been designed as an extension of the WOMAC. The HOOS consists of 5 subscales: pain (10 items), other symptoms (5 items; 3 for symptoms and 2 for stiffness), function in activities of daily living (17 items), function in sport/recreation (4 items), and hip-related quality of life (4 items). Each item is scored on a 5-point Likert scale ranging from 0 to 4 (no, mild, moderate, severe, and extreme). Scores are summarized for each subscale and transformed to a 0–100 scale (0 indicates extreme problems, and 100 indicates no problems).

In a sample of 88 patients with hip OA, Ornetti et al. (2010) found the reliability of the HOOS to be ICC 0.83 (0.70–0.90), 0.84 (0.72–0.91), 0.86 (0.76–0.92), 0.89 (0.80–0.94), 0.86 (0.76–0.92) for the pain, symptoms, function ADL, function sport/recreating, and quality of life domains, respectively. Kemp et al. (2013) found slightly higher values with the ICC ranging from 0.92 to 0.96 for the 5 subscales, but this was in a population that had undergone arthroscopy for a myriad of disorders which might have resulted in the difference. Ornetti et al. (2010) also identified the MDC to be as 15.1 for pain, 10.5 for symptoms, 9.6 for ADLs, 15.5 for sports/recreation and 16.2 for quality of life, which is nearly identical to the findings of Kemp et al. (2013), which ranged between 9 and 17.

This section of the chapter intended to provide a brief insight as to some of the commonly used PROMs for individuals with hip disorders. While the list is not exhaustive, it provides several commonly used PROMs in both the clinical and research setting. Additionally, while the focus here was on individuals with non-arthritic and arthritic hip pain, many of the aforementioned PROMs have also been recommended for use in a population status post total hip arthroplasty (Nilsdotter & Bremander, 2011). For example, Stratford et al. (2009, 2010) examined the measurement properties of the LEFS in individuals with both total hip and total knee replacements. These findings suggest the LEFS exhibits excellent test–retest reliability (r = 0.85–0.90), which is like that in the population with arthritic hip pain.

PROMs for Knee Disorders (Table 9.2)

Many knee PROMs are available for use in clinical and research applications. In addition to hip disorders, the LEFS and WOMAC are also often used for the assessment of the knee. Other common assessments of knee outcomes include the Knee Injury and Osteoarthritis Outcome Score (KOOS), International Knee Documentation Committee Subjective Knee Form (IKDC), Oxford Knee Score (OKS), and Victorian Institute of Sport Assessment Patella Tendinopathy (VISA-P).

The LEFS, as described above, is utilized for many lower extremity conditions and is frequently employed in knee conditions. A systematic review reported strong test–retest reliability (ICC 0.81–0.99) for anterior knee pain, knee OA, total knee arthroplasty, and multiple lower extremity conditions (Mehta et al., 2016). Construct validity for LEFS in knee disorders is supported through a high correlation with both WOMAC and KOOS (Mehta et al., 2016). In a sample of 284 Dutch individuals with knee OA, Hoogeboom et al. (2012) reported moderate to strong correlation (r = 0.60–0.78) between the LEFS and all KOOS subscales. Variability in MDC of 14.1–18.1 has been reported in patients with knee OA (Williams et al., 2012) and 8.0 in patients with anterior knee pain (Watson et al., 2005).

Similar to LEFS, the WOMAC has been used in both hip and knee conditions. A systematic review by Gandek (2015) reported strong test–retest reliability for function (0.92, 95%CI 0.84–0.96), pain (0.85, 95%CI 0.74–0.98), and stiffness (0.80, 95%CI 0.52–0.90) for patients with knee OA. In a sample of 168 patients with knee OA, Williams et al. (2012) reported comparable reliability and responsiveness between WOMAC and LEFS. At two-month follow-up reliability of LEFS and WOMAC were ICC 0.81 (95%CI 0.63–0.91) and 0.90 (95%CI 0.76–0.95) while MDC values were 15.4 and 13.4, respectively. Escobar et al. (2007) reported a similar MDC for patients post total knee arthroplasty in the function subscale (13.1) but greater values for pain (22.4) and stiffness (29.1).

TABLE 9.2 Summary of Patient-reported Outcome Measures (PROMs) for Knee Disorders

PROM	Knee disorder	Domains	Score/interpretation	Examples of measurement properties investigated*
Lower Extremity Functional Scale (LEFS)	Knee pain and knee osteoarthritis	Standing, squatting, walking, lifting, getting in and out of the car, and performing usual activities	20 items (0–80). Higher scores indicate greater levels of function	Sufficient reliability and construct validity
Western Ontario and McMaster Universities Osteoarthritis Index (WOMAC)	Knee osteoarthritis	Pain, stiffness, and physical function	24 items (0–20 for pain, 0–8 for stiffness, and 0–68 for physical function. Higher scores indicate worse outcomes	Sufficient reliability and construct validity
Knee Injury and Osteoarthritis Outcome Score (KOOS)	Knee injuries or osteoarthritis (young to older adults)	Pain, symptoms, activities of daily living, sport and recreation, and knee-related quality of life	42 items (0–100). Higher scores indicate no knee problems	Sufficient reliability, construct validity, and responsiveness
International Knee Documentation Committee Subjective Knee Form (IKDC)	Various knee conditions	Symptoms, sports activities, and function domains	18 items (0–100). Higher scores indicate no limitation or symptoms	Sufficient reliability
Oxford Knee Score (OKS)	Total knee arthroplasty	Individual's activities of daily living and how they have been affected by pain over the preceding four weeks	12 items (12–60). Higher scores indicate more difficulty or severity	Sufficient reliability, construct validity, and responsiveness
Victorian Institute of Sport Assessment Patella Tendinopathy (VISA-P)	Patellar tendinopathy	Symptoms, function, and ability to undertake sport	8 items (0–100). Higher scores indicate higher levels of performance	Sufficient reliability and construct validity

* Interpretation according to the original report.

Another PROM often utilized is the Knee Injury and Osteoarthritis Outcome Score (KOOS), a self-administered PROM intended for young to older adults and individuals with knee injuries or osteoarthritis (Roos et al., 1998). The KOOS, built as an extension of the WOMAC, contains 42 items covering five domains – pain (9 items), symptoms (7 items), activities of daily living (ADL) (17 items), sport and recreation (5 items), and knee-related quality of life (4 items) – each scored separately. Each item is scored from 0 to 4, with higher values representing more severe limitations. The score for each domain is determined by summing the total responses for each answered item divided by the total possible points for answered items then subtracting that value from 100. Final score for each domain ranges from 0, representing extreme knee problems, and 100, representing no knee problems. A systematic review and meta-analysis reported the KOOS has good reliability, construct validity, and responsiveness across knee disorders (Collins et al., 2016). The authors found excellent test–retest reliability for pain (ICC 0.89, 95%CI 0.87–0.91), symptoms (ICC 0.87, 95%CI 0.84–0.89), ADL (ICC 0.90, 95%CI 0.87–0.92), sport and recreation (ICC 0.85, 95%CI 0.80–0.89), and knee-related quality of life (ICC 0.87, 95%CI 0.83–0.90) domains. The smallest detectable change (SDC) ranged from 15.7 for activities of daily living to 25.1 for sport and recreation. The SDC reportedly varied based upon age and diagnosis with greater SDC for older adults and those with knee arthritis compared to younger individuals or those with an anterior cruciate ligament injury. Content validity was reportedly greater for ADL subscale in older adults with sports and recreational subscale for younger adults. These findings suggest individual domains may be more useful in some patients with knee pain than others. For example, the sport and recreation subscale may be appropriate for younger patients but not relevant for older age groups for which the ADL subscale may be better suited.

The International Knee Documentation Committee (IKDC) Subjective Knee Form is intended for various knee conditions containing 18 items covering symptoms, sports activities, and function domains (Grevnerts et al., 2015; Irrgang et al., 2001). Item scoring includes ordinal scales of differing length with lower values representing lowest function or highest symptoms. Individual item scores are summed and transformed with a final score of 0 representing severe limitation and 100 representing no limitation or symptoms. The original validation study identified test–retest reliability ICC of 0.94 (95%CI 0.88–0.97) and SEM of 4.6 (Irrgang et al., 2001).

The measurement properties of IKDC have been investigated in patients with various knee conditions (Kanakamedala et al., 2016). It has excellent test–retest reliability ICC 0.85–0.99 with an MDC of 8.8–16.4 and strong construct validity compared to the various outcomes (Kanakamedala et al., 2016). A systematic review of PROMs in individuals with patellofemoral pain identified adequate measurement

properties for IKDC with ICC ranging from 0.92–0.99 and an MDC of 6.7–13.0 (Esculier et al., 2013). Greco et al. (2010) reported similar reliability (ICC 0.91–0.93) and slightly higher MDC (13.7–15.6) in patients with articular cartilage lesions. In individuals with anterior cruciate ligament rupture, the IKDC demonstrated excellent test–retest reliability ICC 0.93 (95%CI 0.89–0.96) with an SDC of 12.2 (van Meer et al., 2013). Given these findings, the IKDC could be considered a reasonable tool for assessing symptoms, activity limitations, and participation restrictions in patients with knee pain.

While the LEFS, WOMAC, KOOS, and IKDC can be used to assess patients with a variety of conditions, other PROMs are designed for specific patient populations. The Oxford Knee Score (OKS) is designed to assess PRO for patients receiving total knee arthroplasty. This PROM assesses individuals' activities of daily living and how they have been affected by pain over the preceding four weeks (Dawson et al., 1998). It contains 12 items each scored from 1 to 5 and totaled to determine a combined score from 12 to 60, with greater scores representing more difficulty or severity. Dawson et al. (1998) reported good reliability (r = 0.92), construct validity, and responsiveness in the original report. Impellizzeri et al. (2020) reported comparable reliability (ICC 0.91) with an MDC of 6.1 and moderate correlation with WOMAC subscales (r = 0.45–0.67) after total knee arthroplasty. A study of 94,015 patients after total knee replacement resulted in a slightly lesser MDC of 4.15 (Beard et al., 2015). The OKS demonstrated utility in patients after total knee arthroplasty; however, this has not been meaningfully validated in other knee conditions.

The Victorian Institute of Sport Assessment Patellar Tendinopathy (VISA-P) questionnaire was developed to assess symptoms, function, and ability to undertake sport in patients with patellar tendinopathy (Visentini et al., 1998). VISA-P contains 8 items, with 6 items utilizing a 0–10 visual analog scale and 2 items on an ordinal scale. Total scores range from 0 to 100, with greater scores representing higher levels of performance. A systematic review reported strong construct and known group validity, strong reliability (r = 0.96, 95%CI 0.95–0.98), and responsiveness for the VISA-P in patients with patellar tendinopathy (Korakakis et al., 2021). Like the OKS for total knee arthroplasty, the VISA-P demonstrates sufficient measurement properties for the assessment of PROM in patellar tendinopathy.

This section of the chapter presented some of the typical PROMs used in individuals with knee disorders. The measures presented are intended to be a sample of those employed in clinical and research practice. Some knee PROMs (LEFS and WOMAC) demonstrate utility in the hip and other areas of the lower extremity. In comparison, other PROMs (KOOS and IKDC) are useful for a variety of knee disorders or specific knee-related conditions (OKS and VISA-P).

Keys to Successful and Meaningful Clinical Application

Although PROMs have become somewhat ubiquitous in clinical practice, few clinicians optimize their use in the management of patients with hip and knee pain disorders. The following eight suggestions are designed to improve the integration of outcome measures into clinical practice, increase the understanding of the measures, and further the engagement of the patient by anchoring the outcomes to their patient encounter.

Tip One: Capture the Outcomes Before the Patient Encounters and Reads Them

Although most researchers and clinicians have adopted a standardized approach to collecting outcome measures, it is our experience that few clinicians actually *read* the measures before engaging the patient during care. Reading the outcomes does several things. First, it substantiates "why" the patient is completing the document. Keep in mind that the patient is often required to complete a great deal of paperwork and will not see the value in completing an outcome measure realistically if the clinician does not emphasize the importance. Secondly, embed this as a "routine" during the patient encounter (Wu et al., 2014). Patients will easily assume the standard pattern of care if given the opportunity. Lastly, if completing the measure is taking too much time during the clinic visit, schedule the patient earlier for the next visit.

Tip Two: Take the Time and Score the Findings

Most hip and knee outcome measures have measurement values that are meaningful and are designed to give perspective of the severity of the patient's condition. A majority will give perspective regarding the patient change from visit to visit which may be meaningful for prognosis. Measures such as the Short-Form 12 (SF-12) or the Patient-Reported Outcomes Measurement Information System (PROMIS) measures, are t-score based, thus raw scores mean very little (Nwachukwu et al., 2020). Having a conversion chart handy will give the clinician a firmer understanding of how the values are related to the population as a whole.

Tip Three: Develop a Routine Timing for Data Capture

There is no hard and fast rule on how often one should capture outcome measures. Certainly, early in the patient care process, one will see greater changes in the patient's condition. We suggest a weekly capture of data that becomes part of the management sequence of the patient.

Tip Four: Share the Results with the Patient and Follow Up in Areas of Concern

It is also our experience (one that has been shared with others) that few clinicians discuss the scores with their patients (Wu et al., 2014). Most outcome measures include multiple functional activities that may or may not be problematic for the patient. The outcome measures will improve communication, and since content validity is often the weakest element of an outcome measure, having a detailed conversation about "why" the patient scored the instrument the way they did may lead to meaningful intervention choices.

Tip Five: Understand What an Outcome Measure Actually Measures

Most outcome measures measure health status. That said, there are a number of things in addition to the hip and knee problem that may influence the score of the tool. Patients with comorbidities or long-term chronic illnesses will have lower overall region-specific measures. These individuals will often have lower change scores as well since many of the chronic conditions are difficult to change and are not the focus of the care at hand.

Tip Six: Recognize the Strengths and Weaknesses of Minimally Clinically Important Difference Scores

Despite its multiple limitations, a MCID score is a necessary evil in clinical practice (Cook, 2008). It is best used as a conversational measure with the patient. Since MCIDs vary depending on the patient population, their severity, and gender, its best considered a "soft" measure of meaningful change (Young et al., 2009). The patient will be the best person to determine whether their experience is clinically meaningful or not, regardless of what change score you calculate (Fernandez et al., 2017).

Tip Seven: Emphasize Identified Differences Over Time and Address This with the Patient

When one experiences a musculoskeletal problem, it's often difficult to recognize the slow change over time. The outcome measures provide the ability to show change over time and can give context to the changes you see as the treating clinician. On the other hand, the tools can also show the patient when the patient's progress has plateaued and help determine when it's time to try something different (Wu et al., 2014).

Tip Eight: Document, Document and Document

A majority of the change seen in outcome measures for patients with musculoskeletal conditions is related to natural history (or time). Consequently, document the change over time to show steady progress for third-party payer sources or any other regulatory body that requires routine data capture. It also gives one an estimate of the typical prognosis for patient conditions, an element that is complicated and often takes years of understanding.

Conclusion

Clinical measures are more commonly used to quantify and/or describe patients' impairments in body functions and structures. Patient-reported outcome measures are one of many clinical measures widely used in clinical practice. There are several considerations when selecting a PROM for a patient with knee and/or pain disorders, including the pathology, current presentation (acute, subacute, or chronic), outcome of interest, current functional level, baseline sociodemographic, and comorbidity conditions. Beyond patient-related factors the clinician must also consider whether the focus is on generic or disease-specific measures, the method of scoring and interpretation of the results, the respondent burden, the administrative burden, ease of implementation, cost, and the measurement properties. A PROM that has demonstrated sufficient reliability produces stable results over time. A PROM that has demonstrated sufficient validity is said to correctly capture what is supposed to be measured, whereas a responsive PROM has demonstrated the ability to detect change in the phenomenon of interest. Finally, outcome measures are only meaningful when used in a meaningful, routine fashion. Using the eight tips suggested will improve implementation into clinical practice and improve the clinician's ability to provide quality care.

References

Beard DJ, Harris K, Dawson J, et al. Meaningful changes for the Oxford hip and knee scores after joint replacement surgery. J Clin Epidemiol. 2015;68:73–9.

Binkley JM, Stratford PW, Lott SA, Riddle DL. The Lower Extremity Functional Scale (LEFS): scale development, measurement properties, and clinical application. North American Orthopaedic Rehabilitation Research Network. PhysTher. 1999;79:371–83.

Black N. Patient reported outcome measures could help transform healthcare. BMJ. 2013;346:f167.

Chiarotto A. Patient-Reported Outcome Measures: Best is the enemy of good (but what if good is not good enough?). J Orthop Sports Phys Ther. 2019;49:39–42.

Collins NJ, Prinsen CA, Christensen R, et al. Knee Injury and Osteoarthritis Outcome Score (KOOS): systematic review and meta-analysis of measurement properties. Osteoarthritis Cartilage. 2016;24:1317–29.

Cook CE. Clinimetrics Corner: The Minimal Clinically Important Change Score (MCID): A Necessary Pretense. J Man Manip Ther. 2008;16:E82–3.

Dawson J, Fitzpatrick R, Murray D, Carr A. Questionnaire on the perceptions of patients about total knee replacement. J Bone Joint Surg Br. 1998;80:63–9.

Enseki K, Harris-Hayes M, White DM, et al. Nonarthritic hip joint pain. J Orthop Sports Phys Ther. 2014;44:A1–32.

Escobar A, Quintana JM, Bilbao A, et al. Responsiveness and clinically important differences for the WOMAC and SF-36 after total knee replacement. Osteoarthritis Cartilage. 2007;15:273–80.

Esculier JF, Roy JS, Bouyer LJ. Psychometric evidence of self-reported questionnaires for patellofemoral pain syndrome: a systematic review. Disabil Rehabil. 2013;35:2181–90.

Fernandez B, Dore L, Velanovich V. Patient-centered outcomes in surgical research and practice. J Gastrointest Surg. 2017;21:892–5.

Gandek B. Measurement properties of the Western Ontario and McMaster Universities Osteoarthritis Index: a systematic review. Arthritis Care Res. 2015;67:216–29.

Giezen H, Stevens M, van den Akker-Scheek I, Reininga IHF. Validity and reliability of the Dutch version of the Copenhagen Hip And Groin Outcome Score (HAGOS-NL) in patients with hip pathology. PLoS One. 2017;12:e0186064.

Greco NJ, Anderson AF, Mann BJ, et al. Responsiveness of the International Knee Documentation Committee Subjective Knee Form in comparison to the Western Ontario and McMaster Universities Osteoarthritis Index, modified Cincinnati Knee Rating System, and Short Form 36 in patients with focal articular cartilage defects. Am J Sports Med. 2010;38:891–902.

Grevnerts HT, Terwee CB, Kvist J. The measurement properties of the IKDC-subjective knee form. Knee Surg Sports Traumatol Arthrosc. 2015;23:3698–706.

Griffin DR, Parsons N, Mohtadi NG, Safran MR. A short version of the International Hip Outcome Tool (iHOT-12) for use in routine clinical practice. Arthroscopy. 2012;28:611–16

Hawkins M, Elsworth, GR, Osborne RH. Application of validity theory and methodology to patient-reported outcome measures (PROMs): building an argument for validity. Qual Life Res. 2018;27:1695–710

Hoogeboom TJ, de Bie RA, den Broeder AA, van den Ende CH. The Dutch Lower Extremity Functional Scale was highly reliable, valid and responsive in individuals with hip/knee osteoarthritis: a validation study. BMC Musculoskelet Disord. 2012;13:117.

Impellizzeri FM, Jones DM, Griffin D, et al. Patient-reported outcome measures for hip-related pain: a review of the available evidence and a consensus statement from the International Hip-related Pain Research Network, Zurich 2018. Br J Sports Med. 2020;54:848–57.

Irrgang JJ, Anderson AF, Boland AL, et al. Development and validation of the international knee documentation committee subjective knee form. Am J Sports Med. 2001;29:600–13.

Jewell DV. Guide to evidence-based physical therapist practice. Burlington, MA: Jones & Bartlett Publishers, 2014.

Kanakamedala AC, Anderson AF, Irrgang JJ. IKDC Subjective Knee Form and Marx Activity Rating Scale are suitable to evaluate all orthopaedic sports medicine knee conditions: a systematic review. Journal of ISAKOS: Joint Disorders & Orthopaedic Sports Medicine. 2016;1:25–31.

Kemp JL, Collins NJ, Roos EM, Crossley KM. Psychometric properties of patient-reported outcome measures for hip arthroscopic surgery. Am J Sports Med. 2013;41:2065–73.

Korakakis V, Whiteley R, Kotsifaki A, et al. Systematic review evaluating the clinimetric properties of the Victorian Institute of Sport Assessment (VISA) questionnaires for lower limb tendinopathy shows moderate to high-quality evidence for sufficient reliability, validity and responsiveness-part II. Knee Surg Sports Traumatol Arthrosc. 2021;29(9):2765–88.

Marshall S, Haywood K, Fitzpatrick R. Impact of patient-reported outcome measures on routine practice: a structured review. J Eval Clin Pract. 2006;12:559–68.

Martin RL, Kelly BT, Philippon MJ. Evidence of validity for the hip outcome score. Arthroscopy. 2006;22:1304–11.

Martin RL, Philippon MJ. Evidence of validity for the hip outcome score in hip arthroscopy. Arthroscopy. 2007;23:822–6.

Martin RL, Philippon MJ. Evidence of reliability and responsiveness for the hip outcome score. Arthroscopy. 2008;24:676–82.

Mehta SP, Fulton A, Quach C, et al. Measurement properties of the Lower Extremity Functional Scale: A systematic review. J Orthop Sports Phys Ther. 2016;46:200–16.

Mohtadi NG, Griffin DR, Pedersen ME, et al. The development and validation of a self-administered quality-of-life outcome measure for young, active patients with symptomatic hip disease: the International Hip Outcome Tool (iHOT-33). Arthroscopy. 2012;28:595–605

Mokkink LB, de Vet HCW, Prinsen CAC, et al. COSMIN Risk of Bias checklist for systematic reviews of Patient-Reported Outcome Measures. Qual Life Res. 2018;27:1171–9.

Nilsdotter A, Bremander A. Measures of hip function and symptoms: Harris Hip Score (HHS), Hip Disability and Osteoarthritis Outcome Score (HOOS), Oxford Hip Score (OHS), Lequesne Index of Severity for Osteoarthritis of the Hip (LISOH), and American Academy of Orthopedic Surgeons (AAOS) Hip and Knee Questionnaire. Arthritis Care Res. 2011;63:S200–7.

Nwachukwu BU, Beletsky A, Naveen N, et al. Patient-Reported Outcomes Measurement Information System (PROMIS) Instruments correlate better with legacy measures in knee cartilage patients at postoperative than at preoperative assessment. Arthroscopy. 2020;36:1419–28.

Ornetti P, Parratte S, Gossec L, et al. Cross-cultural adaptation and validation of the French version of the Hip disability and Osteoarthritis Outcome Score (HOOS) in hip osteoarthritis patients. Osteoarthritis Cartilage. 2010;18:522–9.

Prinsen CAC, Mokkink LB, Bouter LM, et al. COSMIN guideline for systematic reviews of patient-reported outcome measures. Qual Life Res. 2018;27:1147–57.

Pua YH, Cowan SM, Wrigley TV, Bennell KL. The Lower Extremity Functional Scale could be an alternative to the Western Ontario and McMaster Universities Osteoarthritis Index physical function scale. J Clin Epidemiol. 2009;62:1103–1111.

Roos EM, Roos HP, Lohmander LS, et al. Knee Injury and Osteoarthritis Outcome Score (KOOS)-development of a self-administered outcome measure. J Orthop Sports Phys Ther. 1998;28:88–96.

Ryser L, Wright BD, Aeschlimann A, et al. New look at the Western Ontario and McMaster Universities Osteoarthritis Index using Rasch analysis. Arthritis Care Res. 1999;12:331–5.

Sorensen NL, Hammeken LH, Thomsen JL, Ehlers LH. Implementing patient-reported outcomes in clinical decision-making within knee and hip osteoarthritis: an explorative review. BMC Musculoskelet Disord. 2019;20:230.

Stratford PW, Kennedy DM, Riddle DL. New study design evaluated the validity of measures to assess change after hip or knee arthroplasty. J Clin Epidemiol. 2009;62:347–52.

Stratford PW, Kennedy DM, Maly MR, Macintyre NJ. Quantifying self-report measures' overestimation of mobility scores postarthroplasty. Phys Ther. 2010;90:1288–96.

Terwee CB, Prinsen CAC, Chiarotto A, et al. COSMIN methodology for evaluating the content validity of patient-reported outcome measures: a Delphi study. Qual Life Res. 2018;27:1159–70.

Thorborg K, Holmich P, Christensen R, et al. The Copenhagen Hip and Groin Outcome Score (HAGOS): development and validation according to the COSMIN checklist. Br J Sports Med. 2011;45:478–91.

van Meer BL, Meuffels DE, Vissers MM, et al. Knee injury and Osteoarthritis Outcome Score or International Knee Documentation Committee Subjective Knee Form: which questionnaire is most useful to monitor patients with an anterior cruciate ligament rupture in the short term? Arthroscopy. 2013;29:701–15.

Visentini PJ, Khan KM, Cook JL, et al. The VISA score: an index of severity of symptoms in patients with jumper's knee (patellar tendinosis). J Sci Med Sport. 1998;1:22–8.

Watson CJ, Propps M, Ratner J, et al. Reliability and responsiveness of the lower extremity functional scale and the anterior knee pain scale in patients with anterior knee pain. J Orthop Sports Phys Ther. 2005;35:136–46.

Weldring T, Smith SM. Patient-Reported Outcomes (PROs) and Patient-Reported Outcome Measures (PROMs). Health Serv Insights. 2013;6:61–8.

Williams K, Sansoni J, Darcy M, et al. Patient-reported outcome measures. Literature review.

Sydney: Australian Commission on Safety and Quality in Health Care, 2016.

Williams VJ, Piva SR, Irrgang JJ, et al. Comparison of reliability and responsiveness of patient-reported clinical outcome measures in knee osteoarthritis rehabilitation. J Orthop Sports Phys Ther. 2012;42:716–23.

Wilson I, Bohm E, Lubbeke A, et al. Orthopaedic registries with patient-reported outcome measures. EFORT Open Rev. 2019;4:357–67.

Wu AW, Bradford AN, Velanovich V, et al. Clinician's checklist for reading and using an article about patient-reported outcomes. Mayo Clin Proc. 2014;89:653–61.

Young BA, Walker MJ, Strunce JB, et al. Responsiveness of the Neck Disability Index in patients with mechanical neck disorders. Spine J. 2009;9:802–8.

Sono-anatomy and scanning technique of hip and knee

Suresh Sudula, Benoy Mathew, Alfred Markovits

Introduction

Diagnostic ultrasonography (US) is a non-invasive imaging procedure, which has been gaining in popularity in musculoskeletal (MSK) medicine in the last decade. The earliest use of US application in MSK medicine dates back to 1972 when it was utilized to differentiate Baker's cyst from thrombophlebitis (McDonald & Leopold, 1972). Ultrasound imaging can be performed over an area of concern, providing a dynamic instant image of the structures directly under the transducer. Furthermore, a limb or joint of interest can be moved in various planes to mimic and reproduce symptoms under real-time image analysis as part of the objective evaluation. Unlike other imaging modalities such as X-rays and computed tomography (CT), ultrasound has no contraindications and does not expose the patient to ionizing radiation. Further, it is economically affordable, easily accessible and provides real-time dynamic visualization of muscle, tendons, ligaments, and joints.

The addition of US to the physical examination adds to the sensitivity of the physical examination for identification of pathology and improves clinical diagnostic accuracy in musculoskeletal and rheumatology settings (Ciurtin et al., 2019). Ultrasound in the hands of an experienced user provides excellent image quality of soft tissues. With advances in technology, access to training, cost reduction and availability, it is expected that more clinicians will be utilizing ultrasound in their clinics in the diagnosis and management of MSK disorders. The objective of this chapter is to briefly review the relevant anatomy and scanning technique of the hip and knee region, as part of MSK clinical evaluation. It focuses primarily on the needs of the practicing MSK clinicians who manage patients with hip and knee disorders.

Ultrasound Basics

Ultrasound functions using the principle of reverse piezoelectric effect, where electrical energy passing through a crystal vibrates to create sound waves (Smith & Finnoff, 2009). These waves become attenuated as they pass through human tissue, due to loss of energy. Some waves are absorbed, while others are diverged or deflected. Depending on the type of structure and the depth of the tissue, an appropriate transducer is chosen for MSK evaluation. A high-frequency linear transducer (usually 12 MHz+) has higher resolution and is preferred for the majority of scanning in MSK examination. A low-frequency transducer (5–8 MHz range) is useful for imaging deeper structures, such as the hip, but it compromises image quality with poorer resolutions. Image quality correlates directly with the frequency of the transducer. Therefore, high-frequency waves provide excellent superficial tissue resolution, while low-frequency waves provide better visualization for deeper structures. For smaller areas, such as joints of the hand or foot, a "hockey-stick" probe is useful due to the smaller footprint and ease of access.

Most modern machines have in-built Doppler technology, which is useful to identify blood flow in the tissues and to distinguish fluid moving away and toward the probe. Color Doppler shows directional flow in arteries and veins, whereas power Doppler displays the strength of the Doppler signal in color, rather than the speed and direction information. It has three times the sensitivity of conventional color Doppler for detection of flow (Babcock et al., 1996). This feature is particularly useful for tissues with a low flow such as pathological tendons or picking up hyperemia in areas of inflammation.

Key Terminology

Find below common terms in MSK diagnostic US which are utilized to describe tissue characteristics and imaging findings.

Transducer: The ultrasound probe that converts electrical energy into sound energy and receives back the ultrasound echoes.

Echogenicity: This term refers to the ability of the tissue to reflect ultrasound waves back towards the transducer and produce an echo. The higher the echogenicity, the brighter the structure appears in the ultrasound image (Figure 10.1).

Hyper, Hypo or Iso-echoic: These terms are used when making comparisons between the intensities of the echoes produced by the examined structure and the reference structure. Based on echogenicity, a structure can be termed

CHAPTER TEN

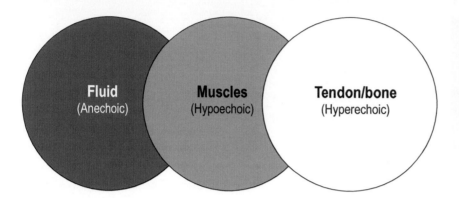

FIGURE 10.1
Echogenicity. Echogenicity refers to brightness of structures. Fluid is considered anechoic, tissues such as muscles can be considered hypoechoic, and tendon/bone on ultrasound is hyperechoic.

hyperechoic (white on the screen, Figure 10.2A) or hypoechoic (grey on the screen, Figure 10.2B). Hyperechoic images are bright and can be visualized at the interfaces between bone and soft tissue as the sound beam is strongly reflected to the transducer. Weak sound reflection leads to hypoechoic or darker images on the screen. Isoechoic is the term to describe a structure that is of similar echogenicity to the adjacent tissues.

Anechoic: Refers to a structure that returns no echoes and is used for any structure that is entirely crossed by the ultrasound beam without any reflection and displayed as a jet-black image on the screen. Typical examples would be a simple cyst and blood vessels. Bone appears anechoic on US, with a bright hyperechoic rim, since the US beam is unable to penetrate the bone. When the sound beam is perpendicular to the bone, the cortex will appear hyperechoic and well defined (Figure 10.2C).

Acoustic Shadowing: Decreased echoes, and thus a darkening of the image, deep to an echogenic structure due to attenuation of the ultrasound beam reaching the deeper structures.

Acoustic Enhancement: It is also called posterior enhancement and refers to the increased echoes, deep to the structures that transmit sound exceptionally well. This is characteristic of fluid-filled structures such as cysts.

Anisotropy: This is a term to describe an artifact encountered in MSK ultrasound, particularly in tendons. It is a phenomenon whereby a structure changes its echogenicity depending on the angle of the transducer relative to the structure. It occurs secondary to the amount of sound beam that is reflected back to the transducer based on the angle of the beam reflected off the structure of interest.

When the ultrasound beam is incident on a fibrillar structure such as a tendon, the organized fibrils may reflect the majority of the sound beam in a direction away from the transducer. When this occurs, the transducer does not receive the returning echo and assumes the corresponding area to be hypoechoic. This may falsely lead to a diagnosis of tendinopathy or tendon tear (Ihnatsenka et al., 2010). Changing the angle as little as 3 to 5 degrees relative to the perpendicular can result in a hyperechoic structure (expected healthy tendon) appearing hypoechoic (pathologic) as fewer sound waves are reflected to the transducer. To minimize the artifact of anisotropy, it is ideal to align the probe perpendicular to the structure of interest.

Probe Position (Short and Long Axis): The position of the ultrasound probe is usually described, relative to the direction of the structure of interest. For example, a long axis of the Achilles tendon would be a sagittal view (Figure 10.3A). A short axis of the Achilles tendon would be a cross-sectional view of the tendon (Figure 10.3B). Ultrasound scanning should include visualizing the target structure in the long axis and short axis when applicable.

Applied Anatomy of the Hip Region

The hip is a ball and socket joint connecting the lower limb to the axial skeleton, which provides both stability and mobility. As a multi-axial ball and socket synovial joint, the hip is capable of motion in all three planes. Control of the hip joint during movement involves complex interactions between the nervous, muscular, and skeletal systems (Ward et al., 2010). The peak contact forces at the hip joint are two to three times the body weight during level walking and more than seven times the body weight during stair climbing

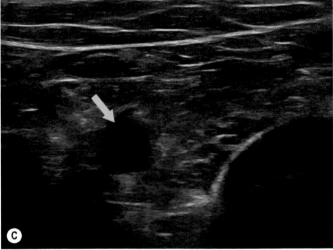

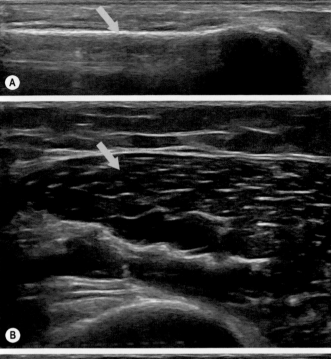

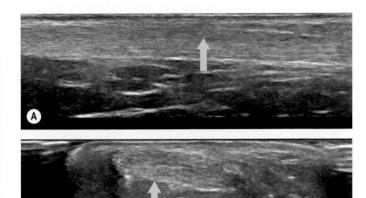

FIGURE 10.3
Long and short axis views. (A) Long axis demonstrating the fibrillar pattern of the tendon (arrow) with parallel hyperechoic line. (B) Short axis demonstrating an ovoid tendon (arrow) containing bright clustered dots.

FIGURE 10.2
Hyper-, hypo- and anechoic. (A) Hyperechoic bony cortex of a metatarsal. (B) Hypoechoic appearance of the vastus medialis muscle. (C) Anechoic appearance of popliteal vessel in the popliteal fossa.

(Bergmann et al., 2001). There are multiple anatomical structures in and around the hip joint and this section will mainly focus on the structures in the anterolateral aspect of the hip in keeping with the scanning protocols outlined in the chapter.

The anterolateral aspect of the hip can be divided into three layers, based on distinct anatomical levels:

1. Joint level (shaded in blue, Figure 10.4)

2. Ilium level (shaded in green, Figure 10.4)

3. Crest level (shaded in yellow, Figure 10.4)

The joint level consists of the joint cartilage, capsule (including the capsular ligaments) and labrum. These structures can be found just inferior to the anterior inferior iliac spine (AIIS) and within the acetabular region and over the neck of the femur. The hip joint capsule is a sleeve-like structure enclosing the hip joint structure originating from the acetabulum and labrum. The anterior aspect of the capsule consists of the strong and thick iliofemoral ligament (Walters et al., 2014). The space between the tight anterior joint capsule and the neck of the femur is called the anterior joint recess (Nestorova et al., 2012). Medially, the anterior aspect of the femoral head that is not in contact with the acetabulum can be seen, overlaid by capsule and the iliopsoas muscles. The structures above are all described in orientation with the angle of the neck of the femur.

The next level up is the ilium level, which is made up of the structures originating on the ilium between the muscles. The long muscles consist of the rectus femoris and hamstrings, which both cross the hip and knee joints. The short muscles consist of the gluteus medius, minimus, iliopsoas, and the six small lateral rotators of the hip.

These muscles all share a common insertion around the proximal femoral neck (Philippon et al., 2014). Starting laterally, the gluteus medius is attached at the ilium under the crest, covering the gluteus minimus and converging into a tendon, inserting on the lateral aspect of the greater trochanter. Deeper and anterior to it, the gluteus minimus originates on the ilium superior to the acetabulum and inserts on the anterior aspect of the greater trochanter. Moving more medially, slightly above the acetabulum, the AIIS is found, giving origin to the rectus femoris.

The iliopsoas is made up of two muscles, the psoas major and the iliacus. These originate on the lumbar and lower thoracic vertebrae and the iliacus originates on the ilium, mirroring the gluteus medius and minimus. They pass under the inguinal ligament and over the head of the femur to insert into the lesser trochanter.

The crest, at the superficial level, consists of structures originating on the ilium crest and the various bony landmarks. Structures originating at this level are relatively easy to follow and tend to stay superficial. The musculature and soft tissue originating at the crest level tend to cross both the hip and knee joint and act on both. Finding one's way around this level is fairly straightforward, by palpating the bony landmarks and following structures to their insertion.

This level consists of the sartorius and tensor fasciae latae (TFL) muscles that originate at the anterior superior iliac spine (ASIS). Sartorius will deviate medially to join the pes anserine tendons, at the medial aspect of the tibia and the TFL will remain laterally and is continuous with the iliotibial tract. This leads us posteriorly to the iliotibial band (ITB) and gluteal fascia that originate as a continuation line on the crest leading to the gluteus maximus originating at the posterior iliac crest, posterior–lateral aspect of the sacrum and coccyx, sacrotuberous ligament, thoracolumbar fascia, and gluteal aponeurosis.

Note that all the above structures, with the exception of the sartorius, blend and attach into the lateral fascia lata and pass over the greater trochanter of the femur forwards to the Gerdy tubercle on the proximal tibia.

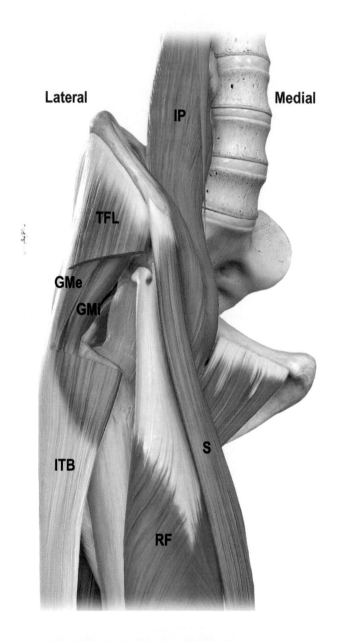

FIGURE 10.4
Applied anatomy of hip. Anterior view of the right hip with blue shading representing the deep capsular level. The structures in green represent the muscles originating at the ilium level. The structures at the crest level are in yellow. IP, Iliopsoas; TFL- Tensor Fasciae Latae, C, Capsule; GMe, Gluteus Medius; GMi, Gluteus Minimus; P, Pectineus; S, Sartorius; RF, Rectus Femoris; ITB, Iliotibial Band.

acetabulum and the iliac crest and under the inguinal ligament. This consists of two muscle groups: the long and short

Sono-anatomy and scanning technique of hip and knee

Ultrasound Evaluation of the Hip Region

Hip joint pathologies have traditionally been imaged with plain radiographs and MRI. However, more recently, innovative imaging techniques such as US have been widely applied to obtain a better understanding of the different soft tissue conditions, involving the hip region.

The clinician's ability to evaluate the hip joint pathologies depends on having expert knowledge of the scanning technique, the various anatomic areas to be examined, as well as optimizing the ultrasound scanner equipment setting. The hip is typically imaged using an intermediate frequency linear transducer (5–8 MHz). However, a curvilinear probe may be preferred to allow deep penetration and a wide depth of field. The highest frequency possible for the depth of the structures should be used. The routine scanning technique for ultrasound examination should consider the anterior, medial, lateral and posterior aspects of the hip as separate quadrants (Pinchcofsky et al., 2012).

For beginners, employing a systematic approach to each quadrant aids understanding of both ultrasound anatomy and scanning technique. To best examine the hip, the patient lies on the examination table with the aspect of the hip to be evaluated adequately exposed. Before starting to examine the patient's hip with ultrasound, two important steps should be considered. Firstly, the clinician should be aware of the essentials of the clinical history and also complete a physical examination to best focus the ultrasound examination on the appropriate structures of the hip. The clinical history should be focused on the duration of symptoms, characteristics of the pain (i.e., inflammatory or mechanical) and associated conditions. Physical examination should focus on differentiation between intra-articular and extra-articular disorders. The main limitation of US in hip evaluation is its partial accessibility to the deeper joint structures. This is due to the inability of the ultrasound beam to penetrate the bony cortex, resulting in frequent difficulties in the complete visualization of the hyaline cartilage.

Indications

Common diagnostic indications of musculoskeletal ultrasound in the anterolateral hip region include (Table 10.1):

- Hip joint effusion/synovitis
- Iliopsoas tendinopathy, bursitis and snapping iliopsoas tendon

TABLE 10.1 Checklist of Structures to Examine on Scanning of the Anterolateral Hip
Anterior Hip
1. Hip joint *(capsule, anterior synovial recess)*
2. Femoral head, femoral neck, acetabular and anterior labrum
3. Iliopsoas muscle, tendon and bursa
4. AIIS and the tendon and muscle of rectus femoris
5. ASIS and the tendons and muscles of sartorius and tensor fasciae latae (TFL)
Lateral Hip
1. Greater trochanter and bursae (if pathological)
2. Gluteus maximus, tensor fasciae latae (TFL) and the fascia lata
3. Gluteus medius muscle and tendon
4. Gluteus minimus muscle and tendon
5. Iliotibial band (ITB)

- Rectus femoris muscle and tendon pathology
- Gluteal medius and minimus tendinopathy and associated bursitis

Scanning Technique of Anterior Hip

The following structures should be evaluated over the anterior hip joint:

- Anterior joint recess and iliopsoas tendon/bursa
- Femoral neurovascular bundle
- Rectus femoris
- Tensor fasciae latae and sartorius

The hip joint is best evaluated in both longitudinal and transverse oblique planes obtained over the femoral neck.

1. Anterior joint recess and iliopsoas tendon/bursa

Patient position: The patient is supine, the hip is in a neutral position, a pillow positioned underneath the knee joint to keep anterior thigh muscles relaxed.

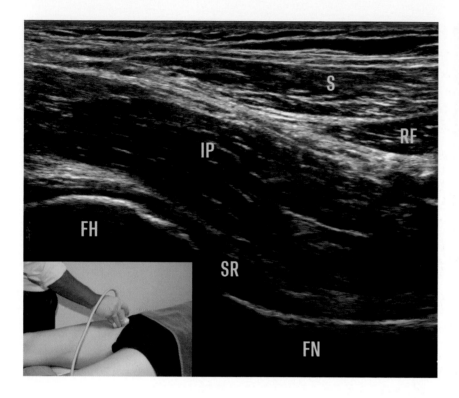

FIGURE 10.5
Longitudinal scan of the anterior recess of the hip joint. FH, femoral head; FN, femoral neck; SR, synovial recess; IP, iliopsoas muscle; S, sartorius; RF, rectus femoris.

Transducer: Place the transducer in an oblique longitudinal plane over the femoral neck to examine the anterior synovial recess, using the femoral head as a landmark (Figure 10.5).

Scanning tip: When examining this recess, care should be taken not to confuse the anterior and posterior layers of the joint capsule with an effusion, because the capsule may appear artifactually hypoechoic when imaging is not perpendicular to the ultrasound beam. Signs of inflammation, such as joint effusion, are not revealed by physical examination, due to the depth of the hip joint. However, with US, even small intra-articular effusion of the hip joint can be detected by measuring the distance between the neck of the femur and the joint capsule. A hip joint effusion is defined as a distance of 7 mm or greater between the femoral neck and the anterior joint capsule (Koski et al., 1989).

In obese or muscular patients, lower frequency probes may help with the examination. Cranial to the anterior recess, the fibrocartilaginous anterior labrum of the acetabulum can be detected as a homogeneously hyperechoic triangular structure (Figure 10.6). The iliofemoral ligament can also be appreciated superficial to the labrum.

Over the joint space and the femoral head, the iliopsoas muscle is identified lateral to the femoral neurovascular bundle. The iliopsoas tendon is found in a deep eccentric position within the posterior and medial part of the muscle belly and lies over the iliopectineal eminence (Martinoli et al., 2012).

Moving the transducer probe proximally in the transverse plane over the femoral head toward the iliac bone can demonstrate the myotendinous junction of the iliopsoas tendon as a bright hyperechoic dot surrounded by iliopsoas muscle against iliac bone. The iliopsoas bursa lies between the tendon and the anterior capsule of the hip joint. In normal subjects, it is collapsed and cannot be detected with ultrasound.

2. Femoral neurovascular bundle

Patient position: Supine with the hip in a neutral position, a pillow positioned underneath the knee joint to keep anterior thigh muscles relaxed.

Transducer: Place the transducer in a transverse plane over the medial edge of the iliopsoas muscle and tendon. Medial to the iliopsoas muscle and tendon, the femoral

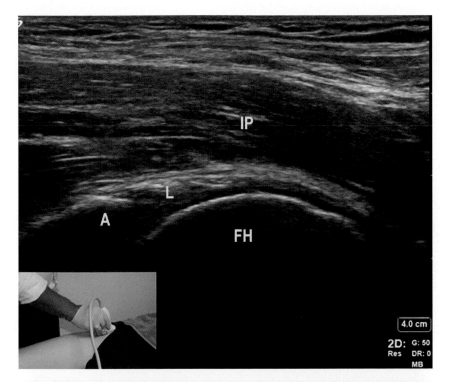

FIGURE 10.6
Longitudinal scan of the anterior hip joint.
FH, femoral head, A, acetabulum; L, labrum;
IP, iliopsoas muscle.

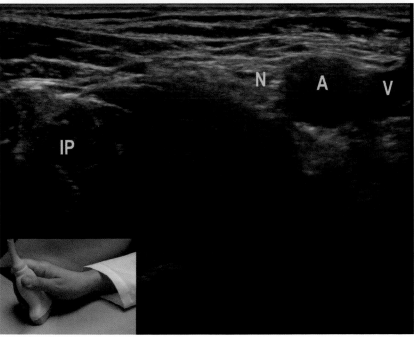

FIGURE 10.7
Transverse scan of the neurovascular
bundle. N, femoral nerve; A, femoral artery;
V, femoral vein; IP, iliopsoas muscle.

nerve (lateral structure), the common femoral artery and the common femoral vein (medial structure) can be visualized (Figure 10.7). The vein is larger than the artery and is compressible with the transducer. Further medially, the pectineus muscle can be seen over the pubis.

3. Rectus Femoris

Patient position: Supine with hip in a neutral position, a pillow positioned underneath knee joint to keep anterior thigh muscles relaxed.

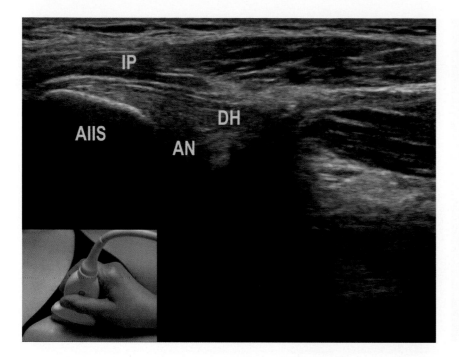

FIGURE 10.8
Longitudinal scan of the rectus femoris direct tendon. AIIS, anterior inferior iliac spine; DH, direct head of rectus femoris; IP, iliopsoas; AN, anisotropy created by indirect head.

Transducer: Place the transducer in a longitudinal plane over the anterior inferior iliac spine (AIIS) to examine the direct tendon of the rectus femoris. The origin can easily be identified as a linear bright structure with posterior acoustic shadowing that related to the indirect tendon of the rectus femoris muscle (Figure 10.8). Moving the transducer downward in the transverse plane can demonstrate the myotendinous junction of the rectus femoris with its muscle fibers that arise from the lateral aspect of the tendon. Further distally, the muscle belly is observed progressively enlarging between the TFL and the sartorius.

4. Tensor Fasciae Latae and Sartorius

Patient position: Supine with the hip in a neutral position, a pillow positioned underneath the knee joint to keep anterior thigh muscles relaxed.

Transducer: Place the transducer in a transverse plane over the ASIS. Just medial to the ASIS, the lateral femoral cutaneous nerve can occasionally be seen as a small tubular structure passing through a tunnel formed by a split in the lateral end of the inguinal ligament. The short tendons of the sartorius (medial) and the TFL (lateral) are visualized in sagittal planes (Figure 10.9). Move the probe down over the muscle bellies; the sartorius can be seen traveling medially to reach the medial thigh over the rectus femoris muscle, whereas the TFL proceeds laterally and caudally to insert into the anterior border of the fascia latae, superficial to the vastus lateralis.

Scanning Technique of Lateral Hip

The following structures should be evaluated over the lateral hip:

- The gluteal muscle and tendons
- Greater trochanter
- Trochanteric bursa
- Iliotibial band

Patient position: Lateral decubitus, affected side up.

Scan 1

Place transducer in longitudinal plane cranially to the greater trochanter, oriented toward the ASIS (Figure 10.10). This allows the visualization of the most superficial layer, which is the TFL or the gluteus maximus if scanned slightly posteriorly followed by gluteus medius and the deepest muscle is the gluteus minimus.

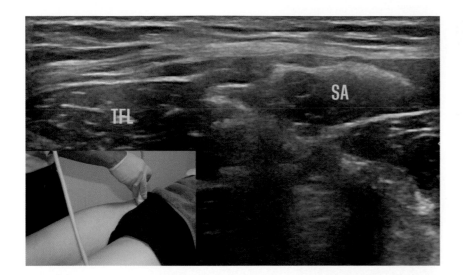

FIGURE 10.9
Transverse scan showing tensor fasciae latae (TFL) and sartorius (SA).

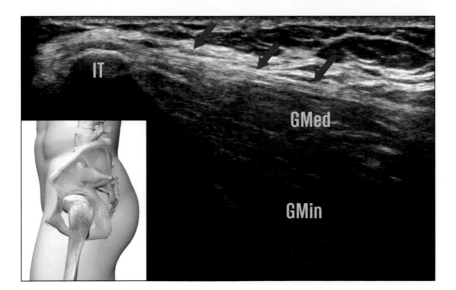

FIGURE 10.10
Longitudinal view of proximal iliotibial band (ITB). The probe is placed in a longitudinal plane over the iliac tubercle to show the normal appearance of the ITB (arrows) at the iliac tubercle (IT). Gmed, gluteus medius; Gmin, gluteus minimus.

Scan 2

Place transducer in the transverse plane over the greater trochanter and parallel to the lateral facet. Slide the transducer anteriorly to visualize the "rooftop" (Figure 10.11) appearance of the anterior and lateral facets and the round profile of the gluteus minimus tendon. On the anterior facet, you will find the gluteus minimus tendon and on the lateral facet gluteus medius tendon attachments. Signs of gluteus medius and minimus tendinopathy including tendon thickening, hypoechogenicity, loss of fibrillar pattern, cortical irregularity or calcifications can be assessed in this view (Klauser et al., 2013). Fluid accumulation or thickening of the bursa between the gluteus maximus and gluteus medius tendons suggests bursal inflammation (Chang et al., 2018).

Scan 3

Lateral hip tendons are best evaluated by placing the probe parallel to their long axis in order to avoid anisotropic effects. Place the transducer in the longitudinal plane over the anterior aspect of the greater trochanter. The gluteus minimus tendon is appreciated anteriorly as a hyperechoic structure that arises from the deep aspect of the muscle to insert into the anterior facet of the greater trochanter. Moving the transducer posteriorly in the longitudinal

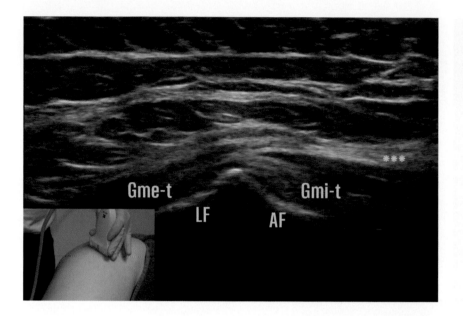

FIGURE 10.11
Roof top view (transverse scan). AF, anterior facet; LF, lateral facet; Gme-t, gluteus medius tendon; Gmi-t, gluteus minimus tendon. *** Iliotibial band (ITB).

plane, the anterior portion of the gluteus maximus muscle can be seen covering the posterior part of the gluteus medius tendon.

Scanning Tips:

1. Gluteal tendons are located superficially and therefore can be evaluated without difficulty. However, evaluation of the gluteal muscles depends on the variable thickness of subcutaneous fat. Therefore, an adequate adjustment of the focal zone is necessary to optimize muscle bellies.

2. Gentle hip rotation while scanning facilitates visualization of the gluteus medius and minimus tendons rotating under the gluteus maximus and TFL.

3. For high BMI or muscular patients, a curvilinear probe (2–6 MHz) may be beneficial for optimal images.

Applied Anatomy of the Knee Area

The knee joint is a synovial bicondylar joint, modified to act as a hinge joint. It is assisted by the patella (largest sesamoid bone in the body) in improving force transmission across the joint axis. The joint is stabilized by the joint capsule, the medial and lateral collateral ligaments and the anterior and posterior cruciate ligaments. The knee has a large range of motion into flexion and extension but also has a limited but critical degree of axial rotation. The knee joint transmits considerable forces through the long moment arms of the tibia and femur during functional tasks (Hartmann et al., 2013).

These high forces and large ranges of motion are sustained, due to the bilateral dynamic and static stability systems across the knee. When examining the structures surrounding the knee joint, a noticeable mirroring pattern of structures can be seen. This applies to most structures crossing the knee joint with the exception of the extensor mechanism.

As this chapter aims to introduce the anatomy and function of the knee for the purpose of ultrasound scanning, the menisci, anterior cruciate ligament (ACL) and posterior cruciate ligament (PCL) will not be discussed.

Passive Knee Stability (shaded in red Figures 10.12–10.13)

The medial collateral ligament (MCL) and the lateral collateral ligament (LCL) both stabilize the medial and lateral femoral condyles respectively. These two ligaments generally maintain a relatively perpendicular position in relation to

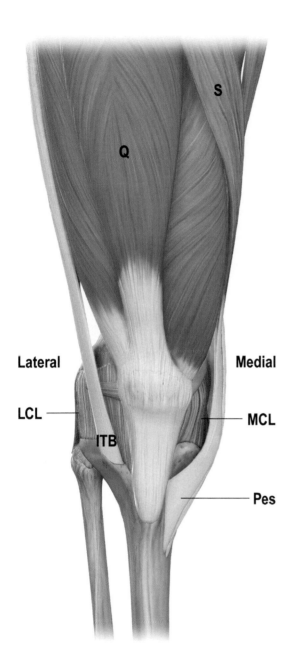

FIGURE 10.12
Applied anatomy of the anterior view of the knee. View of the anterior right knee with the passive stabilizers of the knee shaded in red. The tibial tuberosity collateral system is in yellow and the extensor mechanism is in green.
please add these to the end of the caption:
S, Sartorius; Q- Quadriceps; MCL, Medial Collateral Ligament; LCL, Lateral Collateral Ligament; ITB, Iliotibial Band; Pes, Pes Anserinus.

the tibial plateau throughout the knee range of motion, providing passive stability to the knee joint. This can be helpful to know when trying to scan them separately to the muscular structures and the medial and lateral aspect of the knee.

The MCL is a broad flat sheet that blends in with the joint capsule, making it slightly challenging to distinguish the two structures. Its main bulk originates at the medial femoral epicondyle and inserts just inferior to the medial tibial condyle in a flat sheath (LaPrade et al., 2015). The LCL is slightly more distinguishable and it originates from the lateral femoral epicondyle and inserts into the head of the fibula. It is located more posterior than generally perceived on sonographic evaluation.

Tibial Tuberosity Collateral System (shaded in yellow Figure 10.12)

The ITB is a thick strip of dense connective tissue located on the lateral thigh from the ilium to the tibia. It arises at its proximal end from the tendons of the TFL and gluteus maximus muscles and travels along the lateral side of the thigh to insert in the Gerdy tubercle, a bony prominence between the fibula and tibia tubercle (Landreau et al., 2019).

Pes anserinus is the anatomic name given to the conjoined tendons inserted onto the anteromedial aspect of the proximal tibia. Its name comes from the webbed-foot appearance of the tendons of the sartorius, gracilis, and semitendinosus insertion onto the tibia and plays a significant role as a stabilizer of the medial aspect of the knee joint (Mochizuki et al., 2004).

These two flat and sheet-shaped structures insert into either side of the tibial tuberosity, essentially hugging it from both sides. The ITB inserts into the Gerdy tubercle laterally and the pes anserinus inserts medial to the tibial tuberosity and inferior to the medial condyle of the tibia. This mirroring effect is not only reflected by the insertion shapes or relation to the tibial tuberosity, but also reflected in the forces these structures transmit. Both structures conduct contractile force from muscles situated anterior and posterior to the hip joint. The medial pes anserinus consists of an adductor hip component, while the ITB attaches to an abductor component of the hip.

A brief breakdown of the muscular contributions into the ITB and pes anserine by their orientation relative to

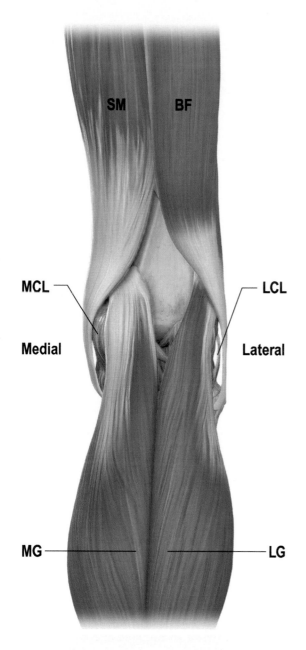

FIGURE 10.13
Applied anatomy of the posterior view of the knee. View of the posterior knee presenting the dynamic cross system with the hamstring muscles crossing over the medial and lateral gastrocnemius muscles shaded in blue. The passive stabilizers of the knee are shaded in red.
SM, Semimembranosus; BF, Biceps Femoris; MCL, Medial Collateral Ligament; LCL, Lateral Collateral Ligament; MG, Medial Gastrocnemius; LG, Lateral Gastrocnemius.

the hip joint is presented. Anterior to the hip axis, the ITB transmits the force from TFL that originates in the ASIS, while the pes anserinus includes sartorius which has a similar origin.

Posterior to the hip axis, the gluteus maximus transmits force through the ITB, while the semitendinosus originates on the ischial tuberosity and joins the pes anserinus. While the ITB transmits forces from the gluteus medius as an abductor through the attachment of the ITB and the gluteal aponeurosis, the pes anserinus consists of the opposing gracilis as an adductor component.

Extensor Mechanism (shaded in green Figure 10.12)

The extensor mechanism runs across the front of the knee and extends from the quadriceps tendon and is composed of three layers formed by the vastus lateralis, vastus intermedius and rectus femoris. The vastus medialis insert into these tendon layers, to collectively transmit force to the base of the patella. Some of the fibers terminate at the insertion into the base of the patella while some of the fibers are forming a flat continuation sheet over the patella and merge into the wide and flat patella tendon attaching to the tibial tuberosity (Pasta et al., 2010).

Underlying this extensor mechanism proximally, the suprapatellar pouch is located on the lateral aspect of the vastus lateralis. Over the patella, the prepatellar bursa is located between the patella and the subcutaneous tissue. Under the patella, between the apex of the patella and the tibial tuberosity deep to the patella tendon, the infrapatellar fat pad is found. The small infrapatellar bursa can sometimes be noticed before arriving at the insertion point of the patellar tendon onto the tibial tuberosity.

Dynamic Cross System (shaded in blue Figure 10.13)

The two X-like structures are made up of the two profound tendons of the gastrocnemius, attaching to the posterior superior aspect of the medial and lateral femoral condyles, respectively, and the two superficial hamstring tendons that cross over them. The medial cross is formed by the tendons of the medial gastrocnemius and the superficial tendon of the semimembranosus. It is between these two tendons where one can identify a Baker's cyst if present. The lateral cross is made up of the superficial tendon of the biceps femoris that crosses over the lateral gastrocnemius tendon.

The knee has been optimally adapted to the forces and loads acting at and through the joint. Generally, each function of the knee is the result of a complex interaction of several anatomical structures (Hirschmann et al., 2015).

Ultrasound Evaluation of the Knee Area

For didactic reasons, the knee can be anatomically divided into four compartments: anterior, medial, lateral and posterior. For a thorough ultrasonographic evaluation of the knee, it is essential to be systematic and follow a sequence beginning anteriorly, then progressing to medial and lateral sides, and finally to the posterior compartment.

A multi-frequency (5–12 MHz) linear probe is suggested with higher frequency (>10 MHz) used to evaluate all compartments of the knee, except the posterior compartment where lower frequencies (5–8 MHz) are optimal. It is important to be aware of the limitations of ultrasound in the evaluation of the knee joint. Intra-articular and deeper structures (menisci, ACL, and PCL) can be difficult to visualize fully by means of ultrasound imaging, and alternate imaging such as magnetic resonance imaging (MRI) should be considered.

The structure of interest should be scanned in both transverse (short axis) and longitudinal (long axis) planes for a comprehensive evaluation. The asymptomatic side can be used for anatomic correlation and for side to-side comparison. In most cases, the knee examination is focused on one compartment only, based on clinical findings.

Indications

Common diagnostic indications of musculoskeletal ultrasound in the knee include (Table 10.2):

- Joint effusion/synovitis
- Quadriceps and patellar tendon pathology
- MCL and LCL pathology
- ITB syndrome
- Bursal pathology (e.g., pes anserinus, infrapatellar)
- Baker's cyst

TABLE 10.2 Checklist of Structures to Examine on Scanning of the Knee

Anterior Knee
1. Bony landmarks (patella and tibial tubercle)
2. Tendons – quadriceps and patellar tendons
3. Hoffa's fat pad
4. Suprapatellar recess
5. Femoral trochlea (articular cartilage)

Medial Knee
1. Medial collateral ligament (include valgus stressing if indicated)
2. Medial compartment joint space
3. Medial meniscus (body, anterior horn)
4. Pes anserinus tendons and bursa

Lateral Knee
1. Lateral collateral ligament (include varus stressing if indicated)
2. IT band
3. Lateral compartment joint space
4. Lateral meniscus (body, anterior horn)
5. Tendons – biceps femoris, popliteus

Posterior Knee
1. Semimembranosus and semitendinosus muscle and tendon
2. Biceps femoris muscle and tendon
3. Medial and lateral gastrocnemius muscles and tendons
4. Popliteal fossa and neurovascular structures
5. Semimembranosus–gastrocnemius bursa *(if present)*

(Note: The knee should be viewed approximately 5 cm proximal and 5 cm distal to the knee.)

Anterior Compartment of the Knee

The following structures should be evaluated over the anterior knee:

- Quadriceps and patellar tendons
- Hoffa's fat pad
- Suprapatellar recess
- Femoral trochlea (articular cartilage)

Patient position: The patient is in supine position with the knee flexed to 20 and 30 degrees. A pillow should be placed below the knees to ensure patient comfort.

Transducer: Begin by placing your transducer (a high-frequency linear array with a large footprint is preferable) longitudinally over the superior aspect of the knee joint in the midline. This should give you a clear view of the quadriceps tendon, the superior aspect of the patella and the suprapatellar space. The transducer should be parallel to the quadriceps tendon to minimize anisotropy. Both the quadriceps and patellar tendons lack a synovial sheath. The quadriceps tendon is hyperechoic and presents with the typical fibrillar pattern, which is characteristic of tendons (Figures 10.14 and 10.15). Ultrasound can differentiate between partial and complete tears of the quadriceps and patellar tendon. Full-thickness tears are visualized as complete disruption of the tendon with separated ends (LaRocco et al., 2008).

The suprapatellar recess (SPR) is a recess that connects with the knee joint and is bounded by the suprapatellar and pre-femoral fat pad. The transducer is placed on the long axis to the femur just on the superior border of the patella. This will reveal the SPR (see Figure 10.15). When there is difficulty in visualizing the recess, applying pressure in the parapatellar space to squeeze the synovial fluid to the SPR may help in the absence of significant effusion. Ultrasound shows high specificity and sensitivity in diagnosing knee joint effusion and could be used in patients who are unable to undergo MRI (Draghi et al., 2015). Further, it has been shown to be superior to clinical examination for evaluation of knee joint effusion (Hauzeur et al., 1999).

A small amount of physiological fluid is commonly seen in the suprapatellar recess. It has been shown in cadaver specimens that the threshold for detecting knee joint effusion by US was 7 ml for synovial fluid and 10 ml for blood (Delaunoy et al., 2003). If you do see an effusion in the suprapatellar space, rotate your probe 90 degrees and take some images in the transverse plane with and without color Doppler.

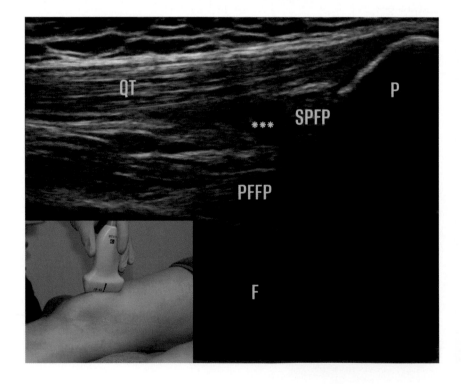

FIGURE 10.14
Longitudinal axis of the quadriceps tendon. PFFP, pre-femoral fat pad; SPFP, suprapatellar fat pad; QT, quadriceps tendon; F, femur; P, patella. ***Suprapatellar recess.

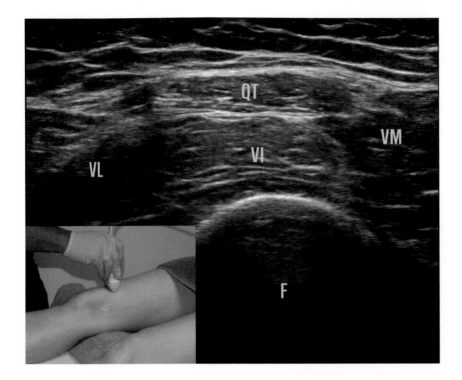

FIGURE 10.15
Transverse view of the distal quadriceps. QT, quadriceps tendon; VL, vastus lateralis; VM, vastus medialis; VI, vastus intermedius; F, femur.

If there is hyperemia and synovial thickening, it should raise suspicion of underlying inflammatory pathology such as rheumatoid arthritis, psoriatic arthritis, gout or pseudo-gout (Vlad & Iagnocco et al., 2012). Excessive knee flexion should be avoided as it will displace the joint fluid away from the SPR and can also compromise assessment with Doppler.

Moving the probe inferiorly below the patella, in the sagittal plane, the patellar tendon is easily identified as a striated hyperechoic tendon (Figure 10.16). The entire patellar tendon must be explored from its proximal patellar attachment to the distal attachment on the tibial tuberosity. Further, the tendon should be examined in the short axis, by rotating the transducer to 90 degrees. Deep to the patellar tendon is the large infrapatellar fat pad of Hoffa with its hypoechoic fat mixed with hyperechoic strands of connective tissue fibers. Follow the patellar tendon till it reaches its attachment at the tibial tuberosity. The deep infrapatellar bursa is located between the posterior surface of the patella tendon and the tibia, proximal to the tuberosity. In most cases, the bursa is difficult to identify unless it is inflamed or pathological.

If the knee is fully flexed, the femoral trochlea can be visualized in the long-axis plane. This allows visualization of the articular cartilage of the trochlea, particularly in the intercondylar notch of the femur. Normal hyaline cartilage appears as a homogeneous, anechoic layer lining the bony cortex of the trochlea. The normal condylar cartilage has a thickness ranging from 2.7 mm to 3.5 mm (Schmidt et al., 2004).

Medial Compartment of the Knee

The following structures should be evaluated over the medial knee:

- Medial collateral ligament
- Medial compartment joint space
- Medial meniscus (body, anterior horn)
- Pes anserinus tendons and bursa

Patient position: The patient is placed in a supine position, slightly tilted toward the affected side. The leg to be scanned is held in external rotation, until the lateral border of the foot touches the examination table.

Transducer: Placing the transducer over the long axis of the MCL will reveal the superficial and deep components of the ligament. The MCL is a flat, quadrilateral ligament that extends from the medial femoral condyle and attaches to the medial tibial metaphysis (Figure 10.17). It appears as a thin hyperechoic band comprising superficial and deep components, which are separated by fibro-adipose tissue which is hypoechoic. The width of the normal MCL at the level of the concavity of the medial femoral condyle varies from 3 to 6 mm (Craig & Fessell, 2012). The MCL must be examined for the entire length and dynamic scanning can also be undertaken with valgus stress to examine for joint space widening and integrity of the ligament. The outer portion of the medial meniscus can be visualized as a hyperechoic triangular structure between the femur and tibia. In knee osteoarthritis, US can detect medial compartment joint space narrowing, cortical irregularities and osteophyte formation.

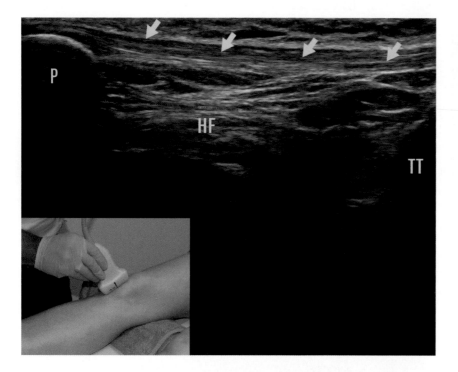

FIGURE 10.16
Longitudinal axis view of the patellar tendon. P, patella; TT, tibial tubercle; HF, Hoffa fat pad. Arrows, patellar tendon.

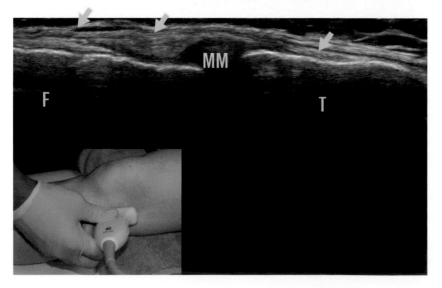

FIGURE 10.17
Longitudinal axis of the medial collateral ligament (MCL). F, femur; T, tibia; MM, medial meniscus. Arrows, medial collateral ligament (MCL).

Note the normal slight thickening proximally of the medial collateral ligament.

Moving the transducer distally and rotating it medially in an oblique position, the tendons of sartorius, gracilis and semitendinosus are seen blended together, forming the pes anserinus complex (Figure 10.18). However, ultrasound cannot easily distinguish the individual tendons. There is a bursa that allows the tendons to slide freely during flexion and extension of the knee. It can be visualized as a thin hypoechoic line in the plane between the MCL and the pes anserine tendons. This bursa can be a source of extra-articular pain in some patients with knee osteoarthritis.

Lateral Compartment of the Knee

The following structures should be evaluated over the lateral knee:

- Lateral collateral ligament
- IT band
- Lateral compartment joint space
- Lateral meniscus (body, anterior horn)
- Tendons – biceps femoris, popliteus

Patient position: The patient is in a lateral decubitus position on the opposite of the knee that needs to be scanned. A pillow should be placed between the knees for patient comfort. For an alternate position, the patient's leg can be rotated internally in the supine position, maintaining a slight knee position.

Transducer: Moving the transducer laterally from the anterior knee long axis at the patellar tendon level, the ITB can be identified as it extends distally to reach the lateral tibial tubercle or the Gerdy tubercle (Figure 10.19). This structure is the distal aponeurosis of the TFL and the gluteus maximus muscle. In asymptomatic individuals, the ITB measures around 2 mm in thickness at the level of the femoral condyle and 3 to 4 mm at the level of the tibial condyle (Goh et al., 2003). ITB syndrome is an overuse injury usually observed in the active athletic population such as runners but can occur in patients with varus deformity and/or lateral compartment osteoarthritis.

The next step is the identification of LCL, which is a narrow band that runs oblique and posterior, bridging between the lateral aspect of the femoral condyle and the head of the fibula (Figure 10.20). It has a similar sonographic appearance to the MCL, although it is thicker in the long axis. Keeping the distal part of the probe at the fibula and rotating the proximal end of the transducer posteriorly, one can identify the distal insertion of the biceps femoris tendon at the fibular head, next to the LCL. To view the popliteus tendon, the probe is placed in the anatomical coronal plane so that it lies along the long axis of the femur over the lateral femoral condyle and lateral knee joint.

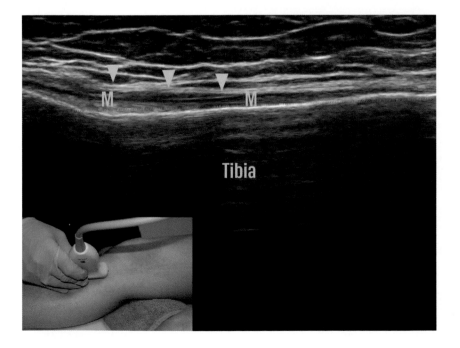

FIGURE 10.18
Longitudinal scan of the pes anserine tendons superficial to the distal medial collateral ligament (MCL). The pes anserine tendons often appear as a single entity at this level. M, medial collateral ligament (MCL). Arrows, pes anserine tendons.

Posterior Compartment of the Knee

The following structures should be evaluated over the posterior knee:

- Semimembranosus and semitendinosus muscle and tendon

- Biceps femoris muscle and tendon

- Medial and lateral gastrocnemius muscles and tendons

- Popliteal fossa and neurovascular structures

- Semimembranosus–gastrocnemius bursa (if present)

Patient position: The patient is placed in the prone position with the knees extended and both feet hanging over the examination table.

Transducer: By placing the transducer longitudinally on the superior–medial border of the popliteal fossa, the medial head of the gastrocnemius muscle can be visualized. Palpate the semitendinosus (ST) tendon by slightly flexing

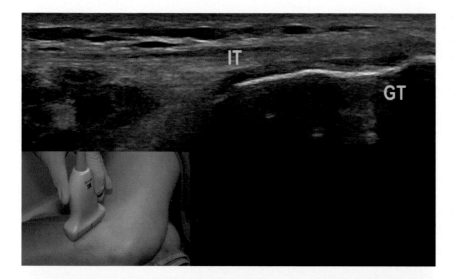

FIGURE 10.19
Longitudinal scan of iliotibial band. IT, iliotibial band; GT, Gerdy tubercle.

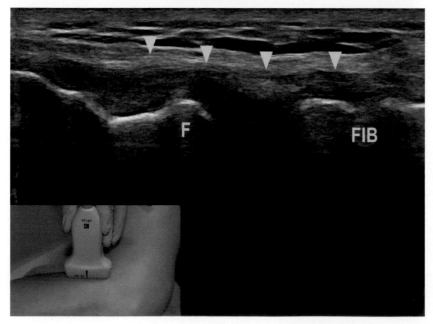

FIGURE 10.20
Longitudinal scan of lateral collateral ligament (LCL). FIB, fibular head; F, femur. Arrows, lateral collateral ligament (LCL).

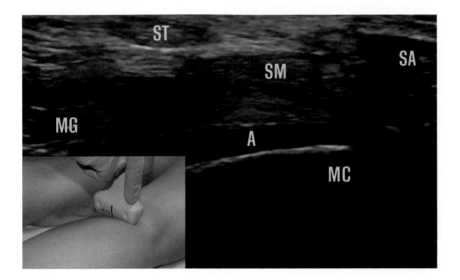

FIGURE 10.21
Transverse view of the semimembranosus tendon. MC, medial condyle of femur; A, articular cartilage; SM, semimembranosus tendon; ST, semitendinosus tendon; MG, medial head of gastrocnemius; SA, sartorius muscle.

the knee. Put the ultrasound probe over the ST tendon and a "cherry on the cake" appearance with the ST tendon as the cherry and semimembranosus as the cake (Figure 10.21). The semimembranosus–gastrocnemius bursa appears between the tendons of the gastrocnemius muscle and semimembranosus. Because of lack of fluid in the normal state, one should apply very light pressure to the ultrasound probe to reveal its presence.

Popliteal cyst or Baker's cyst is commonly located in the posteromedial aspect of the popliteal fossa. Technically, it is a non-malignant, fluid-filled swelling formed by distention of the semimembranosus–gastrocnemius bursa. Ultrasound is extremely sensitive for the detection of Baker's cyst, which is typically visualized as thin-walled fluid collections with occasional debris. The fluid can be anechoic, hypoechoic or of mixed echogenicity (Liao et al., 2010).

Baker's cyst is a common finding and is usually linked with degenerative or inflammatory arthropathies of the knee. The utilization of Power Doppler can be useful to differentiate a small Baker's cyst from a popliteal aneurysm (Park et al., 2020). The majority of Baker's cysts are secondary cysts and associated with degenerative knee joint diseases and meniscal pathologies, whereas primary cysts are less common and occur primarily in children (Alessi et al., 2012). Moving the transducer laterally, the short-axis scan of the popliteal fossa reveals the neurovascular bundle. The biceps femoris muscle and tendon are examined by moving the probe further laterally.

Conclusions

Ultrasound is a valuable diagnostic tool that has gained popularity among MSK clinicians and allows immediate correlation with the patient's symptoms and provides useful information to the clinician. Common clinical indications of the hip area include identification of effusion within the hip joint or its adjacent bursae, whereas clinical indications of the knee would include evaluation of the quadriceps and patellar tendons, muscles, joint effusion and collateral ligament of the knee. The benefits of real-time imaging allow for stress and dynamic maneuvers. Correct positioning of the patient and correct probe placement is essential for optimal imaging of the hip and knee regions. Although sonography may demonstrate tears of the menisci and cruciate ligaments, MRI is the preferred modality for evaluating internal derangements of the knee joint. It is important to emphasize that US complements MSK clinical skills and does not replace them.

References

Alessi S, Depaoli R, Canepari M, et al. Baker's cyst in pediatric patients: ultrasonographic characteristics. J Ultrasound. 2012;15:76–81.

Babcock DS, Patriquin H, LaFortune M, et al. Power Doppler sonography: basic principles and clinical applications in children. Ped Radiol. 1996;26:109–15.

Bergmann G, Deuretzbacher G, Heller M, et al. Hip contact forces and gait patterns from routine activities. J Biomech. 2001;34:859–71.

Chang KV, Wu WT, Lew HL, et al. Ultrasound imaging and guided injection for the lateral and posterior hip. Am J Phys Med Rehab. 2018;97:285–91.

Ciurtin C, Jones A, Brown G, et al. Real benefits of ultrasound evaluation of hand and foot synovitis for better characterisation of the disease activity in rheumatoid arthritis. Eur Radiol. 2019;29:6345–54.

Craig JG, Fessell D. Ultrasound of the knee. Ultrasound Clinics. 2012;7:475.

Delaunoy I, Feipel V, Appelboom T, et al. Sonography detection threshold for knee effusion. Clin Rheumatol. 2003;22:391–2.

Draghi F, Urciuoli L, Alessandrino F, et al. Joint effusion of the knee: potentialities and limitations of US. J Ultrasound. 2015;18:361–71.

Goh LA, Chhem RK, Wang SC, et al. Iliotibial band thickness: sonographic measurements in asymptomatic volunteers. J Clin Ultrasound. 2003;31:239–44.

Hartmann H, Wirth K, Klusemann M. Analysis of the load on the knee joint and vertebral column with changes in squatting depth and weight load. Sports Med. 2013;43:993–1008.

Hauzeur JP, Mathy L, De Maertelaer V. Comparison between clinical evaluation and ultrasonography in detecting hydrarthrosis of the knee. J Rheumatol. 1999;26:2681–3.

Hirschmann MT, Müller W. Complex function of the knee joint: the current understanding of the knee. Knee Surg Sports Trauma Arthroscopy. 2015;23:2780–8.

Ihnatsenka B, Boezaart AP. Ultrasound: Basic understanding and learning the language. Int J Should Surg. 2010;4:55.

Klauser AS, Martinoli C, Tagliafico A, et al. Greater trochanteric pain syndrome. Semin MSK Radiol. 2013;17:43–8.

Koski JM, Anttila PJ, Isomäki HA. Ultrasonography of the adult hip joint. Scand J Rheum. 1989;18:113–7.

Landreau P, Catteeuw A, Hamie F at al. Anatomic study and reanalysis of the nomenclature of the anterolateral complex of the knee focusing on the distal iliotibial band: identification and description of the condylar strap. Orthop J Sports Med. 2019;7:2325967118818064.

LaPrade MD, Kennedy MI, Wijdicks CA, et al. Anatomy and biomechanics of the medial side of the knee and their surgical implications. Sports Med Arthroscopy Rev. 2015;23:63–70.

LaRocco BG, Zlupko G, Sierzenski P. Ultrasound diagnosis of quadriceps tendon rupture. J Emergency Med. 2008;35:293–5.

Liao ST, Chiou CS, Chang CC. Pathology associated to the Baker's cysts: a musculoskeletal ultrasound study. Clin Rheum. 2010;29:1043–7.

Martinoli C, Garello I, Marchetti A, et al. Hip ultrasound. Eur J Radiol. 2012;81:3824–31.

McDonald DG, Leopold GR. Ultrasound B-scanning in the differentiation of Baker's cyst and thrombophlebitis. Br J Radiol. 1972;45:729-32.

Mochizuki T, Akita K, Muneta T, Sato T. Pes anserinus: layered supportive structure on the medial side of the knee. Clin Anat. 2004;17:50-4.

Nestorova R, Vlad V, Petranova T, et al. US of the hip. Med Ultrasound. 2012;14:217–24.

Park GY, Kwon DR, Kwon DG. Clinical, radiographic, and ultrasound findings between simple and complicated baker's cysts. Am J Phys Med Rehabil. 2020;99:7–12.

Pasta G, Nanni G, Molini L, Bianchi S. Sonography of the quadriceps muscle: examination technique, normal anatomy, and traumatic lesions. J Ultrasound. 2010;13:76–84.

Pinchcofsky H, Wansaicheong GK. Ultrasonography of the hip and groin: Sports injuries and hernias. Ultrasound Clin. 2012;7:457–73.

Philippon MJ, Michalski MP, Campbell KJ, et al. Surgically relevant bony and soft tissue anatomy of the proximal femur. Ortho J Sports Med. 2014;2:2325967114535188.

Schmidt WA, Schmidt H, Schicke B, et al. Standard reference values for MSK US. Ann Rheum Dis. 2004;6:988–94.

Smith J, Finnoff JT. Diagnostic and interventional MSK US: Part 1. Fundamentals. PM&R. 2009;1:64–75.

Vlad V, Iagnocco A. US of the knee in rheumatology. Med Ultrasound. 2012;14:318–25.

Walters BL, Cooper JH, Rodriguez JA. New findings in hip capsular anatomy: dimensions of capsular thickness and pericapsular contributions. Arthroscopy. 2014;30:1235–45.

Ward SR, Winters TM, Blemker SS. The architectural design of the gluteal muscle group: implications for movement and rehabilitation. J Orthop Sports Phys Ther. 2010;40:95–102.

Clinical examination of the lumbar spine in patients with hip and knee pain

11

Kyle Adams, Shane Koppenhaver, Timothy Flynn

Introduction

When patients present with hip or knee pain, it is important to determine primary and secondary contributing factors and mechanisms which may be responsible for their symptoms. Symptoms may be a result of local hip or knee tissue impairments, radicular or referred pain from the spine, or even referred pain from non-musculoskeletal structures. As discussed in Chapter 8, taking a thorough patient history and performing a detailed interview enables the clinician to learn about the potential mechanism of injury or mode of onset, duration, history, severity and irritability of symptoms. Gaining knowledge about relevant patient and family past medical history and developing an awareness of possible environmental or biopsychosocial factors that may influence the patient's condition are also key pieces of information that should be acquired. The culmination of this process is the development an initial hypothesis, multiple competing hypotheses, a general prognosis, and determination of a potential pathology or treatment classification, all based on emerging data.

Upon completion of the patient history and interview, a thorough physical examination should be performed, while respecting the patient's severity and irritability, to help further rule up (rule in) or rule down (rule out) the initial and competing hypotheses (Barakatt et al., 2009; Rothstein et al., 2003). Once the initial hypothesis is determined, a more definitive prognosis can be developed, along with a treatment plan based on the examination findings (Rothstein et al., 2003). Along with providing diagnostic and prognostic information, the physical examination has the added benefit of developing the foundation for a trusting relationship and a high-quality therapeutic alliance between the patient and clinician (Phoon, 2000). A thorough physical examination consists of screening the neuromotor and vascular systems via appropriate tests and measures followed by a more focused assessment of local body regions that may be causing or contributing to the patient's symptoms (Rothstein et al., 2003). In the case of individuals with hip or knee pain, evaluating the lumbar spine and neurological structures that can cause lower extremity symptoms is critical to correctly identify potential causes for the patient's symptoms. Only after assessing for the presence of red flag conditions, or more proximal musculoskeletal causes of the patient's symptoms, should the more focused examination be performed (Ross & Boissonnault, 2010). Suspicion of a red flag condition is heightened when the information gathered during the interview and exam findings is inconsistent with common neuromusculoskeletal pathologies. Prior to reviewing the various physical examination tests and measures, it is important to review the key components related to psychometric properties so that the clinician can make informed decisions regarding which assessments to choose and how to interpret the findings.

The appropriate use of diagnostic tests and measures requires an awareness of several important properties, with two of the most important being diagnostic accuracy, and reliability. Diagnostic accuracy measures the ability of a test to detect a condition when it is present, as well as to let us know when it is absent. The diagnostic accuracy of a test is often determined by comparing the test with a reference standard, which is defined as the test, or combination of tests, that are currently considered the best at helping to identify whether or not a condition is present (Bossuyt et al., 2003; Fritz & Wainner, 2001; Jaeschke et al., 1994). The diagnostic accuracy of the reference standard is compared to that of the clinical test being studied to determine the percentage who were appropriately diagnosed with the test being explored. To accurately use a clinical test, it is important to have an awareness of the reference standard for the condition you are assessing, and the patient population that was used to compare the reference standard and the current clinical test. Sensitivity, specificity, and positive and negative likelihood ratios are the terms used to described diagnostic accuracy. Sensitivity (true positive rate) is defined as the ability of a test to correctly identify patients that have a particular disorder (Straus et al., 2019; Portney, 2020). A highly sensitive test is best when negative, as it can help to rule out a particular diagnosis. However, highly sensitive tests frequently have a high number of false positives, meaning the results of the test indicate the patient has the condition we are assessing for when in fact they do not. This is why a positive result with a highly sensitive test is less valuable than a negative result. On the other hand, specificity (true negative rate), is a test's ability to predict individuals that do not have a particular condition (Straus et al., 2019; Portney, 2020). Tests with a high specificity are best for ruling up (or ruling in) a condition. The ideal test would have 100% sensitivity (meaning that it accurately predicts everyone with the condition as having it) and 100% specificity (meaning that it does not predict anyone without the condition as having it).

When comparing sensitivity and specificity with likelihood ratios, the latter tend to be more clinically useful due to their ability to predict the probability of a patient having a specific condition (Hayden & Brown, 1999). Likelihood ratios are calculated by using both the sensitivity and specificity to estimate the likelihood that a condition is present. If the test that is being assessed is positive, the positive likelihood ratio (+LR) is used to determine how likely it is that the patient has the condition. When the test is negative, the negative likelihood ratio (–LR) is used to determine how confident we can be that the patient does not have the condition in question. The following scale is used to determine the significance of +LRs: 10 or greater generates a large and often conclusive shift in the probability that the patient has the condition we are assessing, 5–10 generates moderate shifts in probability, 2–5 indicates small, but occasionally important shifts, and under 2 indicates a rarely important shift in the probability of the patient having the condition (Portney, 2020). With –LRs, less than 0.1 indicates a large shift in probability, 0.1–0.2 demonstrates a moderate shift, 0.2–0.5 indicates a small shift, and 0.5–1 shows a rarely important shift that the patient does not have the condition (Portney, 2020).

The reliability of a test provides information regarding the consistency of results when performing the same test repeatedly with the same sample. Intra-rater reliability is the consistency of multiple measurements taken by the same individual, whereas inter-rater reliability is the consistency of measurements when taken by more than one individual. Reliability is most often measured with reliability coefficients that range from 0 (no agreement) to 1 (perfect agreement). Intra-class correlation coefficients (ICCs) are one of the most common coefficients used for describing reliability of information measured on a continuous scale (e.g., manual muscle test scores). Kappa coefficients (κ), on the other hand, are used for categorical data (e.g., positive or negative tests), and automatically account for chance associations. Here are some general guidelines

for interpreting reliability coefficients: excellent reliability is >0.90, good reliability is anything between 0.75 and 0.90, moderate reliability for anything between 0.50 and 0.75, and poor reliability for anything <0.50 (Portney, 2020).

Clinicians should utilize tests and measures that have strong diagnostic utility while being as reliable as possible. For example, screening tests should be successful at ruling out the likelihood of a particular condition being present. This means they should be highly sensitive and have a small –LR. When assessing a patient using a highly sensitive test with a small –LR, the presence of a negative result can drastically lower the probability that the patient has the condition, thereby allowing us to rule it out. On the other hand, screening tests tend to have an elevated number of false positives. Therefore, when these screening tests are positive, the clinician must utilize other tests and measures to improve confidence regarding the presence or absence of the condition. When attempting to improve the ability to rule in a particular condition, we want to utilize highly specific tests with a large +LR, as they are better designed for ruling in conditions. A solid appreciation of these diagnostic properties is critical for appropriate use and interpretation. Consider a clinician that performs a special test with a high specificity and large +LR on a patient to attempt to rule out the presence of a serious pathology. When the test is negative, the clinician may conclude the condition is not present, which could be very dangerous for the patient. This is due to tests with a high specificity and large +LR having an increased number of false negatives. A different test with a high sensitivity and small –LR should have been selected to appropriately screen the patient for the sinister condition. A good way to keep track of what these terms are best used for is SNOUT (SeNsitive tests help to rule OUT) and SPIN (SPecific tests help to rule IN) (Sackett et al., 1985).

The screening portion of the physical exam for someone with hip or knee pain is our chance to rule out other conditions prior to the region-specific physical exam. As stated previously, these other conditions could be red flag spinal and neurological pathologies that may require referral outside of physical therapy. However, more commonly the screening of related areas identifies key contributing factors that may require physical therapy interventions outside of the hip or knee region to achieve optimal outcomes. This screening process should be a relatively standard and systematic process, with some tests and measures added or removed based on data gathered during the patient history and interview. Here are all of the components that should be considered for the screening examination:

- Observation
- Screening for known and unknown medical diseases or conditions
- Screening for severe injuries to the spine
- Screening for neuropathy
- "Clearing" the spine (removing the lumbar spine from consideration as a primary or secondary contributor to the patient's current symptoms)

Once the screening examination is complete, it is time to dive into the region-specific examination. This should be a systematic assessment that is directed by the information gathered during the patient interview and further modified based on findings obtained during the physical examination that has been performed up to this point. In general, region-specific physical examination should consist of the following activities:

- Active movements
- Passive movements (with and without overpressure)
- Palpation
- Clinical special tests

The focus of this chapter is on the screening portion of the physical examination for identifying conditions related to the lumbar spine that may result in hip or knee pain. It is important to identify spinal conditions that require medical assessment and interventions beyond the scope of physical therapy. In addition, there is evidence pointing to the benefit of manual therapy and exercises/interventions directed at the spine for individuals with hip and knee conditions, and therefore it is important these regions are screened appropriately (Iverson et al., 2008; Sueki et al., 2013; Hoglund et al., 2018). While this screening process is quite standardized from patient to patient, the region-specific examination has more variability depending on the location of primary symptoms and the suspected joints and tissues that may be involved. Those specific examination procedures will be the focus of future chapters within this textbook.

Observation and Screening for Medical Conditions

One of the primary questions that needs to be answered during a physical examination is whether the patient's symptoms are related to a condition that can be effectively treated by the clinician, or perhaps something that needs referral to a medical or surgical specialist. There are many visceral pathologies that can result in pain in the areas of the hip and knee. Screening for these visceral conditions can often be achieved via a thorough patient history and interview, especially for infections and spinal tumors. Combining appropriate questioning with additional information gathered during the physical examination helps to improve the likelihood of identifying a sinister condition, when present (Henschke et al., 2007, 2009; Finucane et al., 2020).

An appropriately performed physical examination should reproduce and/or aggravate the patient's familiar neuromusculoskeletal symptoms. Therefore, the inability to reproduce and/or aggravate a patient's familiar symptoms during the physical examination when symptom intensity is moderate to severe should elevate the clinician's suspicions of an underlying medical pathology.

Observation of the patient during the initial examination is very useful for identifying many non-neuromusculoskeletal pathologies. For this reason, the patient should expose all necessary tissues in the areas of the spine, abdomen and region of symptoms for careful inspection. Macules, papules, patches, wheals, and cysts are some examples of primary skin lesions that can be easily identified during the observation portion of the physical exam (Fernández-de-las-Peñas et al., 2016). Fortunately, most skin lesions are not a sign of life-threatening conditions, but it is important to bring these findings to the attention of the patient and their physician so they can be appropriately addressed. When these lesions are new, changing, and/or with irregular edges and different shades of coloring, it is possible they have a life-threatening condition that requires immediate medical referral (Luttrell et al., 2012).

Shingles, also referred to as herpes zoster, is a viral infection caused by the varicella–zoster virus. This is the same virus that causes chickenpox, which lies dormant in the body after someone has had chickenpox. Occasionally, it reactivates as shingles, sometime several years later.

The initial symptoms of shingles are pain and burning, most commonly on one side of the body. These symptoms are often followed by a painful rash that may be accompanied by fluid-filled blisters, itching, a fever, headache, fatigue, and muscle aches (Saguil et al., 2017; CDC, 2020). Therefore, careful observation is important to identify this condition when it is present, as it may be otherwise misinterpreted as a joint of soft tissue pathology of the spine or lower extremities. If the clinician is suspicious of this condition, the patient should be referred to their physician.

Other possible findings during the observation portion of the exam are abdominal mass, or atraumatic swelling. Atraumatic swelling may be an indicator of an infection or malignant condition, especially when accompanied by a fever. In addition, the palpation of a prominent and frequently nontender yet strong abdominal pulse may be a sign of an abdominal aortic aneurysm (Dargin & Lowenstein, 2011; Mechelli et al., 2008). However, the ability to accurately identify an aneurysm with palpation often depends on the size of the aneurysm, as well as the girth of the patient. Both of these conditions require immediate physician referral due to being life-threatening conditions.

Screening for Severe Injuries to the Spine

Undiagnosed vertebral fractures are one of many conditions that clinicians should be aware of when determining the underlying cause of an individual's back and lower extremity symptoms, particularly after a traumatic incident. In fact, spinal fractures are the most common serious pathology in the spine (Finucane et al., 2020). In this study, Finucane et al. discussed several indicators that, when present, play the biggest role in increasing the possibility of a spinal fracture. They are: history of osteoporosis, corticosteroid use, severe trauma, female sex, older age (>50 years), and previous spinal fractures (Finucane et al., 2020). Another study (Downie et al., 2013) identified older age (>64 years), prolonged steroid use, severe trauma, and contusion or abrasion as factors that increase the probability of a fracture to between 10% and 33%, and when more than one of these is present, the probability of a fracture is increased to between 42% and 90%. Therefore, clinicians should keep the above factors in mind whenever patients presenting with hip or knee pain also report acute pain and tenderness in the lumbar spine.

Screening for Neuropathy

Along with screening for serious neuromusculoskeletal pathologies, clinicians should also screen patients with hip or knee pain for the presence of lumbar radiculopathy. This is a condition that involves compression or irritation of the nerve roots of the lumbar spine, often due to disc herniations or narrowing of the vertebral foramen where the lumbar nerve roots exit the spinal canal (Alexander & Varacallo, 2020). Symptoms are often described as "sharp," "aching," or "burning" sensations that are often present in the low back, buttocks, and one or both lower extremities (Tomić et al., 2009). In addition, radiculopathy commonly results in altered strength, sensation, and/or muscle stretch reflexes related to the involved nerve roots, but the absence of these symptoms does not rule out the presence of radiculopathy (Hoy et al., 2010). It is important to note that symptoms do not follow the specific dermatomal patterns as closely as they do in the cervical spine, with the exception of S1 (Murphy et al., 2009).

Cauda equina syndrome is a rare, but serious neurological condition caused by compression to the cauda equina below the termination of the spinal cord, resulting in disruption of the function of the nerves associated with motor and sensory innervation to the lower extremities, bladder, anus, and perineum (Brouwers et al., 2017; Quaile, 2019). Due to this being an emergency condition, it is important to develop immediate suspicion of cauda equina during the patient history and physical examination. Key indicators are severe back pain, lower motor neuron abnormalities in bilateral lower extremities (often in multiple segments), changes in bowel and/or bladder function, saddle area sensation changes, and sexual dysfunction (Shi et al., 2010; Gardner et al., 2011). When the patient history, interview, and exam lead to elevated suspicion of cauda equina syndrome, immediate surgical referral is necessary.

Screening for Lumbar Radiculopathy

There is a lack of consensus regarding the best way to diagnose someone that fits into the International Classification of Function, Disability, and Health (ICF) categories related to low back pain with radiating pain. When using ICD-10 classification, lumbago with sciatica, also known as lumbar radiculopathy, identifies the closest with the ICF categories mentioned above (Delitto et al., 2012). This lack of consensus is in part due to there being multiple definitions of radiculopathy. Some sources discuss diagnosing radiculopathy via the physical exam only, whereas others recommend utilizing imaging and/or electrophysiologic findings (Rubinstein et al., 2007; van der Windt et al., 2010). Individuals with a lumbar radiculopathy present with a wide variety of symptoms, which adds another level of complexity when trying to diagnose them (Murphy et al., 2009; Tomić et al., 2009; van der Windt et al., 2010; Tawa et al., 2017). Radiculopathy from the L1 to L3 nerve roots is the most relevant to be aware of for accurate differential diagnosis in individuals with hip pain, and even an L5 radiculopathy may refer pain into the buttock and lateral hip area, whereas radiculopathy from the L3 nerve roots may most closely mimic someone with knee pain (Hirabayashi et al., 2009; Buckland et al., 2017). As per a Cochrane review, the best approach for a clinician to diagnose a lumbar radiculopathy for someone with complaints of hip or knee pain is to use multiple screening tests and combine findings due to the limitations of each test when used in isolation (van der Windt et al., 2010).

Nerve Root Examination

The typical neurologic screening exam in a musculoskeletal setting consists of sensation, muscle stretch reflex, and manual strength (myotome) testing. Evidence regarding the clinical utility of the neurologic testing is limited, and the available evidence is mixed (Tawa et al., 2017). As a result, it is recommended that all three assessments be performed regularly during every musculoskeletal examination. This is particularly true when the patient intake and interview reveal symptoms that may be neurological in nature or whenever symptoms are present distal to the gluteal fold. Sensation, muscle stretch reflex and manual strength assessment, despite their limitations, are considered the standard for physical examination of the neurological system while also providing legal/ethical value for the patient and clinician. In addition, data obtained from the screening examination can be used as objective outcome measures to monitor changes in the patient's status during and between treatment sessions. Finally, a detailed neurological examination is another way to increase patient confidence that they are being thoroughly evaluated by a competent, compassionate provider, which can have positive therapeutic benefits.

1. Sensation

While light touch and pinprick are the most common testing procedures, sensation can be assessed using other techniques, such as 2-point discrimination, localization, graphesthesia, vibration, and temperature testing. Figure 11.1 illustrates a dermatome map with key sensory points, although it is important to note that there are individual differences that may deviate from what is shown in these images (American Spinal Injury Association, 2008; Lundy-Ekman, 2018). Light touch and pin-prick procedures are best performed by gently touching a localized segment of tissue in the appropriate place for the desired dermatome and comparing side to side to determine if the sensation is present, absent, or abnormal. It is important to avoid brushing against the skin, as brushing provides worse precision and potentially activates other nerve pathways that may alter the accuracy of the findings. Sensation related to L1 to L3, and L5 are most relevant to individuals with hip or knee pain who are being screened to determine if their symptoms are being caused by a primary spine condition. A Cochrane review reported sensitivity for sensory testing from 0.39 to 0.68, and specificity from 0.62 to 0.89 (van der Windt et al., 2010). As stated earlier in this chapter, it is important for screening assessments to have higher sensitivity than specificity to enable clinicians to confidently rule out conditions when the test results are negative. Since this is not the case with sensation testing, it is important to interpret results with caution due to the possibility of false negatives. However, sensation loss should be used to guide further testing, hypothesis development, and can serve as a baseline assessment that can be monitored while working with a patient. This can be achieved by not only identifying potential dermatomes with sensation loss, but via more in-depth mapping of areas with sensation impairments to determine if they represent a neuroanatomically plausible distribution (Finnerup et al., 2016).

2. Myotomes

Manual strength testing techniques are described using various procedures, but they share in common the goal of identifying whether strength deficits are present. Typically, strength is assessed with the joint in a mid-range or close to end-range position, depending on various factors related to muscle length–tension relationships and joint mechanics (Magee, 2014). Many of these positions mimic those used

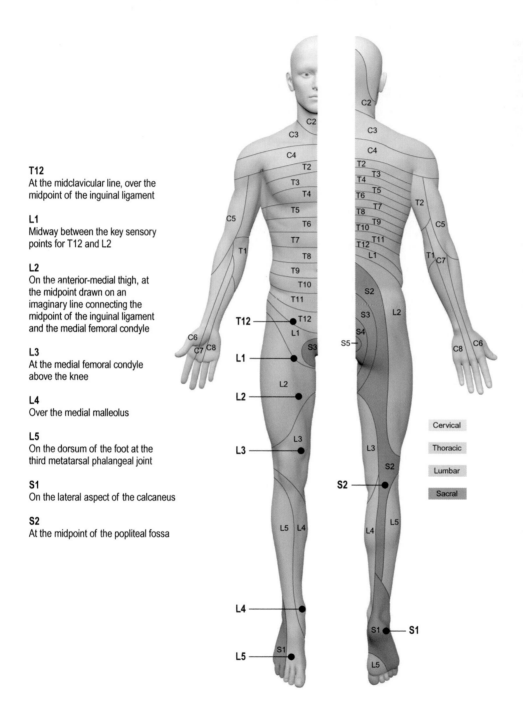

FIGURE 11.1
Key sensory points for lower extremity dermatomes.

T12
At the midclavicular line, over the midpoint of the inguinal ligament

L1
Midway between the key sensory points for T12 and L2

L2
On the anterior-medial thigh, at the midpoint drawn on an imaginary line connecting the midpoint of the inguinal ligament and the medial femoral condyle

L3
At the medial femoral condyle above the knee

L4
Over the medial malleolus

L5
On the dorsum of the foot at the third metatarsal phalangeal joint

S1
On the lateral aspect of the calcaneus

S2
At the midpoint of the popliteal fossa

Cervical

Thoracic

Lumbar

Sacral

with manual muscle testing (Avers & Brown, 2018). During this procedure, the instructions provided are "do not let me move you" as the clinician provides enough force to overcome (break) the patient's ability to provide maximal isometric resistance to maintain the desired position (Avers & Brown, 2018). With true manual muscle testing, strength is often graded on a scale from 0 to 5 (see below), with some clinicians providing + or – to further highlight small differences in strength (Avers & Brown, 2018). However, manual strength testing for the purpose of screening for neurological integrity typically involves grading an individual's strength as normal or abnormal, and in this instance, L1 to L3, and L5 are the most important for screening individuals presenting with hip or knee pain. Analysis of the diagnostic utility of

TABLE 11.1 Strength Testing for Lumbosacral Nerve Roots

Nerve Root	Primary Innervated Muscle	Test Procedure
L2	Hip flexors	The patient will be sitting with hip flexed so that the thigh is not resting on the table. The examiner applies a force to the distal anterior thigh to resist further flexion of the hip.
L3	Knee extensors	The patient will sit with thigh resting on table and knee extended to slightly less than full extension. The examiner stabilizes the posterior aspect of the patient's distal thigh with one hand while the other hand applies pressure on the distal anterior tibia to resist knee extension.
L4	Ankle dorsiflexors	The patient sits with ankle dorsiflexed and slightly inverted. The examiner stabilizes the distal tibia with one hand while the other hand applies pressure on the dorsum of the foot to resist dorsiflexion and inversion.
L5	Great toe extensors	The great toe is placed into extension. The examiner stabilizes the foot with one hand while the other hand applies pressure on the dorsum of the distal phalanx of the big toe to resist extension of the 1st metatarsophalangeal joint.
S1	Ankle plantarflexors	The patient stands and rises up and down onto toes repeatedly. The inability to do so, or more difficulty on one side vs the other, may be indicative of involvement of the S1 nerve root. The patient can be provided with assistance for balance, as needed, as long as it does not compromise the ability to accurately assess plantarflexion strength.
S2	Knee flexors	The patient sits with the knee in a flexed position. The examiner stabilizes the anterior aspect of the patient's distal thigh with one hand while the other hand applies pressure on the distal posterior tibia to resist knee flexion.

myotome testing for predicting a disc herniation, which is often, but not always associated with lumbar radiculopathy, includes sensitivity ranging from 0.29 to 0.62 and specificity from 0.50 to 0.89 (van der Windt et al., 2010). This again highlights the limitations of strength testing as an individual screening test for lumbar radiculopathy. Table 11.1 lists the various muscles that are tested to screen the various lumbar nerve roots, and Figures 11.2 to 11.7 provide illustrations of the testing for each muscle (Dutton, 2016).

- 5 (Normal): Full AROM against gravity, can hold against maximum resistance.
- 4 (Good): Full AROM against gravity, only able to hold against moderate resistance.
- 3 (Fair): Full AROM against gravity, unable to hold against more than mild resistance.
- 2 (Poor): Full active range of motion with gravity minimized.
- 1 (Trace): Slight muscle contraction detected (visually or by palpation).
- 0 (Zero): No evidence of muscle contraction (visually or by palpation).

3. Reflexes

Diminished muscle stretch reflexes (MSRs) are indicators of lower motor neuron impairments, most commonly within the spinal nerve roots (i.e., radiculopathy). On the other hand, a single hyperactive muscle stretch reflex and multiple increased responses (clonus) are a sign of upper motor neuron lesions. Patellar and Achilles MSRs are the most common means for assessing lumbar nerve roots, with the patellar MSRs being the one that would be the focus of someone with hip or knee pain that may be caused by a lumbar radiculopathy. These are shown in Figures 11.8 and 11.9. Similar to the findings regarding sensation and myotome

233

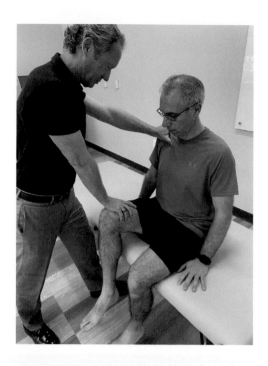

FIGURE 11.2
Hip flexion (L2).

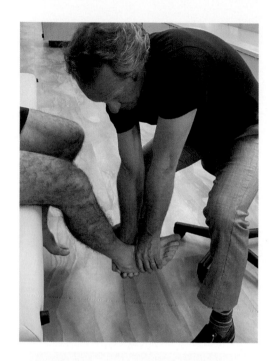

FIGURE 11.4
Ankle dorsiflexion (L4).

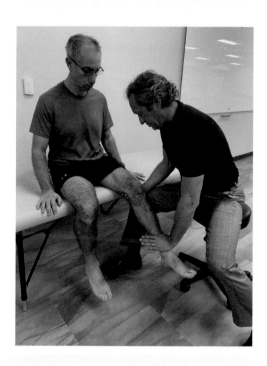

FIGURE 11.3
Knee flexion (L3).

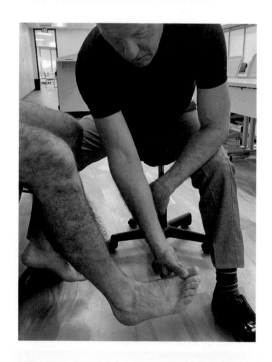

FIGURE 11.5
Great toe extension (L5).

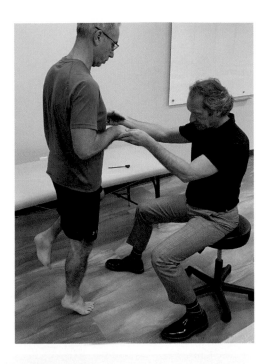

FIGURE 11.6
Ankle plantarflexion (S1).

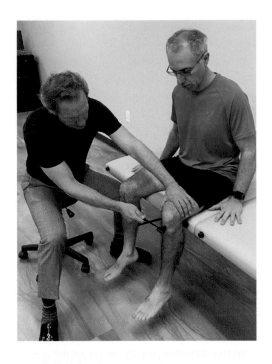

FIGURE 11.8
Patellar muscle stretch reflex (L3).

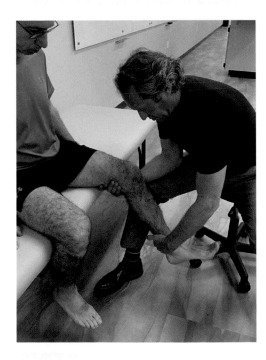

FIGURE 11.7
Knee flexion (S2).

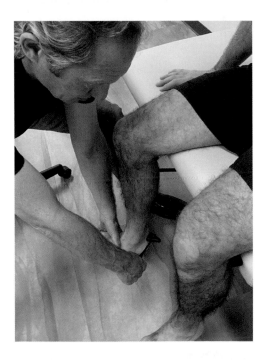

FIGURE 11.9
Achilles muscle stretch reflex (S1).

testing, MSRs have typically been shown to have better specificity than sensitivity values for identifying lumbar disc herniations and radiculopathy (Lauder et al., 2000; van der Windt et al., 2010). Van der Windt et al. (2010) reported it was too difficult to develop meaningful conclusions regarding patellar MSRs due to the great variability found in their diagnostic utility values (van der Windt et al., 2010). This same review analyzed multiple studies, seven of which revealed sensitivity ranging from 0.31 to 0.62, and specificity ranging from 0.60 to 0.89. One might think the aforementioned lack of evidence would be reason to avoid using sensation, myotome, and muscle reflex testing, but they are still highly recommended for all patients with spine and lower extremity disorders due to the lack of an approach that is better supported by the evidence.

Neurodynamic Assessment

In addition to assessing sensation, muscle stretch reflexes, and manual strength testing, there are other screening tests that should be part of the examination for individuals with low back and lower extremity symptoms. An assessment used to identify radiculopathy of the middle/upper lumbar spine is the slump knee bend test. This test is performed by having the patient lie on their uninvolved side with lumbar, thoracic, and cervical spines flexed while holding the uninvolved knee with the hip and knee flexed. The examiner supports the uppermost hip so that it is in neutral abduction/adduction and rotation, passively flexes the knee, and then extends the hip as far as tolerated (Figure 11.10). Reproduction of familiar symptoms in the patient's back, buttocks or lower extremity that are reduced with cervical extension, or loss of expected motion are indicators of a positive test. In a pilot study, sensitivity was determined to be 1.0, specificity was 0.98, the +LR was 6.0, –LR was 0, and kappa coefficient was 0.71 (Trainor & Pinnington, 2011). False positive tests are not uncommon in individuals with shortened iliopsoas or rectus femoris muscles or decreased hip extension range of motion, and should be considered with further assessment (Nadler et al., 2001). The straight leg raise (SLR) is good for ruling down lumbar radiculopathy of the lower lumbar levels due to disc herniation. To perform the straight leg assessment in its simplest form, the patient starts in the supine position with both lower extremities resting flat on the treatment table. The clinician slowly flexes the patient's involved hip while

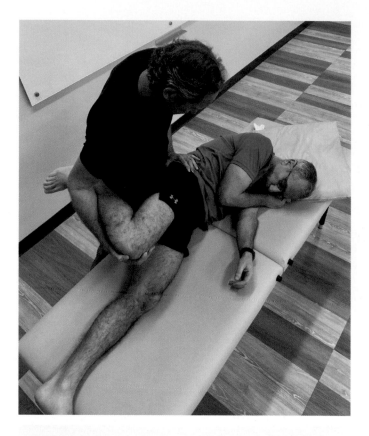

FIGURE 11.10
Slump knee bend test.

keeping the knee extended, ankle in 0 degrees dorsiflexion, and hip in neutral position of rotation and abduction/adduction (Figure 11.11). A positive test is reproduction of symptoms at 40 degrees or less. Pooled estimates from a systemic review revealed a sensitivity of 0.91, and specificity of 0.28 (van der Windt et al., 2010). This high sensitivity reveals that there is a strong likelihood that a negative test indicates there is no radiculopathy. On the other hand, a pooled estimate for the crossed straight leg raise has a sensitivity of 0.28 and specificity of 0.90 (van der Windt et al., 2010). This test is performed in the same manner as the straight leg raise, but on the uninvolved lower extremity. The seated slump test is another option for ruling down lumbar radiculopathy in the lower lumbar segments. It is performed by having the patient sitting upright on the edge of a table with hips and knees flexed 90 degrees. Next, the patient is asked to relax their spine into a slumped

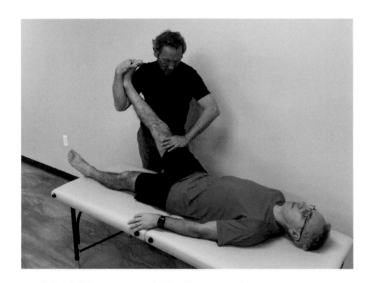

FIGURE 11.11
Straight leg raise test.

position, followed by addition of cervical flexion. Then, the clinician rests their forearm and hand on the patient's upper thoracic spine and head to maintain the slump and asks the patient to extend a knee followed by dorsiflexion of the ankle as far as tolerated (Figure 11.12). The test is considered positive if the patient's familiar symptoms are elicited during these maneuvers. It has a sensitivity of 0.84 and +LR of 4.94 (Majlesi et al., 2008).

Neurodynamic assessments, while primarily discussed related to their ability to diagnose lumbar radiculopathy, can also be used to assess for general mechanosensitivity of the nerves of the lower extremities (Boyd et al., 2009). An important consideration when differentiating between neurodynamic and local tissue (muscle or joint structures) irritation is moving joints in a manner that rules down the likelihood that the symptoms can be explained by local tissues. For example, if a patient presents with anterior hip, thigh, or knee pain and symptoms are reproduced during the slump knee bend test, have the patient extend their cervical spine while keeping all other positions the same, and reassess the patient's symptoms. If symptoms change, suspicion of neurodynamic involvement relative to local structures should increase, as cervical spine movements should not change the stress on local hip, thigh, or knee structures. In addition, when a patient experiences buttocks or posterior thigh symptoms during a straight leg raise, the

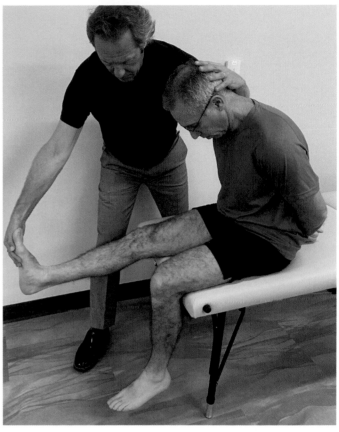

FIGURE 11.12
Seated slump test.

examiner should change the amount of ankle dorsiflexion while keeping the hip and knee in the same position, and reassess symptoms. If symptoms change, suspicion of neurodynamic involvement relative to local structures should increase, as ankle movements should not have any impact on local hip thigh muscles/joints. For individuals presenting with posterior knee symptoms and a positive straight leg raise, increased symptoms with the addition of dorsiflexion could be explained by gastrocnemius impairments. However, if changing dorsiflexion did not change symptoms prior to flexing the hip, there is less likelihood that altered gastrocnemius flexibility alone is the cause of the posterior knee symptoms. Other sensitizing maneuvers can be combined with neurodynamic testing, but those are beyond the scope of this discussion.

Upper Motor Neuron Examination

While not necessary for every patient, there are times when additional neurologic examination may be warranted based on the patient interview and physical exam. For example, patient reports of bilateral lower extremity neurologic involvement, history of neck trauma, incontinence or sexual dysfunction, as well as problems with balance or walking should elicit the clinician to perform an upper motor neuron examination. Observations that would prompt the upper motor neuron examination are gait incoordination and clonus during muscle stretch reflex testing. The typical response to muscle reflex testing in the presence of nerve root irritation is a diminished response, whereas involvement of upper motor neurons results in reflexes that are hyperreflexic (Zayia & Tadia, 2021). Studies have examined the diagnostic utility of several tests for their usefulness for ruling up/down upper motor neuron conditions, mostly as they pertain to the cervical spine. One such study identified a cluster of tests that had a sensitivity of 0.94 and specificity of 0.31 when one out of five tests were positives, and a sensitivity of 0.19 and specificity of 0.99 when three of five tests were positive (Cook et al., 2010). This demonstrates the ability of these tests, when used together, to rule up and rule down cervical myelopathy. The five assessments used in this cluster are: (1) gait deviation; (2) >45 years of age; (3) inverted supinator sign; (4) Babinski reflex; and (5) Hoffmann's reflex. Let us discuss how to perform these and other tests that have been traditionally used to identify the various upper motor neuron abnormalities.

Inverted supinator sign (Figure 11.13) is performed with the patient sitting. The examiner provides quick strikes with a reflex hammer to the area of the radial styloid process near the insertion of the brachioradialis tendon while the patient's arm is relaxed over the clinician's forearm in moderate elbow flexion and slight forearm pronation. This should be a familiar description, as it is the same as that used for the brachioradialis muscle reflex test. The difference is identification of finger flexion or slight elbow extension with a positive inverted supinator sign (Cook et al., 2009).

Babinski reflex (or sign) (Figure 11.14) is tested with the patient supine. The clinician stabilizes the foot and ankle in a neutral resting position and strokes the bottom of the foot from the lateral heel up along the lateral foot and over

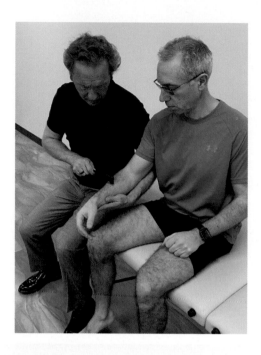

FIGURE 11.13
Inverted supinator sign.

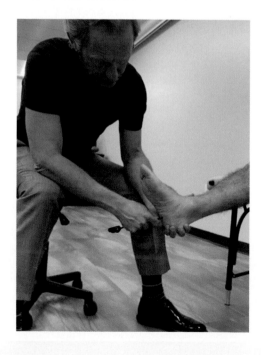

FIGURE 11.14
Babinski reflex (or sign).

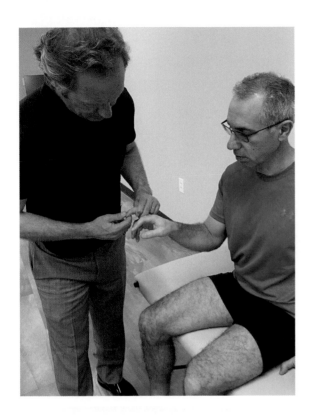

FIGURE 11.15
Hoffman's reflex (or sign).

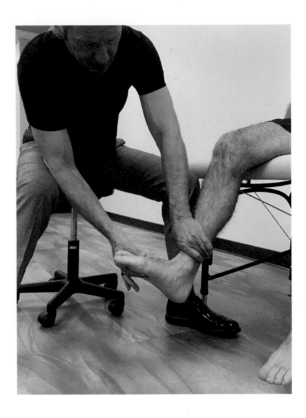

FIGURE 11.16
Clonus.

to the medial forefoot with the use of a blunt object that can be sanitized afterwards. The reflex is considered present if the great toe extends and other toes fan outward, and is indicative of an upper motor neuron abnormality (Cook et al., 2009).

Hoffman's reflex (or sign) (Figure 11.15) is assessed with the patient standing or sitting and holding the hand and middle finger in a way that the thumb and index finger are hanging freely. The examiner then flicks the dorsal aspect of the distal phalanx of the middle finger into flexion. A positive test is flexion of the interphalangeal joint of the thumb, with or without flexion of the index finger (Cook et al., 2009).

Clonus (Figure 11.16) is typically assessed with the patient seated with feet off the ground. The examiner provides a quick stretch of the Achilles tendon via rapid ankle dorsiflexion. A positive test is repetitive (at least 3) twitches of the foot in and out of dorsiflexion (Cook et al., 2009).

Clearing the Spine

When patients present with lower extremity complaints and the above screening procedures are negative, there is still potential for symptoms to originate from the lumbar spine. This reinforces the need to examine the lumbar spine for anyone with complaints of symptoms in the hip or knee regions. The clinician should assess lumbar range of motion in all directions, including flexion, extension, bilateral side-bending, bilateral rotation, and combined motions involving extension, rotation, and side-bending (extension quadrant). The goal is to determine if the patient's primary complaints are altered with spinal movements. If all motions are pain-free the examiner should add overpressure to each motion to further screen them for potential involvement (Figures 11.17–11.20).

Another component of clearing the lumbar spine as the primary or secondary contributor to the patient's current complaints is central posterior-to-anterior accessory

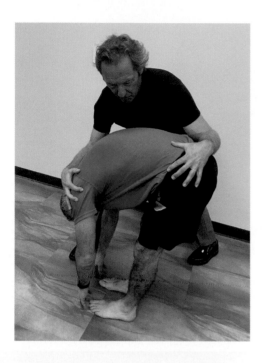

FIGURE 11.17
Lumbar flexion with overpressure.

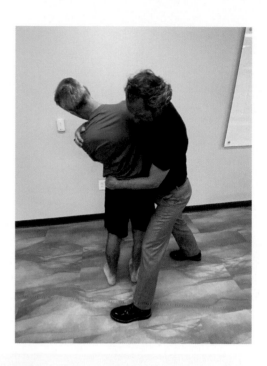

FIGURE 11.19
Lumbar side-bending with overpressure.

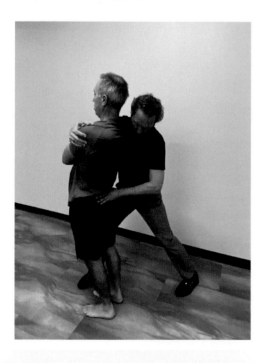

FIGURE 11.18
Lumbar extension with overpressure.

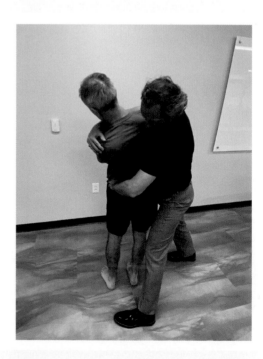

FIGURE 11.20
Combined lumbar extension, rotation, and side-bending with overpressure (extension quadrant).

mobility testing. This is used to assess for provocation of symptoms and relative segmental movement of the vertebrae. When testing posterior-to-anterior mobility of the lumbar spine, the patient will be positioned in a comfortable prone position, which sometimes involves placement of a pillow under the stomach to decrease the lordotic curvature of the lumbar spine. The clinician will place the hypothenar eminence of their hand over the spinous process, and will perform a slight twist of the hand over that spinous process in order to take up the skin slack. Next, the examiner will place the carpal tunnel region of the other hand over the scaphoid region of the hand that is contacting the spine (Figure 11.21A). At this point, make sure elbows are extended and shoulders are aligned directly over the vertebra that is being assessed. The clinician will use their body to apply slow posterior to anterior oscillations while gradually increasing the force to appreciate the amount of mobility and determine if the patient's familiar pain is reproduced, whether in the spine or the lower extremities (Figure 11.21B). The available mobility is rated as hypomobile, normal, or hypermobile. This assessment should be performed at every level of the lumbar spine, the sacrum, and the lower couple vertebrae of the thoracic spine. A recent systematic review assessed the diagnostic utility of accessory mobility testing (Stolz et al., 2020). The use of accessory mobility testing to identify individuals with non-traumatic lumbar instability, as identified by flexion–extension radiography, has a relatively high specificity (0.81 and 0.95), whereas the sensitivity is rather poor (0.17 and 0.46) (Stolz et al., 2020). Reliability of mobility testing for detecting hypomobile and hypermobile segments is poor, as per most studies, and their ability to detect painful segments has poor to moderate reliability (Stolz et al., 2020). Therefore, caution should be used when using these tests in isolation for ruling out instability and for general assessment of joint mobility or pain in the lumbar spine.

The final component of clearing the lumbar spine as the primary or secondary contributor to the patient's symptoms involves careful palpation of the joint and muscle structures in the lumbar spine region. Specifically, palpating for trigger points that may refer pain distally is important. Two such muscles that should be assessed when working with someone with hip pain are the quadratus lumborum and psoas major, as they can refer into the buttocks and anterior hip/groin area, respectively (Figures 11.22 and 11.23)

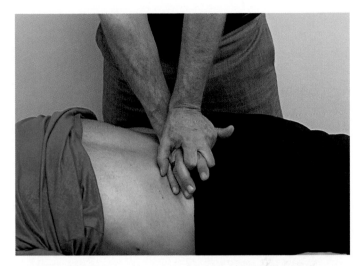

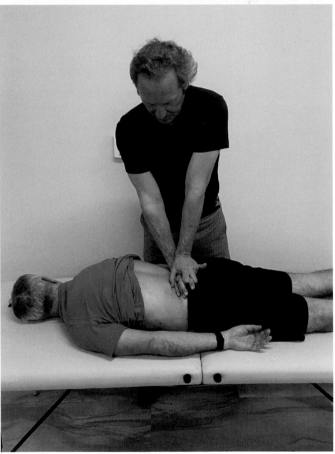

FIGURE 11.21
(A) Hand positioning for lumbar posterior-to-anterior mobility assessment. (B) Posterior-to-anterior mobility assessment.

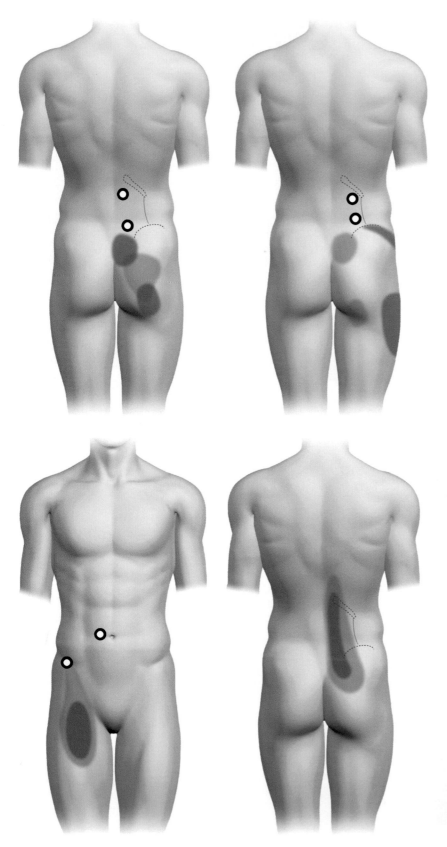

FIGURE 11.22
Pain referral pattern from quadratus lumborum myofascial trigger points.

FIGURE 11.23
Pain referral pattern from psoas major muscle myofascial trigger points.

(Fernández-de-las-Peñas et al., 2016). See also Chapter 17 of this textbook for more data on muscle referred pain.

Upon completion of the clearing exam for the spine, the information gathered will help the examiner conclude if the lumbar spine is likely to be a contributor to the patient's familiar hip and/or knee pain, at which point a more thorough region-specific exam should be performed during the initial visit to determine the best course of treatment for the patient. On the other hand, if impairments are identified that may be secondary contributors to the patient's distal symptoms, the clinician may focus initially on treating the identified hip and knee impairments and perform more detailed spinal examination and treatment at subsequent visits.

Conclusion

In this chapter, the importance of examining the region of the lumbar spine in individuals complaining of hip or knee pain was discussed. The chapter focused on screening the lumbar spine to identify conditions or impairments that may result in hip or knee pain. This included observation and specific screening techniques that can be used identifying for known and previously unknown medical diseases or conditions, severe lumbar spine injuries, and neuropathy. In addition, a standardized "clearing" process for the lumbar spine was presented that can be used to assist in removing the lumbar spine from being considered as the primary or secondary contributor to the patient's current symptoms.

References

Alexander CE, Varacallo M. Lumbosacral radiculopathy. Treasure Island, FL: StatPearls Publishing; 2020.

American Spinal Injury Association. International Standards for the Classification of Spinal Cord Injury: Key Sensory Points [Internet]. 2008. Available from: https://asia-spinalinjury.org/wp-content/uploads/2016/02/Key_Sensory_Points.pdf.

Avers D, Brown M. Daniels and Worthingham's Muscle Testing: Techniques of Manual Examination and Performance Testing. 10th edition. St Louis, MO: Saunders; 2018.

Barakatt ET, Romano PS, Riddle DL, et al. An exploration of maitland's concept of pain irritability in patients with low back pain. J Man Manip Ther. 2009;17:196–205.

Bossuyt PM, Reitsma JB, Bruns DE, et al. The STARD statement for reporting studies of diagnostic accuracy: explanation and elaboration. Ann Int Med. 2003;138:W1–12.

Boyd BS, Wanek L, Gray AT, Topp K. Mechanosensitivity of the lower extremity nervous system during straight-leg raise neurodynamic testing in healthy individuals. J Orthop Sports Phys Ther. 2009;39:780–90.

Brouwers E, van de Meent H, Curt A, et al. Definitions of traumatic conus medullaris and cauda equina syndrome: a systematic literature review. Spinal Cord. 2017;5:886–90.

Buckland AJ, Miyamoto R, Patel RD, et al. Differentiating hip pathology from lumbar spine pathology: Key points of evaluation and management. J Am Acad Orthop Surg. 2017;25:e23–e34.

Centers for Disease Control and Prevention (CDC). Shingles (Herpes Zoster). Atlanta, GA: CDC; 2020. Available from: https://www.cdc.gov/shingles/about/symptoms.html.

Cook C, Roman M, Stewart KM, et al. Reliability and diagnostic accuracy of clinical special tests for myelopathy in patients seen for cervical dysfunction. J Orthop Sports Phys Ther. 2009;39:172–8.

Cook C, Brown C, Isaacs R, et al. Clustered clinical findings for diagnosis of cervical spine myelopathy. J Manual Manipul Ther. 2010;18:175–80.

Dargin JM, Lowenstein RA. Ruptured abdominal aortic aneurysm presenting as painless testicular ecchymosis: the scrotal sign of Bryant revisited. J Emerg Med. 2011;40:e45–8.

Delitto A, George SZ, Van Dillen L, et al. Low Back Pain: Clinical Practice Guidelines Linked to the International Classification of Functioning, Disability, and Health from the Orthopaedic Section of the American Physical Therapy Association. J Orthop Sports Phys Ther. 2012;42:A1–A57.

Downie A, Williams C, Henschke N, et al. Red flags to screen for malignancy and fracture in patients with low back pain: systematic review. BMJ. 2013;347:f7095.

Dutton M. Dutton's Orthopaedic Examination, Evaluation, and Intervention. 4th edn. New York: McGraw-Hill Medical; 2016. Available at: https://accessphysiotherapy-mhmedical-com.ezproxy.baylor.edu/content.aspx?bookid=1821&sectionid=127518037.

Fernández-de-las-Peñas C, Cleland J, and Dommerholt J. Manual therapy for musculoskeletal pain syndromes: an evidence-and clinical-informed approach. London: Elsevier; 2016.

Finnerup NB, Haroutounian S, Kamerman P, et al. Neuropathic pain: an updated grading system for research and clinical practice. Pain. 2016;157:1599–606.

Finucane LM, Downie A, Mercer C, et al. International framework for red flags for potential serious spinal pathologies. J Orthop Sports Phys Ther. 2020;50:350–72.

Fritz JM, Wainner RS. Examining diagnostic tests: an evidence-based perspective. Phys Ther 2001;81:1546–64.

Gardner A, Gardner E, Morley T. Cauda equina syndrome: a review of the current clinical and medico-legal position. Eur Spine J. 2011;20:690-7.

Hayden SR, Brown MD. Likelihood ratio: A powerful tool for incorporating the results of a diagnostic test into clinical decision-making. Ann Emerg Med. 1999;33:575–80.

Henschke N, Maher CG, Refshauge, KM. Screening for malignancy in low back pain patients: a systematic review. Eur Spine J. 2007;16:1673–9.

Henschke N, Maher C, Refshauge KM, et al. Prevalence of and screening for serious spinal pathology in patients presenting to primary care settings with acute low back pain. Arthritis Rheumatism. 2009;60:3072–80.

Hirabayashi H, Takahashi J, Hashidate H, et al. Characteristics of L3 nerve root radiculopathy. Surgical Neurology. 2009;72:36–40.

Hoglund LT, Pontiggia L, Kelly JD. A 6-week hip muscle strengthening and lumbopelvic-hip core stabilization program to improve pain, function, and quality of life in persons with patellofemoral osteoarthritis: a feasibility pilot study. Pilot Feasibility Studies. 2018;4:70.

Hoy D, Brooks P, Blyth F, Buchbinder R. The epidemiology of low back pain. Clin Rheumatol. 2010;24:769–81.

Iverson CA, Sutlive TG, Crowell MS, et al. Lumbopelvic manipulation for the treatment of patients with patellofemoral pain syndrome: development of a clinical prediction rule. J Orthop Sports Phys Ther. 2008;38:297–309.

Jaeschke RZ, Guyatt GH, Sackett DL. Users' guides to the medical literature. III. How to use an article about a diagnostic test. B. What are the results and will they help me in caring for my patients? The Evidence-Based Medicine Working Group. JAMA. 1994;271:703–7.

Lauder TD, Dillingham TR, Andary M, et al. Effect of history and exam in predicting electrodiagnostic outcome among patients with suspected lumbosacral radiculopathy. Am J Phys Med Rehabil. 2000;79:60–8.

Lundy-Ekman L. Neuroscience Fundamentals for Rehabilitation. 5th edn. St Louis, MO: Elsevier; 2018.

Luttrell MJ, McClenahan P, Hofmann-Wellenhof R, et al. Laypersons' sensitivity for melanoma identification is higher with dermoscopy images than clinical photographs. Br J Dermatol. 2012;167:1037–41.

Magee DJ. Orthopedic physical assessment. 6th edn. St Louis, MO: Elsevier; 2014.

Majlesi J, Togay H, Unalan H, Toprak S. The sensitivity and specificity of the Slump and the Straight Leg Raising tests in patients with lumbar disc herniation. J Clin Rheumat. 2008;14:87–91.

Mechelli F, Preboski Z, Boissonnault WG. Differential diagnosis of a patient referred to physical therapy with low back pain: abdominal aortic aneurysm. J Orthop Sports Phys Ther. 2008;38:551–7.

Murphy DR, Hurwitz EL, Gerrard JK, Clary R. Pain patterns and descriptions in patients with radicular pain: does the pain necessarily follow a specific dermatome? Chiropractic Osteopathy. 2009;17:9.

Nadler SF, Malanga GA, Stitik TP, et al. The crossed femoral nerve stretch test to improve diagnostic sensitivity for the high lumbar radiculopathy: 2 case reports. Arch Phys Med Rehabil. 2001;82:522–3.

Phoon CK. Must doctors still examine patients? Perspect Biol Med. 2000;43(4):548–61.

Portney LG. Foundations of clinical research: applications to evidence-based practice. 4th Edition. Philadelphia, PA: F.A. Davis Company; 2020.

Quaile A. Cauda equina syndrome-the questions. International Orthopaedics. 2019;43:957–61.

Ross MD, Boissonnault WG. Red flags: To screen or not to screen? J Orthop Sports Phys Ther. 2010;40:682–4.

Rothstein JM, Echternach JL, Riddle DL. The hypothesis-oriented algorithm for clinicians II (HOAC II): A guide for patient management. Phys Ther. 2003;83:455–70.

Rubinstein SM, Pool JJ, van Tulder MW, et al. A systematic review of the diagnostic accuracy of provocative tests of the neck for diagnosing cervical radiculopathy. Eur Spine J. 2007;16:307–19.

Sackett D, Haynes R, Guyatt G, Tugwell P. Clinical Epidemiology: A Basic Science for Clinical Medicine. Boston, MA: Little, Brown and Company; 1985.

Saguil A, Kane SF, Mercado MG, Lauters R. Herpes zoster and postherpetic neuralgia: prevention and management. Am Family Phys. 2017;96:656–63.

Shi J, Jia L, Yuan W, et al. Clinical classification of cauda equina syndrome for proper treatment. Acta Orthop. 2010;81:391–5.

Stolz M, von Piekartz H, Hall T, et al. Evidence and recommendations for the use of segmental motion testing for patients with LBP – a systematic review. Musculosk Sci Pract. 2020;45:12.

Straus SE, Glasziou P, Richardson WS, Haynes RB. Evidence-based medicine: how to practice and teach EBM. 5th Edition. Edinburgh: Elsevier; 2019.

Sueki DG, Cleland JA, Wainner RS. A regional interdependence model of musculoskeletal dysfunction: research, mechanisms, and clinical implications. J Manual Manipul Ther. 2013;21:90–102.

Tawa N, Rhoda A, Diener I. Accuracy of clinical neurological examination in diagnosing lumbo-sacral radiculopathy: a systematic literature review. BMC Musculoskeletal Disorders. 2017;18:93.

Tomić S, Soldo-Butkovic S, Kovac B, et al. Lumbosacral radiculopathy--factors effects on its severity. Collegium Antropologicum. 2009;33:175–8.

Trainor K, Pinnington M. Reliability and diagnostic validity of the slump knee bend neurodynamic test for upper/mid lumbar nerve root compression: a pilot study. Physiother. 2011;97:59–64.

van der Windt DA, Simons E, et al. Physical examination for lumbar radiculopathy due to disc herniation in patients with low-back pain. Cochrane Database Syst Rev. 2010;2:CD007431.

Zayia LC, Tadi P. Neuroanatomy, Motor Neuron. [Internet]. Treasure Island, FL: StatPearls Publishing; 2021. Available from: https://www.ncbi.nlm.nih.gov/books/NBK554616/.

Clinical examination of the hip and knee

12

Benoy Mathew, Elizabeth Marlow, Martin Thomas, Madhan K. Ramanathan

Subjective Examination of the Hip

Introduction

Hip pain is a common presentation in musculoskeletal and sports medicine clinics and can affect patients of all ages. An adult presenting with hip pain often presents a diagnostic dilemma. Identifying the etiology of a painful hip is challenging due to the inherent complexity of the anatomy of the lumbopelvic region with multiple referral patterns (Bizzini, 2011). Clinical examination of the hip requires a meticulous and systematic approach, while taking the patient's history and choosing appropriate physical examination techniques.

Non-traumatic hip pain in any age group is often a clinical challenge to diagnose as the potential source of pain may arise from multiple areas including the lumbar spine, sacroiliac joint, visceral referral and lower abdomen pathologies. Hip pathologies can be broadly divided into intra-articular, extra-articular and non-musculoskeletal pathologies. A patient's age, sex and activity levels can often give the clinician appropriate clues to the nature of pathologies, encountered in hip pain (Plante et al., 2011).

It is important to consider atypical presentations and red flags while assessing a patient with hip pain. The onset of pain, nature and distribution of pain, duration of pain, associated other symptoms, aggravating and relieving factors, the 24-hour pattern of the pain, previous history of the same presentation, past medical history, family history, and psychosocial history all are important factors to consider in the evaluation process (Reiman & Thorborg, 2014).

This chapter will outline the approach to hip pain with a focus on intra-articular pathologies. Conditions that present predominantly with groin pain (e.g., osteitis pubis, adductor tendon disorders) are not addressed here.

History of Symptoms

An appropriate history will guide the physical examination, appropriate clinical tests and, ultimately, decision-making. The differential diagnosis is vast for hip pain and can be caused by a wide spectrum of pathologic conditions (Table 12.1). It is important to acknowledge that many non-orthopedic conditions such as hernia, ovarian cyst, pelvic inflammatory disease, hydrocele can present with hip pain.

Age, history of trauma and duration of symptoms are the primary factors that direct the examination process. Acute onset of hip and groin pain, especially during sporting activity, is likely to be musculotendinous in origin, whereas chronic dull pain may correspond to intra-articular origin (Trofa et al., 2017).

The main goals of the clinical history should be to:

1. Rule out any alarming sources of hip pathology such as infection, malignancy, systemic disorders and inflammatory pathologies.

2. Differentiate between intra-articular and extra-articular sources of hip pain.

3. Narrow the differential diagnosis to a few, to perform a focused physical examination.

Screening for Serious Pathology (Red Flags)

Previous history of cancer should be screened in the initial appointment and may warrant early referral for imaging, since prostate cancer in men and breast cancer in women are likely to metastasise to the spine and hip joint (Henschke et al., 2007). The tumor that metastasizes to the hip and pelvic region with the greatest frequency is carcinoma of the breast (Horowitz & Berman, 1999).

The following areas must also be addressed in the initial evaluation: past injuries, childhood or adolescent hip disease, history of inflammatory pathologies and risk factors of avascular necrosis. Inflammatory arthritis commonly exhibits early morning stiffness and more symmetrical patterns in pain. An acute change in hip pain and inability to bear weight should raise concern for serious hip pathology and prompt an urgent orthopedic referral.

Stress fractures in the hip and pelvis region (femoral neck, pubis, sacrum and ischium) are most common in female runners and should not be missed as a possible differential diagnosis of hip and groin pain (Robertson & Wood, 2017). Typically, the pain is diffuse around the

CHAPTER TWELVE

TABLE 12.1 Differential Diagnosis of Hip Pain		
Articular Pathologies	**Extra-articular Pathologies**	**Referred Pain (Hip Mimickers)**
• Hip osteoarthritis • Femoroacetabular impingement • Hip dysplasia • Acetabular labral tears • Osteochondral lesions • Femoral malversion (excessive anteversion or retroversion) • Ligamentum teres tears and rupture • Hip joint instability • Loose bodies • Femoral neck stress fracture • Avascular necrosis • Transient osteoporosis of the hip • Synovitis and inflammatory disorders • Septic arthritis • Osteomyelitis • Paget disease • Osteoid osteoma	• Adductor-related groin pain • Hip flexor-related groin pain • Gluteus medius tendinopathy and tears • Rectus abdominis strain • Pubic-related groin pain (osteitis pubis) • Snapping hip syndrome (external and internal) • Athletic pubalgia (sports hernia) • Groin hernias (inguinal hernia, femoral hernia, obturator hernia) • Stress fractures of the pelvis	• Lumbar spine pathology (e.g., disc, pars injuries, facet arthropathy) • SIJ disorders • Intra-abdominal pathologies (aneurysm, diverticulosis, inflammatory bowel disease) • Genitourinary disorders (urinary tract infection, testicular torsion, nephrolithiasis) • Uro-gynecological pathologies (endometriosis, pelvic inflammatory disease) • Abdominal muscle strains • Nerve entrapment syndromes (ilioinguinal, femoral, lateral femoral cutaneous, obturator, pudendal)

groin, anterior hip, and proximal thigh. The pain typically worsens with impact activities and worsens over time. In advanced cases, it may progress to night pain and even limping during walking (Harris & Chahal, 2015). In female runners, history comprising amenorrhea, reduced calorie intake, and previous bone stress injuries should raise the suspicion and prompt investigation of a stress fracture (Lodge et al., 2020).

The mnemonic "SAM" (Stress fractures, Avascular necrosis and Metastasis or primary bone tumor) can be helpful in remembering the important red flags of the hip and groin region (Table 12.2).

Layer Approach to Hip Evaluation

A comprehensive evaluation of the hip pain requires detailed knowledge and assessment of four distinct layers of the hip joint: osteochondral, capsule–labral, musculotendinous, and neurovascular (Table 12.3).

The layer concept as described by Draovitch et al. (2012) is a systematic means of determining which structures about the hip are the source of the patient's symptoms and how to best plan treatment. A clinical approach of the hip that incorporates this layered concept is likely to lead to an accurate diagnosis in a timely manner.

Nature of Pain

The nature of pain is of great importance in subjective history. Many patients with chronic hip pain may find it difficult to characterize their pain clearly or localize it accurately. Low-grade dull, aching pain is likely to signify a degenerative pathology, especially if the patient is more than forty years of age. Stiffness about the hip, especially

TABLE 12.2 Screening for Serious Pathology of the Hip (Mnemonic – SAM)

Red Flags	Guiding Questions
Stress fractures	1. History of bone stress injuries 2. Osteoporosis, low vitamin D 3. Spike in training load 4. Worsening symptoms and unable to run 5. *Female patients:* Screen for low BMI, low-calorie intake, delayed menarche and menstrual disorders
Avascular necrosis	1. Long-term oral steroids 2. Excess alcohol intake 3. Substance abuse, IV drug user 4. Sickle cell anemia 5. History of radiotherapy for cancer treatment
Metastatic cancer or primary bone tumor	1. Previous history of cancer 2. Unremitting pain and unable to sleep properly due to night pain 3. Constitutional symptoms such as fever, unexplained weight loss, night sweats, lethargy, malaise 4. Lump or growth around the hip, groin or buttock region

TABLE 12.3 The Layer Concept

Layer	Name	Structure	Purpose
1	Osteochondral	Femur Acetabulum Innominate	Joint congruence Arthro-kinematic Movement
2	Inert	Capsule Labrum Ligaments Ligamentum teres	Static stability
3	Contractile	Musculature crossing hip Lumbosacral muscles Pelvic floor	Dynamic stability
4	Neuromechanical	Thoracolumbar mechanics Lower extremity mechanics Neurovascular structures referring to the hip	Kinetic chain

after prolonged inactivity, is suggestive of hip osteoarthritis (Cibulka & Threlkeld, 2004). It is important to inquire about the presence of associated low back pain and any radicular complaints to the ipsilateral leg or foot. The mnemonic "SOCRATES" can be helpful in ensuring that a thorough pain history is taken (Table 12.4).

The presence of sharp, stabbing, pinching pain may indicate a mechanical cause such as labral tears, which commonly coexist in pathologies such as femoroacetabular impingement (FAI) and hip dysplasia (Burnett et al., 2006). Patients with snapping hip syndrome or anterior rim damage often describe feelings of catching, clicking or popping sensation, arising deep in the hip (Lee et al., 2013). External snapping hip syndrome originating from the iliotibial band is frequently described as the "hip coming out of the joint" by the patient, as the iliotibial band slips over the greater trochanter and spontaneously reduces (Spina, 2007). In female patients, it is important to investigate whether the hip and groin pain is cyclical and fluctuates with menstruation, as it could be a sign of gynecological disorders such as endometriosis (Rana et al., 2001).

TABLE 12.4 Hip Pain History (Mnemonic – SOCRATES)		
	Component	**Guiding Questions**
S	Site	Where exactly is the pain? (e.g., anterior, lateral, groin, pubic region, lower abdomen, anterior thigh)
O	Onset	When did the pain start? How long ago? Was it sudden or gradual? History of trauma?
C	Character	What does the pain feel like? (e.g., ache, deep, sharp, shooting, throbbing)
R	Radiation	Does the pain travel anywhere else? (e.g., thigh, leg, buttock, knee)
A	Associated symptoms	Are there any other signs/symptoms associated with the pain? (e.g., limping, weakness of legs, fever, pins and needles, numbness)
T	Timing	Does the pain follow a pattern? Any variation with day and night? When does your hip bother you the most?
E	Exacerbating and relieving symptoms	Does anything make it better or worse? Effect of rest and painkillers? Does it affect your ability to manage your daily life, climb stairs, do sports, gym work?
S	Severity	How severe is the pain? Rate it. Visual analog scale: 0 to 10 (0, no pain; 10, worst pain)

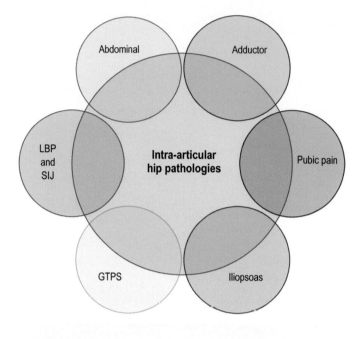

FIGURE 12.1
Overlap in hip pathologies. GTPS, greater trochanteric pain syndrome; LBP, low back pain; SIJ, sacroiliac joint.

In many patients with chronic hip pain, it is common to have a mixed clinical presentation (Figure 12.1) due to overlap of multiple pathologies, with two or more diagnoses present in 27%–90% of patients (Lovell et al., 1995). Essential questions that aid the diagnostic process during the history taking are outlined in Table 12.5.

Inciting Activities

Specific activities which aggravate the patient's symptoms should be investigated in detail. The clinician should explore aggravating activities by asking open-ended questions such as "When do you experience pain?" or "When does your hip bother you the most?" Activities of daily living are often affected by intra-articular hip pathologies and these include ascending/descending stairs, reaching to put on shoes and socks, getting in and out of a car and sitting/rising from a low chair.

It is important to enquire about the occurrence of limp following sporting activities, or one that develops the next day, which is highly suggestive of intra-articular pathology (Bassett & Tjoumakaris, 2019). More pain with sitting than

TABLE 12.5 Essential Subjective Evaluation of the Hip

Clinical History	Current Symptoms

• History of trauma including long bone fractures of the lower limb
• Childhood hip disorders such as developmental dysplasia, Perthes disease, slipped capital femoral epiphysis, and any associated surgery
• Family history of early hip osteoarthritis in parents or siblings
• *Female Patients:* Uro-gynecological disorders such as endometriosis, pelvic inflammatory disease. Does the hip or groin pain fluctuate during menstruation? Do they have hip pain during sex?
• *Current Sporting History:*
  – Pivoting and shifting sports
  – Heavy weight-training
  – Flexibility-based training such as yoga, ballet, or martial arts
	• *Location of Pain:* anterior hip, lateral hip, buttock pain, low back pain, or anterior thigh pain
	• C-Sign, triangulation sign, or deep pointer sign
	• Radiating leg pain with associated pins and needles or numbness
	• History of limping during pain
	• Mechanical symptoms such as clicking, catching, clunking. Is it associated with pain?
	• History of hypermobility or pain in multiple joints
	• Early morning stiffness around the low back, pelvis, or hip region
	• *Any pain or discomfort during these following activities*
	  – Prolonged sitting, especially in low chairs or sofas
	  – Pulling on shoes and socks
	  – Getting in and out of the car
	  – Deep squats or lunges during weight-training
	  – Stretching pain during yoga, ballet, or martial arts, especially during end-range hip flexion or rotation

walking may suggest the presence of FAI, whereas osteoarthritis and adult hip dysplasia patients may present with increased pain during activities such as prolonged standing and walking (Stubbs & Howse, 2017). Deep hip flexion is usually painful in clients with FAI syndrome and also change of direction during contact sports such as football, rugby or basketball (Egger et al., 2016). Features that are suggestive of intra-articular hip pathology (Byrd & Jones, 2004; Frangiamore et al., 2017) are outlined in Table 12.6.

In certain patients, symptoms may only be present during sporting activities or whilst training in the gym. Common triggers in the athletic population include deep squat during weight training, running uphill or on uneven ground, twisting, pivoting or kicking activities in contact sports like football and rugby. The severity of hip pain must be quantified and it is important to differentiate between pain that only interferes with sporting activity versus pain during normal daily activities. Relieving factors should be explored along with usage of analgesia or anti-inflammatories and pattern of usage.

TABLE 12.6 Symptoms Suggestive of Intra-articular Hip Pathology

1. Insidious onset of activity-related hip/groin pain
2. Vague, deep and poorly localized symptoms (C-sign, triangulation sign, deep pointer sign)
3. Mechanical symptoms such as clicking, catching or popping
4. History of limping during or after inciting activities
5. Pain with prolonged sitting, especially in low chairs and sofas. Pain and catching sensation, during rising from seated position.
6. Pain or discomfort during rotational activities (e.g., twisting, pivoting, cutting, change of direction activities); activities on level surface and straight-line activities are relatively well tolerated
7. Stiffness around the hip and groin region following sporting activities (can last for a few hours to few days)
8. Difficulty or discomfort with putting on shoes and socks

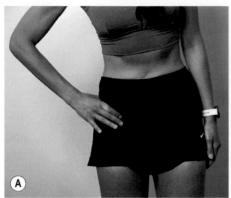
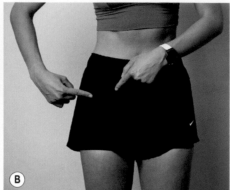
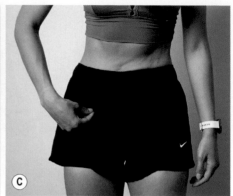

FIGURE 12.2
Clinical signs often presented by patients with intra-articular hip pathologies. (A) Trochanteric C-sign. (B) Triangulation sign. (C) Deep pointer sign.

In intra-articular hip pathologies, the patient often localizes pain by cupping the anterolateral hip with the thumb and forefinger in the shape of "C" known as the C-sign (Wilson & Furukawa, 2014). Other common clinical signs performed by patients with intra-articular hip pathologies are the triangulation sign and deep pointer sign (Figure 12.2). The presence of a limp, groin pain or restricted internal rotation predicts intra-articular hip pathologies, as opposed to referral from the spine (Brown et al., 2004).

Quantification of hip pain, function and severity of symptoms can be scored using one or more of the following validated questionnaires: Harris Hip Score (HHS), Hip Outcome Score (HOS), the Copenhagen Hip and Groin Outcome Score (HAGOS) and Non-Arthritic Hip Score (NAHS) and the International Hip Outcome Tool (iHOT-33) (Ramisetty et al., 2015).

Social history should be reviewed to determine the current use of alcohol, steroid and drug use, which might place the patient at risk of avascular necrosis (Shah et al., 2015). The history is not complete without gathering information on previous treatments that the patient had undergone to treat their hip and also any relevant investigations, organized by previous clinicians.

Finally, the clinician should ask the patient what he or she believes is causing their symptoms. Further, the patient's goals and expectations of the encounter should be discussed and the opportunity should be given to ask questions or raise specific concerns regarding their symptoms.

Clinical Pain Conditions of the Hip

To create uniformity on the diagnosis of hip and groin pain, the Doha consensus was agreed by international experts (Weir et al., 2015). These definitions and terminology are based on history and physical examination findings to categorize patients in a simple and clinical way that is also suitable for research purposes (Table 12.7). Further, the group also recommended avoiding the use of the following popular terms while describing hip and groin pain: adductor and iliopsoas tendinitis or tendinopathy, athletic groin pain, athletic pubalgia, biomechanical groin overload, Gilmore's groin, groin disruption, hockey goalie syndrome, hockey groin, osteitis pubis, sports groin, sportsman's groin, sports hernia and sportsman's hernia.

Physical Examination of the Hip

The hip can be difficult to examine due to its deep structure and thick soft-tissue envelope. To ease in the clinical evaluation of possible aetiologies of hip pain, it is helpful to divide the hip and pelvis into anterior, medial, lateral, and posterior regions. The purpose of this section is to introduce an evidence-based examination for individuals with hip joint-related pain. A systematic approach during the physical examination will enable the clinician to narrow the differential diagnosis made from the subjective history.

The key to the physical examination is to determine if the hip and groin pain originates from the intra-articular or

TABLE 12.7 Clinical Pain Conditions of the Hip (Adapted from DOHA Consensus)

Nomenclature	Symptoms	Signs
Adductor-related groin pain	Pain around the insertion of the adductor longus tendon at the pubic bone. Pain may radiate distally along the medial thigh	• Adductor tenderness • Pain on resisted adduction testing
Iliopsoas-related groin pain	Pain in the anterior part of the proximal thigh, more laterally located than adductor-related groin pain	• Iliopsoas tenderness (either supra-inguinal or infra-inguinal) • Pain on resisted hip flexion or pain on hip flexor stretching
Inguinal-related groin pain	Pain in the inguinal region that worsens with activity. If pain is severe, often inguinal pain occurs when coughing or sneezing or sitting up in bed	• Pain in the inguinal canal and inguinal canal tenderness, or pain with Valsalva maneuver, coughing, and/or sneezing • No palpable inguinal hernia found, including on invagination of the scrotum to palpate the inguinal canal
Pubic-related groin pain	Pain in the region of the symphysis joint and the immediately adjacent bone	Local tenderness of the pubic symphysis and the surrounding bone
Hip-related groin pain	Pain in hip and groin region with consistent aggravating factors and reproduced by hip provocative tests on physical examination	Clinical suspicion that the hip joint is the source of groin pain, either through history or clinical examination

extra-articular pathology and to confirm that the hip pain is not referred from other structures, e.g., the spine, lower abdomen or genitourinary system. Extra-articular pathologies will typically be aggravated by resisted muscular contraction or pain to manual palpation. Pain with contraction or passive stretch may indicate a muscle pathology or tendinopathy. Passive accessory and physiological examination are also a critical component of the hip exam (see Chapter 15 of this textbook).

A positional approach (Martin et al., 2017) is recommended to minimize patient discomfort, in which examinations are performed with the patient in standing, seated, supine, lateral and prone positions (Table 12.8).

Clinical assessment of the hip complex should incorporate standard screening of the lumbosacral spine and neurovascular testing of the lower extremities (see Chapter 11). The clinician should be cognizant that accurate diagnosis can be challenging, due to overlapping symptoms between the hip and lumbar spine pathologies (Buckland et al., 2017).

Standing Evaluation (Figure 12.3)

The patient must be exposed adequately for the physical examination and a chaperone should be offered to the patient, due to the intimate nature of the examination process. At first, the patient is instructed to demonstrate the pain location by pointing with one finger.

If the pain is localized at a specific location (e.g., greater trochanter), then it is likely that the source of symptoms is extra-articular. However, if the patient holds their hand in

TABLE 12.8 Hip Physical Examination in Five Different Positions

Standing	Seated	Supine	Lateral	Prone
General:	Neurological assessment	Limb length discrepancy	*Palpation:*	*Palpation:*
Posture, habitus, laxity	Peripheral circulation	*Palpation:*	Greater trochanter	Sacroiliac joint
Gait:	*Range of Motion:*	Adductor origin, pubic tubercle, lower abdominals	*Tests:*	*ROM:*
Antalgic gait, Trendelenburg gait	Hip internal and external rotation		• Abduction strength test	Hip internal and external rotation
Foot progression angle	*Test:*	*ROM:* Flexion, abduction, adduction, internal, and external rotation	• Gluteus medius Contracture	Hip extension
Spine:	Flexion strength test		• Snapping hip	*Tests:*
ROM, scoliosis, lordosis, pelvis symmetry		*Tests:*		• Ely's test
Tests:		• Log roll		• Craig test
Trendelenburg, squat, single-leg squat step-down test		• Adductor squeeze		• Active hip extension
		• FADIR		
		• FABER		
		• Stinchfield		
		• Thomas		

the characteristic C-sign or points to the groin region, it may be indicative of an intra-articular problem (Byrd, 2021).

The spine should be inspected from behind for scoliosis, excessive lordosis or kyphosis. Spinal obliquity and symmetry should be assessed by placing hands on the shoulder and iliac crests. Active range of motion of the spine should be evaluated to assess spinal limitation and the presence of pain referral to the limbs. At this stage, joint laxity is screened as per Beighton's criteria.

The patient should be observed for at least 6 to 8 strides to evaluate the gait pattern (Martin et al., 2010). The clinician should observe for gait abnormalities such as antalgic gait, Trendelenburg gait and foot progression angle (excessive in-toeing or out-toeing). An antalgic gait could be an indication of either hip or low back pathology (Braly et al., 2006). Many patients with hip pain may demonstrate an antalgic gait with a shortened stance and the trunk shifting towards the affected side.

A useful test to be included in the gait assessment is the Foot Progression Ankle Walk Test (FPAW) as described by Ranawat et al. (2017). The patient is instructed to internally

rotate the foot 15 degrees from their baseline pattern and the gait pattern is then evaluated. The test is repeated with the foot in 15 degrees of external rotation (Figure 12.4).

The presence of hip pain during this test raises the clinical suspicion of FAI or hip instability. The Trendelenburg test is performed by asking the patient to stand on one leg and hold the position for at least five seconds. A drop in the pelvis towards the non-weight-bearing side is indicative of the weakness of the hip abductors (Plante et al., 2011).

The single-leg squat and step-down tests can assess for kinematic and biomechanical deficiencies in individuals with non-arthritic hip pain (McGovern et al., 2018). Clinical assessment of performance on the single-leg squat test is a reliable tool that is useful to identify patients with hip abductor muscle function (Crossley et al., 2011).

The patient capability to deep squat is assessed in the standing position. A positive test is the reproduction of a patient's symptoms or inability to perform the test due to pain (Ayeni et al., 2014). Any other provocative activities identified during the subjective exam should also be assessed.

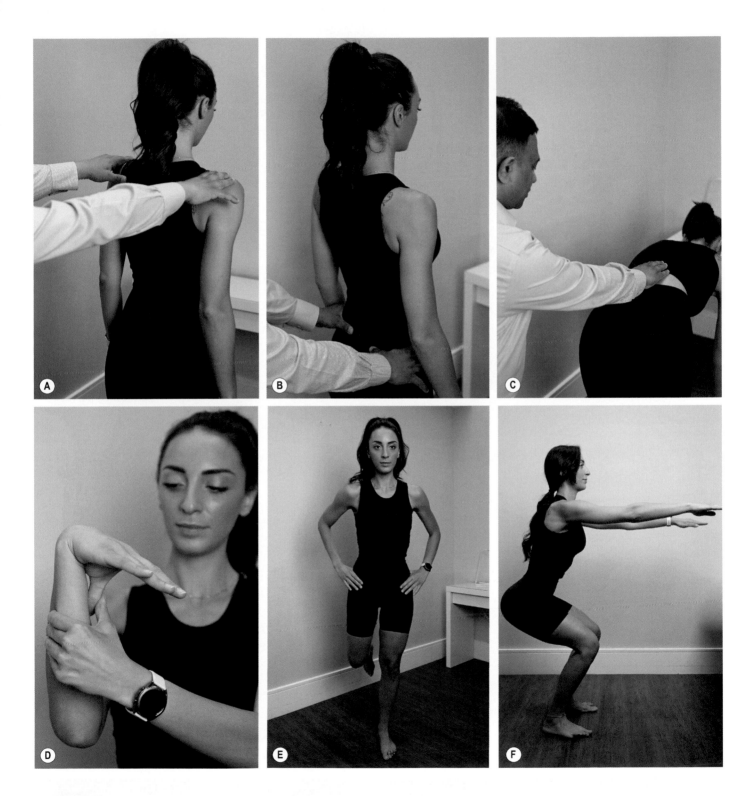

FIGURE 12.3
Standing evaluation. (A–B) Shoulder and iliac crest heights are examined. (C) The degree of full spinal flexion is noted. (D) Laxity of the thumb. (E) Single-leg stance test. (F) Squat test.

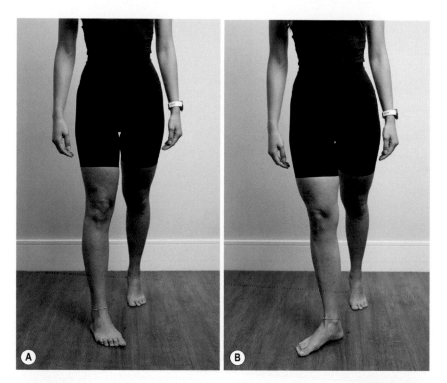

FIGURE 12.4
Foot Progression Angle Walking (FPAW) Test. (A) Internally rotate the foot 15 degrees. (B) Externally rotate the foot 15 degrees.

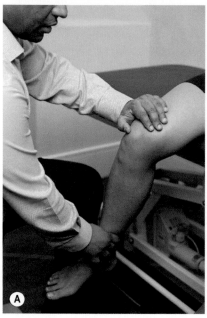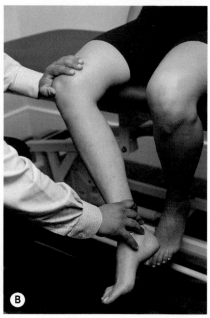

FIGURE 12.5
Sitting evaluation. (A) Internal rotation. (B) External rotation. Passive internal and external rotation testing are compared from side to side.

Sitting Evaluation (Figure 12.5)

One of the common complaints of a patient suffering from hip pathology is pain and discomfort with prolonged sitting (Clohisy et al., 2009). Therefore, examination of hips must include assessing hips in the sitting position. Observe for sitting posture, pelvic alignment over the lumbar spine and antalgic posturing while sitting. Alteration in pelvic tilt and reduction in seated hip flexion range could indicate compensatory lumbopelvic adaptation due to potential hip pathology. Neurological evaluation (including sensation, motor and reflexes) and peripheral circulation should be evaluated in the sitting position. Vascular assessment

TABLE 12.9 Normal Hip Range of Motion		
Range of Motion Assessment	Range (Degrees)	Abnormal (Degrees)
Seated internal rotation	20–35	<20
Seated external rotation	30–45	<30
Supine hip flexion	100–110	<100
Supine hip adduction	20–30	<20
Supine hip abduction	>45	<45
(Adapted from Martin et al. 2017.)		

includes inspection of the skin, swelling of the leg and posterior tibial pulse.

In the seated position, the pelvis is stabilized with both the ischia square with the table, while the hips and knees are flexed to 90 degrees. A key assessment in the seated position is passive hip internal and external rotation and this should be compared side to side for variations (Table 12.9). For optimal walking, there should be at least 10 degrees of internal rotation at the mid-stance phase of gait and a value less than 20 degrees is considered abnormal (Perry & Burnfield, 2010).

Excessive range of motion compared to the contralateral hip or normal anticipated range may indicate generalized ligamentous laxity or capsular laxity, whereas reduced range of motion (ROM) can be a sign of soft-tissue contracture, bony impingement or osteoarthritis of the hip. An increased internal rotation combined with a decreased external rotation may indicate femoral anteversion (Srimathi et al., 2012). The strength of the iliopsoas can be assessed in the seated position by asking the patient to lift their knee off the examination table against resistance.

Supine Evaluation

The supine examination begins with an inspection of both the limbs for any abnormality such as soft-tissue changes, discoloration, anterior thigh muscle bulk, symmetry of the whole lower limb and obvious leg length discrepancy. Leg length discrepancy can be assessed by comparing the distances between the anterior superior iliac spine and the medial malleolus (Sabharwal & Kumar, 2008).

Active and passive range of hip flexion, abduction and rotation must be evaluated as a part of the supine assessment. The patient should be encouraged to demonstrate provocative movements during active range of motion (ROM) test in the supine position to understand the potential etiology for their symptoms. The clinician should pay attention to audible clicking and clunking and crepitus during active range of motion, which could indicate snapping hip or coxa saltans (Byrd, 2005). The asymptomatic hip should be assessed prior to the symptomatic side and if bilateral symptoms present, the less symptomatic side assessed first.

While pain during active movements in this position mostly alludes to contractile elements as the source of the patient's symptoms, passive range of motion assessment will help to evaluate the articular involvement. Maximum hip flexion, abduction, internal and external rotation in 90 degrees of flexion should be recorded.

Palpation for localized tenderness is an important part of the supine examination. Initial palpation of the lower abdomen region to check for fascial hernias or masses is important to rule out gastrointestinal or genitourinary sources of pain. We recommend a sequential palpation, starting from the bony pelvis (ASIS, symphysis pubis, identifying the anterior border of greater trochanter), to the palpation of attachments of rectus abdominis and adductor muscle group.

Hip provocation pain maneuvers have relatively high sensitivity but relatively low specificity for detecting intra-articular hip pathology (Maslowski et al., 2010). With all provocative tests, the patient is asked if the specific maneuver recreates their typical symptoms, rather than simply asking if the pain is present during the test (Table 12.10).

1. Log Roll Test (Figure 12.6)

The patient is supine with the leg extended. The examiner passively moves the patient's lower extremity through the maximal available range of hip internal and external rotation. The log roll test is specific for hip joint pathologies,

TABLE 12.10 Hip Provocation Tests		
Test	Sensitivity	Specificity
FADDIR	99%	7%
FABER	82%	25%
Stinchfield	59%	32%
(Adapted from Maslowski et al., 2010; Reiman et al., 2015.)		

since it moves the femoral head in relation to the acetabulum and the capsules, but does not stress any of the surrounding extra-articular structures (Byrd et al., 2021).

2. Adductor Squeeze Tests (Figure 12.7)

When adductor-related groin pain is suspected from the history, adductor squeeze tests are performed (Serner et al., 2016). In the long-lever position, the examiner stands at the end of the table with the hands between the patient's feet and the patient is asked to press together with maximal force. In the short-lever position, the hips are flexed to 45 degrees

and the patient is asked to press both the thighs together with maximal force. The tests are considered positive if the patient experiences focal pain in the proximal part of the adductor muscles (Hölmich et al., 2004).

3. FADDIR Test (Figure 12.8)

The Flexion Adduction Internal Rotation (FADDIR) is performed in supine with hip flexion to 90 degrees, adduction and internal rotation of the hip, trying to reproduce the patient's symptoms. This test is highly sensitive and if negative, an intra-articular hip problem is less likely (Reiman et al., 2015). It is recommended that the FADDIR test is performed last, since it is typically the least comfortable for the patient (Lad & Kropf, 2019).

4. FABER Test (Figure 12.9)

The Flexion Abduction External Rotation (FABER) test is performed with the extremity placed in figure-of-4 position with the hip flexed to 45 degrees, abduction and external rotation and ankle resting on the contralateral knee. From this position, the examiner places gentle downward pressure on the tested knee. It should be noted that the FABER test can elicit symptoms resulting from pathology involving the hip joint, sacroiliac joint or iliopsoas tendon (Bagwell et al., 2016).

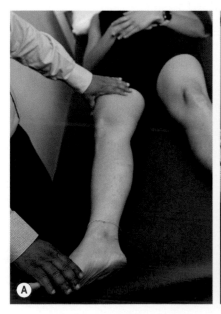 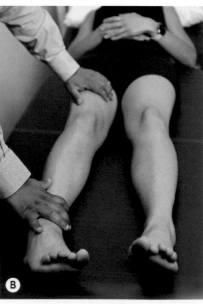

FIGURE 12.6
Log roll test. The patient is supine with the hip in neutral flexion. The entire extremity is log rolled back and forth to internal (A) and external rotation (B).

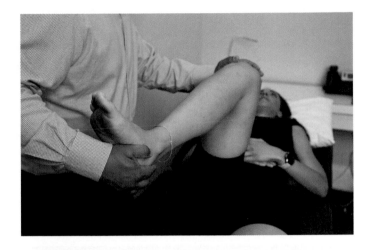

FIGURE 12.8
The Flexion Adduction Internal Rotation (FADDIR) Test. The FADDIR or anterior impingement test is performed in the supine position with flexion to 90 degrees, adduction and internal rotation of the hip, bringing the anterior femoral neck in contact with the anterior rim of the acetabulum, trying to reproduce the patient's symptoms thus indicating a positive test.

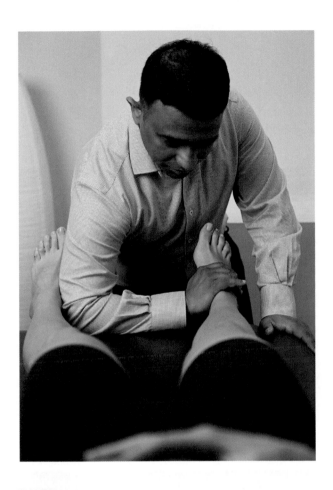

FIGURE 12.7
Adductor squeeze test. There are several adductor squeeze tests. The most sensitive is performed with the patient in the supine position. The clinician stands at the end of the examination table with hands and lower arms between the patient's feet holding them apart. The patient is asked to press the feet together with maximal force with the feet pointing straight up. A positive test accounts for pain reproduced from the common adductor insertion site. Another common version of the test is performed with the hips flexed to 45 degrees.

5. Stinchfield Test (Figure 12.10)

The Stinchfield test, or resisted straight leg raise, is performed with the clinician directing a downward force just proximal to the knee, with the leg in active hip flexion from 30 to 45 degrees for the reproduction of hip pain or weakness. This test evaluates both iliopsoas and intra-articular pathology, as the psoas muscle puts pressure on the anterolateral labrum (Poultsides et al., 2012).

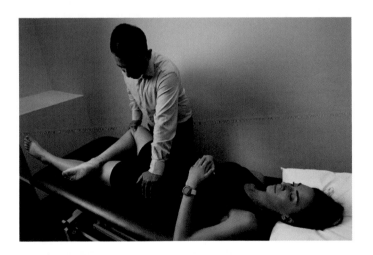

FIGURE 12.9
The Flexion Abduction External rotation (FABER) Test. The FABER test stands for flexion, abduction, and external rotation. It is considered positive for intra-articular hip pain if it reproduces the patient's typical groin symptoms.

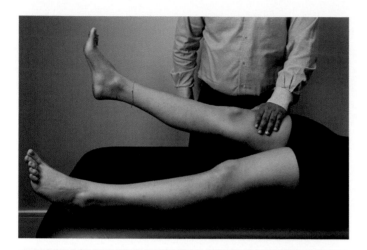

FIGURE 12.10
Stinchfield test. The examiner places a downward force on the proximal thigh just above the knee, as the patient forcefully flexes the hip to 45 degrees, with an extended knee.

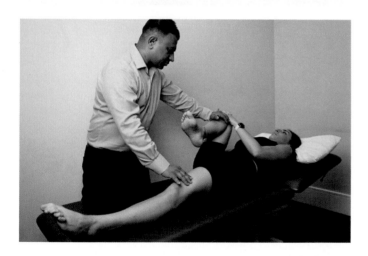

FIGURE 12.11
Thomas test or hip flexion contracture test. Zero set point of the pelvis is achieved by having the patient hold the contralateral leg in full flexion, thus establishing neutral pelvic inclination. The examined hip is passively extended toward the table. Both hips are evaluated for side-to-side comparison.

6. Thomas Test (Hip Flexion Contracture Test) (Figure 12.11)

The patient is instructed to flex both the knee and hip joint on the unaffected side and pull the leg to the chest.

A positive test would be indicated by passive flexion of the contralateral straight leg lifting off the exam test (McCarthy & Busconi, 1995). It is a useful screening test for iliopsoas tightness and hip flexion contracture.

Side-Lying Evaluation (Figure 12.12)

The side-lying evaluation is performed with the patient lying on the unaffected side. In this position, all the facets

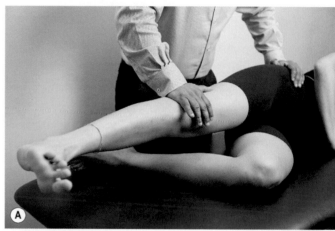

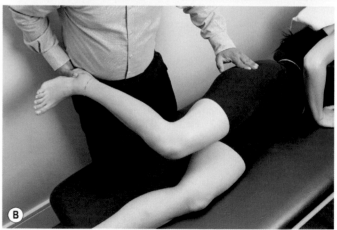

FIGURE 12.12
Side-lying evaluation of the hip. (A) Abductor strength assessment. The patient actively abducts the limb against the examiner, who utilizes his body weight as force of resistance. (B) Bicycle test. This test determines the presence of external hip snapping, by having the patient actively cycle the affected extremity from flexion to extension while lying in the lateral decubitus position. A palpable snap or clunk over the greater trochanter is confirmatory for this diagnosis.

of the greater trochanter (anterior, lateral, supero-posterior and posterior) are palpated and the gluteus medius is also palpated along its course. This is a common site of tenderness in greater trochanteric pain syndrome. The overall abductor strength is tested with the knee in extension and graded with a standardized 5-point scale. The passive adduction test in side-lying (the gluteus medius contracture test) is performed by the examiner supporting the limb in a neutral position, the knee in flexion and passively adducting the hip towards the examination table, to assess for tightness of the lateral hip structures (Cirdi et al., 2019).

External snapping is caused by a thickened or tight iliotibial band snapping over the greater trochanter and the patient often complains of the feeling that their hip is giving out or feeling unstable (Lewis, 2010). The patient is usually able to actively reproduce the snapping. Alternatively, it can also be reproduced by asking the patient to perform the bicycle test in side-lying, where the motion of a bicycle pedalling pattern is recreated as the examiner monitors for audible snap or clunk over the greater trochanter (Anderson, 2016).

Prone Evaluation (Figure 12.13)

Passive internal and external rotation of the hip should also be tested in the prone position. Hip rotation measured in three different positions (seated, supine, prone) can help the clinician to differentiate active versus passive structures that could cause a rotational range of motion restriction. It is important to be aware that the values of hip rotations can vary up to 10 degrees in different positions due to the ligamentous function and lumbopelvic interactions (Martin et al., 2017). A 20-degree difference between hip internal and external rotation range of motion would be suggestive of an abnormal femoral version (Uding et al., 2019). Active hip extension for gluteus maximus function is assessed by having the patient extend the hip and lift the whole leg off the table. In patients with suspected hip osteoarthritis, evaluation of passive hip extension range of motion is useful to identify any restriction.

Tenderness of the piriformis muscle and sacroiliac joint can be assessed in this position. The rectus contracture test (also known as Ely test) to assess muscle length of rectus femoris muscle can be done by passively flexing the knee and comparing it to the contralateral side. The upward motion of the pelvis indicates a positive test, which suggests contracture of the rectus femoris, since this muscle crosses both the hip and knee joints (Margo et al., 2003).

The femoral anteversion test (traditionally known as Craig's test) is also performed in prone position to assess the degree of femoral anteversion/retroversion. The examiner flexes the knee to 90 degrees and palpates the greater trochanter to keep it in its most lateral position by internally and externally rotating the hip (Souza & Power, 2009a). The degree of femoral anteversion can be estimated

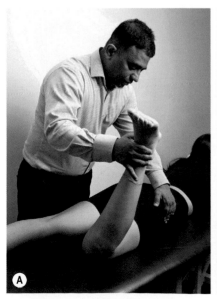
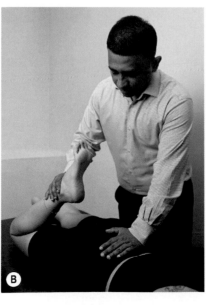

FIGURE 12.13
Prone evaluation of the hip. (A) The femoral anteversion test. The knee is flexed to 90 degrees and the examiner manually rotates the leg while palpating the greater trochanter. The examiner positions the greater trochanter so that it protrudes most laterally, noting the angle between the axis of the tibia and an imaginary vertical. (B) Rectus contracture test. The lower extremity is flexed toward the gluteus maximus. Any raise of the pelvis or restriction of knee flexion motion is indicative of rectus femoris muscle tightness/contracture.

using a goniometer with one arm perpendicular to the floor and the other arm to the angle of the leg; the normal range is between 10 and 20 degrees (Ruwe et al., 1992).

Subjective Examination of the Knee

Introduction

A comprehensive examination of the painful knee requires in-depth knowledge of anatomy, biomechanics and physiology, all of which are vital for optimal knee function. The clinician should have a thorough understanding of how injury and pathology influence knee health and therefore relate to the clinical presentation. This starts with careful and sensitive questioning, followed by the selection of relevant physical tests which help to support or negate a clinical hypothesis. This section will focus on the clinical examination of the most common traumatic and non-traumatic knee disorders, with consideration of the available evidence and current best practice.

History of Symptoms

A thorough knee assessment should always begin with a detailed subjective history, exploring the key components as listed in Table 12.11. The clinician should listen carefully to the patient's story, as it will provide vital clues regarding the possible diagnosis and whether urgent escalation of care is required, for example, if a significant intra-articular injury is suspected. When taking a clinical history, it is important to establish the patient's main concerns and their perception of the injury, as these factors will need to be addressed and may influence patient engagement and long-term prognosis.

Screening for Serious Knee Pathology

Serious knee pathologies include fractures, infections, inflammatory arthropathies and malignant processes such as a primary bone tumor or secondary metastases. Traumatic knee fractures typically occur following high energy trauma in the young, or low energy trauma in the elderly and individuals with compromised bone health. Common sites for knee fractures include the patella, distal femur and tibial plateau. Patients typically present with significant pain, swelling, difficulty weight-bearing and point tenderness. The Ottawa knee rules is a clinical decision-making tool to help clinicians determine which patients require

TABLE 12.11 Subjective History of the Knee	
Traumatic Injuries	**Atraumatic Injuries**
• Mechanism of injury • Initial symptoms, e.g., audible pop, ability to weight bear, ability to continue playing	• Onset of symptoms, e.g., sudden, gradual • Recent change in activity or load
General Knee History	
• Location and behavior of symptoms • Swelling onset, behavior, location and severity • Mechanical signs, e.g., clicking, locking, giving way • Aggravating and easing factors • Affected functional tasks and/or sport • Previous significant injuries • Previous interventions and response • Other joint involvement • General health, relevant medical conditions and medications • Patient beliefs, expectations and goals	

TABLE 12.12 Ottawa Knee Rules
A knee radiograph should be requested for patients with acute knee injuries who meet one or more of the following criteria: 1. Age 55 years or older 2. Point tenderness at the fibular head 3. Point tenderness at the patella 4. Inability to flex the knee to 90 degrees 5. Inability to bear weight immediately and in the emergency department (four steps)

radiographic imaging in acute knee injuries (Table 12.12). Given that these rules have high sensitivity and a low negative likelihood ratio, clinicians can be reasonably confident in excluding a fracture if the patient is negative on the Ottawa knee rules (Sims et al., 2020).

Septic arthritis is a joint infection that most commonly manifests in the knee, and it is a medical emergency.

Patients may present with sudden onset of a red, hot, swollen knee. Around 60% of patients present with systemic features such as fever (Weston et al., 1999). Risk factors include recent intra-articular corticosteroid injection, surgery, intravenous drug use, immunosuppressive medication, rheumatoid arthritis and diabetes mellitus. Gout is a crystal arthropathy that commonly manifests in the knee. It is caused by the build-up of uric acid in the blood, leading to the deposition of urate crystals in the joint. Patients typically present with acute onset of severe pain, swelling, erythema and heat. Associated factors include male sex, age 30–50 years, genetic predisposition and high purine diet (meat, shellfish, beer). Osteosarcoma is the most common primary bone tumor, occurring most frequently in the distal femur (Mirabello et al., 2009). Associated factors include age under 24 years or between 60 and 85 years, previous history of cancer, genetic predisposition, radiation therapy and Paget's disease (Mirabello et al., 2009).

Screening for Traumatic Knee Injuries

The knee is the largest and one of the most commonly injured joints. The rising popularity of sports such as skiing, snowboarding, basketball and football has resulted in an increasing number of traumatic knee injuries. During tasks that involve cutting, pivoting and twisting movements, the knee is often caught between the fixed foot and the moving torso, making it vulnerable to a variety of different injuries. The knee is also exposed to direct impact from opponents, as well as the environment. The most common traumatic knee injuries are detailed here (Figure 12.14).

Acute Meniscal Injuries

The medial and lateral menisci are crescent-shaped fibrocartilaginous structures that deepen the contour of the tibial plateaus and play an essential role in tibiofemoral joint stability, shock absorption and cartilage protection (Greis et al., 2002; Fox et al., 2015).

Acute meniscal tears typically occur in young adults when an excessive force is applied to an otherwise normal and healthy meniscus. According to an epidemiological study by Stanley et al. (2016), acute meniscal injury rates amongst collegiate and high school athletes are 0.53 per 10,000 athletic exposures for females and 0.68 per 10,000 athletic exposures for males. In this cohort, acute meniscal injury rates are highest in soccer and more common in males.

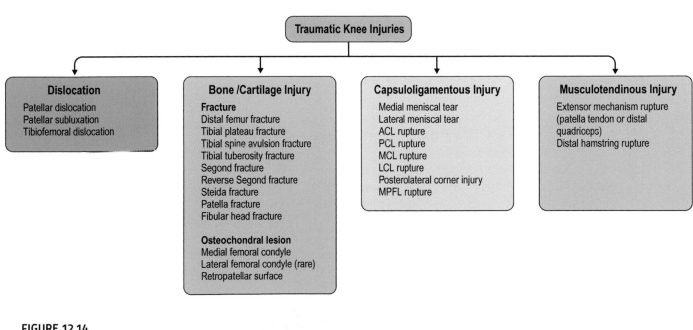

FIGURE 12.14
Traumatic Knee Injuries.

Acute meniscal injuries usually occur during cutting or pivoting tasks, when the foot is fixed and the femoral condyles rotate on a partially flexed knee. This creates a combination of shear and compressive load on the meniscal tissue (Hayes et al., 2000). Whilst meniscal injuries can occur in isolation, they are more commonly associated with a variety of osteochondral and ligamentous injuries (Brindle et al., 2001). In a cohort of 1104 patients undergoing anterior cruciate ligament (ACL) reconstruction, 65% demonstrated concurrent meniscal injuries; 26% of these involved both menisci, 52% involved the lateral meniscus, and 22% involved the medial meniscus (Slauterbeck et al., 2009).

Patients with an acute meniscal tear will often describe a twisting mechanism of injury associated with sudden pain and a possible tearing sensation deep inside the knee. They may also describe mild to moderate swelling that develops from 6 to 24 hours post-injury. Patients may describe clicking or catching with certain movements. True mechanical locking occurs when a displaced tear flips into the joint space and blocks extension, for example, during a bucket handle tear. Patients with true mechanical locking are unable to fully extend the knee unless the tear flips back into position. All patients with a locked knee require urgent referral to an orthopedic knee surgeon.

Anterior Cruciate Ligament (ACL) Injuries

The ACL is a complex structure extending from the distal femur to the proximal tibia. Functionally, the ACL is formed of anteromedial and posterolateral bundles, which are described according to their attachment to the tibia. The ACL is one of the main stabilizers of the tibiofemoral joint, providing primary restraint to anterior translation of the tibia (Petersen & Zantop, 2007), and playing a key role in resisting rotational forces (Andersen & Dyhre-Poulsen, 1997). ACL injuries are common in sports that have a high demand for landing, pivoting and cutting. Gornitzky et al. (2016) reported an overall incidence rate of 0.062 injuries per 1000 exposures in high school athletes participating in high-risk sports such as football, soccer and basketball. According to a recent study by Della Villa et al. (2020), 88% of ACL injuries in professional male football occur without any direct contact to the knee; however, around half of these injuries may involve some form of indirect contact, for example, to the upper body or pelvis. Approximately

---

> **TABLE 12.13 Key Subjective Features of an Anterior Cruciate Ligament (ACL) Injury**
>
> 1. Knee flexion, valgus and tibial internal rotation mechanism of injury
> 2. Audible "pop" or "snap" at time of injury
> 3. Significant knee effusion within 1–2 hours
> 4. Giving way during or after injury
> 5. Inability to continue playing
> 6. Poorly localized pain

12% of ACL injuries are attributed to a direct contact mechanism. Non-contact ACL injuries typically occur during deceleration tasks when the foot is fixed, and there is a combination of knee flexion, dynamic valgus and tibial internal rotation. Direct contact ACL injuries often result from an external valgus force to a flexed knee. Hyperextension ACL injuries are less common but may occur when a direct force is applied to the anterior aspect of the extended knee.

A thorough history is essential for diagnosing ACL injuries, and patients usually report typical features listed in Table 12.13. The "LIMP index" was proposed by Ayre et al. (2017) to support the early identification of patients with ACL injuries. The following features require careful consideration:

- **L**eg giving way (at the time of injury)
- **I**nability to continue activity immediately after injury
- **M**arked effusion (within six hours of injury)
- **P**op (either heard or felt at the time of injury)

According to Ayre et al. (2017), 95.8% of patients with a confirmed ACL injury report at least two features on the LIMP index. Therefore, patients with a score of two or more should be referred to a knee specialist without hesitation. This may reduce the potential delay to diagnosis and any consequences associated with this, such as secondary meniscal or osteochondral injuries.

Medial Collateral Ligament (MCL) Injuries

The MCL is arranged in layers with multiple attachment points. The superficial MCL is the largest structure on the medial side of the knee, and its deeper fibres blend with the medial joint capsule and posterior oblique ligament (POL) (LaPrade et al., 2007). The superficial MCL provides primary restraint to valgus knee loads, contributing to around 78% of the valgus knee restraint at 25 degrees knee flexion (Grood et al., 1981). The MCL is one of the most commonly injured ligaments of the knee, with an overall injury rate of 1.07 per 10,000 athletic exposures for female athletes and 1.16 per 10,000 athletic exposures for male athletes (Stanley et al., 2016). MCL injuries can occur through contact and non-contact mechanisms. Contact injuries to the MCL typically occur when a valgus force is applied to the lateral aspect of the knee (Andrews et al., 2017). Non-contact MCL injuries typically occur during cutting, pivoting or twisting, when the knee is in slight flexion and a valgus load is combined with tibial external rotation. MCL injury patterns have been studied in professional male football players and are suggested to occur most commonly near the proximal attachment (54%), followed by the middle third (31%) and less commonly the distal attachment (15.1%) (Lundblad et al., 2019). Grade III medial knee injuries are associated with ACL ruptures and can result in anteromedial rotational instability (AMRI), which occurs when the medial tibial plateau rotates anteriorly and laterally on the distal femur.

Patients with isolated MCL injuries usually report localized pain along the medial aspect of the knee joint line. They may also report localized swelling without significant hemarthrosis, unless there are concomitant injuries such as an ACL rupture. Patients may describe a side-to-side feeling of instability, especially with tasks that involve cutting and change of direction.

Screening for Non-traumatic Knee Pathologies

The key musculoskeletal sources of non-traumatic knee pain and their typical pain distributions are illustrated in Figure 12.15. Patellar tendinopathy and knee osteoarthritis are discussed in Chapters 6 and 4, respectively; therefore, these topics will not be discussed in this section.

Degenerative Meniscal Pathology

Degenerative meniscal tears develop gradually throughout adulthood and can be considered an early feature of knee osteoarthritis. Degenerative meniscal tears are frequently seen on imaging, with a prevalence of 30% in asymptomatic sedentary adults (Horga et al., 2020) and 31% in asymptomatic athletes (Beals et al., 2016). The cause of degenerative meniscal tears is often multifactorial and can include

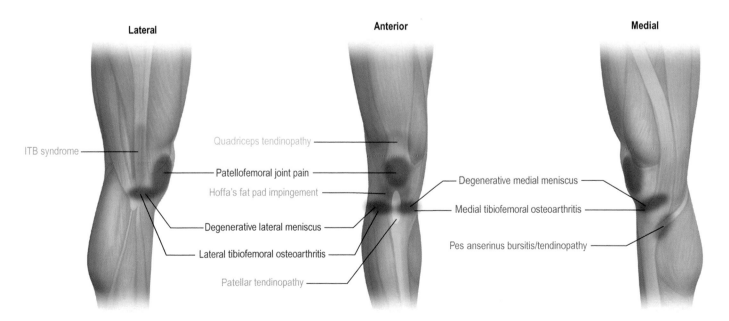

FIGURE 12.15
Common causes of non-traumatic knee pain and gross representation of the area of pain.

CHAPTER TWELVE

repeated micro-trauma, advancing age, high BMI and genetic predisposition.

Patients with symptomatic degenerative meniscal tears typically report a gradual onset of pain, which may be localized to the tibiofemoral joint line or felt diffusely around the whole knee joint. Pain is usually worse with weight-bearing, especially deep knee flexion or twisting movements. There may be some localized joint line swelling. Symptoms may initially improve with rest, but as the condition progresses, patients often report pain and stiffness after prolonged periods of inactivity, including up to 10 minutes of early morning stiffness. Patients may report painful clicking, but they rarely describe true mechanical locking, which is associated with acute bucket-handle meniscal tears.

Patellofemoral Pain (PFP)

PFP is a common source of anterior knee pain, affecting people of all ages and activity levels. PFP has an overall incidence of around 25% for sporting and military populations (Callaghan & Selfe, 2007). The annual prevalence of PFP is 22.7% in the general adult population (female 29.2%, male 15.5%), and 28.9% in adolescents (Smith et al., 2018). The differential diagnosis of anterior knee pain is extensive (Table 12.14); therefore, it is important to exclude other relevant conditions before making a diagnosis of PFP. The etiology of PFP is well described in Chapter 3 of this textbook.

Patients with PFP usually describe an insidious onset of poorly localized peri-patellar or retro-patellar pain, which is worse with activities that load the patellofemoral joint (PFJ), such as squatting, prolonged sitting and stairs.

TABLE 12.14 Differential Diagnosis of Patellofemoral Pain (PFP)

- Patellofemoral osteoarthritis
- Patellar tendinopathy
- Quadriceps tendinopathy
- Hoffa's fat pad impingement
- Meniscal pathology
- Patellar stress fracture
- Tibiofemoral osteoarthritis

Patients may also report additional symptoms such as crepitus, grinding and peripatellar swelling. Pseudo-giving way is sometimes reported during activities like descending stairs. This "break phenomenon" is believed to occur following reflex inhibition of the quadriceps, to avoid further pain associated with PFJ stress (Anderson & Herrington, 2003).

Iliotibial Band Syndrome (ITBS)

The iliotibial band (ITB) is a lateral thickening of the fascia lata of the thigh, which passes distally over the lateral femoral epicondyle (Fairclough et al., 2006), attaching onto the lateral surface of the patella and Gerdy's tubercle. Between the ITB and the lateral femoral epicondyle is a highly vascularized and richly innervated fat pad (Fairclough et al., 2006). The ITB is an important stabilizer of the anterolateral knee and it is suggested to provide primary restraint to tibial internal rotation from 30 to 90 degrees knee flexion (Kittl et al., 2016). The ITB is firmly anchored to the distal lateral femur via strong, oblique fibrous strands which prevent friction or sheering over the lateral epicondyle. It is suggested that the ITB is drawn medially towards the epicondyle at 30 degrees of flexion, which compresses the intervening fat pad (Fairclough et al., 2006). ITBS is the most common cause of lateral knee pain in runners (Van der Worp et al., 2012), but it also affects endurance athletes like rowers and cyclists. These sports involve repeated flexion and extension of the knee, resulting in high cumulative loads which compress the ITB fat pad, and over time may be sufficient to trigger a local inflammatory response. Runners with ITBS may demonstrate excessive femoral adduction and tibial internal rotation, which is suggested to exacerbate compressive loads beneath the distal ITB (Noehren et al., 2007). Around a third of runners with ITBS demonstrate varus knee alignment (Taunton et al., 2002), which is suggested to increase strain at the distal ITB when running.

Pain is localized to the lateral femoral epicondyle and is usually worse with activities such as downhill running or stair descent. Patients with ITBS often describe a recent increase or change in training load. During the early stages of ITBS, lateral knee pain occurs towards the end of a run or cycle, but as the condition progresses, pain is experienced earlier into the activity and can eventually become problematic at rest.

Hoffa's Fat Pad Syndrome

The infrapatellar fat pad (IFP) is a highly vascularized collection of adipose tissue that is richly innervated with nerve endings (Dragoo et al., 2012). This large, dynamic structure is believed to play several essential roles, including lubrication, movement facilitation, biomechanical support, and neurovascular supply to neighboring tissues (Gallagher et al., 2005). The IFP is a common source of anterior knee pain that is often overlooked and frequently misdiagnosed as PFP pain. The IFP can become pathological following mechanical overload, direct trauma, or penetrating injury from arthroscopy portals. These events trigger a local inflammatory response, which can lead to an edematous and enlarged fat pad, therefore exacerbating further compression, and affecting PFJ mechanics. Over time, chronic fat pad inflammation can lead to hypertrophy, fibrosis, scarring and persistent pain. Metabolic factors such as obesity can exacerbate the proinflammatory cascade in fat pad pathology (Chuckpaiwong et al., 2010).

Patients with Hoffa's fat pad syndrome typically report infrapatellar pain that is worse with prolonged standing, especially if the knees are hyperextended. Symptoms are generally eased with flexion and therefore better when wearing heels. Swelling is a common feature and patients may report a history of direct trauma to the front of the knee, or previous knee arthroscopy.

Physical Examination of the Knee

Physical examination of the painful knee should follow a systematic process to ensure that all relevant aspects are considered. It can be useful to perform the most provocative tests at the end of the examination, to reduce the risk of a false positive test occurring once painful structures have become sensitized or irritated. The following sections offer a general guide, but the significance of each section will depend on the history and main clinical suspicions.

Observation

The patient's lower limbs should be exposed sufficiently to allow for detailed observation of alignment and consideration of any relevant contributing factors both proximally and distally. When observing the lower limbs, it can be useful

TABLE 12.15 Observation of the Knee Area		
Standing	**Gait**	**Supine**
Weight-bearing symmetry	Antalgic (time in stance)	Resting knee position
Femoral ante/retroversion	Trendelenburg	Swelling/erythema
Genu valgum/varum	Hyperextension	Skin quality/integrity
Genu recurvatum	Reduced extension	Muscle wasting
Swelling/erythema	Quadriceps activation	Patella position/tilt
Muscle wasting	Varus thrust	
Tibial rotation or torsion	Excessive pronation	
Pes planus/cavus		

to adopt a top-down or bottom-up approach, to ensure that important information is considered (Table 12.15).

Functional Assessment

In the absence of significant knee trauma that compromises the patient's ability to weight bear and achieve normal movement, it can be useful to perform a functional assessment. This should explore key functional tasks such as walking, squatting, single-leg stance, single-leg squat and, where appropriate, jumping, landing and hopping. The clinician should consider local, proximal, and distal factors that may influence knee loads. For example, patients with patellofemoral pain have demonstrated strength and control deficits around the hip and pelvis when compared to pain-free controls (Dierks et al., 2008; Souza & Powers, 2009b, 2009c; Willson & Davis, 2009). Functional movements can also be used as pain provocation tests, and this provides an objective marker that can be re-assessed following a specific treatment intervention.

Swelling Assessment

Clinical assessment of knee effusion is an essential part of the examination. When combined with a thorough history, it can provide useful information regarding the possible underlying pathology. Careful consideration should be made regarding the potential causes of knee effusion, which include traumatic, systemic, inflammatory, infective, and degenerative pathologies.

Following acute knee trauma, the severity and timing of swelling can assist in establishing a diagnosis. Acute traumatic hemarthrosis may indicate a significant internal derangement of the knee and should therefore raise suspicion of the injuries listed in Table 12.16. Non-traumatic causes of knee joint effusion include osteoarthritis, inflammatory arthropathy, crystal deposition, infection, and neoplastic disease, examples of which are listed in Table 12.17. There is no gold standard method for quantifying knee joint effusion, and no single test is sufficiently reliable or accurate (Maricar et al., 2016). The clinical examination should therefore include careful observation of the normal knee contours, which are often lost around the extensor mechanism and patella.

The sweep test is considered a quick and easy way of assessing knee joint effusion (Figure 12.16). If a small bulge of fluid is detected on the medial aspect of the knee following the downward sweep, this is suggestive of intra-articular swelling. A simple grading scale can be used (Table 12.18), which is considered a reliable method of quantifying intra-articular swelling (Sturgill et al., 2009). The patellar tap/ballottement test is widely used to assess knee effusion, but it has demonstrated questionable inter-rater reliability (Fritz et al., 1998), therefore results should be interpreted with caution.

TABLE 12.16 Traumatic Knee Effusion

Acute Traumatic Hemarthrosis	Traumatic Localized Swelling
ACL rupture	Meniscal tear
PCL rupture	MCL tear
Significant meniscal tear	LCL tear
Tibial plateau fracture	Quadriceps muscle tear
Femoral condyle fracture	Hamstring muscle tear
Patellar dislocation	
Patellar fracture	

TABLE 12.17 Non-traumatic Knee Effusion

Musculoskeletal	Other
Degenerative meniscal pathology	Inflammatory arthropathy
Osteoarthritis	Gout
Suprapatellar bursitis	Calcium pyrophosphate deposition (CPPD)
Prepatellar bursitis	Infection, e.g., septic arthritis, osteomyelitis
Infrapatellar bursitis	
Pes anserinus bursitis	Pigmented villonodular synovitis (PVNS)
Stress fracture	Hemophilia
Spontaneous insufficiency fracture	Primary bone tumor, e.g., osteosarcoma
	Metastases
	Charcot arthropathy

Manual Palpation

Palpation can provide useful diagnostic information regarding pain, swelling or changes in temperature. Knee palpation should follow a structured approach, with careful consideration of the underlying anatomy, including soft tissue and bony landmarks (Figure 12.17). With the patient lying supine, the clinician carefully palpates along the length of the quadriceps and patella tendons, followed by the MCL, LCL, ITB and pes anserine. Bony landmarks such as the medial and lateral femoral condyles, patella, tibial tubercle, and fibular head should also be palpated. The knee should then be flexed to around 80 degrees, to allow palpation of the anteromedial and anterolateral tibiofemoral joint lines. Posterior structures such as the distal hamstring tendons can be palpated in prone. The clinician should identify whether palpation of each structure elicits the patient's symptoms.

Active and Passive Range of Motion

Knee active range of motion testing can be useful to establish the severity of symptoms and the patient's willingness to move, but it does not provide information about the strength or the full available range of motion at the knee

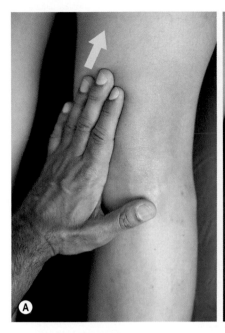
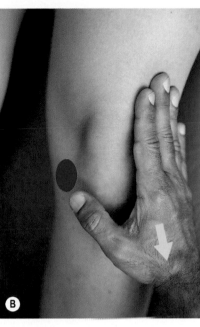

FIGURE 12.16
The sweep test. The patient lies supine with their legs relaxed and the clinician gently sweeps upwards over the medial aspect of the knee (A), attempting to move the effusion from the medial joint capsule into the suprapatellar pouch. If the fluid disappears, the clinician then sweeps downwards across the lateral aspect of the knee (B).

TABLE 12.18 Sweep Test Grading Scale	
0	No fluid wave produced with a downward stroke
Trace	Small fluid wave produced on the medial side with a downward stroke
1+	Large fluid wave produced on the medial side with a downward stroke
2+	Medial fluid spontaneously returns immediately after upward stroke (no downward stroke necessary)
3+	Effusion makes it impossible to stroke the fluid out of the medial aspect of the knee

joint. Passive range of movement testing, both accessory and physiological, provides invaluable information regarding local joints and soft tissues which may be painful, restricted or hypermobile. This information adds to the overall clinical reasoning process and provides a baseline for future assessment, treatment and rehabilitation. The clinician should begin by exploring passive knee movements slowly and gently, whilst considering the range of motion

available, any symptoms provoked, and the tissue resistance felt. Once the full available range is reached, the clinician should apply gentle overpressure to explore the "end feel," a phenomenon that was first described by Cyriax in 1975 (Cyriax, 1975). Certain anatomical structures will have a characteristic resistance that may be appreciated by the clinician (Table 12.19). Therefore, any deviations from normal may provide information regarding potential underlying injury or pathology. Goniometric measures of knee movement are considered more reliable than visual estimates (Watkins et al., 1991), with inter-rater reliability scores ranging from acceptable to excellent (van Trijffel et al., 2010). Smartphones can also be used to measure the passive range of movement by installing a simple goniometric application, which is considered as reliable as standard goniometers (Dos Santos et al., 2017).

Strength

Muscle strength testing forms an integral part of the knee examination. In an acute setting, it can raise or lower clinical suspicion of a significant muscle or tendon injury. It can also provide useful baseline information, which can inform future assessment and rehabilitation. Historically, manual muscle testing scales have been used to manually quantify knee muscle strength (Brigadier et al., 1943). The application of manual muscle testing to musculoskeletal practice

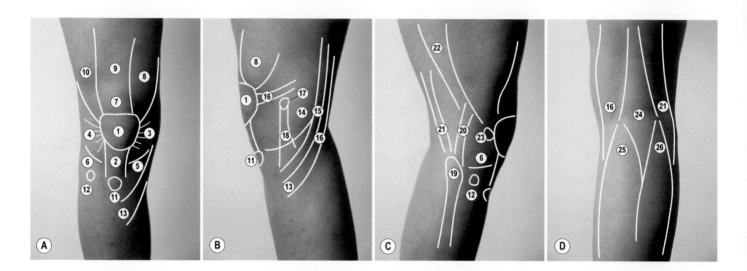

1	Patella	8	Vastus medialis oblique	15	Gracilis	22	Iliotibial band
2	Patellar tendon	9	Vastus intermedius	16	Semitendinosus	23	Iliopatellar band attachment
3	Medial patella retinaculum	10	Vastus lateralis	17	Medial femoral epicondyle	24	Popliteal fossa
4	Lateral patella retinaculum	11	Tibial tuberosity	18	Medial collateral ligament	25	Medial head of gastrocnemius
5	Medial tibiofemoral joint line	12	Gerdy's tubercle	19	Fibular head	26	Lateral head of gastrocnemius
6	Lateral tibiofemoral joint line	13	Pes anserinus	20	Lateral collateral ligament		
7	Quadriceps tendon	14	Sartorius	21	Biceps femoris		

FIGURE 12.17
Knee surface anatomy and general knee palpation.

TABLE 12.19 Knee Passive Range of Motion and Characteristic End-feel

Movement	Normal PROM	Primary Restraints	Normal End-feel	Abnormal End-feel
Flexion	135–140 degrees	Contact between posterior leg and thigh muscles	Soft-tissue approximation	Bony or hard end-feel may indicate osteoarthritis, loose body or bony injury
Extension	Up to 10 degrees of hyperextension is normal if equal to the uninjured side	Cruciate ligaments, oblique popliteal ligament, fabellofibular ligament, posterior joint capsule	Capsular restriction	Soft end-feel or excessive laxity may indicate capsuloligamentous injury, e.g., ACL rupture

has been criticized because large muscle groups such as the quadriceps are capable of producing significant internal forces, which are difficult to overcome by the clinician. Manual muscle testing has also been shown to lack sensitivity and diagnostic accuracy when compared to hand-held dynamometry (HHD) for identifying impairments in knee extensor strength (Bohannon, 2005). Given that manual muscle testing cannot detect subtle changes in

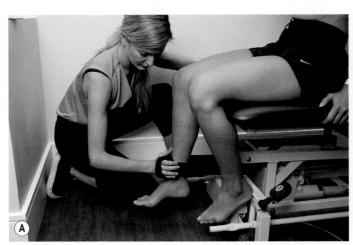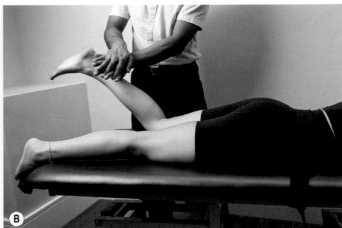

FIGURE 12.18
Isometric strength testing using HHD. (A) Quadriceps. (B) Hamstrings.

strength, it should only be used to detect signs of significant clinical weakness, for example following a suspected tendon rupture, or peripheral nerve injury. Following acute knee trauma, the ability to perform an active straight leg raise and seated knee extension can assist in excluding a significant extensor mechanism injury (McGrory, 2003). Further information on muscle and tendon injuries of the hip and knee can be found in Chapter 6 of this textbook.

HHD testing is affordable, portable and easily accessible to clinicians, providing rapid results that are reliable, reproducible and correlated with isokinetic values (Muff et al., 2016). HHD has demonstrated good intra-rater reliability when assessing lower extremity strength (Kelln et al., 2008), but it relies on the adequate force-generating capacity of the clinician, which may be difficult to achieve with young and active patients. The addition of an external belt removes the need for clinician applied forces and has demonstrated acceptable inter-rater reliability (Thorborg et al., 2013) (Figure 12.18).

Specific Tests

Meniscal Tests

There is no gold standard clinical test for diagnosing acute meniscal injuries. The clinician should therefore combine physical assessment findings with a carefully collated history. Lowery et al. (2006) developed a composite score that can be used to predict patients who are likely to have a meniscal injury. The composite score consists of five key elements: history of catching or locking, pain with forced hyperextension, pain with maximum flexion, pain or an audible click with McMurray's test, and joint line tenderness on palpation. A score of five points is suggested to have a positive predictive value of 92.3%, and a score of three or more is suggested to have a positive predictive value of >75%.

The most commonly used clinical tests for identifying meniscal injuries are McMurray's, Thessaly's and joint line palpation (Table 12.20). McMurray's test was first described in 1942 (McMurray, 1942), and several adaptations of this test are widely used in clinical practice. McMurray's test is

TABLE 12.20 Clinical Tests for Meniscal Injuries

Test	Sensitivity (%)	Specificity (%)
McMurray	61	84
Thessaly	75	87
Joint line palpation	83	83
(From Smith et al., 2015.)		

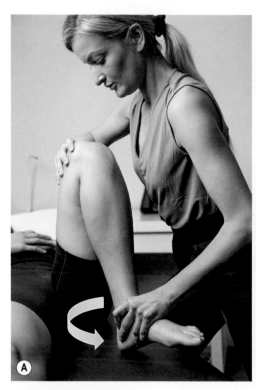
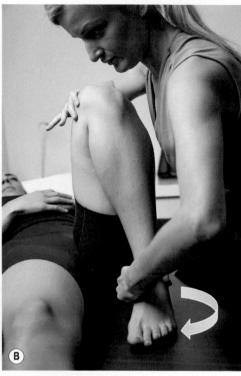

FIGURE 12.19
McMurray's test. (A) With the patient's knee fully flexed, the tibia is externally rotated, engaging the posterior horn of the medial meniscus under the medial femoral condyle. The knee is then extended, stressing the medial meniscus. (B) The clinician repeats the test with the tibia internally rotated, stressing the lateral meniscus.

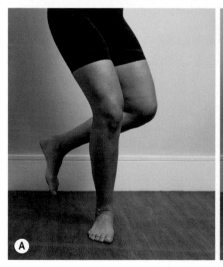
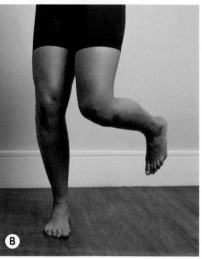

FIGURE 12.20
Thessaly's test. (A) Swivelling to the left. (B) Swivelling to the right. The patient stands on one leg and the clinician lightly supports their hands to assist with balance. Alternatively, the patient can rest their hands on a plinth for support. The patient flexes the knee to 20 degrees and rotates their body over the fixed foot three times from left to right. The other knee is flexed to avoid contact with the floor. Patient-reported pain at the medial or lateral joint line is a positive finding.

suggested to compress the posterior horn of the meniscus directly beneath its respective femoral condyle during knee flexion (Figure 12.19). The test is considered positive if a palpable clunk is reproduced together with pain at the joint line. Thessaly's test was originally described by Karachalios et al. (2005). Thessaly's test is performed in weight-bearing to reproduce axial joint loads combined with rotation, which are suggested to stress meniscal tissue (Figure 12.20).

The test is considered positive if joint line pain with or without clicking is reproduced. This test has moderate diagnostic utility, but may be less useful in an acute setting when significant swelling and pain are likely to produce false positives. Finally, joint line palpation is a quick and simple test, which is considered the most sensitive test for identifying meniscal injuries (Smith et al., 2015) (Figure 12.21).

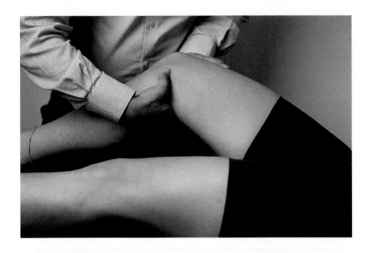

FIGURE 12.21
Joint line palpation. The patient lies supine with their knee flexed to around 80 degrees to expose the anterior tibiofemoral joint line. The clinician palpates along each joint line from the edge of the patellar tendon, as far back as can be reached. The test is considered positive if the patient's familiar pain is reproduced.

Anterior Cruciate Ligament (ACL) Tests

When assessing patients with suspected ACL injuries, it is important to combine elements from the history with key examination findings, using a combination of sensitive and specific tests (Table 12.21). The clinical utility of special tests for ACL ruptures has been extensively investigated, with varied results depending on factors such as rupture severity, associated injuries, clinician experience and whether the patient was awake or anesthetized. The three main tests for ACL injuries are the Lachman test, the anterior drawer test and the pivot shift test. More recently, the lever sign (also known as Lelli's test) has gained some popularity (Lelli et al., 2016). The Lachman test (Figure 12.22) and the anterior drawer test (Figure 12.23) are designed to identify anteroposterior laxity of the tibia. As the tibia is thrust anteriorly, a soft or absent endpoint compared to the uninjured side may suggest an ACL injury, whereas a definite or hard endpoint suggests an intact ACL. The Lachman test is considered the most sensitive ACL test in the fully conscious patient. The pivot shift test is the only ACL test that uses an

TABLE 12.21 Clinical Tests for Anterior Cruciate Ligament (ACL) Injuries

Test	Sensitivity	Specificity	Limitations
Lachman	89% (all ruptures) 96% (complete ruptures) 68% (partial ruptures) (Leblanc et al., 2015) 80%–99% (Malanga et al., 2003)	95% (Malanga et al., 2003)	Difficult to perform if the clinician has small hands or the patient has large legs False negatives – acutely swollen knee, unstable meniscal tear, protective hamstrings spasm False positives – PCL injury
Anterior Drawer	22%–95% (Malanga et al., 2003)	>97% (Malanga et al., 2003)	Less sensitive in awake patients. False negatives – acutely swollen knee, protective hamstrings spasm, meniscal wedging False positives – PCL injury
Pivot Shift	Awake: 79% (all ruptures) 86% (complete ruptures) 67% (partial ruptures) (Leblanc et al., 2015) Anesthetized 98% (Malanga et al., 2003)	>98% (Malanga et al., 2003)	Requires expert handling skills Less sensitive in awake patients

(Continued)

TABLE 12.21 *(Continued)*			
Test	**Sensitivity**	**Specificity**	**Limitations**
Lever Sign/Lelli test	68% (awake) 86% (anesthetized) (Jarbo et al., 2017)	96% (awake) 85% (anesthetized) (Jarbo et al., 2017)	Novel test which requires further scientific validation in different patient populations

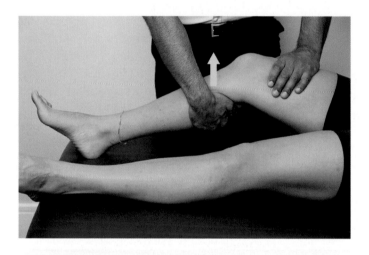

FIGURE 12.22
Lachman test. The patient lies supine, and the clinician stabilizes the distal femur with one hand, whilst holding the proximal tibia with the other hand. The knee should be in about 30 degrees of flexion. If handling is too difficult, the clinician may place their thigh underneath the patient's knee for support. The clinician applies a firm anterior force to the posterior tibia in an attempt to draw it anteriorly on the femur. The clinician observes and feels for excessive anterior tibial displacement compared to the uninjured side.

additional rotatory force to assess the ability of the ACL to resist anterior tibial translation, combined with knee valgus and tibial internal rotation. This test may reproduce rotatory and translatory instability of the tibia in an ACL deficient knee, which occurs when the tibia subluxes on the femur and then suddenly reduces at 30–40 degrees of knee flexion. The pivot shift test demands expert therapeutic handling skills, which require years of clinical experience; therefore, it is not widely used outside of specialist knee clinics. The test also lacks sensitivity in fully conscious patients, and so

may be more useful when performed on the operating table. Lever sign (Lelli's test) is a novel clinical test that uses the clinician's fist as a fulcrum to assess the lever mechanism of the ACL (Figure 12.24). A ruptured ACL will result in the tibia sliding anteriorly on the femur when the downward force is applied to the anterior thigh. The test is considered positive if the knee remains in flexion and the heel does not lift off the plinth. An intact ACL will limit anterior translation of the tibia, therefore when a downward force is applied to the distal femur, the leg acts as a complete lever and the knee is forced into extension, lifting the heel off the plinth. This test is easy to perform, and it is generally well tolerated by patients, therefore reducing the risk of pain or spasm influencing the overall result.

Medial Collateral Ligament (MCL) Tests

The clinician should observe for signs of localized swelling or valgus knee deformity in standing. Palpation along the entire length and width of the MCL may help to identify the location of superficial MCL injuries, but it is difficult to localize injuries to the deep MCL or POL. The valgus stress test is the main clinical test for identifying MCL injuries (Figure 12.25).

Historically, MCL injuries are graded according to the amount of valgus laxity demonstrated at 30 degrees of flexion, when compared to the uninjured side (Hughston et al., 1976) (Table 12.22). There is significant variation in the literature regarding the classification and grading of MCL injuries, which creates understandable confusion amongst clinicians and makes it difficult to establish an appropriate clinical diagnosis. A controlled laboratory study used stress radiographs to quantify medial knee gapping in cadaver knees and found that complete sectioning of the proximal superficial MCL produced 3.2 mm of medial compartment gapping

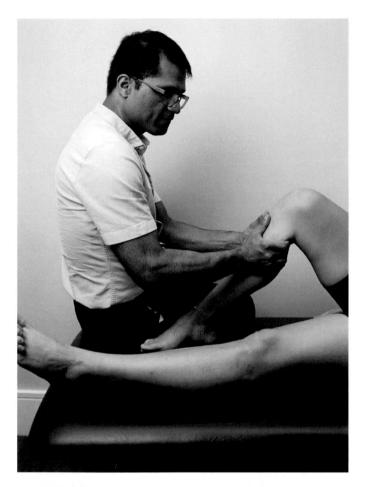

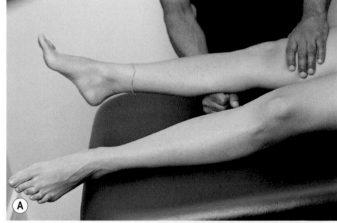

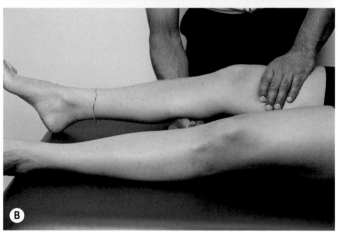

FIGURE 12.23
Anterior drawer test. The patient lies supine with their knee flexed to 90 degrees. The clinician stabilizes the patient's foot by perching gently on it and holding the proximal tibia in both hands, keeping both thumbs on the front of the joint line to palpate for signs of laxity. The clinician applies an anterior force to the proximal tibia, whilst observing and feeling for excessive anterior tibial displacement compared to the uninjured side, which may suggest an ACL injury.

FIGURE 12.24
Lever sign (Lelli's test). (A) Negative test. (B) Positive test. The patient lies supine with the knees relaxed in extension. The clinician places a closed fist under the proximal third of the calf, causing the knee to flex slightly. With the other hand, the clinician applies a downward force to the distal femur and observes the position of the heel.

at 20 degrees of flexion, whilst sectioning of all medial knee structures produced 9.8 mm of medial knee gapping at 20 degrees of flexion (LaPrade et al., 2010). These findings suggest that a valgus stress test may provide false reassurance to the clinician if the deep MCL fibers remain intact. The presence of valgus knee laxity in extension may indicate concurrent injury of one or both cruciate ligaments. However, medial compartment gapping has also been demonstrated with isolated MCL injuries (LaPrade et al., 2010). Therefore,

the presence of valgus laxity in full knee extension should always be correlated with the assessment of anteroposterior laxity, as well as a thorough clinical history.

Patellofemoral Joint Tests

There is no single clinical test that can reliably or accurately diagnose PFP (Nunes et al., 2013). The diagnosis should therefore be based on a cluster of signs and symptoms that

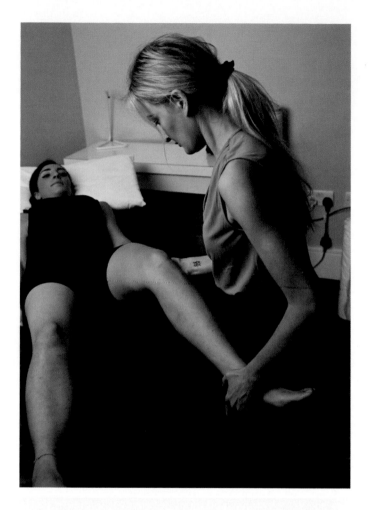

FIGURE 12.25
Valgus stress test. The patient lies supine and the clinician applies a valgus force to the knee in both 0 and 30 degrees of flexion.

TABLE 12.22 Medial Collateral Ligament (MCL) Injury Grading and Severity		
Grade I	<5 mm medial separation	Mild, minimal disruption
Grade II	6–10 mm medial separation	Moderate disruption
Grade III	>10 mm medial separation	Complete failure, significant laxity with a soft endpoint
(Originally described by Hughston et al., 1976.)		

anteversion, knee hyperextension and pes plano-valgus, all of which may be associated with PFP. Local observations should include muscle bulk, swelling, and resting patella position. The clinician should observe the patient performing specific loading tasks that can help to identify movement-related factors that may influence PFJ loads. A double- and single-leg squat can be useful pain provocation tests, but they can also be used to identify local, proximal, and distal factors that may be associated with symptoms. A qualitative scale can be used when evaluating the single-leg squat test, to provide clinicians with a reliable and standardized assessment of limb alignment and movement control (Almangoush et al., 2014). Palpation can be used to identify painful patellar and peripatellar structures, which may inform the diagnosis.

The lateral patella tilt test aims to detect tightness in the lateral peripatellar soft tissues (Figure 12.26). The test is considered positive if the clinician is unable to tilt the lateral edge of the patella when a downward force is applied to the medial surface of the patella in 20 degrees flexion of the knee. This is suggested to occur due to significant restriction from the lateral retinaculum and other lateral peripatellar soft tissues. The test is considered normal if the lateral edge of the patella tilts around 20 degrees above horizontal. According to Haim et al. (2006), this test has a sensitivity of 43% and a specificity of 92% when used on a cohort of infantry soldiers with patellofemoral pain. Therefore, a positive test may have some relevance in a

support a diagnosis of PFP, as well as a battery of clinical tests that exclude other conditions. The diagnostic criteria for PFPS were recently described by Willy et al. (2019).

1. Retropatellar or peripatellar pain.

2. Retropatellar or peripatellar pain reproduced with PFJ loading, e.g., squatting, stairs, prolonged sitting or other activities loading the PFJ in a flexed position.

3. Exclusion of all other conditions that may cause similar symptoms.

The clinician should observe the patient in standing and consider lower limb alignment including femoral

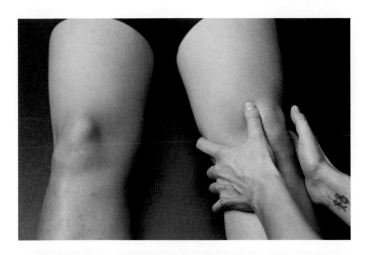

TABLE 12.23 Differential Diagnosis of Lateral Knee Pain

- ITBS
- Lateral patellofemoral joint pain
- Lateral meniscal pathology
- Lateral compartment osteoarthritis
- Lateral collateral ligament sprain
- Hoffa's fat pad impingement
- Distal biceps femoris tendinopathy
- Distal lateral femur bone stress injury

FIGURE 12.26
Lateral patella tilt test. The patient lies supine with the knees relaxed and supported on a pillow or towel in around 20 degrees of flexion. In this position, it is normal for the lateral edge of the patella to be tilted inferiorly in the horizontal plane by up to 10 degrees. The clinician attempts to lift the lateral edge of the patella by applying a downward force to the medial surface of the patella with their thumb.

small subgroup of patients but should always be combined with a cluster of tests.

Accessory glides of the patella can be useful to identify hyper- or hypomobility which may be unidirectional or multidirectional. Assessment of patella mobility has been shown to have moderate reliability and diagnostic accuracy in patients with PFP and may add useful information to the clinical reasoning process, but it should never be used in isolation (Sweitzer et al., 2010). Accessory glides should include lateral, medial, caudad, and cephalad directions. Anteroposterior compression can also be applied to the patella, which forces it into the trochlear groove and may reproduce retro-patellar pain. Clarke's test is commonly used as a pain provocation test for PFP. This highly provocative test has questionable diagnostic utility (Cook et al., 2012), therefore it is unlikely to add value to the assessment of PFP.

Iliotibial Band (ITB) Tests

There are currently no reliable or valid clinical tests for ITBS; therefore, the diagnosis should be based on a thorough clinical history and exclusion of other potential sources of lateral knee pain (Table 12.23). The clinician should observe standing lower extremity alignment and consider the influence of anatomical factors such as genu varum, internal tibial torsion and pes planus, which may be associated with ITBS. There may be mild swelling localized to the lateral femoral epicondyle. The lateral femoral epicondyle is often tender to palpate approximately 3 cm proximal to the knee joint. Knee range of motion is usually pain-free and unrestricted. The Ober test has historically been used to assess ITB tightness. However, a recent cadaver study has challenged this long-held assumption by demonstrating that outcomes of the Ober test did not significantly change following complete transection of the ITB (Willett et al., 2016). The validity of this clinical test for diagnosing ITBS should therefore be questioned.

Renne's test was first described by Renne in 1975 and it involves performing a single-leg squat to around 30–40 degrees of knee flexion (Renne, 1975). This position is suggested to compress the distal ITB against the lateral femoral epicondyle and therefore irritate the intervening fat pad. The Noble compression test was originally described by Noble in 1979 (Noble, 1979) and involves applying compression to the lateral femoral epicondyle, whilst passively extending the knee (Figure 12.27). Both these tests are considered positive if the patient's lateral knee pain is produced over the lateral femoral epicondyle when the knee is at around 30–40 degrees of flexion. Neither of these tests is well validated and their use in clinical practice is largely based on anecdotal evidence.

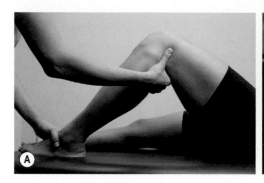
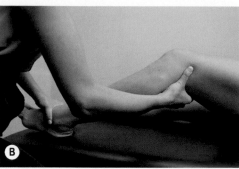

FIGURE 12.27
Noble compression test. The patient lies supine with the knee flexed to 90 degrees (A). The clinician applies and maintains compression to the lateral femoral epicondyle whilst extending the knee. The test is considered positive if the patient complains of pain over the lateral femoral epicondyle at approximately 30 degrees of knee flexion (B), when compressive forces are suggested to be the highest.

Hoffa's Fat Pad Tests

The clinician should observe the anterior knee for diffuse infrapatellar swelling. The patient may experience pain when standing with hyperextended knees and may have poor inner range quadriceps control when walking or negotiating stairs. Passive range of movement may reveal subtle loss of terminal knee extension, which is often associated with pinching pain (Hoffa's test). When palpated, the fat pad may be tender, thickened or enlarged. The patella may be stiff, especially with inferior glides because the fat pad can restrict the patella from descending into the trochlear groove.

A comprehensive examination should always start with a thorough history, which should form a significant part of the clinical reasoning process. Arriving at a clinical diagnosis is a complex process that combines significant elements of the history with key physical tests, to help rule in a clinical hypothesis and rule out any alternative diagnoses. Clinicians must maintain a broad differential during the evaluation process. This chapter outlines the importance of correct handling skills and interpreting physical tests within the context of the clinical history and other examination findings. Understanding these steps will support the clinician in developing excellent examination skills.

Conclusion

Hip and knee pain are common complaints among patients presenting to outpatient musculoskeletal clinics.

References

Almangoush A, Herrington L, Jones R. A preliminary reliability study of a qualitative scoring system of limb alignment during single leg squat. Phys Ther Rehabil. 2014;1:2.

Andersen HN, Dyhre-Poulsen P. The anterior cruciate ligament does play a role in controlling axial rotation in the knee. Knee Surg Sports Traumatol Arthrosc. 1997;5:145–9.

Anderson CN. Iliopsoas: Pathology, diagnosis, and treatment. Clin Sports Med. 2016;35:419–33.

Anderson G, Herrington L. A comparison of eccentric isokinetic torque production and velocity of knee flexion angle during step down in patellofemoral pain syndrome patients and unaffected subjects. Clin Biomech. 2003;18:500-4.

Andrews K, Lu A, McKean L, et al. Medial collateral ligament injuries. J Orthop. 2017;14:550–4.

Ayeni O, Chu R, Hetaimish B, et al. A painful squat test provides limited diagnostic utility in CAM-type femoroacetabular impingement. Knee Surg Sports Traumatol Arthrosc. 2014;22:806–11

Ayre C, Hardy M, Scally A, et al. The use of history to identify anterior cruciate ligament injuries in the acute trauma setting: the 'LIMP index'. Emerg Med J. 2017;34:302–7.

Bagwell JJ, Bauer L, Gradoz M, et al. The reliability of FABER test hip range of motion measurements. Int J Sports Phys Ther. 2016;11:1101–5

Bassett AJ, Tjoumakaris FP. Femoroacetabular impingement. Oper Tech Orthop. 2019;29:100735.

Beals CT, Magnussen RA, Graham WC, et al. The prevalence of meniscal pathology in asymptomatic athletes. Sports Med. 2016;46:1517–24.

Bizzini M. The groin area: the Bermuda Triangle of sports medicine? Br J Sports Med. 2011;45:1.

Bohannon RW. Manual muscle testing: does it meet the standards of an adequate screening test? Clin Rehabil. 2005;19:662–7.

Braly BA, Beall DP, Martin HD. Clinical examination of the athletic hip. Clin Sports Med. 2006;25:199–210.

Brigadier G, Riddoch M, Brigadier W, et al. Aids to the examination of the peripheral nervous system. London: Crown Copyright; 1943:70.

Brindle T, Nyland J, Johnson DL. The meniscus: review of basic principles with application to surgery and rehabilitation. J Athl Train. 2001;36:160–9.

Brown MD, Gomez-Marin O, Brookfield KFW, et al. Differential diagnosis of hip disease versus spine disease. Clin Orthop Related Res. 2004;419:280–4.

Buckland AJ, Miyamoto R, Patel RD, et al. Differentiating hip pathology from lumbar spine pathology: Key points of evaluation and management. J Am Acad Orthop Surg. 2017;25:e23–34.

Burnett RSJ, Della Rocca GJ, Prather H, et al. Clinical presentation of patients with tears of the acetabular labrum. J Bone Joint Surg Am. 2006;88:1448–57.

Byrd JWT. Snapping hip. Oper Tech Sports Med. 2005;13:46–54.

Byrd JWT. Make the right diagnosis: My pearls for working up hip-related pain. Sports Med Arthrosc Rev. 2021;29:2–8.

Byrd JWT, Jones KS. Diagnostic accuracy of clinical assessment, Magnetic Resonance Imaging, Magnetic Resonance arthrography, and intra-articular injection in hip arthroscopy patients. Am J Sports Med. 2004;32:1668–74.

Callaghan MJ, Selfe J. Has the incidence or prevalence of patellofemoral pain in the general population in the United Kingdom been properly evaluated? Phys Ther Sport. 2007;8:37–43.

Chadayammuri V, Garabekyan T, Bedi A, et al. Passive hip range of motion predicts femoral torsion and acetabular version. J Bone Joint Surg Am. 2016;98:127–34.

Chuckpaiwong B, Charles HC, Kraus VB, et al. Age-associated increases in the size of the infrapatellar fat pad in knee osteoarthritis as measured by 3T MRI. J Orthop Res. 2010;28:1149–54.

Cibulka MT, Threlkeld J. The early clinical diagnosis of osteoarthritis of the hip. J Orthop Sports Phys Ther. 2004;34:461–7.

Cırdı YU, Ergün S, Karahan M. Physical examination and imaging of the painful athletic hip. Hip and Groin Pain in the Athlete: Springer; 2019:1–31.

Clohisy JC, Knaus ER, Hunt DM, et al. Clinical presentation of patients with symptomatic anterior hip impingement. Clin Orthop Related Res. 2009;467:638–44.

Cook C, Mabry L, Reiman MP, et al. Best tests/clinical findings for screening and diagnosis of patellofemoral pain syndrome: a systematic review. Physiother. 2012;98:93–100.

Crossley KM, Zhang WJ, Schache AG, et al. Performance on the single-leg squat task indicates hip abductor muscle function. Am J Sports Med. 2011;39(4):866–73.

Cyriax J. Textbook of Orthopaedic Medicine, 6th edn. London: Baillière Tindall; 1975.

Delahunt E, Kennelly C, McEntee BL, et al. The Thigh Adductor Squeeze Test: 45° of hip flexion as the optimal test position for eliciting adductor muscle activity and maximum pressure values. Man Ther. 2011;16:476–80.

Della Villa F, Buckthorpe M, Grassi A, et al. Systematic video analysis of ACL injuries in professional male football (soccer): injury mechanisms, situational patterns and biomechanics study on 134 consecutive cases. Br J Sports Med. 2020;54:1423–32.

Dierks TA, Manal KT, Hamill J, et al. Proximal and distal influences on hip and knee kinematics in runners with patellofemoral pain during a prolonged run. J Orthop Sports Phys Ther. 2008;38:448–56.

Dos Santos RA, Derhon V, Brandalize M, et al. Evaluation of knee range of motion: Correlation between measurements using a universal goniometer and a smartphone goniometric application. J Bodywork Mov Ther. 2017;21:699–703.

Dragoo JL, Johnson C, McConnell J. Evaluation and treatment of disorders of the infrapatellar fat pad. Sports Med. 2012;42:51–67.

Draovitch P, Edelstein J, Kelly BT. The Layer Concept: Utilization in determining the pain generators, pathology and how

structure determines treatment. Current Rev Musculoskeletal Medicine. 2012;5:1–8.

Egger AC, Frangiamore S, Rosneck J. Femoroacetabular impingement: a review. Sports Med Arthroscopy Rev. 2016;24:e53–8.

Fairclough J, Hayashi K, Toumi H, et al. The functional anatomy of the iliotibial band during flexion and extension of the knee: implications for understanding iliotibial band syndrome. J Anatomy. 2006;208:309–16.

Fox AJS, Wanivenhaus F, Burge AJ, et al. The human meniscus: a review of anatomy, function, injury, and advances in treatment. Clin Anat. 2015;28:269–87.

Frangiamore S, Mannava S, Geeslin AG, et al. Comprehensive clinical evaluation of femoroacetabular impingement: Part 1, Physical Examination. Arthroscopy Techn. 2017;6:e1993—2001.

Fritz JM, Delitto A, Erhard RE, et al. An examination of the selective tissue tension scheme, with evidence for the concept of a capsular pattern of the knee. Phys Ther. 1998;78:1046–56.

Gallagher J, Tierney P, Murray P, et al. The infrapatellar fat pad: anatomy and clinical correlations. Knee Surgery Sports Traumatol Arthroscopy. 2005;13:268–72.

Gornitzky AL, Lott A, Yellin JL, et al. Sport-specific yearly risk and incidence of anterior cruciate ligament tears in high school athletes: a systematic review and meta-analysis. Am J Sports Med. 2016;44:2716–23.

Greis PE, Bardana DD, Holmstrom MC, et al. Meniscal injury: I. Basic science and evaluation. JAAOS. 2002;10:168–76.

Grood ES, Noyes FR, Butler DL, et al. Ligamentous and capsular restraints preventing straight medial and lateral laxity in intact human cadaver knees. JBJS. 1981;63:1257–69.

Haim A, Yaniv M, Dekel S, et al. Patellofemoral pain syndrome: validity of clinical and radiological features. Clin Orthop Related Res. 2006;451:223–8.

Harris JD, Chahal J. Femoral neck stress fractures. Oper Tech Sports Med. 2015;23:241–7.

Hayes CW, Brigido MK, Jamadar DA, et al. Mechanism-based pattern approach to classification of complex injuries of the knee depicted at MR imaging. Radiographics. 2000;20:S121–34.

Henschke N, Maher CG, Refshauge KM. Screening for malignancy in low back pain patients: a systematic review. Eur Spine J. 2007;16:1673–9.

Hölmich P, Hölmich LR, Bjerg AM. Clinical examination of athletes with groin pain: an intraobserver and interobserver reliability study. Br J Sports Med. 2004;38:446–51.

Horga LM, Hirschmann AC, Henckel J, et al. Prevalence of abnormal findings in 230 knees of asymptomatic adults using 3.0 T MRI. Skeletal Radiol 2020;49:1099–107

Horowitz SM, Berman AT. Metastatic Disease of the Hip. In: Horowitz SM, Berman AT (editor). Revision Total Hip Arthroplasty. Springer, New York, NY; 1999. Pp 498-504

Hughston JC, Andrews JR, Cross MJ, et al. Classification of knee ligament instabilities. Part I. The medial compartment and cruciate ligaments. JBJS. 1976;58:159–72.

Jarbo KA, Hartigan DE, Scott KL, et al. Accuracy of the lever sign test in the diagnosis of anterior cruciate ligament injuries. Orthop J Sports Med. 2017;5(10):2325967117729809.

Karachalios T, Hantes M, Zibis AH, et al. Diagnostic accuracy of a new clinical test (the Thessaly test) for early detection of meniscal tears. JBJS. 2005;87:955–62.

Kelln BM, McKeon PO, Gontkof LM, et al. Hand-held dynamometry: reliability of lower extremity muscle testing in healthy, physically active, young adults. J Sport Rehabil. 2008;17:160–70.

Kittl C, El-Daou H, Athwal KK, et al. The role of the anterolateral structures and the ACL in controlling laxity of the intact and ACL-deficient knee. Am J Sports Med. 2016;44:345–54.

Lad N, Kropf EJ. Hip pathology evaluation and imaging. Operative Techniques in Orthopaedics. 2019;29:100734.

LaPrade RF, Engebretsen AH, Ly TV, et al. The anatomy of the medial part of the knee. JBJS. 2007;89:2000–10.

LaPrade RF, Bernhardson AS, Griffith CJ, et al. Correlation of valgus stress radiographs with medial knee ligament injuries: an in vitro biomechanical study. Am J Sports Med. 2010;38:330–8.

Leblanc MC, Kowalczuk M, Andruszkiewicz N, et al. Diagnostic accuracy of physical examination for anterior knee instability: a systematic review. Knee Surg Sports Traumatol Arthrosc. 2015;23(10):2805–13.

Lee KS, Rosas HG, Phancao JP. Snapping hip: imaging and treatment. Semin Musculoskelet Radiol. 2013;17(3):286–94.

Lelli A, Di Turi RP, Spenciner DB, et al. The "Lever Sign": a new clinical test for the diagnosis of anterior cruciate ligament rupture.

Knee Surgery Sports Traumatol Arthros. 2016;24:2794–7.

Lewis CL. Extra-articular snapping hip: a literature review. Sports Health. 2010;2:186–90.

Lodge CJ, Sha S, Yousef ASE, et al. Stress fractures in the young adult hip. Orthopaedics Trauma. 2020;34:95–100.

Lovell G. The diagnosis of chronic groin pain in athletes: a review of 189 cases. Austral J Sci Med Sport. 1995;27:76–9.

Lowery DJ, Farley TD, Wing DW, et al. A clinical composite score accurately detects meniscal pathology. Arthroscopy. 2006;22:1174–9.

Lundblad M, Hägglund M, Thomeé C, et al. Medial collateral ligament injuries of the knee in male professional football players: a prospective three-season study of 130 cases from the UEFA Elite Club Injury Study. Knee Surgery Sports Traumatol Arthrosc. 2019;27:3692–8.

Malanga GA, Andrus S, Nadler SF, et al. Physical examination of the knee: a review of the original test description and scientific validity of common orthopedic tests. Arch Phys Med Rehabil. 2003;84(4):592–603.

Margo K, Drezner J, Motzkin D. Evaluation and management of hip pain: an algorithmic approach. J Family Practice. 2003;52:607–17.

Maricar N, Callaghan MJ, Parkes MJ, et al. Clinical assessment of effusion in knee osteoarthritis: A systematic review. Semin Arthritis Rheum. 2016;45:556–63.

Martin HD. Clinical examination of the hip. Oper Tech Orthop. 2005;15:177–81.

Martin HD, Shears SA, Palmer IJ. Evaluation of the hip. Sports Med Arthroscopy Rev. 2010;18:63–75.

Martin RL, Davenport TE, Paulseth S, et al. Ankle stability and movement coordination impairments: ankle ligament sprains: clinical practice guidelines linked to the international classification of functioning, disability and health from the orthopaedic section of the American Physical Therapy Association. J Orthop Sports Phys Ther. 2013;43:A1–40.

Martin HD, Palmer IJ, Hatem M. Essential findings in the clinical exam. In: Hip Joint Restoration. New York: Springer; 2017:145–55.

Maslowski E, Sullivan W, Harwood JF, et al. The diagnostic validity of hip provocation maneuvers to detect intra-articular hip pathology. PM R: 2010;2:174–81.

McCarthy JC, Busconi B. The role of hip arthroscopy in the diagnosis and treatment of hip disease. Canadian J Surg. 1995;38:S13–7.

McGovern RP, Martin RL, Christoforetti JJ, et al. Evidence-based procedures for performing the single leg squat and step-down tests in evaluation of non-arthritic hip pain: a literature review. Int J Sports Phys Ther. 2018;13(3):526.

McGrory JE. Disruption of the extensor mechanism of the knee. J Emerg Med. 2003;24:163–8.

McMurray TP. The semilunar cartilages. Br J Surg. 1942;29:407–14.

Mirabello L, Troisi RJ, Savage SA. Osteosarcoma incidence and survival rates from 1973 to 2004: data from the Surveillance, Epidemiology, and End Results Program. Cancer: 2009;115:1531-43.

Muff G, Dufour S, Meyer A, et al. Comparative assessment of knee extensor and flexor muscle strength measured using a hand-held vs. isokinetic dynamometer. J Phys Ther Science. 2016;28:2445–51.

Noble CA. The treatment of iliotibial band friction syndrome. Br J Sports Med. 1979;13:51-4.

Noehren B, Davis I, Hamill J. ASB. Prospective study of the biomechanical factors associated with iliotibial band syndrome. Clin Biomech. 2007;22:951–6.

Nunes GS, Stapait EL, Kirsten MH, et al. Clinical test for diagnosis of patellofemoral pain syndrome: Systematic review with meta-analysis. Phys Ther Sport. 2013;14:54–9.

Perry J, Burnfield JM. Gait analysis. Normal and pathological function 2nd ed. Thorofare, NJ: Slack; 2010.

Petersen W, Zantop T. Anatomy of the anterior cruciate ligament with regard to its two bundles. Clin Orthop Related Res. 2007;454:35–47.

Plante M, Wallace R, Busconi BD. Clinical diagnosis of hip pain. Clin Sports Med. 2011;30:225–38.

Poultsides LA, Bedi A, Kelly BT. An algorithmic approach to mechanical hip pain. HSS J. 2012;8(3):213–24

Ramisetty N, Kwon Y, Mohtadi N. Patient-reported outcome measures for hip preservation surgery: A systematic review of the literature. J Hip Preservation Surg. 2015;2:15–27.

Rana S, Stanhope RC, Gaffey T, et al. Retroperitoneal endometriosis causing unilateral hip pain. Obstet Gynecol. 2001;98:970–2.

Ranawat AS, Gaudiani MA, Slullitel PA, et al. Foot progression angle walking test: A dynamic diagnostic assessment for femoroacetabular impingement and hip instability. Orthop J Sports Med. 2017;5:2325967116679641.

Reiman MP, Thorborg K. Clinical examination and physical assessment of hip joint-related pain in athletes. Intern J Sports Phys Ther. 2014;9:737–55

Reiman MP, Mather RC, Cook CE. Physical examination tests for hip dysfunction and injury. Br J Sports Med. 2015;49:357–61.

Renne JW. The iliotibial band friction syndrome. JBJS. 1975;57:1110–1.

Robertson GA, Wood AM. Femoral neck stress fractures in sport: A current concepts review. Sports Med Internat Open. 2017;1:E58–68.

Rosenthal MD. Clinical testing for extra-articular lateral knee pain. A modification and combination of traditional tests. North Am J Sports Phys Ther. 2008;3:107–9.

Ruwe PA, Gage JR, Ozonoff MB, et al. Clinical determination of femoral anteversion. a comparison with established techniques. J Bone Joint Surg Am. 1992;74:820–30.

Sabharwal S, Kumar A. Methods for assessing leg length discrepancy. Clin Orthop Rel Res. 2008;466.2910–22

Serner A, Weir A, Tol JL, et al. Can standardised clinical examination of athletes with acute groin injuries predict the presence and location of MRI findings? Br J Sports Med. 2016;50:1541–7.

Shah KN, Racine J, Jones LC, et al. Pathophysiology and risk factors for osteonecrosis. Current Rev Musculoskeletal Med. 2015;8:201–9

Sims JI, Chau MT, Davies JR. Diagnostic accuracy of the Ottawa Knee Rule in adult acute knee injuries: a systematic review and meta-analysis. Eur Radiol. 2020;30:4438–46.

Slauterbeck JR, Kousa P, Clifton BC, et al. Geographic mapping of meniscus and cartilage lesions associated with anterior cruciate ligament injuries. JBJS. 2009;91:2094–103.

Smith BE, Thacker D, Crewesmith A, et al. Special tests for assessing meniscal tears within the knee: a systematic review and meta-analysis. BMJ. 2015;20:88–97.

Smith BE, Selfe J, Thacker D, et al. Incidence and prevalence of patellofemoral pain: a systematic review and meta-analysis. PloS One. 2018;13:e0190892.

Souza RB, Powers CM. Concurrent criterion-related validity and reliability of a clinical test to measure femoral anteversion. J Orthop Sports Phys Ther. 2009a;39:586–92.

Souza RB, Powers CM. Differences in hip kinematics, muscle strength, and muscle activation between subjects with and without patellofemoral pain. J Orthop Sports Phys Ther. 2009b;39:12–19.

Souza RB, Powers CM. Predictors of hip internal rotation during running: an evaluation of hip strength and femoral structure in women with and without patellofemoral pain. Am J Sports Med. 2009c;37:579–87.

Spina AA. External coxa saltans (snapping hip) treated with active release techniques®: a case report. J Canadian Chiropractic Assoc. 2007;51:23.

Srimathi T, Muthukumar T, Anandarani VS, et al. A study on femoral neck anteversion and its clinical correlation. J Clin Diagn Res. 2012;6:155–8.

Stanley LE, Kerr ZY, Dompier TP, et al. Sex differences in the incidence of anterior cruciate ligament, medial collateral ligament, and meniscal injuries in collegiate and high school sports: 2009-2010 through 2013-2014. Am J Sports Med. 2016;44:1565–72.

Stubbs AJ, Howse EA. Clinical evaluation of hip function: essential features in the history. In: McCarthy JC, Noble PC, Villar RN (Eds). Hip Joint Restoration. New York: Springer; 2017:139–43.

Sturgill LP, Snyder-Mackler L, Manal TJ, et al. Interrater reliability of a clinical scale to assess knee joint effusion. J Orthop Sports Phys Ther. 2009;39:845–9.

Sweitzer BA, Cook C, Steadman JR, et al. The inter-rater reliability and diagnostic accuracy of patellar mobility tests in patients with anterior knee pain. Physician Sports Med. 2010;38:90–6.

Taunton JE, Ryan MB, Clement DB, et al. A retrospective case-control analysis of 2002 running injuries. Br J Sports Med. 2002;36:95-101.

Thorborg K, Bandholm T, Hölmich P. Hip-and knee-strength assessments using a hand-held dynamometer with external belt-fixation are inter-tester reliable. Knee Surg Sports Traumatol Arthrosc. 2013;21:550–5.

Trofa DP, Mayeux SE, Parisien RL, et al. Mastering the physical examination of the athlete's hip. Am J Orthopedics. 2017;46:10–16.

Uding A, Bloom NJ, Commean PK, et al. Clinical tests to determine femoral version category in people with chronic hip joint pain and asymptomatic controls. Musculoskel Science Pract. 2019;39:115.

Van der Worp MP, van der Horst N, de Wijer A, et al. Iliotibial band syndrome in runners. Sports Med. 2012;42:969–92.

Van Trijffel E, van de Pol RJ, Oostendorp RAB, et al. Inter-rater reliability for measurement of passive physiological movements in lower extremity joints is generally low: a systematic review. J Physiother. 2010;56:223–35.

Watkins MA, Riddle DL, Lamb RL, et al. Reliability of goniometric measurements and visual estimates of knee range of motion obtained in a clinical setting. Phys Ther. 1991;71:90–6.

Weir A, Brukner P, Delahunt E, et al. Doha agreement meeting on terminology and definitions in groin pain in athletes. Br J Sports Med. 2015;49:768–74.

Weston VC, Jones AC, Bradbury N, et al. Clinical features and outcome of septic arthritis in a single UK Health District 1982–1991. Annals Rheum Dis. 1999;58:214–9.

Willett GM, Keim SA, Shostrom VK, et al. An anatomic investigation of the Ober test. Am J Sports Med. 2016;44:696–701.

Willson JD, Davis IS. Lower extremity strength and mechanics during jumping in women with patellofemoral pain. J Sport Rehabil. 2009;18:76-90.

Wilson JJ, Furukawa M. Evaluation of the patient with hip pain. Am Family Physician. 2014;89:27–34.

Willy RW, Hoglund LT, Barton CJ, et al. Patellofemoral pain: clinical practice guidelines linked to the international classification of functioning, disability and health from the Academy of Orthopaedic Physical Therapy of the American Physical Therapy Association. J Orthop Sports Phys Ther. 2019;49(9):CPG1–95.

Sacroiliac joint pain diagnosis in patients with hip and knee pain

Kenneth E. Learman, David W. Griswold

Introduction

Pain in the lower quarter can arise from any known pain generators distal to the ribcage. A comprehensive clinical examination must consider any and all of these potential pain generators as part of the screening process. The focus of this chapter is on the relationship between pathology stemming from the sacroiliac joint (SIJ) and its contribution to pain syndromes of the hip and knee.

Regional interdependence describes the relationship between impairments in one area of the body that may contribute to pain and dysfunction in another. These impairments may seem either directly or indirectly related to the patient's primary symptomology (Sueki et al., 2013). The notion of regional interdependence is more complex than strictly involving the musculoskeletal system as there are additional physiological systems that may contribute (Bialosky et al., 2008) or be involved with the treatment response (Bialosky et al., 2009; Bishop et al., 2015). In this chapter, we are focusing on how the SIJ may present with a pain pattern that might suggest hip or knee pathology.

The idea of the SIJ causing low back and leg pain has been supported for more than 100 years (Goldthwait & Osgood, 1905). Bogduk (2005) postulated that in order to be a pain generator, the SIJ must: (1) have a nerve supply; (2) cause clinical pain in asymptomatic subjects if provoked; (3) be susceptible to an injury or disease process that could cause pain; and (4) diagnostic techniques should be able to confirm that the SIJ causes pain (Bogduk, 2005). The SIJ is innervated, but the exact nature of that innervation is not conclusively well known (Bogduk, 2005). When the SIJ of asymptomatic volunteers was injected with contrast media, subjects experienced pain in the medial buttock (Fortin et al., 1994a). Beyond provocation with contrast media, the SIJ has been shown to experience disease and injury. A study of 484 lumbar CT exams of people aged 18–40 presenting with low back pain (LBP) found 150 SIJ imaging alterations comprised of suspected sacroiliitis (10.2%); definite sacroiliitis (3.3%); osteitis–condensans–ilii (7.8%); diffuse idiopathic skeletal hyperostosis (5%); degenerative changes (4.5%); accessory SIJ (4.5%); and tumor (<1%) (Klang et al., 2017). Finally, intra-articular injections (IAI) have been shown to reduce pain that arises from the SIJ, fulfilling Bogduk's postulates of sacroiliac joint pain (Bogduk, 2005).

Lower Quarter Differentiation

The SIJ and lumbar spine share a near-identical referral, from the thoracolumbar line to the foot, complicating differentiation of low back from SIJ; however, there are a number of subjective and objective assessments that should make parsing the conditions possible. Sacroiliac joint pain (SIJP) can share the same distribution as a herniated disk following the path of sciatic nerve distribution (Fortin et al., 1994a, 1994b). A study including 234 subjects with diagnosed disc herniations assessed for sacroiliac joint dysfunction (SIJD) and 33.3% were found to have a positive diagnosis of SIJP (Telli et al., 2020). This may be secondary to the branches of innervation from the lower lumbar segments. Those with SIJD had higher proportions of neuropathic pain, as measured by the Leeds Assessment of Neuropathic Symptoms and Signs Pain Scale (LANSS), depression (Beck Depression Inventory), lower overall function and higher kinesiophobia (Tampa Scale) (Telli et al., 2020), suggesting those with SIJP may also have relatively high rates of psychosocial factors perpetuating their pain syndromes. A sample of patients with persistent pain following lumbar fusion were examined for SIJP. Of the 130 patients, 52 (40%) had subjective histories that might include SIJ pathology and 21/52 were found to have SIJP as identified by a dual IAI (Liliang et al., 2011).

An examination for spinal pathology should include a neurological examination as needed to ensure buttock pain is not radiculopathic regardless of imaging (Weksler et al., 2007). Active and passive physiological movements, sustained positions and repeated movements, and special tests help determine if lumbar pathology may be present and to rule out centralization phenomenon.

Sacroiliac Joint and Hip Pain

A painful SIJ should be differentiated from primary hip pathology. The comprehensive examination of the hip is covered in a previous chapter. Pathology arising from the hip joint can refer proximally into the low back, as well as refer into the groin, and distally into the thigh, knee, or the entire lower extremity and must be differentially diagnosed as part of the comprehensive examination. Likewise, the SIJ can refer to the posterior, lateral, and anterior hip as well as cover all the areas just stated as referral patterns for the hip. These overlapping referral patterns from the hip and SIJ may require differentiation of these structures' contributions to the anticipated hip problem. Numerous studies have suggested that when examining hip pain, particularly posterior hip pain, one should rule out the SIJ as a source of symptoms (Cibulka & Delitto, 1993; Margo et al., 2003; Wilson & Furukawa, 2014). All these studies failed to use the current diagnostic gold standard for identifying SIJ, but all encouraged the use of pelvic asymmetry and just a single provocation test such as the FABER test.

One study demonstrated that 76% of subjects with SIJP had radiographic abnormalities of the hip, including femoroacetabular impingement (Morgan et al., 2013). More recent evidence suggests that in patients with femoroacetabular impingement (FAI) syndrome severe enough to warrant surgical intervention, more than 25% of those patients had concomitant SIJ pathology on imaging including joint surface erosion, subchondral sclerosis, joint space narrowing, pseudo-widening, bone marrow edema, and ankylosis (Krishnamoorthy et al., 2019). Those patients also experienced less successful outcomes following hip surgery (Krishnamoorthy et al., 2019). Because this was a retrospective comparative study, one must interpret these findings with caution (Morgan, 2019) since we know there isn't a strong correlation between radiographic changes and pain. The gold standard for SIJ dysfunction was not employed with this cohort (Morgan, 2019), but interestingly, this study demonstrates the complexity of differential diagnosis of lumbopelvic–hip pathology.

One study found that in the presence of SIJP, subjects had tight hamstrings accompanied by weaker gluteal muscles (Massoud Arab et al., 2011). This finding would suggest the possibility that there may be asymmetrical functioning of the hips secondary to strength differences that could create different forces through the hips of the subjects with SIJP.

Sacroiliac Joint and Knee Pain

Symptoms referred from the SIJ to the knee area should be differentiated from primary knee pathology. The comprehensive examination of the knee is also covered in a previous chapter of this textbook. Patients who have primary knee pain rarely experience pain proximal to mid-thigh so the knee can be effectively ruled out if the primary pain includes the proximal limb, groin, abdomen, or low back.

A case report examined the impact of SIJ manipulation and Kinesiotaping on anteromedial knee pain (Bucek, 2019). The author found that gait-limiting knee pain with no known mechanism of injury was unrelated to all lower extremity examinations. After ruling out neurological involvement, the subject was found to have SIJD as defined by Gillet's and Nachlas' test (Bucek, 2019). A muscle energy technique to modify innominate rotational position and Kinesiotaping to the knee were used along with Kinesiotaping and muscle strengthening for the weak ipsilateral gluteus medius muscle. The author attributes the improvement to correcting the pelvic imbalance identified by the SIJ testing, but since taping has been shown to reduce knee pain and strengthening of the gluteus medius has also shown an association with knee pain, it is not possible to conclude that the proposed SIJD was the reason for the pain. However, while the validity of the Gillet and other palpatory tests have been questioned (Palsson et al., 2019), this case study does bring up the question of whether or not knee pain could come from SIJD.

Suter et al. (1999) explored the relationship between SIJD and inhibition of the quadriceps muscle in subjects with anterior knee pain. In this single group observational study, subjects with anterior knee pain were examined for signs and symptoms of SIJD through posture, motion palpation, and SIJ provocation tests. Manipulation of the ipsilateral SIJ reduced the inhibition of the quadriceps muscle as well as increased knee extension torque. Of the 18 subjects tested, 12 had symptomatic SIJs and 6 had SIJD without symptoms. This study lacked a control group to enhance internal validity. A follow-up to this study involved a randomized clinical trial that sought to control for the limitations of the previous study and found the manipulation was more effective than control in reducing inhibition but there were no significant between-group differences in quadriceps recruitment or torque produced. All subjects had either symptomatic or asymptomatic SIJD on the ipsilateral side of anterior knee pain (Suter et al., 2000). Interestingly, both studies combined found that every single patient with anterior knee pain had SIJD. This may imply that either SIJD is universal in anterior knee pain, recruitment was limited to those that had SIJD, or that bias may be involved.

A primary limitation of each of these studies is that the diagnostic standard for SIJP was not used to verify the presence of SIJD. It is possible that asymmetry of pelvic landmarks is associated with muscle imbalance across the lower quarter and that contributes to the knee pain without actual SIJD. This problem presents a very interesting conundrum for the clinician. The historical methods of diagnosing SIJ has been the presence of asymmetry of bony landmarks or sulci based on palpatory tests or perceived movement dysfunction of the pelvis based on movement tests. It is possible that these abnormalities are assessing problems associated with imbalances in length and/or tension of surrounding musculature that impact the pelvic girdle. If this is indeed correct, assessment of these tests could be used to determine potential treatment options for these muscle impairments regardless of their relationship to SIJP.

Prevalence of Sacroiliac Joint Pain

If we are to differentiate SIJP from LBP, hip, or knee pathology, it would be advantageous to know prevalence to provide a pre-test probability of the disorder. The true prevalence of SIJP remains unknown because there isn't a clinical gold standard to reliably identify SIJP and because of the heterogeneity in research sampling strategies. Currently, the prevailing, but not universally accepted, diagnostic standard is a predetermined response to a fluoroscopic guided IAI (Chou et al., 2004). Diagnostic studies suggest that SIJP occurs in 15%–30% of chronic low back pain (CLBP) (Klerx et al., 2020). Remarkably, little is known of the prevalence of SIJP in the acute and subacute stages since the majority of prevalence studies have focused on differentiating the SIJ in samples with CLBP. It doesn't seem reasonable to subject patients with acute to IAI.

A study of 54 patients with chronic unilateral LBP consistent with SIJ found that 18.5% (95%CI 9%–26%) responded to an SIJ double IAI (Maigne et al., 1996). Schwarzer et al. (1995) found that 30% of CLBP may be the result of the SIJ with a more conservative estimate of at least 13%. Young et al. (2003) found 22 of 81 (27%) patients with CLBP responded to an IAI of the SIJ. Visser et al. (2013) examined 158 patients with CLBP and found that 26.6%

responded well to a dual IAI and that 41% of all patients with back and leg pain had mechanical SIJP. A study that employed a single IAI block had a 53% rate from 85 subjects with possible SIJP (Dreyfuss et al., 1996). Manchikanti et al. (2001) used broad inclusion criteria and found a remarkably low prevalence rate of 2% but an incidence of 10%. More recently, Sulieman et al. (2018) found that 22% of CLBP met the criteria for SIJP. These studies clearly show the variability of prevalence estimates based on the type of injection response used.

Using diagnostic imaging to identify patients with potential SIJP has yielded variable yet similar results. In fact, 31.7% of 315 who mostly had CLBP (n = 213) showed radiographic findings consistent with spondyloarthropathies or DJD of the SIJ (O'Shea et al., 2010). Madani et al. (2013) performed a cross-sectional study that found 72.3% of subjects with imaging-confirmed herniated disc pathology also displayed clinical signs and symptoms consistent with SIJ pathology. The study suggests that multifactorial conditions are prevalent and corresponds to Laslett's determination that subjects with a centralization phenomenon, usually associated with discogenic back pain, also test positive for the test item cluster (Laslett et al., 2003).

We know the SIJ can cause pain; we also know that abnormalities in the joint are common; therefore, it has been easy to jump to the conclusion that radiographic abnormalities are the cause of the pain. Further studies suggest that imaging abnormalities are common amongst asymptomatic individuals in the low back (Brinjikji et al., 2015), SIJ (Eno et al., 2015), and hip (Tresch et al., 2017). Eno et al. (2015) found that there was a steady progression of radiographic pathology in the SIJ with increasing age where 16% of subjects <20 years of age had degeneration, 30% in their 20s, and 91% of people in their 80s had DJD of the SIJ. Articular degradation occurs over time mostly with little to no discomfort in people, potentially implying that the degradation is simply a physiological adaptation to aging (Sizer et al., 2002).

Several studies have attempted to determine prevalence rates from the clinical examination alone. A study identified that 20.1% of pregnant Danish women at ~33 weeks' gestation had pelvic girdle pain (PGP) (Albert et al., 2002). The authors further attempted to categorize the 293 women with PGP into homogeneous groups and settled on the following four discrete categories: single-sided SIJ pain (5.5%), bilateral SIJ pain (6.3%), symphysiolysis (2.3%), and a combination PGP syndrome (pain in all three pelvic joints: 6.0%), and a general miscellaneous category of mixed presentation. A cross-sectional study reports a higher prevalence of PGP related to pregnancy at 60.4%, with an alarming 20% of the subjects reporting severe pain of >5 on the numeric pain rating scale (Mens et al., 2012).

Economic Impact

The economic burden of SIJP to society is essentially unknown because of the lack of precise prevalence estimates. Depending on the data used, it is possible to estimate SIJP being approximately 15% of the 29% of adults in the US with CLBP or roughly 10 million people (Cher et al., 2014). With total costs of CLBP in the US conservatively estimated at over $100 billion (Katz, 2006), SIJP may exceed $15 billion annually. Beyond the economic cost of SIJP is the burden of disease to the patient that is worse than many common chronic diseases but similar to those orthopedic conditions that require surgical intervention (Cher et al., 2014).

The Sacroiliac Joint

Anatomy

The sacroiliac joint (SIJ) is the largest axial joint of the body, ranging from 10.7 to 18.0 cm^2 (Vleeming et al., 2012) with a ligamentous area of 22.3 cm^2 (Miller et al., 1987), allowing the transference of forces between the lumbar spine and the lower extremity (Cohen, 2005). The SIJ is considered a diarthrodial cartilaginous joint containing synovial fluid with two distinct parts: a syndesmotic and articular section (Prassopoulos et al., 1999). The bony composition of the SIJ involves articulation between the sacrum and ilium bilaterally with ventral and dorsal joint surfaces at 1–2 mm thickness. The sacral side of the joint is covered with denser hyaline cartilage compared with more ventrally located fibrocartilaginous ligamentous tissue (Foley & Buschbacher, 2006). The sacrum medially and the two innominates laterally comprise the pelvic ring. There are five sacral levels with the sacral articular surfaces occurring at the S1 through S3 levels (Vleeming et al., 2012). The innominate is made up of separate ilium, ischium, and pubis bones at birth that fuse between puberty and the third decade of life. The innominates articulate anterior through a strong fibrocartilaginous joint, the pubic symphysis. Posteriorly, the wedge-shaped sacrum acts as a keystone between the innominates with the weight of the trunk and upper body creating form closure. The anterior, synovial portion of the joint starts with flat articular surfaces that eventually develop furrows and ridges that serve to further stabilize movement within the joint. These furrows and ridges are variable and irregular and begin to develop during the second decade and continue throughout life. Stability can be further enhanced through the development of bony bridges that occur on the joint anteriorly as some people age (Dar et al., 2008). The posterior component of the SIJ is syndesmotic and strong ligaments extend from the sacrum to the iliac tuberosities.

Ligaments contribute to the stability and limit the mobility of the SIJ. Ligamentous structures are classified as either intrinsic or extrinsic (Cuppett & Paladino, 2001) and are the strongest in the body (Vleeming & Schuenke, 2019). Intrinsic ligaments consist of the anterior and posterior sacroiliac ligaments (ASL/PSL), interosseous ligament, and long posterior sacral ligament (LPSL). Extrinsic ligaments consist of the sacrospinous (SSL), iliolumbar (ILL), and sacrotuberous ligaments (STL). The ASL connects the anterior surface of the sacrum to the ilium and is thinner and weaker compared to the PSL. The PSL consists of cranial and caudal running fibers located on the posterior aspect of the articulating surface. The multiband PSL attaches from the lateral edge of the dorsal half of the sacral ala to the ridge on the ilium. The interosseous ligament connects the sacrum to the ilium at the S1–2 levels. The LPSL consists of several bundles connecting the lateral surface of the sacrum to the posterior superior iliac crest (PSIS). The sacrospinous ligament connects from the sacrum and coccyx to the spine of the ischium and resides posterior to the sacrotuberous ligament. The sacrotuberous ligament is located on the posterolateral side of the joint connecting the lateral sacrum to the ischial tuberosity. Finally, the iliolumbar ligaments connect the 4th and 5th lumbar vertebrae to the iliac crest (Vleeming et al., 2012).

There is morphologic variability in the SIJ (Prassopoulos et al., 1999) and asymmetries in pelvic bony landmarks (Badii et al., 2003). A study of cadavers found that angles created from bony landmark differed (Preece et al., 2008), confirming a previous study that assessed angles using instrumented palpation (Petrone et al., 2003). A straight line drawn from the ASIS through the PSIS and a straight line from the anterior pubis through the ASIS was measured and found to vary between specimens by up to 23 degrees (Preece et al., 2008). Preece et al. (2008) also identified up to an 11-degree difference within specimen when compared bilaterally with up to a 16-mm difference in innominate height. These findings question whether or not symmetry can be expected during palpation and movement-based special tests of the SIJ.

Although the SIJ is surrounded by some of the largest and strongest muscles of the body that act on the lumbar spine and hip, no specific muscle appears to act directly on the SIJ. This fact suggests the driving force for SIJ movement must be force attenuation. The regional muscles that contribute to force closure include the iliacus, psoas, erector spinae, quadratus lumborum, gluteal, abdominal oblique, hamstrings, and pelvic floor muscles (Vleeming & Schuenke, 2019). The hamstrings attach to the sacrotuberous ligament and add posterior tension, the psoas crosses the joint ventrally, the transversus abdominis and latissimus dorsi both tighten the thoracolumbar fascia across the back of the SI creating tension. The pelvic floor serves as a functional stabilizer acting with the transversus abdominis for the SIJ and may be a method to retrain stabilization deficits in SIJD (Pel et al., 2008).

The innervation of the SIJ is multisegmental, complex, and variable across human studies (Vleeming et al., 2012). This complexity likely explains the various pain patterns that exist. It has been reported that nerve fibers extend from the ventral rami of the L4–L5, superior gluteal nerve, and the dorsal rami of L5–S3, to the SIJ (Nakagawa, 1966). Other authors report that the ventral part of the joint is innervated by segments L4–S2 (occasionally S3) and the sacral plexus, while the dorsal portion is innervated by lateral branches of the dorsal rami of segments L5–S4. Conflicting studies have shown the SIJ is strictly innervated by the dorsal rami of the sacral plexus (Grob et al., 1995; Fortin et al., 1999). Communicating branches also exist between the SIJ and nearby nerve structures, including the L5 radicular sheath and lumbosacral plexus (Fortin et al., 2003).

A comprehensive review of the literature reported that blood flow to the SIJ is supplied by the median sacral artery and lateral sacral branches of the internal iliac artery (Poilliot et al., 2019). These arise from the posterior sacral iliac blood supply from the gluteal arteries. Likewise, venous drainage occurs through branches that flow into the internal iliac veins (Poilliot et al., 2019).

Mechanics

The SIJs have 6 degrees of freedom as they rotate and translate around 3 distinct axes with an instantaneous axis of rotation midway between the PSISs (Smidt et al., 1995). The transverse X-axis runs side to side through the PSISs whereby sagittal plane nutation and counternutation of the sacrum occur. The vertical Y-axis allows the sacrum to rotate in the transverse plane as anterior translation of one SIJ with posterior translation for the contralateral SIJ. The sagittal Z-axis runs anterior to posterior through the mid sacrum for frontal plane rotation. Additionally, the right and left oblique axes have been proposed and serve as the theoretical basis for SIJD categories such as sacral torsions (Mitchell, 1958). There currently are no imaging data that validate these theories and DeStefano acknowledges that their biomechanics are unknown and their existence is largely hypothetical and useful for descriptive purposes (DeStefano, 2017).

A systematic review of the literature concluded that the SIJ has minimal movement (Goode et al., 2008). Seven manuscripts confirmed that rotational movements were −1.1/2.2 degrees of movement along the X-axis, −0.8/4.0 degrees along the Y-axis and −0.5/8.0 degrees along the Z-axis and corresponded to translation of −0.3/8.0 mm in the X-axis, −0.2/7.0 mm in the Y-axis and −0.3/6.0 mm in the Z-axis (Goode et al., 2008). Roentgen stereophotogrammetric analysis (RSA), the most reliable and valid measurement technique, favors ranges and translations on the lower end of these reports. Movement of the SIJ is lessened in weight-bearing (Sturesson et al., 2000) and may be the result of additional compressive loads of the trunk enhancing form and force closure (Pool-Goudzwaard et al., 1998). As an individual moves in function, the pubic symphysis shears and the innominates deform (Pool-Goudzwaard et al., 2012), which may complicate the ability to identify mechanical and positional abnormalities, if they exist.

The pelvic joints provide an avenue for force translation and dissipation between the legs and trunk because of their mobility dictated by passive forces (Snijders et al., 1993a). It has been hypothesized that the pelvis would fracture if the small amount of available movement wasn't there. Sacral insufficiency fractures have occurred in people who have reduced natural movement through age and weakened bony structures of the sacrum (Grasland, 1996) such as postmenopausal women and those with highly repetitive loading on a weakened sacrum (Myburgh et al., 1990), e.g., high-mileage female runners lacking sufficient nutritional support (Wentz et al., 2011).

Pelvic ring stabilization occurs through two mechanisms, form and force closure (Vleeming et al., 1990a, 1990b; Snijders et al., 1993a, 1993b). Form closure consists of passive structures working together to create stabilization. The sacrum is a wedge-shaped bone acting as a keystone as gravity and body weight force it down between the ilia. The SIJs have reduced movement in weight-bearing because of this effect (Sturesson et al., 2000). The sacral facets that articulate with the inferior L5 facets are posteriorly facing to reduce the anterior shearing of the lumbar spine on a nutated sacrum. Many strong ligaments previously described hold the ilia together as the sacrum tries to force them apart while the medially facing necks of the femurs translate ground reaction forces to the ilia forcing them together to stabilize the pubic symphysis. Stability should be maximized with equal, bilateral weight-bearing but the highest forces translated into the kinematic chain occur during unilateral jumping and landing, necessitating another mechanism to enhance stabilization of the pelvic ring.

External stabilization to the SIJs and pelvic ring through muscular tension is called force closure. Numerous muscles attach with either the thoracolumbar fascia or stabilizing ligaments of the SIJ or pubic symphysis to enhance the stability of the SIJ. Vleeming et al. (1995) have reported that there are two slings, the anterior and posterior slings. The posterior sling comprises the hamstrings and gluteus maximus muscles on one side with the multifidi and latissimus dorsi on the contralateral side, whereas the anterior sling is the transversus abdominis and internal oblique on the homolateral side with the contralateral adductors. These two slings work in concert to create additional tension in the SIJ as needed with the diagonal patterning assisting during unilateral stance in functional movements such as gait. A co-contraction of the multifidi and the transversus abdominis will stiffen the SIJ to a greater extent than a targeted diagonal pattern of the pelvic slings (Richardson et al., 2002); however, the additional force for stabilization through the anterior (Richardson et al., 2002) and posterior slings (van Wingerden et al., 2004) is there as part of the natural system to provide force closure. Form and force closure are interdependent because those muscular attachments into the stabilizing ligaments create additional tension to stabilize the pelvis.

Pathomechanics

The theories of alternate axes for the SIJs have served as a foundational basis for numerous pathologies whereby the SIJ is thought to get "stuck" in positions that are not normal. These positional faults are thought to cause pain and altered movement and are classified as dysfunctions. These dysfunctions include upslips, downslips, inflares, ouflares, forward or backward sacral torsions. Despite the fact that they are theoretically possible, there is no evidence to suggest that they typically occur in everyday life outside of circumstances of extreme trauma. Radiographic examination has never verified the existence of positional faults. The use of these positional faults as a model to examine and treat dysfunction of the SIJ, clinically speaking, is no longer relevant and should be abandoned (Palsson et al., 2019).

Clinically, it is not uncommon to find asymmetries in the positions of the ASISs and PSISs relative to one another that would give the appearance of validity to these theories of dysfunction. But the asymmetries identified clinically may not correspond to movement at the SIJ as measured through RSA techniques. The best example of this dissonance of clinical versus radiographic reality was identified by Tullberg et al. (1998). In this study, 10 patients were examined by three expert clinicians and found to have pelvic asymmetries, before receiving a manipulative treatment. These patients also had radiographic assessment of pelvic position as identified by RSA. Following the manipulative treatment, the clinicians found that the position of the pelvis had normalized by their clinical assessment; however, the RSA techniques found no change in the position of the SIJs. This study suggests that something other than the SIJ would account for the observed relationship of the bony landmarks clinically. It is far more likely that muscular influences alter the perception of the positional fault than actual SIJ patho-mechanics.

Motor control appears to be associated with the development of PGP (Aldabe et al., 2012). De Groot et al. (2008)

reported that a sample of subjects with PGP had increased muscle activity with less force production during the active straight leg raise test. Wu et al. (2008) found that a sample of patients with PGP had rotational differences compared to subjects without PGP during a gait analysis. More recent evidence suggests that the pelvic floor does not fire in a feedforward manner on the ipsilateral leg during the active straight leg raise test (Sjödahl et al., 2016). Despite motor control differences, even in severe protracted PGP, the active straight leg raise test only results in small amounts of SIJ rotation and nearly no translation as measured by RSA techniques (Kibsgård et al., 2017). This reinforces previous work from a sample of 163 women that those with moderate to severe pelvic pain didn't have significantly different laxity than those that had mild or no pain but that side-to-side symmetry in laxity was different (Damen et al., 2001). However, greater muscular recruitment may be required by subjects to perform the active straight leg raise test than those without pain (de Groot et al., 2008; Beales et al., 2009) with a greater perception of effort to complete the task (de Groot et al., 2008).

Diagnosis

The first question addressed in the assessment of lower quarter pain should be whether or not the presumed musculoskeletal pathology is an underlying medical condition that may not be suited for rehabilitation care (Murphy & Hurwitz, 2007). Only after appropriate medical screening can we move onto our follow-up questions of specific tissue diagnosis, and potential psychosocial involvement (Huijbregts, 2004; Sizer et al., 2007).

Many medical conditions can cause SIJP and should be ruled out before a course of rehabilitation treatment is begun. These pathologies can be divided up into rheumatologic versus non-rheumatologic ailments (Gupta, 2009). Examples of conditions that can produce SIJ pain include but are not limited to spondyloarthropathies, infectious, neoplastic, or metabolic disorders (Gupta, 2009). Depending on the age and condition of the patient, local fractures can also be a differential diagnosis.

To make a clear diagnosis of SIJP, three features must exist according to the International Association for the Study of Pain (IASP). The primary concordant pain should be in the general region of the SIJ, either directly over the PSIS or the medial buttock; there should be positive tests of provocation for pain in the SIJ region pain; and the pain must be alleviated by IAI (Merskey & Bogduk, 1994). These criteria are difficult to accomplish clinically since the vast majority of patients with suspected SIJ pathology fail to receive the confirmatory IAI, especially in the acute phase of pain. But the first two criteria are easily implemented in the clinical examination. These criteria are routinely referenced as the gold standard for SIJP; they are not universally accepted by all disciplines or researchers.

Pain patterning is not always consistent. Most studies have found that the primary pain is unilateral, below the L5 spinous process and in the region of the PSIS. There may be inconsistent pain referral patterns from the primary site that may include but are not limited to a span ranging from the upper lumbar spine to the foot. It has also been documented through injection studies that the SIJ can be accompanied by sciatica including both numbness and tingling extra-segmentally through those distribution patterns as well with only 6% showing a consistent dermatomal pattern (Murakami et al., 2017). Therefore, the clinician needs to be mindful of the full array of symptoms associated with SIJP.

Diagnostic blocks may be the best method of diagnosing pain of SIJ origin but they are invasive, aren't without difficulties in performance and interpretation, and are not routinely available for clinical use (Simopoulos et al., 2012). The region of periarticular structures infiltrated may determine the region of pain or vice versa. The area of pain may suggest which region of the periarticular structures are symptomatic (Kurosawa et al., 2015). Murakami et al. (2007) found that periarticular injections were more effective than intra-articular and they suggested that periarticular should be tried initially. As an alternative to fluoroscopically guided IAI, diagnostic ultrasound can also be used to guide the IAI, which may help avoid vessels but also reduces the accuracy from 98.2% to 87.3% (Jee et al., 2014). The final clinical criteria will be addressed in the next section.

Clinical Examination of the Sacroiliac Joint

The first step in the clinical examination should be to screen for other possible causes of pain from the lumbar spine, hip and knee, as previously stated. Once the clinician is satisfied that the spine is not the primary pain generator, provocation tests can be undertaken for the SIJ.

Sacroiliac pathology is often identified using tests of postural symmetry, symmetry of movement patterns and tests of pain provocation. The reliability of special tests is a requirement to establish validity. The pain provocation tests advocated for the diagnosis of SIJP have been studied for reliability by numerous authors, and while variable, have been found to have acceptable intra-rater reliability (Telli et al., 2018) and inter-rater reliability (Kokmeyer et al., 2002; Robinson et al., 2007; Laslett & Williams, 1994; van der Wurff et al., 2000a). However, one study (van Tilburg et al., 2017) found low levels of inter-rater agreement amongst four physicians in tests for SIJ, facet, or discogenic pathology with values ranging from chance agreement to 0.91. These differences suggest that variable results are possible if clinicians do not consistently apply the tests.

Numerous authors have examined the validity of provocation tests and combinations of these tests to determine their diagnostic accuracy (Laslett et al., 2003, 2005; van der Wurff, 2006; Ozgocmen et al., 2008). Laslett et al. (2003) combined the distraction test, compression test, thigh thrust test, sacral thrust, and Gaenslen's test (Figure 13.1), and found that the presence of at least 3 of 5 positive tests had a positive likelihood ratio (LR+) of 4.16 that increased to 6.97 when centralization was ruled out, with a negative likelihood ratio (LR–) of 0.11. Laslett et al. (2005) found that if Gaenslen's test was eliminated from the cluster and a positive result was defined as 2 of 4 positive tests, the LR+ dropped to 4.00 with an LR– of 0.16. Van der Wurff et al. (2006) replaced the sacral thrust test from Laslett's cluster with the Patrick's sign (FABER test) and found that when 3 of 5 tests were positive, the LR+ was 4.02 with an LR– of 0.19. Ozgocmen et al. (2008) clustered Gaenslen's test, Mennell's test, and the thigh thrust test for the identification of sacroiliitis and found that 2 of 3 positive yielded an LR+ of 3.44 and an LR– of 0.52. Laslett also determined that pain moving from sitting to standing with a positive TIC increased the odds ratio to 20 times more likely to have SIJP (Laslett, 2008). Based on the available evidence, Laslett's composite is the best available clinical diagnostic rule (Petersen et al., 2017) and maybe the acceptable gold

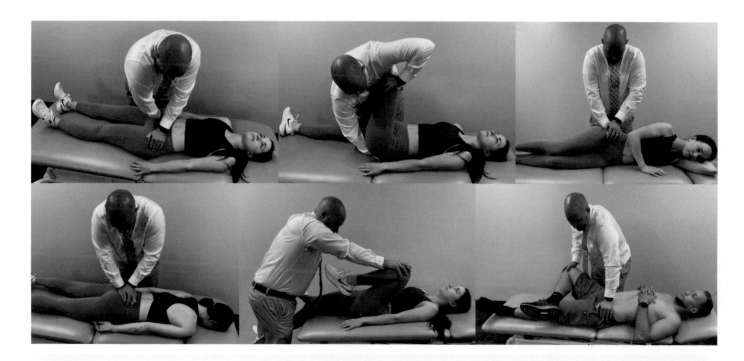

FIGURE 13.1
Sacroiliac joint provocation test item cluster: distraction test, thigh thrust test, compression test, sacral thrust, Gaenslen's test and Patrick's test (FABER).

standard for diagnostic validity without the need to verify with IAI. Here we briefly described this cluster of tests as described in Figure 13.1:

- *Distraction test*: The patient is supine, and the examiner applies an equal force posteriorly through both ASISs.

- *Thigh thrust test*: The patient is supine with the hip on the painful side flexed to 90 degrees and adducted sufficiently to control hip rotation. The examiner places one hand under the sacrum avoiding the PSIS of the testing side and places a force posteriorly through the thigh to stress the SIJ.

- *Compression test*: The patient is side-lying with hips and knees comfortably flexed for stability. The examiner applies a downward force through the uppermost iliac crest.

- *Sacral thrust*: The patient is prone while the examiner performs a posterior to anterior force through the center of the sacrum.

- *Gaenslen's test*: The patient is supine with one leg in maximum hip and knee flexion and the other hip in extension. Pelvic torsion is created with overpressure through both legs. This test is repeated on the contralateral side.

- *Patrick's test (FABER)*: In supine, the patient places their lateral ankle on the contralateral distal thigh, and the examiner places pressure toward the table on the bent knee and contralateral ASIS. A positive test is the reproduction of the chief complaint (see Figure 13.1).

Following provocative testing, a movement examination may prove useful. Rotate the painful innominate posteriorly into the end range to determine if that provokes pain. If provocative, repeatedly perform to establish a direction of preference and provide a possible movement-based treatment. If there is no change in symptoms from the position, the repeated movements do not alter symptom production or the symptoms are worsened, the assessment process can be repeated toward anterior rotation (Figure 13.2). If a direction of preference has been established, possible treatments could include mobilization, manipulation, muscle energy techniques, repeated stretching movements, and/or self-mobilization in that direction as a clinic and home program.

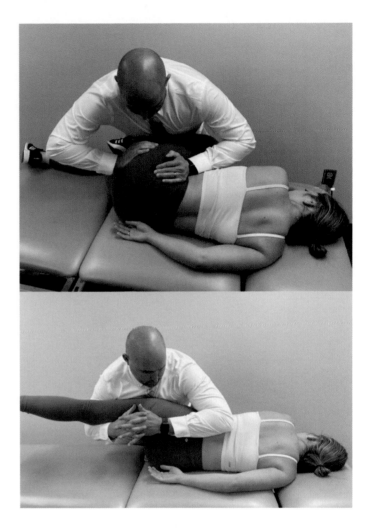

FIGURE 13.2
Posterior and anterior rotation of the innominates.

The physical assessment may include the Active Straight Leg Raise Test (ASLR) to determine if pressure applied to the symphysis pubis through the shear on the hip flexors and adductors may provoke symptoms. A positive ASLR (Figure 13.3) may indicate altered stabilization through insufficient force closure of the symphysis pubis and may warrant external stabilization through a sacroiliac belt or stabilization exercises. Additionally, palpation for tenderness on periarticular structures such as the posterior sacroiliac and sacrotuberous ligaments may also be useful (Figure 13.4).

Tests of postural symmetry have not been found to be consistently reliable; therefore, their clinical utility for

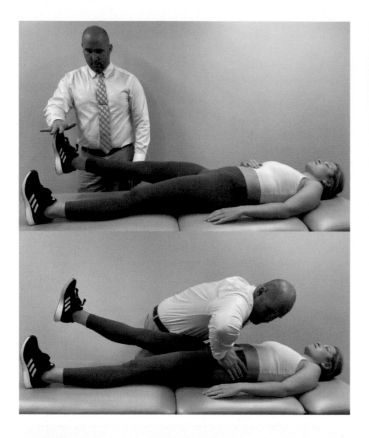

FIGURE 13.3
Active Straight Leg Raise test.

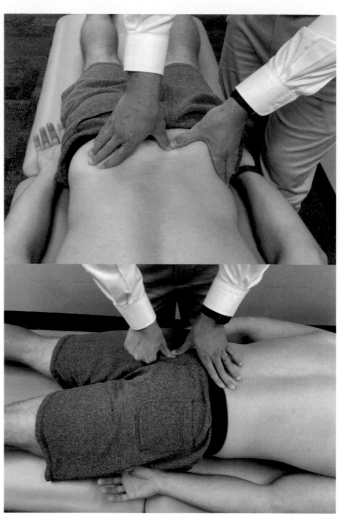

FIGURE 13.4
Long dorsal sacroiliac and sacrotuberous ligament palpation.

identifying SIJD is questioned (van der Wurff et al., 2000a, 2000b). Soleimanifar et al. (2017) found no strong association between motion palpation tests and pain provocation tests either individually or in composites. A more recent review explored the reliability and validity of positional and movement tests for SIJ and found that there is no new compelling information to suggest that this classification of the test is worthwhile to pursue (Klerx et al., 2020). A recent review article for diagnosis and treatment of the SIJ has further emphasized that it is time for a new approach to the examination and management of this condition (Palsson et al., 2019). However, an alternate hypothesis may be that these tests indicate muscle imbalances around the pelvis that may be addressed through stretching and strengthening as appropriate without indicating that SIJP is the actual underlying pathology.

Clinical Examination Proposal

Perform an examination to rule out low back, hip, and knee pathology. History questions to enhance the likelihood of SIJP are summarized within Table 13.1. The strongest likelihood of identifying SIJP is a combination of pain provocation tests advocated by Laslett et al. (Petersen et al., 2017).

A primary concern in the diagnosis of SIJ pathology is an understanding of the limitations of the diagnostic tests involved. This is eloquently stated, "Diagnostic noise begets therapeutic noise" (Bogduk, 2015). Even with tests that

TABLE 13.1 Subjective History Findings Consistent with Sacroiliac Joint Disorders

Subjective Examination	Reference
Pain location	
Below L5 spinous process	Fortin et al., 1994a
Along the PSIS and distal in the medial buttock	Dreyfuss et al., 1996
Unilateral, not midline	Young et al., 2003
No centralization phenomenon	Young et al., 2003
Having pain rising from sitting (shared with disc pathology)	Young et al., 2003

have relatively strong psychometric properties, there still is uncertainty in the outcome. Clinical utility is not perfect and test metrics can be misleading (Cook & Décary, 2020).

One of the major problems with SIJP is that it is diagnosed by pain provocation tests. This merely informs the clinician that there is pain sensitivity in the SIJ; it does not, however, give the clinician any indication of what may be the problem with the structures around the joint (Palsson et al., 2019). There are circumstances where the problem may be asymmetry of stability as in pregnancy and perhaps some cumulative trauma pathologies, but we have no reliable and valid way to make this determination. The lack of specificity in most SIJP has likely driven the general lack of understanding of the best way to provide interventions that work well and consistently.

Prognosis

Dengler et al. (2017) combined data from three RCTs comparing conservative management with minimally invasive fusion. Regression analysis revealed that no baseline measures predicted outcomes from conservative management. However, they found that predictors of success with fusion included older age and longer duration of symptoms, whereas current smoking and use of opioids reduced the benefits.

Few studies have focused on the prognosis for SIJP. Studies that have addressed the prognosis of LBP in general report that most LBP resolves satisfactorily in a relatively short period of time. Many studies that have addressed SIJP have sampled subjects with CLBP, indicating a poorer prognosis since the condition has already become persistent.

Treatment Approaches

Exercise Therapy

Exercise therapy takes on many forms when applied to the care of SIJP. The type of exercise applied should be dependent on the suspected problem. If the clinician thinks there is an abnormal postural or positional issue involving the SIJ, a corrective exercise could be employed. If instability or asymmetrical stability is perceived, stabilization could be used. In cases where weakness is surmised, a strengthening program can be used. With it being difficult to determine if a mechanical issue actually occurs in the SIJ, one might question this form of intervention. Nevertheless, therapeutic exercise is often used successfully in the treatment of SIJP and the literature has demonstrated variable treatment effects.

Movement-based exercises are used to stretch the innominate into end range one direction or another to improve mobility and energy load transfer. Clinical examples of specific exercises determined from assessment display a direction of preference, either anterior or posterior rotation of the innominate (Horton & Franz, 2007). While this study is low-level evidence as a case report, it does highlight a possible manner in which exercise therapy can be applied to patients that do display a specific movement pattern. As part of the examination process, the examiner can rotate the innominate posteriorly to see if it provokes the pain. If it does, repeated posterior rotation can be undertaken to see if the painful responses change at all. If it lessens, exercises that create posterior rotation can be used in the clinic and as part of a home exercise program (Figures 13.5 and 13.6). If posterior rotation does not provoke or fails to centralize the pain, anterior innominate rotation can be undertaken in the same fashion to determine its possible clinical utility.

Stabilization exercises are used to enhance force closure of the SIJ by creating tension across the thoracolumbar fascia (Richardson et al., 2002). Any exercise that creates tension

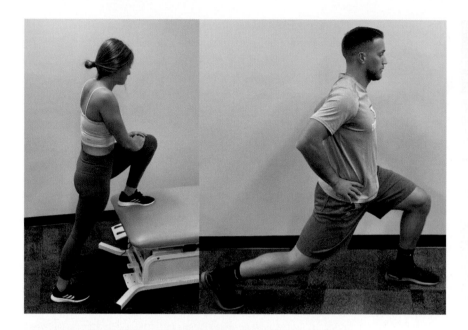

FIGURE 13.5
Standing rotational self-correction stretches.

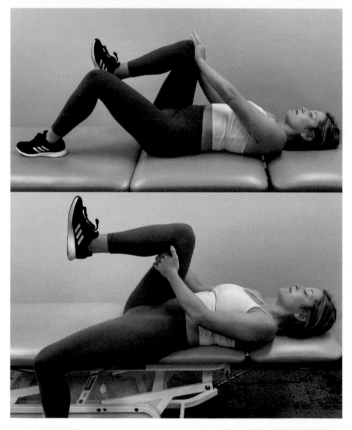

FIGURE 13.6
Supine muscle energy technique for innominate rotation.

in the thoracolumbar fascia could be incorporated. Almousa et al. (2018) concluded that there is limited evidence to substantiate the use of stabilization in treating peripartum pelvic pain. The component studies revealed the following results. Specific recruitment of the transversus abdominis and the multifidi progressively from side-lying to standing to retrain functional movement has been shown to be effective immediately post rehabilitation as compared with strengthening and acupuncture alone for up to one week (Elden et al., 2005). This study also found that acupuncture was as effective as stabilization exercises (Elden et al., 2005). Mens et al. (2000) found no differences for an exercise program that emphasized the diagonal muscle patterns of the anterior sling versus one that did not. Since the diagonal muscles fire bilaterally during straight plane movement, one might question why one would expect the between-group outcomes to be different.

Kordi et al. (2013) found that stabilization exercises were more effective than a patient education control group at 6-week follow-up but patient education with an SI belt was superior to the exercise group. Nilsson-Wikmar et al. (2005) found no between-group differences in study groups at any follow-up time point up to one year. Stuge et al. (2004a) incorporated an exercise program that began with training of the transversus abdominis and multifidi and then progressed to larger prime movers in treating 81 patients with PGP (Figure 13.7). In this study, the stabilization group experienced significantly improved outcomes that were

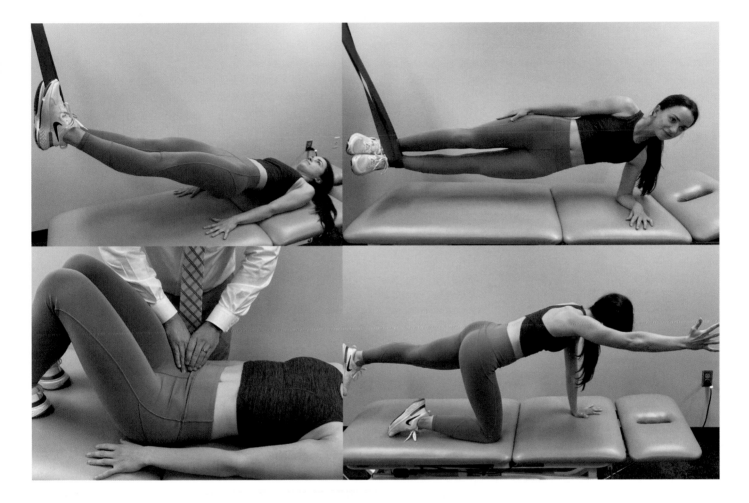

FIGURE 13.7
Stabilization exercises.

maintained at the one year (Stuge et al., 2004a) and two year (Stuge et al., 2004b) follow-ups. A comparison between the contradictory results identified several key differences in the methods. The most compelling evidence in favor of stabilization used exercises specifically designed to recruit transversus abdominis and multifidi (Stuge et al., 2006). As previously stated, a study identified that an isolated contraction of transversus abdominis and the multifidi produced greater stiffening of the SIJ than the other identified stabilizers of both the anterior and posterior pelvic slings (Richardson et al., 2002). Numerous authors (Stuge et al., 2004a; Elden et al., 2005; Kordi et al., 2013) emphasized the isolated muscle group training, whereas Mens et al. (2000) focused on the anterior sling muscles only and Nilsson-Wikmar et al. (2005) used strengthening exercises.

When examining stabilization exercise for SIJP in non-pregnancy-related PGP, the evidence is less prolific. Kamali et al. (2019) found that stabilization exercise that focused on a progressive routine based around local stabilizers progressing to global stabilizers working into function found a significant reduction in pain and enhanced function but the differences were not better than spinal manipulation alone.

Aurelio et al. (2018) published a case series where subjects with clinically diagnosed SIJP demonstrated weaker ipsilateral gluteus maximus muscles compared with asymptomatic normal subjects. Following a 5-week training program, the weakness and pain significantly improved. A previous study (Elden et al., 2005) failed to show demonstrable improvement in patients with PGP using a strengthening program for the gluteals and abdominals; however, there were methodological differences between these studies. Sample sizes were different, the RCT was controlled, and was used in a pregnant population (Elden et al., 2005).

It is reasonable to examine the effects of exercise on CLBP because one-third may be from SIJP. A systematic review with meta-analysis found that there were small but significant effects in favor of stabilization exercise over the control group (SMD 0.47), strengthening exercise over control (SMD 0.50), and combination exercises over control (SMD 0.16), but no significant effect for control over cardio-respiratory exercises (SMD 0.04) in the treatment of CLBP (Searle et al., 2015). We may not be able to extrapolate these results to SIJP but there currently is no compelling reason to believe that CLBP of either lumbar or SIJ origin behaves differently in response to exercise.

Part of the problem with the current stabilization exercise theory is the method used to train them. Many of the studies that have examined the efficacy of stabilization exercise fail to train the muscles in positions of function or at intensity levels required to adequately stimulate a strengthening response. Many training programs perform many exercises in supine where form closure is weakest and target the transversus abdominis in a manner inconsistent with normal function. It would seem more reasonable to perform stabilization in weight-bearing to maximize form closure and enhance training effects that carry over to normal function and to provide a dosage that would create a strengthening response. Most stabilization programs also tend to emphasize isometric holds of the trunk or a neutral posture through the program which is inconsistent with the way the body moves during normal function. Form and force closure must work through a normal range of trunk motion as in functional movement that can be expected to be encountered on a daily basis.

Additionally, the entire theory of stabilization should be questioned and considered carefully. There is little compelling evidence that selectively training specific muscles results in enhanced clinical outcomes. The idea that selectively training the transversus abdominis and multifidi is a theory based on observed altered recruitment in subjects with LBP (Richardson et al., 2002). An alternate theory to selective recruitment has been the overall abdominal brace theory (McGill, 2001). This is based on the conceptual framework that stiffening the trunk will result in greater support and

enhanced function. Stiffening the trunk may make patients overexert the muscles required to stabilize creating undue fatigue and increased pain throughout the day. It also may foster the idea that the spine is somehow inadequate in its current form requiring muscle guarding to protect, and so causing a loss of confidence in one's ability to heal. We are not advocating the abandonment of stabilization exercises; they clearly have clinically worked for many people. The point we are trying to make is that the clinician needs to be careful in how the need for exercise is portrayed to the patient so that wording is carefully considered to avoid the fear of movement or catastrophizing but to enhance movement, functional restoration, confidence and self-efficacy.

A previous examination of exercise for CLBP found that a bilateral leg lift from flexion to hyperextension, a prone trunk hyperextension and pulldowns behind the neck resulted in a substantial reduction in pain and disability that was maintained at 1-year follow-up as long as the subjects continued the program at least once per week (Manniche et al., 1991). A follow-up study found that the hyperextension maneuver was not required to obtain satisfactory outcomes (Manniche et al., 1993). Additionally, bilateral leg lifts from the flexed position to horizontal with a 5-second isometric hold was superior to stabilization alone in increasing the cross-sectional area of the multifidi muscles (Danneels, 2001).

Manual Therapy

There are two main categories of manual therapy: thrust (manipulation) and non-thrust (mobilization) techniques. Manipulation is a high-velocity, low-amplitude thrust at or near the end of the available range of motion. Mobilization involves using a graded oscillatory force or sustained force anywhere in range and for as long as deemed appropriate by the treating clinician. Marshall & Murphy (2006) reported manipulation produces profound and significant normalization of feed-forward activity of the transversus abdominis and multifidi. As previously stated in the exercise section, the clinical impact of this neurophysiological influence is unclear.

If a SIJ manipulation is warranted, the lumbar spine should be positioned in tension with side-bending toward the manipulative side in order to reduce unwanted motion in the lumbar region and to reduce tension on the ipsilateral iliolumbar ligament (Sizer et al., 2002). A lumbosacral manipulative technique has been described in the

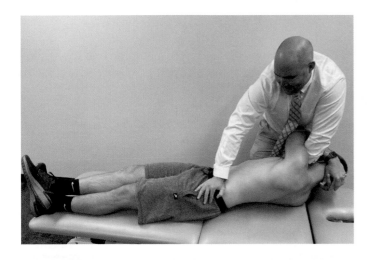

FIGURE 13.8
Sacroiliac thrust manipulation.

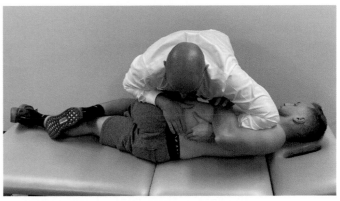

FIGURE 13.9
Rotational neutral gapping manipulation.

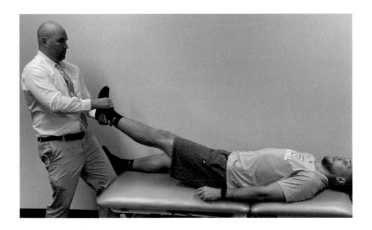

FIGURE 13.10
Long-leg distraction manipulation.

literature to reduce pain symptoms and disability (Flynn et al., 2002; Childs et al., 2004) (Figure 13.8). This technique places the lumbar spine in ipsilateral side bending and contralateral rotation to minimize lumbar motion to direct the thrust into the painful SIJ. Flynn et al. (2002) performed a thorough lumbopelvic examination to determine predictors of success with this treatment and no test of SIJ position, symmetry of movement or general special tests were found. Lumbar hypomobility and having at least one hip with internal rotation of at least 35 degrees were predictive. This finding further challenges the belief that SI mobility can be readily examined clinically and the results of the findings can be used to predict who may do well with a treatment designed to alter SI mobility. Nevertheless, this manipulative technique has been found to be clinically effective for people with LBP and should be considered as an available treatment option. Additional manipulative techniques that may be substituted for the aforementioned technique could include the neutral gapping manipulation technique (Figure 13.9) and the long axis distraction technique (Figure 13.10).

Anterior pelvic pain in the symphysis pubis can be treated using a shotgun muscle energy approach (Figure 13.11), where multiple 3- to 5-second sustained isometric holds are performed into resisted hip abduction in supine followed by multiple isometric holds into hip adduction from the same position. Often, the symphysis pubis will create an audible click and the patient will experience significant pain relief.

If the patient is peripartum, the use of an SIJ belt following treatment is often warranted. Pain in the region of the pubic symphysis or through the groin may also indicate athletic groin pain and should be assessed for this as well. If it does not resolve with conservative care, it may warrant surgical intervention.

Sacroiliac Belts

External force through SIJ belts, applied between the greater trochanter and ASISs, helps reduce pain and dysfunction in SIJ-related pain. A systematic review with meta-analysis suggests that SIJ belts contribute a moderate treatment

CHAPTER THIRTEEN

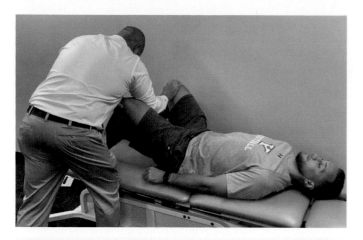

FIGURE 13.11
Pelvic shotgun muscle energy technique.

effect to exercise alone post-intervention at 4–6 weeks (SMD –0.45) and at 3-months (SMD –0.51) (Cates, 2015). The use of the SIJ belt has been associated with altered EMG activity of the hip extensors, increasing the gluteus and reducing the hamstrings (Jung et al., 2013). A systematic review found that SIJ belts reduced laxity and altered neuromotor control (Arumugam, 2012). They reduce the muscular effort needed to perform the ASLR in healthy control subjects (Hu et al., 2012) and in women with pregnancy-related pelvic pain (Hu et al., 2010). Additionally, the belts reduced the muscular effort required during treadmill walking (Hu et al., 2010). These studies might suggest that patients with SIJP may benefit from the application of a belt to enhance motor control and reduce pain irrespective of the clinical exam, suggesting that hypermobility or instability is present.

Patient Education

Studies have incorporated patient education into the treatment programs for SIJP (Elden et al., 2005). Many programs provide information on the anatomy and biomechanics of the SIJ as well as advice to stay physically active and maintain as normal activity levels as possible. Details of how this is covered are generally lacking.

There is a growing body of evidence to suggest that when working with patients, particularly those with chronic conditions, it is crucial to explain the condition in a manner that does not reinforce negative belief systems and promote maladaptive coping. Rather, it presents material in a way that encourages self-efficacy in the management of the condition via adaptive coping methods. We should explain the healing process to the patient, including the neurological basis for the pain response and expectation for a graded reduction in pain over time. We must also reinforce the concept that pain does not equal damage and the correlation, especially when dealing with chronic pain, is minimal at best. While muscular strength adaptations may take up to 3 months to show effect, it is important for the patient to understand the role of changes in perceptions, and that improvements in pain modulation and improved muscular coordination are likely attributed with early responses. The importance of lifestyle change should be emphasized in a way that fosters adaptive coping, including a reduction in kinesiophobic or fear-avoidance beliefs which may be inhibiting improvement. Chronic pain conditions relate more to the emotional and psychological state than to true nociception/mechanical contributors; therefore, it is crucial that these factors be incorporated into our treatment plans to promote healing. This should include education of patients and acknowledgment of the frustration which is often experienced due to the persistence of symptoms. These emotions need to be acknowledged and managed by astute observation and empathic communication. Healing communication is the therapist's superpower in the chronic state and has shown a positive effect of a therapeutic alliance, improved patient compliance, improved self-efficacy, and improved overall outcomes when it comes to chronic musculoskeletal pain. Patients' beliefs have been shown to align with their providers' beliefs and furthermore to influence pain modulatory pathways, which can foster an improved ability to participate in activities and exercise. Readers are referred to Chapter 20 of this textbook for pain neuroscience education.

Many patients diagnosed with SIJP have had the condition for a significant period of time and now have transitioned to a chronic pain state. As stated previously these patients may involve complex psychological and emotional characteristics contributing to their pain experience. We must acknowledge that oftentimes these individuals may have failed previous rehabilitation and therefore must provide patient-centered care, identify what has and has not worked for these patients, and promote a well-rounded and patient-specific multimodal treatment plan. This aligns with the recommendations present for addressing other chronic pain conditions such as chronic low back pain.

A recent systematic review found educational strategies to be superior to waitlisting but similar to other interventional strategies (Barbari et al., 2020). One study compared patient education to activity intervention based on the treatment-based classification system with centralizers performing specific exercise, those in the instability group receiving stabilization exercises and those in the stable group receiving intense back strengthening previously described (Sorensen et al., 2010). The authors reported similar outcomes between the active intervention group (comprised of all three exercise groups) and the patient education group in pain, activity limitations, ability to work and the Back Beliefs Questionnaire; however, the education group had superior outcomes in the Fear Avoidance Beliefs Questionnaire at all time points up to one year (Sorensen et al., 2010). While these studies are not specific to SIJP, rather CLBP in general, with diagnostic limitations and knowing the prevalence of SIJP in CLBP, it is likely that we can extrapolate the results to chronic SIJP.

Conclusions

What we know is examination and treatment of the SIJ are still hard to interpret. There is no universally accepted diagnostic gold standard. The gold standard that we do have has not been applied to a large sample of patients with acute and subacute LBP, making it difficult to ascertain the prevalence rates in this group of patients. The tests clinically used to diagnose SIJP do not necessarily provide guidance in how to treat the condition and the postural palpation and motion tests have been found to be unreliable and invalid to determine the problem is SIJP. There is no evidence to suggest that positional faults in the SIJ exist and whether or not looking for them assists in clinical reasoning or treatment selection. The evidence is lacking for which treatments to use in SIJP because few well-done trials have been performed in each stage of the condition and no very well done, large-scale trials have been published to date.

References

Albert HB, Godskesen M, Westergaard JG. Incidence of four syndromes of pregnancy-related pelvic joint pain. Spine. 2002;27:2831–4.

Aldabe D, Milosavljevic S, Bussey MD. Is pregnancy related pelvic girdle pain associated with altered kinematic, kinetic and motor control of the pelvis? A systematic review. Eur Spine J. 2012;21:1777–87.

Almousa S, Lamprianidou E, Kitsoulis G. The effectiveness of stabilising exercises in pelvic girdle pain during pregnancy and after delivery: A systematic review. Physiother Res Int. 2018;23:e1699.

Arumugam A. Effects of external pelvic compression on form closure, force closure, and neuromotor control of the lumbopelvic spine: A systematic review. Man Ther. 2012:17:275–84.

Aurelio MN, de Freitas DG, Kasawara KT, et al. Strengthening the gluteus maximus in subjects with sacroiliac dysfunction. Int J Sports Phys Ther. 2018;13:114–20.

Badii M, Shin S, Torreggiani WC, et al. Pelvic bone asymmetry in 323 study participants receiving abdominal CT scans. Spine. 2003;28(12):1335–9.

Barbari V, Storari L, Ciuro A, Testa M. Effectiveness of communicative and educative strategies in chronic low back pain patients: A systematic review. Patient Educ Couns. 2020;103:908–29.

Beales DJ, O'Sullivan PB, Briffa NK. Motor control patterns during an active straight leg raise in chronic pelvic girdle pain subjects. Spine. 2009;34(9):861–70.

Bialosky JE, Bishop MD, George SZ. Regional interdependence: a musculoskeletal examination model whose time has come. J Orthop Sports Phys Ther. 2008;38:159–60.

Bialosky JE, Bishop MD, Price DD, et al. The mechanisms of manual therapy in the treatment of musculoskeletal pain: a comprehensive model. Man Ther. 2009;14:531–8.

Bishop MD, Torres-Cueco R, Gay CW, et al. What effect can manual therapy have on a patient's pain experience? Pain Manag. 2015;5:455–64.

Bogduk N. Clinical anatomy of the lumbar spine and sacrum. 4th ed. Edinburgh, UK: Elsevier; 2005:186.

Bogduk N. Commentary on King W, Ahmed S, Baisden J, Patel N, MacVicar J, Kennedy DJ. Diagnosis of posterior sacroiliac complex pain: A systematic review with comprehensive analysis of the published data. Pain Med. 2015;16:222–4.

Brinjikji W, Luetmer PH, Comstock B, et al. Systematic literature review of imaging features of spinal degeneration in asymptomatic populations. Am J Neuroradiol. 2015;36:811.

Bucek DW. Reduction of knee pain in a 45-year-old woman after pelvic manipulation and Kinesiology taping: A case report. J Chiropr Med. 2019;18:236–41.

Cates C. Effectiveness of a therapeutic exercise program with a sacroiliac joint belt compared to a therapeutic exercise program alone to reduce sacroiliac joint-related pain and improve function: a meta-analysis. Published online 2015. Available at: Scholarworks.calstate.edu/downloads/0c483k72j

Cher D, Polly D, Berven S. Sacroiliac joint pain: burden of disease. Med Devices Auckl NZ. 2014;7:73–81.

Childs JD, Fritz JM, Flynn TW, et al. A clinical prediction rule to identify patients with low back pain most likely to benefit from spinal manipulation: A validation study. Ann Intern Med. 2004;141:920–8.

Chou LH, Slipman CW, Bhagia SM, et al. Inciting events initiating injection-proven sacroiliac joint syndrome. Pain Med. 2004;5:26–32.

Cibulka MT, Delitto A. A Comparison of two different methods to treat hip pain in runners. J Orthop Sports Phys Ther. 1993;17:172–6.

Cohen SP. Sacroiliac joint pain: A comprehensive review of anatomy, diagnosis, and treatment. Anesth Analg. 2005;101:1440–53.

Cook CE, Décary S. Higher order thinking about differential diagnosis. Braz J Phys Ther. 2020;24:1–7.

Cuppett M, Paladino J. The anatomy and pathomechanics of the sacroiliac joint. Athl Ther Today. 2001;6:6–14.

Damen L, Buyruk HM, Güler-Uysal F, et al. Pelvic pain during pregnancy is associated with asymmetric laxity of the sacroiliac joints: Pregnancy-related pelvic pain. Acta Obstet Gynecol Scand. 2001;80:1019–24.

Danneels LA. Effects of three different training modalities on the cross-sectional area of the lumbar multifidus muscle in patients with chronic low back pain. Br J Sports Med. 2001;35:186–91.

Dar G, Khamis S, Peleg S, et al. Sacroiliac joint fusion and the implications for manual therapy diagnosis and treatment. Man Ther. 2008;13:155–8.

de Groot M, Pool-Goudzwaard AL, Spoor CW, Snijders CJ. The active straight leg raising test (ASLR) in pregnant women: differences in muscle activity and force between patients and healthy subjects. Man Ther. 2008;13:68–74.

Dengler J, Duhon B, Whang P, et al. Predictors of outcome in conservative and minimally invasive surgical management of pain originating from the sacroiliac joint: A pooled analysis. Spine. 2017;42:1664–73.

DeStefano LA. Pelvic girdle dysfunction. In: Greenman's Principles of Manual Medicine. 5th ed. Philadelphia, PA: Wolters Kluwer; 2017:317.

Dreyfuss P, Michaelsen M, Pauza K, et al. The value of medical history and physical examination in diagnosing sacroiliac joint pain. Spine. 1996;21:2594–602.

Elden H, Ladfors L, Olsen MF, et al. Effects of acupuncture and stabilising exercises as adjunct to standard treatment in pregnant women with pelvic girdle pain: randomised single blind controlled trial. BMJ. 2005;330:761.

Eno J-JT, Boone CR, Bellino MJ, Bishop JA. The prevalence of sacroiliac joint degeneration in asymptomatic adults. J Bone Jt Surg. 2015;97:932–6.

Flynn T, Fritz J, Whitman J, et al. A clinical prediction rule for classifying patients with low back pain who demonstrate short-term improvement with spinal manipulation. Spine. 2002;27:2835–42.

Foley BS, Buschbacher R. Sacroiliac joint pain: Anatomy, biomechanics, diagnosis, and treatment. Am J Phys Med Rehabil. 2006;85:997–1006.

Fortin JD, Dwyer AP, West S, Pier J. Sacroiliac joint: pain referral maps upon applying a new injection/arthrography technique. Part I: Asymptomatic volunteers. Spine. 1994a;19:1475–82.

Fortin JD, April CN, Ponthieux B, Pier J. Sacroiliac joint: pain referral maps upon applying a new injection/arthrography technique. Part II: Clinical evaluation. Spine. 1994b;19:1483–9.

Fortin J, Kissling R, O'Connor B, Vilensky J. Sacroiliac joint innervation and pain. Am J Orthop. 1999;28:687–90.

Fortin JD, Vilensky JA, Merkel GJ. Can the sacroiliac joint cause sciatica? Pain Physician. 2003;6:269–71.

Goldthwait JE, Osgood RB. A consideration of the pelvic articulations from an anatomical, pathological and clinical standpoint. Boston Med Surg J. 1905;152:593–601.

Goode A, Hegedus EJ, Sizer P, Brismee J-M, Linberg A, Cook CE. Three-dimensional movements of the sacroiliac joint: A systematic review of the literature and assessment of clinical utility. J Man Manip Ther. 2008;16:25–38.

Grasland A. Sacral insufficiency fractures: An easily overlooked cause of back pain in elderly women. Arch Intern Med. 1996;156:668.

Grob KR, Neuhuber WL, Kissling RO. [Innervation of the sacroiliac joint of the human]. Z Rheumatol. 1995;54:117–22.

Gupta AD. Sacroiliac joint pathologies in low back pain. J Back Musculoskelet Rehabil. 2009;22:91–7.

Horton SJ, Franz A. Mechanical Diagnosis and therapy approach to assessment and treatment of derangement of the sacro-iliac joint. Man Ther. 2007;12:126–32.

Hu H, Meijer OG, van Dieën JH, et al. Muscle activity during the active straight leg raise (ASLR), and the effects of a pelvic belt on the ASLR and on treadmill walking. J Biomech. 2010;43:532–9.

Hu H, Meijer OG, Hodges PW, et al. Understanding the Active Straight Leg Raise (ASLR): An electromyographic study in healthy subjects. Man Ther. 2012;17:531–7.

Huijbregts P. Sacroiliac joint dysfunction: evidence-based diagnosis. Orthop Div Rev. 2004;8:18–44.

Jee H, Lee JH, Park KD, et al. Ultrasound-guided versus fluoroscopy-guided sacroiliac joint intra-articular injections in the noninflammatory sacroiliac joint dysfunction: A prospective, randomized, single-blinded study. Arch Phys Med Rehabil. 2014;95:330–7.

Jung HS, Jeon HS, Oh DW, Kwon OY. Effect of the pelvic compression belt on the hip extensor activation patterns of sacroiliac joint pain patients during one-leg standing: A pilot study. Man Ther. 2013;18:143–8.

Kamali F, Zamanlou M, Ghanbari A, et al. Comparison of manipulation and stabilization exercises in patients with sacroiliac joint

dysfunction patients: A randomized clinical trial. J Bodyw Mov Ther. 2019;23:177–82.

Katz JN. Lumbar disc disorders and low-back pain: Socioeconomic factors and consequences. J Bone Jt Surg. 2006;88:S21–4.

Kibsgård TJ, Röhrl SM, Røise O, et al. Movement of the sacroiliac joint during the Active Straight Leg Raise test in patients with long-lasting severe sacroiliac joint pain. Clin Biomech. 2017;47:40–5.

Klang E, Lidar M, Lidar Z, et al. Prevalence and awareness of sacroiliac joint alterations on lumbar spine CT in low back pain patients younger than 40 years. Acta Radiol. 2017;58:449–55.

Klerx SP, Pool JJM, Coppieters MW, et al. Clinimetric properties of sacroiliac joint mobility tests: A systematic review. Musculoskelet Sci Pract. 2020;48:102090.

Kokmeyer DJ, van der Wurff P, Aufdemkampe G, Fickenscher TCM. The reliability of multitest regimens with sacroiliac pain provocation tests. J Manipulative Physiol Ther. 2002;25:42–8.

Kordi R, Abolhasani M, Rostami M, et al. Comparison between the effect of lumbopelvic belt and home based pelvic stabilizing exercise on pregnant women with pelvic girdle pain; a randomized controlled trial. J Back Musculoskelet Rehabil. 2013;26:133–9.

Krishnamoorthy VP, Beck EC, Kunze KN, et al. Radiographic prevalence of sacroiliac joint abnormalities and clinical outcomes in patients with femoroacetabular impingement syndrome. Arthrosc J Arthrosc Relat Surg. 2019;35:2598–605.

Kurosawa D, Murakami E, Aizawa T. Referred pain location depends on the affected section of the sacroiliac joint. Eur Spine J. 2015;24:521–7.

Laslett M. Evidence-based diagnosis and treatment of the painful sacroiliac joint. J Man Manip Ther. 2008;16:142–52.

Laslett M, Williams M. The reliability of selected pain provocation tests for sacroiliac joint pathology. Spine. 1994;19:1243–9.

Laslett M, Young SB, April CN, McDonald B. Diagnosing painful sacroiliac joints: A validity study of a McKenzie evaluation and sacroiliac provocation tests. Aust J Physiother. 2003;49:89–97.

Laslett M, April CN, McDonald B, Young SB. Diagnosis of sacroiliac joint pain: Validity of individual provocation tests and composites of tests. Man Ther. 2005;10:207–18.

Liliang PC, Lu K, Liang CL, et al. Sacroiliac joint pain after lumbar and lumbosacral fusion:

findings using dual sacroiliac joint blocks. Pain Med. 2011;12:565–70.

Madani SP, Dadian M, Firouznia K, Alalawi S. Sacroiliac joint dysfunction in patients with herniated lumbar disc: A cross-sectional study. J Back Musculoskelet Rehabil. 2013;26:273–9.

Maigne JY, Aivaliklis A, Pfefer F. Results of sacroiliac joint double block and value of sacroiliac pain provocation tests in 54 patients with low back pain. Spine. 1996;21:1889–92.

Manchikanti L, Singh V, Pampati V, et al. Evaluation of the relative contributions of various structures in chronic low back pain. Pain Physician. 2001;4:308–16.

Manniche C, Lundberg E, Christensen I, et al. Intensive dynamic back exercises for chronic low back pain: a clinical trial. Pain. 1991;47:53-63.

Manniche C, Asmussen K, Lauritsen B, et al. Intensive dynamic back exercises with or without hyperextension in chronic back pain after surgery for lumbar disc protrusion. A clinical trial. Spine. 1993;18:560–7.

Margo K, Drezner J, Motzkin D. Evaluation and management of hip pain: an algorithmic approach. J Fam Pract. 2003;52:607–17.

Marshall P, Murphy B. The effect of sacroiliac joint manipulation on feed-forward activation times of the deep abdominal musculature. J Manipulative Physiol Ther. 2006;29:196–202.

Massoud Arab A, Reza Nourbakhsh M, Mohammadifar A. The relationship between hamstring length and gluteal muscle strength in individuals with sacroiliac joint dysfunction. J Man Manip Ther. 2011;19:5–10.

McGill SM. Low back stability: From formal description to issues for performance and rehabilitation. Exerc Sport Sci Rev. 2001;29:26-31.

Mens JM, Snijders CJ, Stam HJ. Diagonal trunk muscle exercises in peripartum pelvic pain: A randomized clinical trial. Phys Ther. 2000;80:1164–73.

Mens JMA, Huis in 't Veld YH, Pool-Goudzwaard A. Severity of signs and symptoms in lumbopelvic pain during pregnancy. Man Ther. 2012;17:175–9.

Merskey H, Bogduk N. Sacroiliac joint pain (XXVII-10). In: Classification of chronic pain: descriptions of chronic pain syndromes and definitions of pain terms. 2nd ed. Seattle, WA: IASP Press; 1994:191–2.

Miller JAA, Schultz AB, Andersson GBJ. Load-displacement behavior of sacroiliac joints. J Orthop Res. 1987;5:92–101.

Mitchell FS. Structural pelvic function. Yearbook of the American Academy of Osteopathy. Carmel, CA: American Academy of Osteopathy; 1958:71–90.

Morgan PM. Editorial Commentary: Consider the sacroiliac joint: imaging a source of pain can feel compelling. Orthopaedists would do well to remain skeptical. Arthrosc J Arthrosc Relat Surg. 2019;35:2606–7.

Morgan PM, Anderson AW, Swiontkowski MF. Symptomatic sacroiliac joint disease and radiographic evidence of femoroacetabular impingement. Hip Int. 2013;23:212–17.

Murakami E, Tanaka Y, Aizawa T, et al. Effect of periarticular and intraarticular lidocaine injections for sacroiliac joint pain: prospective comparative study. J Orthop Sci. 2007;12:274–80.

Murakami E, Aizawa T, Kurosawa D, Noguchi K. Leg symptoms associated with sacroiliac joint disorder and related pain. Clin Neurol Neurosurg. 2017;157:55–8.

Murphy DR, Hurwitz EL. A theoretical model for the development of a diagnosis-based clinical decision rule for the management of patients with spinal pain. BMC Musculoskelet Disord. 2007;8:75.

Myburgh KH, Hutchins J, Fataar AB, Hough SF, Noakes TD. Low bone density is an etiologic factor for stress fractures in athletes. Ann Intern Med. 1990;113:754–9.

Nakagawa T. [Study on the distribution of nerve filaments over the iliosacral joint and its adjacent regio n in the Japanese]. Nihon Seikeigeka Gakkai Zasshi. 1966;40:419–30.

Nilsson-Wikmar L, Holm K, Öijerstedt R, Harms-Ringdahl K. Effect of three different physical therapy treatments on pain and activity in pregnant women with pelvic girdle pain: A randomized clinical trial with 3, 6, and 12 months follow-up postpartum. Spine. 2005;30:850–6.

O'Shea FD, Boyle E, Salonen DC, et al. Inflammatory and degenerative sacroiliac joint disease in a primary back pain cohort. Arthritis Care Res. 2010;62:447–54.

Ozgocmen S, Bozgeyik Z, Kalcik M, Yildirim A. The value of sacroiliac pain provocation tests in early active sacroiliitis. Clin Rheumatol. 2008;27:1275–82.

Palsson TS, Gibson W, Darlow B, et al. Changing the narrative in diagnosis and management of pain in the sacroiliac joint area. Phys Ther. 2019;99:1511–19.

Pel JJM, Spoor CW, Pool-Goudzwaard AL, Hoek van Dijke GA, Snijders CJ. Biomechanical analysis of reducing sacroiliac joint shear load by optimization of pelvic muscle and ligament forces. Ann Biomed Eng. 2008;36:415–24.

Petersen T, Laslett M, Juhl C. Clinical classification in low back pain: best-evidence diagnostic rules based on systematic reviews. BMC Musculoskelet Disord. 2017;18:188.

Petrone MR, Guinn J, Reddin A, et al. The accuracy of the Palpation Meter (PALM) for measuring pelvic crest height difference and leg length discrepancy. J Orthop Sports Phys Ther. 2003;33:319–25.

Poilliot AJ, Zwirner J, Doyle T, Hammer N. A systematic review of the normal sacroiliac joint anatomy and adjacent tissues for pain physicians. Pain Physician. 2019;22:E247–74.

Pool-Goudzwaard AL, Vleeming A, Stoeckart R, et al. Insufficient lumbopelvic stability: a clinical, anatomical and biomechanical approach to "a-specific" low back pain. Man Ther. 1998;3:12-20.

Pool-Goudzwaard A, Gnat R, Spoor K. Deformation of the innominate bone and mobility of the pubic symphysis during asymmetric moment application to the pelvis. Man Ther. 2012;17:66–70.

Prassopoulos PK, Faflia CP, Voloudaki AE, Gourtsoyiannis NC. Sacroiliac Joints: Anatomical Variants on CT. J Comput Assist Tomogr. 1999;23:323–7.

Preece SJ, Willan P, Nester CJ, et al. Variation in pelvic morphology may prevent the identification of anterior pelvic tilt. J Man Manip Ther. 2008;16:113–17.

Richardson CA, Snijders CJ, Hides JA, et al. The relation between the transversus abdominis muscles, sacroiliac joint mechanics, and low back pain. Spine. 2002;27:399–405.

Robinson HS, Brox JI, Robinson R, et al. The reliability of selected motion- and pain provocation tests for the sacroiliac joint. Man Ther. 2007;12:72–9.

Schwarzer AC, Aprill CN, Bogduk N. The sacroiliac joint in chronic low back pain. Spine. 1995;20:31–7.

Searle A, Spink M, Ho A, Chuter V. Exercise interventions for the treatment of chronic low back pain: a systematic review and meta-analysis of randomised controlled trials. Clin Rehabil. 2015;29:1155–67.

Simopoulos TT, Manchikanti L, Singh V, et al. A systematic evaluation of prevalence and diagnostic accuracy of sacroiliac joint interventions. Pain Physician. 2012;15:E305-44.

Sizer PS, Phelps V, Thompsen K. Disorders of the sacroiliac joint. Pain Pract. 2002;2:17–34.

Sizer PS, Brismée J-M, Cook C. Medical screening for red flags in the diagnosis and management of musculoskeletal spine pain. Pain Pract. 2007;7:53–71.

Sjödahl J, Gutke A, Ghaffari G, et al. Response of the muscles in the pelvic floor and the lower lateral abdominal wall during the Active Straight Leg Raise in women with and without pelvic girdle pain: An experimental study. Clin Biomech. 2016;35:49–55.

Smidt GL, McQuade K, Wei SH, Barakatt E. Sacroiliac kinematics for reciprocal straddle positions. Spine. 1995;20:1047–54.

Snijders CJ, Vleeming A, Stoeckart R. Transfer of lumbosacral load to iliac bones and legs Part 1: Biomechanics of sefl-bracing of the sacroiliac joints and its significance for treatment and exercise. Clin Biomech 1993a;8:285–94.

Snijders CJ, Vleeming A, Stoeckart R. Transfer of lumbosacral load to iliac bones and legs Part 2: Loading of the sacroiliac joints when lifting in a stooped posture. Clin Biomech. 1993b;8:295–301.

Soleimanifar M, Karimi N, Arab AM. Association between composites of selected motion palpation and pain provocation tests for sacroiliac joint disorders. J Bodyw Mov Ther. 2017;21:240–5.

Sorensen PH, Bendix T, Manniche C, et al. An educational approach based on a non-injury model compared with individual symptom-based physical training in chronic LBP. A pragmatic, randomised trial with a one-year follow-up. BMC Musculoskelet Disord. 2010;11:212.

Stuge B, Lærum E, Kirkesola G, Vøllestad N. The efficacy of a treatment program focusing on specific stabilizing exercises for pelvic girdle pain after pregnancy: A randomized controlled trial. Spine. 2004a;29:351-359.

Stuge B, Veierød MB, Lærum E, Vøllestad N. The efficacy of a treatment program focusing on specific stabilizing exercises for pelvic girdle pain after pregnancy: A two-year follow-up of a randomized clinical trial. Spine. 2004b;29:e197–203.

Stuge B, Mørkved S, Dahl HH, Vøllestad N. Abdominal and pelvic floor muscle function in women with and without long lasting pelvic girdle pain. Man Ther. 2006:10:287–96.

Sturesson B, Uden A, Vleeming A. A radiostereometric analysis of the movements of the sacroiliac joints in the reciprocal straddle position. Spine. 2000;25:214–17.

Sueki DG, Cleland JA, Wainner RS. A regional interdependence model of musculoskeletal dysfunction: research, mechanisms, and clinical implications. J Man Manip Ther. 2013;21:90–102.

Suleiman Z, Kolawole I, Okeyemi A. Fluoroscopic-guided sacroiliac joint injections for treatment of chronic axial low back pain in a tertiary Hospital in Nigeria: a preliminary study. Ghana Med J. 2018;52:153–7.

Suter E, McMorland G, Herzog W, Bray R. Decrease in quadriceps inhibition after sacroiliac joint manipulation in patients with anterior knee pain. J Manipulative Physiol Ther. 1999;22:149–53.

Suter E, McMorland G, Herzog W, Bray R. Conservative lower back treatment reduces inhibition in knee-extensor muscles: a randomized controlled trial. J Manipulative Physiol Ther. 2000;23:76–80.

Telli H, Telli S, Topal M. The validity and reliability of provocation tests in the diagnosis of sacroiliac joint dysfunction. Pain Physician. 2018;21:E367–76.

Telli H, Hüner B, Kuru Ö. Determination of the prevalence from clinical diagnosis of sacroiliac joint dysfunction in patients with lumbar disc hernia and an evaluation of the effect of this combination on pain and quality of life. Spine. 2020;45:549–54.

Tresch F, Dietrich TJ, Pfirrmann CWA, Sutter R. Hip MRI: Prevalence of articular cartilage defects and labral tears in asymptomatic volunteers. A comparison with a matched population of patients with femoroacetabular impingement: Hip Defects in Asymptomatic Volunteers. J Magn Reson Imaging. 2017;46:440–51.

Tullberg T, Blomberg S, Branth B, Johnsson R. Manipulation does not alter the position of the sacroiliac joint: A Roentgen Stereophotogrammetric Analysis. Spine. 1998;23:1124–8.

van der Wurff P. Clinical diagnostic tests for the sacroiliac joint: motion and palpation tests. Aust J Physiother. 2006;52:308.

van der Wurff P, Hagmeijer RHM, Meyne W. Clinical tests of the sacroiliac joint. Man Ther. 2000a;5:30–6.

van der Wurff P, Meyne W, Hagmeijer RHM. Clinical tests of the sacroiliac joint. Man Ther. 2000b;5:89–96.

van der Wurff P, Buijs EJ, Groen GJ. A multitest regimen of pain provocation tests as an aid to reduce unnecessary minimally invasive sacroiliac joint procedures. Arch Phys Med Rehabil. 2006;87:10–14.

van Tilburg CWJ, Groeneweg JG, Stronks DL, Huygen FJPM. Inter-rater reliability of diagnostic criteria for sacroiliac joint-, disc- and facet joint pain. J Back Musculoskelet Rehabil. 2017;30:551-7.

van Wingerden JP, Vleeming A, Buyruk HM, Raissadat K. Stabilization of the sacroiliac joint in vivo: verification of muscular contribution to force closure of the pelvis. Eur Spine J. 2004;13:199–205.

Visser LH, Woudenberg NP, de Bont J, et al. Treatment of the sacroiliac joint in patients with leg pain: a randomized-controlled trial. Eur Spine J. 2013;22:2310–17.

Vleeming A, Pool-Goudzwaard AL, Stoeckart R, et al. The posterior layer of the thoracolumbar fascia. Its function in load transfer from spine to legs. Spine. 1995;20:753–8.

Vleeming A, Schuenke M. Form and force closure of the sacroiliac joints. Phys Med Rehabil. 2019;11:S24–31.

Vleeming A, Stoeckart R, Volkers AC, Snijders CJ. Relation between form and function in the sacroiliac joint. Part I: Clinical anatomical aspects. Spine. 1990a;15:130–2.

Vleeming A, Volkers AC, Snijders CJ, Stoeckart R. Relation between form and function in the sacroiliac joint. Part II: Biomechanical aspects. Spine. 1990b;15:133–6.

Vleeming A, Schuenke MD, Masi AT, et al. The sacroiliac joint: an overview of its anatomy, function and potential clinical implications. J Anat. 2012;221:537–67.

Weksler N, Velan GJ, Semionov M, et al. The role of sacroiliac joint dysfunction in the genesis of low back pain: the obvious is not always right. Arch Orthop Trauma Surg. 2007;127:885–8.

Wentz L, Liu P-Y, Haymes E, Ilich JZ. Females have a greater incidence of stress fractures than males in both military and athletic populations: A systemic review. Mil Med. 2011;176:420–30.

Wilson JJ, Furukawa M. Evaluation of the patient with hip pain. Am Fam Physician. 2014;89:27–34.

Wu WH, Meijer OG, Bruijn SM, et al. Gait in pregnancy-related pelvic girdle pain: amplitudes, timing, and coordination of horizontal trunk rotations. Eur Spine J. 2008;17:1160–9.

Young S, April C, Laslett M. Correlation of clinical examination characteristics with three sources of chronic low back pain. Spine J Off J North Am Spine Soc. 2003;3:460–5.

When are foot and ankle impairments important for hip and knee disorders?

Fraser McKinney, Rachel Koldenhoven Rolfe, Benoy Mathew

14

Introduction

The foot and ankle form the distal end of the lower limb and comprise 28 bones with 33 differently shaped joints, which are anatomically unique to each person. Motions of the foot and ankle are produced by 34 different muscles, 13 extrinsic and 21 intrinsic. The complexity of this structure should not be underestimated, and the integral role it plays in the biomechanics of the hip and knee complex should not be undervalued. The aim of this chapter is to guide the reader through our current understanding of the foot and ankle complex and its fundamental relationship to the hip and the knee.

The human foot has evolved to support us during a variety of tasks such as upright standing, walking, gentle locomotion, and running at higher speeds. These activities may occur linearly or require multidirectional movements as during sporting activities. Each of these activities requires variation in foot control and stiffness whilst adapting the function relative to variations in the environment. The foot must quickly adapt to changes in the surface type and task demand.

The interaction between the foot and ankle complex and the ground is not one single response but should be considered as multiple mini-interactions. Interactions between the joints are interdependent and influence each other, which gives the foot and ankle complex the functionality to act as both shock absorber and stable base to propel our body through space. Several congenital malformations, as well as structural and musculoskeletal (MSK) injuries, can also occur within the foot and ankle complex.

The following section will focus on anatomical structure as it pertains to biomechanics and MSK injuries and their potential impact on the functioning of the hip and knee joints.

Anatomy

Functional anatomy is a combination of bones and passive and active tissue intertwined with neural and vascular elements.

Bones

The ankle joint is formed by three bones – the tibia, fibula, and talus – while the foot is often divided into three distinct collections of its 27 bones – the forefoot, midfoot, and rearfoot (Figure 14.1). The forefoot contains the phalanges and metatarsals, while the midfoot is made up of the navicular, cuboid, and three cuneiform bones. The rearfoot or hindfoot is made up of the talus and calcaneus. The calcaneus

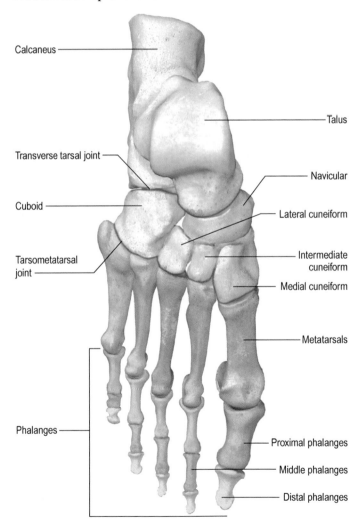

FIGURE 14.1
Osteology of the foot.

is the largest bone of the foot and projects posteriorly past the tibia, which allows it to act as a short lever for the forces transmitted through the ankle joint.

The forefoot includes the metatarsals and phalanges one to five, and is described as having medial and lateral arches joined by a transverse arch. These arches allow for the transmission of forces derived from contractile or inertial energy created by the body. It is proposed that if the 5th metatarsal is displaced inferiorly, the 1st metatarsal is displaced superiorly and vice versa. As we approach late stance and the foot moves to a more supinated position, this motion becomes synchronized with the osseous compression offering stability to the foot.

Joints

The ankle joint is made up of three articular surfaces, the talocrural joint (tibiotalar), the subtalar joint (talocalcaneal), and the transverse tarsal joint (talocalcaneonavicular). The talocrural joint (TCJ) is formed between the distal tibia, fibula, and talus, which creates a crescent-shaped mortise with the curved talar dome resting in the mortise, which allows for motions of dorsiflexion and plantarflexion to occur. The subtalar joint formed between the talus and calcaneus is made of three separate articulations, the anterior, middle, and posterior. The subtalar joint is unique in that motion occurs about an oblique, a tri-planar axis due to the shape of the bones. The anterior and middle facets of the calcaneus are concave, while the posterior facet is convex. This allows for rotational and translatory motion to occur which, when combined, are termed pronation (subtalar eversion/forefoot abduction/ankle dorsiflexion) or supination (subtalar inversion/forefoot adduction/ankle plantarflexion).

The talocalcaneonavicular joint, often termed talonavicular joint, appears to work in synchronization with the calcaneocuboid joints, with the exact method and outcome unclear but current theory points towards a joint-locking mechanism. As the rearfoot moves into valgus, a shift of forces transmits through the talonavicular and calcaneocuboid joints placing their axis of rotation in parallel, which removes the potential for a compressive locking of the joints allowing a more flexible foot to absorb forces. As the foot moves back into supination, the joint axis now moves to oppose each other offering a mutual compressive force giving stability to the midfoot.

Ligaments

The individual bones of the foot and ankle are held together by ligaments and, broadly speaking, these can be divided into anterior, posterior, medial and lateral ligaments (Figure 14.2). The relative contributions towards their impact on both offering stability to a joint and guiding its motion vary depending upon the location of the ankle, foot, or a combination of both.

Muscles

The extrinsic muscles of the lower leg produce many motions for the foot and ankle. There are 12 extrinsic muscles located in 4 compartments (anterior, lateral, deep posterior, and superficial posterior) of the lower leg that produce movements such as ankle dorsiflexion, plantarflexion, inversion and eversion, and toe flexion and extension. In addition, 11 intrinsic foot muscles play a role in stabilizing the foot and have been referred to as the "foot core" (Hogan et al., 2020). On the plantar aspect, there are four layers of intrinsic muscles and on the dorsal aspect, there is one layer.

Nerves

The foot receives its nerve supply from the superficial peroneal nerve, deep fibular nerve, tibial nerve, sural nerve, and saphenous nerve all arising from the L4 to S3 nerve root (Tang et al., 2021). The tibial nerve offers sensory information from the back of the leg and plantar surface of the foot while also supplying the muscles of the posterior compartment and the intrinsic foot muscles. The other main nerve, the common peroneal, divides into two: the superficial peroneal nerve, which is responsible for the muscle contraction of the peroneus longus and peroneus brevis, and the deep peroneal nerve supplying the extensor group, which includes the tibialis anterior and extensor hallucis longus.

Biomechanics of the Foot on Knee and Hip Regions

Biomechanics encapsulates the study of movement, including how muscles, tendons, bones, and ligaments work to produce, promote and guide movement. Analysis of human biomechanics can be viewed as external, a force that

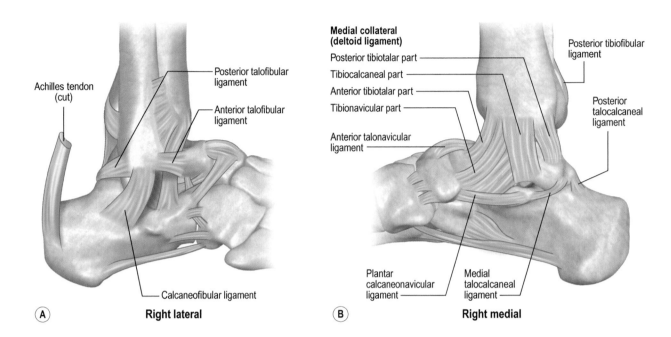

Achilles tendon (cut)

Posterior talofibular ligament

Anterior talofibular ligament

Calcaneofibular ligament

(A) **Right lateral**

Medial collateral (deltoid ligament)
Posterior tibiotalar part
Tibiocalcaneal part
Anterior tibiotalar part
Tibionavicular part

Anterior talonavicular ligament

Posterior tibiofibular ligament

Posterior talocalcaneal ligament

Plantar calcaneonavicular ligament

Medial talocalcaneal ligament

(B) **Right medial**

FIGURE 14.2
Ligaments of the ankle and foot. (A) Lateral view. (B) Medial view.

originates from outside the body, or internal, one that is generated by the body's tissues. This analysis of movement where we consider motion and the forces that created this motion is termed *kinetics*, while the description of motion in the absence of consideration of those forces is termed *kinematics*. Kinematics requires the knowledge of the location of motion, the direction, magnitude, and rate of that motion (displacement), something therapists frequently observe and utilize for treatment purposes. As we expand and consider the impact of this single joint upon its neighboring body segments, a process described as the "kinetic chain," we can now begin to realize the importance of each segment upon distal or proximal segments.

The foot and ankle complex consists of a collection of 33 differently shaped joints with each bone and its articulations fulfilling a specific purpose. To assist in this process each bone is held in place by a series of ligaments – there are over 30 separate ligaments – that guide and restrict motion and support transmission of forces. The specifics of these mechanical processes are poorly described in the literature, understandably given their complexity and potential to be different in each individual. Therefore, a broader approach is described here, with the authors interpreting

the published literature to enable readers to understand the foot and ankle complex relative to its function, the impact of injuries, and the concurrent effects on other joints, particularly the hip and knee. The aim of this section is not to challenge or champion any specific narrative or beliefs but to offer a clinically applicable summary of the current literature. The authors recognize that specific foot types, congenital malformations, or structural factors will vary between individuals and impact the mechanics described.

The foot/ankle complex is the first point of contact with the ground and initially absorbs the forces which are then transmitted up the kinetic chain. The hip acts on the foot and ankle in that it produces proximal movements that influence the position of the foot and ankle when contacting the ground during a variety of tasks.

This relationship between the ankle, knee and hip can be seen when we examine the kinetic chain during common daily tasks. Insufficient ankle dorsiflexion during the stance phase of gait leads to adaptations and compensation in other areas of the kinetic chain, namely the foot, knee or hip. A common change can be seen with greater internal rotation of the foot, tibia and femur influencing the relative contributions of the hip joint and those muscles controlling hip motion. Other common patterns are an early heel lift-off to limit the requirement to dorsiflex or hyperextension of the knee to allow the pelvis to transfer forward over the ankle joint.

The squatting motion during sit to stand in those with limited ankle dorsiflexion requires greater control of the hip range of motion. Specifically, it requires eccentric control to compensate for the loss in range and control of the body's center of mass (CoM) and accompanied by greater knee valgus displacement (Bell et al., 2012). Reduced ankle dorsiflexion may restrict the ability to pass the leg forward over the foot and to lower the CoM during squatting movements. This could lead to compensation, via excessive subtalar and midfoot pronation (Tweed et al., 2008).

If we look at the ability to come downstairs or a lateral step down where a greater range in ankle dorsiflexion is required, greater knee valgus and hip kinematics occur to promote continued completion of tasks (Rabin & Kozol, 2010). Restricted ankle dorsiflexion has been associated with knee injuries such as ACL (Wahlstedt & Rasmussen-Barr, 2015) and patellar tendinopathy (Malliaras et al., 2006). It has been hypothesized that reduced ankle flexibility may alter movement patterns during landing and increase landing forces. Restricted dorsiflexion and the associated reduction in hip and knee flexion could increase ground reaction forces, as the reduced joint excursion causes increased stiffness (Fong et al., 2011).

A systematic review by Mason-Mackay et al. (2017) has highlighted that reduced ankle dorsiflexion range of motion alters lower-extremity landing mechanics in a manner which predisposes athletes to injury. Therefore, screening athletes for ankle flexibility may assist in identifying those at an increased risk of injury. However, further studies are needed to investigate the effect of dorsiflexion restriction on mechanical patterns rather than on individual mechanical variables, and to investigate sport-specific landing tasks.

Clinical Evaluation of Ankle Dorsiflexion Range of Motion

In clinical practice, there are several methods and tools available to measure ankle dorsiflexion range of motion in both non-weight-bearing and weight-bearing positions.

Weight-bearing measures are regarded as more accurately reflecting the available range of motion during functional activities such as walking, running, or stair ambulation, and are more reliable than measures obtained in a non-weight-bearing position (Venturini et al., 2006). Commonly utilized methods to measure ankle dorsiflexion range of motion in weight-bearing include weight-bearing lunge position using a standard goniometer, digital inclinometer, and a tape measure using the distance-to-wall technique (Figure 14.3). All three techniques have good reliability and low measurement error, with the distance-to-wall technique using a tape measure and inclinometer methods resulting in higher reliability, compared to the goniometer (Konor et al., 2012).

Gait

Gait is the word used to describe a manner, pattern, or sequence of walking or moving on the foot. Movements of the foot in individuals during walking in a normal population show significant variation in sequencing, ranges of motion, and speed of motion but they all have one thing in common: for the vast majority of people they "work."

A useful approach to biomechanical assessment and movement analysis of the foot and ankle categorizes the complex into three different sections: the rearfoot, midfoot and forefoot during the swing and stance phase.

Gait Cycle

The *gait cycle* describes the process of walking from the time your heel/foot hits the ground and ends when the same heel/foot hits the ground again. On average this takes around 1 second with 60% termed stance phase, when the foot is in contact with the ground, and 40% swing phase, after toe-off when the foot is not in contact with the ground. This indicates that the time a single leg spends on the ground, i.e., ground contact time, is 0.6 seconds (Chapman et al., 2012). During the stance phase, the foot is required to both absorb energy and offer a stable base to ensure any energy created is transferred efficiently and effectively into the ground to propel our CoM in the direction requested.

The gait cycle can be further divided into three different descriptions of motion based around motion in the sagittal plane, called rockers. The first rocker describes the

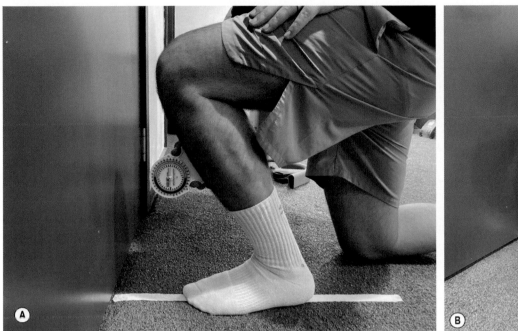
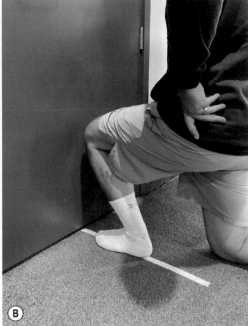

FIGURE 14.3
Weight-bearing measurement of ankle dorsiflexion. (A) Inclinometer placement at the tibial tuberosity along the anterior tibial crest. (B) The patient places the test foot on a tape measure perpendicular to the wall and lunges forward so the knee touches the wall.

heel strike of the calcaneus upon the ground and includes the motion of the ankle joint pivoting around this point of contact until the foot rests flat on the floor. The second rocker mid-foot starts from the flat foot and describes the transition of the tibia over the ankle joint. While the third rocker occurs as the heel lifts off the ground making the 1st metatarsal (MTP) joint the main pivot point until toe-off. Breaking the motion down into these simpler phases allows us to focus on the key moving parts at each stage.

To function with a "normal" gait, a range of motion at the hip, knee, and ankle has to be achieved. The relationship between the foot, ankle, hip and knee is best illustrated when describing combinations of movement, often termed joint coupling. Joint coupling is the movement of one segment around a joint axis in relation to the movement of another segment around a different joint axis (Miller et al., 2010). During the first and second rockers of walking, calcaneal motion occurs as a combination across three planes of motion, termed pronation. Calcaneal motion dominates around the frontal plane relating to eversion and is coupled

with tibial axial internal rotation around the transverse plane. A recent hypothesis suggests that, during gait, increased variability of joint coupling between the shank and rearfoot provides a mechanism for protecting the ankle against variations in terrain, speed of motion, and task (Herb & Hertel, 2015). Increased variability in joint coupling is considered to be essential in offering options and time to select appropriate motion strategies, although this is subconscious.

If we describe the hip in relation to joint coupling, changes to performance in the hip muscles lead to changes in femoral adduction and internal rotation during gait (Leetun et al., 2004). This change to femoral motion results in tibial internal rotation, which is followed by the coupled movement of subtalar abduction into the forefoot resulting in pronation (Mackinnon & Winter, 1993). This concept highlights the contributions of the proximal segments on axial tibial rotation (Bellchamber & Van Den Bogert, 2000) and foot pronation.

There remains some debate around what controls the motion of the tibia around the transverse plane, the rear foot, or proximal hip musculature. The authors suggest it is a combination of both, given that frontal plane control in normal situations is regulated by varying degrees of input from both the subtalar joint and hip joint. Between them, they contribute to controlling the location of our head on the trunk, trunk on the pelvis, and pelvis motion around the lower limb. The dynamic system theory describes a process of central adaptation to achieve a given task whereby the body balances the constraints of each individual segment (ankle, hip, trunk, and head), environmental constraints, and task-required constraints (Davids et al., 2003).

As we develop and grow, our ability to explore and learn to control the variability of joint coupling allows us to optimize our output (McKeon et al., 2008). A significant determinant of this control is the sensorimotor system, cognitive interpretation, but most importantly the capability of our muscles to deliver the control of this coupled relationship. Any variation in the contribution of each component of a segment will influence and determine the requirements of the other segment, for example, the strength of the ankle dorsiflexors will influence ankle rotation and control.

One aspect often taught describes uncontrolled pronation, plantarflexion of the 1st ray, and its relationship in changing the location of the load applied to the joint actions of the subtalar joint and this relationship with the knee. This motion generates early knee flexion, coupled with the motion of tibial internal rotation, causing greater knee valgus. This type of motion is often accompanied by greater femoral internal rotation, which is counterbalanced by contralateral pelvic drop and ipsilateral trunk side flexion and extension (Figure 14.4). A combination of this type of pattern is considered to result in greater hip compression forces. Following injury, the force coupling relationship of lower limb joints is considered very fragile in nature; for example, those with long-standing ankle injuries display a decreased variability in rearfoot to shank joint coupling during walking tasks (Lilley et al., 2018). It is considered that this change in variability is a reflection of the sensorimotor system's attempt to ensure completion of task while ensuring limited exposure to further injury risk. Where the sensorimotor system might find difficulty in controlling the variability of this coupled movement, a safe option is

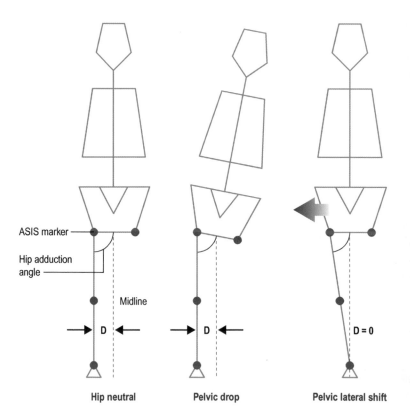

FIGURE 14.4
Contribution of position of pelvis on femur to hip adduction angle and foot position. ASIS, anterior superior iliac spine; D, distance to mid-line.

ASIS marker

Hip adduction angle

Midline

D   D   D = 0

Hip neutral   Pelvic drop   Pelvic lateral shift

to limit exposure to the motion utilizing internal tibial rotation to prevent exposure of the rear foot to inversion. Examining ankle inversion sprains that occur in the frontal and transverse plane of motion allows us to consider the complexity of these variables during our attempt to guide and control joint coupling.

Hip Dynamics

Hip extension driven by the gluteus maximus occurs in the sagittal plane, while those muscles controlling hip and pelvis trajectory occur in the frontal plane, such as the gluteus medius during the first to second rocker (MacKinnon & Winter, 1993) or the hip adductors' role to initiate lateral pelvic tilt in response to displacement of the CoM of the body, arms, and trunk during early stance. This adaptation to femoral orientation following pre- and post-heel strike can be seen with lower EMG of the gluteus medius (Azevedo et al., 2009), decreased short-latency reflex (Hubbard et al., 2007), early activation of gluteus medius (Beckman & Buchanan, 1995) and general lower muscle activation in the lower limb (Wikstrom et al., 2010; Feger et al., 2014).

If we look at this rearfoot to shank relationship in more detail, the concept of rockers discussed the forces based around the foot and its interaction with the ground, implying control of these would be the main drivers to motion. A reverse concept suggests that a reduction in the ability to resist the ground reaction force would lead to a shift in the location of where those forces are resisted. Changes to shank rotation following ankle injury appear to be centrally driven, shifting the coupled relationship of the shank to the proximal joints of the knee and hip to adapt to the constraints of the ankle. This concept elevates the relative contribution of the hip strategy in controlling the tasks of balance, gait, stairs, running, and change of direction (Kuo et al., 2005); interestingly this also increases the metabolic demands of the hip through increased energy consumption. In turn, this may influence the physical status and fatigue levels which will affect force output and delivery of the dynamic system to optimize control.

If we consider the proximal contribution with changes to pelvis position due to gluteus medius weakness during the stance phase, its potential to impact the location of the swinging leg in space most likely leads to medial foot placement error. This is thought to create a greater inversion moment and lateral displacement of the center of gravity causing the lateral border of the foot to act as a fulcrum during the first to second rockers. It is considered this will have two likely outcomes: (1) a positioning of the CoM lateral to the subtalar joint axis of rotation causing an ankle inversion sprain or repeated sprain, or (2) a hip strategy is used to manipulate lateral sway, often assisted via pelvis drop, trunk side flexion and greater arm movements.

Foot and ankle injuries can impact the relationship between muscles of the foot and the hip and knee. For example, following an ankle injury, a relative change in sensorimotor input and force output influences the ankle's relative contribution towards the dynamic system theory. Persistent deficits are considered to lead to reorganization of the sensory processing in the central nervous system resulting in changes to the muscle activation patterns as delivered via the feedforward mechanism of control (Doherty et al., 2015). These changes particularly affect muscles that assist in controlling pronation, which demonstrates reduced output along with those that control hip motion and pelvis stability, gluteus medius and adductors specifically. The individual contributions of these muscles will be considered within the strength session of this chapter.

As we progress into the second rocker, one important situation where ankle movement directly impacts the hip is when there is limited ankle dorsiflexion, which is associated with decreased hip extension. Ankle dorsiflexion is dependent on the talus being able to glide around the joint allowing the body to travel over the foot. It has been shown that those with a long-standing ankle injury with a loss of ankle dorsiflexion have decreased hip extension during the propulsive phase of gait (Doherty et al., 2016a). At slow walking speeds from the propulsive to early swing, changes in femoral adduction and internal rotation occur in the hip (Leetun et al., 2004; Koldenhoven et al., 2019), which may drive increased tibial internal rotation, an action that drives a coupled movement of subtalar abduction resulting in triplane motion of pronation, suggesting pronation is under the control of the proximal muscles of the hip (Bellchamber & Van Den Bogert, 2000). Any limitation to talus dorsiflexion or drive towards excessive pronation will limit the ability of the foot to elongate, with midtarsal joints unable to progress to their loose-packed position, thus limiting force absorption through the foot. Given that our force into the ground will be roughly constant, the absorption of force has to occur somewhere; if a restriction exists in the foot and ankle, the hip is the next best placed to absorb those forces. A second effect here will be the ability of the foot to return to a supinated position in late stance to offer a stiffer foot to promote force transmission through the ankle plantarflexors.

The third rocker also shows changes to foot hypomobility leading to elevated hip muscle activation (Kuo, 2002). As the body weight travels over the ankle joint or, more specifically, the tibia begins to tilt anteriorly, an increase in tension exists in the muscles around the posterior calf and ankle. These, along with the stored elastic energy from the plantar aponeurosis, generate tension that is sufficient to support and draw the forefoot back towards the rearfoot, a process that results in re-supination of the midfoot. The re-supination motion results in the navicular moving towards dorsiflexion and external rotation, a motion that appears to offer structural stability through congruency of the joints offering a solid base to the foot during late stance. As we continue through the gait cycle, our heel lifts off the ground and to ensure stability remains within the foot, tension must be maintained in the muscles and plantar aponeurosis. A key component of the stability is created by the aponeurosis, which through its attachments around the metatarsal phalangeal joints ensures tension is maintained during the 1st to 5th metatarsal phalangeal joint dorsiflexion. The plantar aponeurosis just proximal to insertion splits itself around the side of the joint, a mechanism that is hypothesized to ensure that once the heel lifts off the ground, tension remains in the medial arch to continue to offer a stable base. This is known as the windlass mechanism, as proposed by Hicks (1954). Emerging literature has challenged this long and staunchly held theory and it is now clear this system alone cannot offer complete stability; rather, optimal function is a combination of the windlass mechanism and the intrinsic plantar muscles of the foot, which are required to generate the stability of the midfoot and metatarsal phalangeal joint (Bolga & Malone, 2004).

The plantar intrinsic muscles of the foot appear to play a dominant role not in force absorption but in foot stability during the late stance phase. Any reduction in the work of the foot plantar intrinsic muscles during late stance appears to reduce the stiffness of the MTP joint leading to issues around the force-generating capacity of the foot during late stance in all conditions from walking to fast running (Farris et al., 2019). This deficiency in the foot leads to greater positive work completed by the hip and improved stride frequency.

Finally, in the swing phase of gait, the speed of the foot at toe-off directly impacts hip flexion. A slower toe-off has the potential to generate greater hip extension as the pelvis continues to move forward while ultimately requiring the femur to move faster ensuring its ability to achieve hip flexion prior to heel strike. It is known that errors in foot placement can be corrected by motions at the subtalar joint and hip joint. However, for those with limitations in this system adapted strategies will have to be brought into play. The pre-location of the foot prior to landing is critical to the sequence of motion and this is determined by the stability of the hip's relationship with the contralateral stance leg and control of pelvis location. A contralateral hip drop on the stance leg will place the swinging leg in greater external femoral rotation generating greater ankle inversion moment on foot contact.

The ankle/hip coupling during walking can be influenced by age. Self-selected walking speeds are not age-dependent but how speed is achieved does vary with age (Santana da Silva et al., 2020). As we age, where we generate the force to promote movement is redistributed, with joint torque moving from distal to proximal. In younger adults during the stance phase, the foot and ankle (along with shoes) contribute up to 60%–70% of the force transmission in gait (Honert & Zelik, 2019). Aging causes a reduction in the elastic properties of the non-contractile tissue (Özdemir et al., 2004), thereby reducing force-generating capacity in the plantarflexors, which in turn restricts the foot and ankle's ability to control force absorption and production. This means that to maintain selected walking speeds, there is a shift to the hip to compensate for the loss of elasticity in the foot and ankle.

A common injury to the foot and ankle is the lateral ankle sprain; while this will be discussed in more detail in another section, here we will highlight its key impacting on the gait cycle. According to the findings of Son et al. (2019), "patients with chronic ankle instability (CAI) appear to use a hip-dominant gait strategy for power production (i.e., concentric energy) by re-weighting joint power from distal (ankle and knee) to the proximal (hip) joint." It has been shown those suffering long-term effects following a lateral ankle sprain display up to a 13% decrease in eccentric control of the ankle and 38% decrease at the knee eccentric control during heel strike. The impact of this results in greater vertical ground reaction forces, while the hip remains in 2.0 degrees more hip flexion throughout the stance phase and significantly around a 54% increase in hip concentric power to compensate.

It appears the presence of CAI results in a common foot positional pattern of landing in greater inversion at heel strike. This inversion occurs at initial contact and throughout the swing phase at a variety of walking speeds which appeared to increase as walking speed increased (>120% preferred walking speeds). Interestingly, it could be that, in those with CAI, walking faster than their preferred speed places them at greater risk of ankle inversion sprain. Those with CAI had greater hip abduction and adduction moments at heel strike and greater peak hip adduction during the swing phase of gait. A common tool to address ankle stability utilizes balance or proprioceptive training; this has been shown to demonstrate little carry-over into meaningful changes in gait pattern and hip moments during the gait cycle. The combination of balance and visual biofeedback training during gait significantly increases ankle plantarflexion range of motion, greater ankle inversion, first toe flexion and hip abduction strength but with little change to balance as an outcome measure (Koldenhoven et al., 2021).

Running

Running involves moving faster than walking by taking longer and more powerful strides, i.e., our legs move through the air quicker. As we run faster, say around 3.49 $m.s^{-1}$ (12.56 kmph), the foot is in contact with the ground for approximately 0.243sec (+/ 0.022) while the higher speeds of 5.17 $m.s^{-1}$ (18.61 kmph) = ground contact time of 0.188 sec (+/- 0.015) and with super-high speeds of 6.96 $m.s^{-1}$ (24.08 kmph) this is reduced to 0.145 sec (+/- 0.009) (Dorn et al., 2012). This means to run faster you can exert more force in a short time-frame during the stance phase which would increase stride length; this pattern becomes impossible to maintain due to shorter and shorter time-frames at higher speeds limiting the time to produce the force. At around 7.0 m/s the gastrocnemius and soleus peak force capacity is reached and to run faster an increase in stride frequency is needed to offset limitation in power. To achieve this peak, hip flexor and hip extensor movements

must increase to promote the acceleration of our legs with the peak force of gluteus maximus nearly doubling during the terminal swing phase to accommodate these increases in speed (Dorn et al., 2012).

Muscle anatomy and physiology vary between individuals and for those with weaker or lower force-producing capabilities in the ankle plantarflexors, increasing speed achieved through increased stride frequency places a greater reliance upon the hip muscles. To illustrate, high-level sprinters have significantly longer gastrocnemius muscle fiber length and small pennation angle within the soleus muscle, which enhances their ability to generate force at higher shortening velocities (Abe et al., 2000; Kumagai et al., 2000).

Running is considered one of the best ways to train the muscles around the foot and ankle to generate peak force and improve strength. Ground contact time for walking is around 600 milliseconds while the average runner (Garmin database) will have a ground contact time of 160–300 milliseconds, less than half that of walking (Mooses et al. 2021). This can be seen in the maximum moments increase for the ankle from walking with 1.9 Nm/kg and 4.3 W/kg to running (4 m/s = 14.4 kmph) 3.1 Nm/kg and 13.8 W/kg (Grimmer et al., 2020). To put this into context the same study indicated in young non-athletic males a maximum isometric contraction of the ankle plantarflexors 1.6 Nm/kg.

One of the main contributors to ankle plantarflexion during running is the soleus muscle, which is reported to produce up to 50% of the force involved in the vertical translation of the CoM (Dorn et al., 2012). This motion is achieved through both plantarflexion of the ankle and extension of the knee. Ankle plantarflexion against an immovable object or the ground generates a reverse of ankle plantarflexion and involves the tibia moving into a vertical location which creates ankle plantarflexion. This vertical positioning is also known as knee extension, resulting in straightening of the knee and elevation of our pelvis vertically and consequently the CoM.

Change of Direction

The ability to abruptly change direction is essential to activities of daily living as well as sports performance. Performing these direction changes at high speeds in addition to the complexity of reacting to an opponent or live game situation provides further challenges to the musculoskeletal system. The individual must move their body appropriately to avoid potential injury. It has been hypothesized that following an ankle injury the mechanical laxity and deficits in sensorimotor systems around the ankle result in the body searching for a replacement mechanical advantage to control motor function (Park, 2017; Son et al., 2017). During cutting and landing tasks there is greater utilization of the hip joint, specifically an increase in stiffness with a greater flexion angle, which results in a greater hip extension moment increasing the reliance on the gluteus maximus muscle.

Those with long-standing ankle injury often present with significantly greater uncontrolled variability in joint coupling strategies, between the ankle and the hip, to stabilize in both the frontal and sagittal planes. It is possible that variability arises from changes to tibial motion, as soleus muscle activity is reduced following landing (Brown et al., 2004), which is compensated by less hip flexion pre-landing and abduction post-landing (Brown et al., 2012).

Any loss of ankle dorsiflexion will influence the location and control of forces during cutting movements. One strategy to attenuate these forces is to increase the firing of medial gastrocnemius and peroneus longus muscles. This change from their primary role is likely to lead to muscle fatigue, change in joint stability and joint coupling, and increase in joint loading forces. These forces appear to be transferred to the hip, so during a cutting task hip flexion in the sagittal plane increases by up to 2.2 degrees and hip adduction in the frontal plane by up to 1.5 degrees (Son et al., 2019). This pattern may help to control the downward motion of the CoM in the sagittal plane prior to cutting to the contralateral side (Son et al., 2019), with this position requiring less ankle evertor and hip abductor muscle forces to maintain an upright pelvis and trunk (Son et al., 2017).

Stairs

Climbing stairs is an important part of everyday life, with the average person estimated to climb 47–66 stairs a day (Grimmer & Seyfarth, 2014), although this comprises only a small proportion of daily strides (7000–13,000) (Tudor-Locke & Myers, 2001). Descending stairs requires a greater range of ankle dorsiflexion compared to ascending, which results in increased ankle inversion and plantarflexion prior

to landing. This compromised ankle position impacts the hip, which compensates by increasing hip adduction and flexion angles during loading (Cao et al., 2020). If the landing forces remain constant, this indicates a transition from ankle force absorption to a hip-dominant strategy to accommodate the load. The process of landing during the descent of stairs can be likened to a simplified version of a drop landing, a specific movement that has been researched following an ankle injury and has implications for hip function. Following an ankle injury, the feed-forward mechanism of dynamic motor control, mediated by the spinal or supraspinal mechanisms, displays impairment through a selection of inappropriate or adapted movement strategies, such that in subjects following landing from a height of 32–40 cm, those with CAI displayed significantly longer time to stabilize the CoM in all directions. At the same time, these subjects displayed greater ankle dorsiflexion and inversion pre-landing to post-landing with a coordinated greater knee flexion angle 20 ms prior to landing (Caulfield & Garrett, 2002). This adaptation continues up to the hip, with greater hip flexion and internal rotation from pre-landing to post-landing (Doherty et al., 2016a). Unlike stairs, where the utilization of a hip strategy is sufficient to ensure ground reaction force (GRF) remains constant, drop landing in those following CAI displays a significantly greater GRF and this is produced in a shorter time-frame (Monaghan et al., 2006), further accentuating the impact forces. Interestingly the adoption of greater ankle dorsiflexion post-landing is likely a strategy used to offer stability to the joint, something that would be a centrally driven motor pattern (Brown et al., 2008).

In summary, following ankle injury the control of vertical and horizontally orientated forces utilizes different strategies. The horizontal motion requires stiffer landings with less hip and knee flexion while vertical forces occurring during drop landing used greater hip and knee flexion.

Hopping

Hopping on the spot and hopping in varying directions impacts the stabilizing muscles of the foot and ankle joints. The hopping propulsive phase in a horizontal direction generates forces of which 42.8% are produced by the ankle and 44.3% within the hip (Kotsifaki et al., 2021), while the landing phase is dominated by the knee taking 64.7% of the forces. Interestingly, vertical hopping in both propulsion and landing the production and attenuation of landing is shared equally by the hip, knee, and ankle. In an athletic population of collegiate athletes with CAI following a hop stabilization program over 6 weeks, subjects showed altered jump landing technique with improved hip, knee, and ankle motions all with the benefit of greater control of and reduction in ground reaction forces (Ardakani et al., 2019). This type of training also showed significant improvements in preparatory muscle activation and reactive muscle activation with the added benefit of self-reported improved function (Minoonejad et al., 2019).

Hopping Tests

Hop tests are widely used in a clinical setting to assess the functional performance of an injured leg. Performance during vertical and horizontal hops measures different aspects of the hip, knee, and ankle function during the propulsive and landing phases. Horizontal hop performance is primarily a function of the hip and ankle with the knee contribution limited to 13%, whereas the vertical hop is relatively equally apportioned to the hip, knee, and ankle joints (Kotsifaki et al., 2021). Therefore, the horizontal hop distance should be considered a poor discriminator of knee function and performance.

Foot and Ankle Injuries

Ankle Sprain

Ankle sprains are the most common musculoskeletal injury among athletes, military personnel, and other physically active populations. Of ankle sprain injuries, lateral ankle sprains are the most frequent. Typically, a lateral ankle sprain is the result of sudden ankle inversion, plantarflexion, and/or internal rotation. This may occur in several situations such as stepping on an opponent's foot during competition, stepping off of a curb, or landing with the foot in a compromised position. Lateral ankle sprains most commonly cause damage to the anterior talofibular ligament and the calcaneofibular ligament. This injury can have long-lasting effects if not treated properly. Unfortunately, many individuals view ankle sprains as being an innocuous injury and do not seek treatment which may contribute to the high recurrence rate for subsequent ankle sprains. Lack of proper treatment could lead also to the development of further problems and CAI.

Chronic Ankle Instability (CAI)

Roughly 40% of individuals who sprain their ankle will develop CAI (Doherty et al., 2016b). This condition is described as having residual symptoms, feelings of giving way or instability, decreased self-reported function, and recurrent ankle sprains for at least one year following the index injury. Individuals with CAI have demonstrated decreased hip strength and altered knee flexion angles during functional tasks. These alterations of proximal joints within the kinetic chain should be assessed and rehabilitated by clinicians working with patients who have CAI.

Measurement of Dynamic Postural Control

Dynamic postural control is an intrinsic risk factor, linked with lower extremity injury (Murphy et al., 2003). The Star Excursion Balance Test (SEBT, Figure 14.5) is a low-cost reliable instrument used in clinical practice as a means of evaluating dynamic postural control (Plisky et al., 2006).

Also, SEBT performance can be improved through an appropriate intervention program (Filipa et al., 2010). Aberrant movement of the knee during the SEBT anterior reach appears to be the most reliable and demonstrated the highest specificity for SEBT at-risk outcome when compared to the trunk and pelvis (Ness et al., 2015). The SEBT is thought to better represent functional activity over other postural control assessments because it incorporates a combination of strength, flexibility, and neuromuscular control while testing the limits of postural stability (Gribble et al., 2012).

Muscle Strength of the Lower Extremity Musculature

Hip Musculature

A growing area of research indicates that following an ankle injury the strength of the hip muscle and the coordination of the muscular contraction impact function, specifically around the pelvis, trunk and ankle (McCann et al., 2017).

It has been shown in youth male football (soccer) players that reduced hip extension muscle strength was an independent risk factor for lateral ankle sprains (De Ridder et al., 2017). A meta-analysis in those who developed CAI showed decreased hip external rotation, abduction, and extension strength (DeJong et al., 2020). Further, following

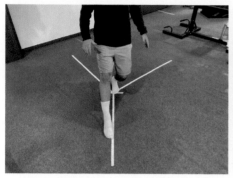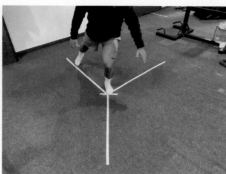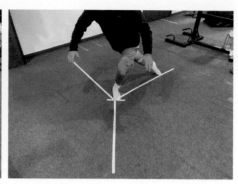

FIGURE 14.5
The Star Excursion Balance Test (SEBT). (A) Anterior reach direction. (B) Posterior–medial reach direction. (C) Posterior–lateral reach direction. The support foot must stay flat on the ground. The patient reaches with the other foot as far as possible in one direction and lightly touches the line before returning back to the starting position.

an acute ankle sprain, hip muscle abductors on the involved side were significantly weaker with no difference shown to hip extension (Friel et al., 2006). In CAI, this pattern continued with evidence indicating no significant change to gluteus maximus activity (DeJong et al., 2020).

It appears important how we collect our information regarding muscle strength, specifically hip extension muscles. The research is limited with those who investigated strength using an isometric test appearing to show a link with future injury, while when using an isokinetic through range testing protocol showed no associations with performance or injury risk (Steinberg et al., 2017).

It could be considered that isometric contractions are more closely related to a muscle's ability to produce force maximally. Greater muscular force production is linked to a muscle's ability to absorb and attenuate those forces not just initially but over time. An interpretation of this concept suggests those with stronger muscles and greater isometric force production will be able to attenuate the impact forces of landing within the contractile tissue of the muscle, thereby reducing the transfer of forces onto the osseous structures. This offers a possible description of why isometric strength is linked to load-based injuries, specifically hip abductor weakness is linked with medial tibial stress syndrome injuries (Verrelst et al., 2014). While a through range motion requires control of those forces and as with the ankle injury, the link with control shows a greater association with gluteus medius muscle.

Taking a closer look at those with CAI, they display a smaller gluteus medius muscle thickness during gait relative to

its resting thickness, called an activation ratio (DeJong et al., 2020). Extrapolating from other areas of the body it might be reasonable to assume changing the size of the hip muscle cross-sectional area will assist in its force-generating capacity and should impact both hip and pelvis motion (Neumann, 2010). It's also important to consider the activation patterns of gluteus medius with its activity required to control hip motion and avoid excessive pelvis drop and rotation (Neptune & McGowan, 2016; Neumann, 2010). It has been shown through a comprehensive program specifically targeting the gluteus medius and maximus muscles that the control of pelvic location, femoral rotation, and trunk position can be adapted.

Interestingly, and not conclusively, it appears when performing rehabilitation for the hip and knee muscles it is important to consider the type of task being performed. Those requested to complete voluntary tasks, such as balancing on a single leg and reacting showed later onset and earlier offset of gluteus medius and maximus muscles, while unexpected reaction to a stimulus such as those unexpected perturbations results in earlier onset of the gluteus medius and maximus muscles. The introduction of unexpected perturbations should be integrated with caution and form part of a progressive program, allowing the therapist to consider the most appropriate environment vs. challenge to maximize the target outcome within minimal injury risk. Examples might be a single-leg standing progressed to the addition of a light lateral push or pull via a stretch band to challenge the hip strategy to react in the horizontal plane. More active motion might be a progression from walking on a foam surface to walking over a wobble board or very active individuals who have progressed appropriately jumping with perturbation laterally or in a forward direction, requiring an adjustment to their landing strategy, trying to avoid posterior perturbation.

Triceps Surae Muscles

The biomechanical descriptions of gait and running indicated the importance of the foot and ankle in producing vertical and horizontal forces, of which strong calf muscles should be considered critical. The ability to resist the ground reaction force acting upon the body and the dynamic coupling strategy we select appears to determine the metabolic demands of our body. An increase in ankle push-off mid to late stance decreases the total work required from the hip muscle (Lewis & Ferris, 2008), while a reduction in push-off through the foot and ankle drives increased utilization of the hip muscles to compensate, a fact that leads to increased metabolic demands of the hip muscles (Kuo et al., 2005).

As we age, healthy adults display a reduction in push-off with up to 29% less ankle power throughout the gait cycle. When we reach the age of 60 the effects of age start to become apparent and we get an increase in soft-tissue stiffness, decrease in joint ROM, and decreased strength, which appears to impact changes in balance, gait, and falls. Age-related changes and strength deficits appear to impact gait speed, less efficient and stable walking with worsening quality of life (Santana da Silva et al., 2020). It appears this decline in calf strength can be addressed with a simple intervention, with one study utilizing 100 calf raises a day to influence a change in the outcomes. They did not need to be completed all at once but rather across the entire day and the benefits were seen in those who adhered to the long-term plan. It is a common sight to see people attempt to increase the work on a treadmill in the gym by adding a 1%–2% incline; in older adults the effect shown in step duration tends to be 10% shorter and up to 19% less ankle peak power but a compensatory 98% more hip peak power (Franz & Kram, 2014). While this might assist the capacity of the hips to continue to produce force, it does not solve the issues of reduced calf strength.

To optimize strength training of the soleus muscle we must apply sufficient load to stress the tissue and result in adaptation. While running is considered an exercise, its focus is the consistent load of our mass in the shortest time and if our focus is to make the muscle stronger, we must focus on longer duration and heavier load. The most successful programs apply a consistent increase in load over 6- to 12-week programs targeting slow and heavy, greater than 1.5× body weight for 3–5 sets for 6–12 repetitions.

Tibialis Anterior Muscle

This muscle of the lower limb is extremely underrated, with its activation linked with controlling forefoot plantarflexion during the first rocker. Changes to this process are associated with reduced force production of the calf muscles during the second to third rockers. This suggests while it might not be directly linked, the force output of this muscle appears to influence the sequence and activation of the foot impacting the other muscles. This is highlighted when we examine those with CAI, who display a greater drive to activate ankle plantarflexors and decreased tibialis anterior activation (Dundas et al., 2014).

To train this muscle, little evidence exists but appears it can occur over 15 sessions over a 5-week period of isometric training. Completion of 5 repetitions maximum effort for 5 sets (Dragert & Zehr, 2011) showed gains of up to 15% increase in ankle dorsiflexion strength.

The authors of this chapter suggest that while the tibialis muscle does not cross the knee, reverse dynamics indicate it influences knee flexion and consequently would impact the hip. Therefore, a progression in rehabilitation would be to learn to utilize ankle dorsiflexion during knee flexion, such as forefoot lifts and holds during sit to stand or forefoot holds as leaning back against a wall prior to a step-up (Figure 14.6).

Flexor Hallucis Longus (FHL) Muscle

One of three deep muscles within the posterior compartment, the flexor hallucis longus has a varied role. Primarily, as its name suggests, it flexes the big toe, while it is also a contributor to ankle plantarflexion and inversion in an open chain and supports mid-foot resupination in a closed chain.

It has been shown that post-training the muscle fascicle length and force output of the FHL showed little change during slow or fast walking, while the contraction speed increased significantly during push-off (Peter et al., 2017), supporting the idea that the FHL plays a role in the dynamic stability of the forefoot and first MTP during the late stages of gait.

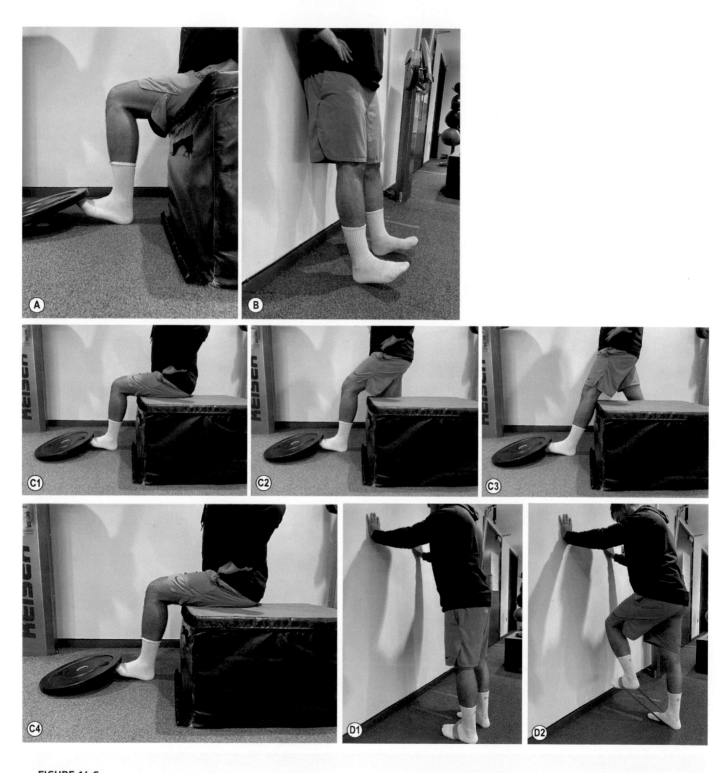

FIGURE 14.6
Tibialis anterior muscle exercises. (A) Isometric hold in sitting. (B) Isometric hold in standing. (C 1–4) Sit to stand version of isometric hold. (D 1–2) Tibialis anterior lift with hip flexion.

A toe flexor strength program greater than seven weeks showed improved gluteus maximus output, 50 meter sprint times and isometric strength by up to 80% (Goldmann et al., 2013; Hashimoto & Sakuraba, 2014). Change of direction shown via the pro-agility test and 3-cone test positively correlated to vertical jump height (Yamauchi & Koyama, 2020) and greater horizontal jump distance (Goldmann et al., 2013). These programs often used isometric muscle action with the ankle in dorsiflexion and first MTP in dorsiflexion focusing on metatarsal phalangeal flexion with 5 repetitions of 3–5 sets using 3-sec on/off.

Tibialis Posterior Muscle

Another muscle located deep within the posterior compartment, the tibialis posterior assists in talocrural joint plantarflexion, subtalar joint inversion, and medial arch support. As discussed, these motions have an impact on hip mechanics and therefore would be reasonable to assume hip flexibility would impact the tibialis posterior muscle. Performing tibialis posterior strength exercises (Figure 14.7) with anterior hip flexibility exercise of stretching ×3 a week for 6 weeks showed improved outcomes around balance, navicular drop, and muscle EMG activity (Alam et al., 2019).

The methodology on how to train this muscle is clear – high eccentric load or high progressive tolerance to load (capacity). An isolated eccentric program performed twice a day for 10–12 weeks led to significant improvements in force production, while similar results were found with a collection of exercises incorporating eccentric tibialis posterior with calf strength, foot core, and general capacity-based movements.

Peroneus Longus and Peroneus Brevis Muscles

The action of peroneus longus is regularly considered in its open-chain effect, while its primary role occurs during closed chain as occurs following heel strike. Due to its long tendon wrapping around the lateral malleolus and traveling around the cuboid to its insertion on the first metatarsal and cuneiform bone, its effect is to pull from the insertion point towards its pulley, the cuboid. This action results in plantarflexion of the 1st ray. The timing and sequence of this motion impacts tibial rotation and consequently a corresponding change in gluteus medius activation (Feger et al., 2014).

The peroneus brevis is considered the biggest limiter to rearfoot inversion during stance due to its tendon supporting the lateral aspect of the calcaneus. This same concept also suggests that while it can block inversion, overactivity might promote rearfoot eversion, pre-heel strike through to late stance.

Foot Intrinsic Musculature

The role of the foot intrinsics has only recently been significantly understood. It appears that, contrary to popular belief, the foot intrinsics contribute minimally to supporting the arch of the foot during walking or running. They remain important contributors to forefoot stiffness (Farris et al., 2019), which appears to be the main driver that links intrinsic activation and enhanced triceps surae muscle force output during push-off (Kelly et al., 2014; Farris et al., 2019). A consequence following a manufactured reduction in force output of the intrinsics led to an increase in the stride rate and power production from the hip muscles (Farris et al., 2019).

The foot core system, a new paradigm for understanding intrinsic foot muscle function, is the integration of active, passive, and neural structures (Figure 14.8) within the foot to provide dynamic foot control during functional activities (McKeon et al., 2015).

Training the foot muscles through a progression of isolation to integration provides a means to increase the functional variability of the foot core system in dynamic foot control (McKeon & Fourchet, 2015). Whilst the various intrinsic foot muscles, including the flexor digitorum brevis and interosseous muscles, contribute to arch support during gait, the abductor hallucis has lately received considerable attention. EMG studies have shown that abductor hallucis contracts to support the medial longitudinal arch and control pronation during static stance (Headlee et al., 2008). Preliminary evidence has shown that neuromuscular recruitment of the plantar intrinsic foot muscles may have value in dynamically supporting the medial longitudinal arch during functional tasks (Mulligan & Cook, 2013).

Effects of a 4- to 6-week intrinsic foot program led to improvements in motor performance (Fraser & Hertel, 2019), improved balance and function in CAI patients (Lee & Choi, 2019), and improved stair ascent and descent in healthy adults (Goo et al., 2016).

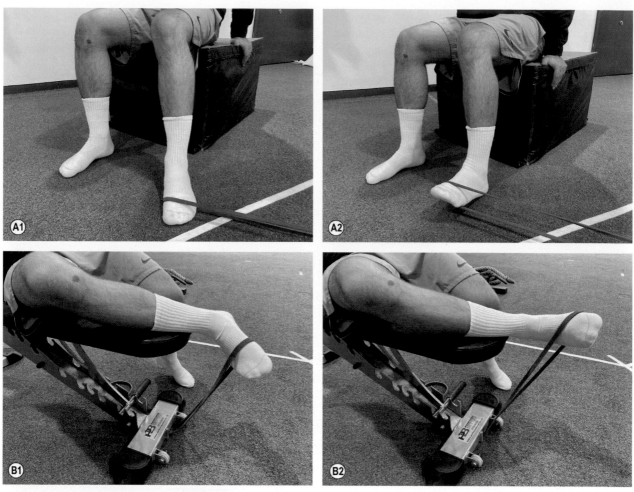

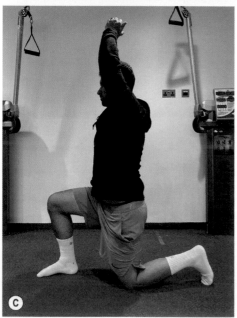

FIGURE 14.7
Tibialis posterior muscle exercises. (A 1-2) Seated with knee in 90 degrees, resistance band around fore-foot and controlled external and internal tibial rotation. (B 1-2) This exercise can be isometric or through range. The ankle travels from eversion to inversion while tibia is fixed on the bench. (C) Combination of tibial posterior exercises with an anterior hip stretch.

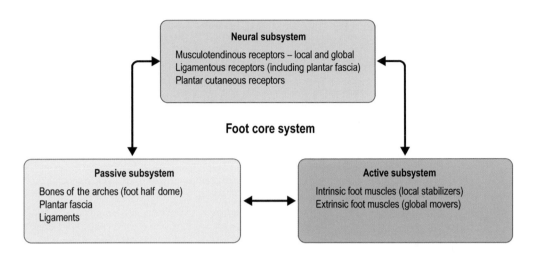

FIGURE 14.8
Foot core system.
(Adapted from McKeon et al., 2015.)

Plyometric Training

This type of training is made up of three phases, eccentric pre-stretch (loading), amortization (coupling), and concentric (rebound) phase. Plyometric training aims to perform an exercise with the intent of exerting maximum force in the shortest time, with the goal of increasing power (speed-strength). Strength training can increase the peak torque, which is the amount of force a muscle can produce, while plyometric training aims to optimize power, which is the maximum force produced in a short time-frame (Chmielewski et al., 2006).

Plyometric training is impacted by the velocity and direction of forces. Plyometric training such as vertically orientated programs over time increase ankle dorsiflexion and decrease ankle inversion during unilateral drop landing tasks (Huang et al., 2014). Horizontally directed hopping drills with a focus on controlling deceleration at the end-stage appear to promote greater control of the knee and hip flexion. This highlights that any rehabilitation must target the maladapted strategy as in this case vertical training could limit the influence on controlling horizontal forces and vice versa.

Conclusion

The highly complex anatomy and functioning of the foot and ankle, as summarized above, is integral to the functional anatomy of the hip and knee. An injury or pathology in the foot and ankle can have repercussions on the hip and knee joints and vice versa. Therefore, a holistic approach to joint problems of the lower limb will have benefits, particularly in the differential diagnosis and management of hip and knee injuries.

References

Abe T, Kumagai K, Brechue WF. Fascicle length of leg muscles is greater in sprinters than distance runners. Med Sci Sport Exerc. 2000;32:1125–9.

Alam F, Raza S, Ali Moiz J, et al. Effects of selective strengthening of tibialis posterior and stretching of iliopsoas on the navicular drop, dynamic balance and lower limb muscle activity in pronated feet: a randomized clinical trial. Phys Sportsmed. 2019;47:301–11.

Ardakani MK, Wikstrom E, Minoonejad H, et al. Hop stabilization training and landing biomechanics in athletes with chronic ankle instability: a randomized controlled trial. J Athl Train. 2019;54:1296–303.

Azevedo LB, Lambert MI, Vaughan CL, et al. Biomechanical variables associated with Achilles tendinopathy in runners. Br J Sports Med. 2009;43:288–92.

Beckman SM, Buchanan TS. Ankle inversion injury and hypertrophy: effect on hip and ankle muscle electromyography onset latency. Arch Phys Med Rehabil. 1995;76:1138–43.

Bell DR, Vesci BJ, DiStefano LJ, et al. Muscle activity and flexibility in individuals with medial knee displacement during the overhead squat. Athletic Training Sports Health Care. 2012;4:117–25.

Bellchamber TL, Van Den Bogert AJ. Contributions of proximal and distal moments to axial tibial rotation during walking and running. J Biomech. 2000;3:1397–403.

Bolgla LA, Malone TR. Plantar fasciitis and the windlass mechanism: a biomechanical link to clinical practice. J Athl Train. 2004;39:77–82.

Brown C, Ross S, Mynark R, et al. Assessing functional ankle instability with joint position sense, time to stabilization and electromyography. J Sport Rehab. 2004;13:122–34.

Brown C, Padua D, Marshall SW, et al. Individuals with mechanical ankle instability exhibit different motion patterns than those with functional ankle instability and ankle sprain copers. Clin Biomech. 2008;23:822–31.

Brown C, Bowser B, Simpson KJ. Movement variability during single-leg jump landings in individuals with and without chronic ankle instability. Clin Biomech. 2012;27:52–63.

Browne MG, Franz JR. The independent effects of speed and propulsive force on joint power generation in walking. J Biomech. 2017;55:48–55.

Cao W, Chen C, Hu H, et al. Effect of hip assistance modes on the metabolic cost of walking with a soft exoskeleton. IEEE Transactions Automation Sci Engineering. 2020;18:426–36.

Caulfield BM, Garrett M. Functional instability of the ankle: differences in patterns of ankle and knee movement prior to and post landing in a single leg jump. Int J Sports Med. 2002;23:64–8.

Chapman RF, Laymon AS, Wilhite DP, et al. Ground contact time as an indicator of metabolic cost in elite distance runners. Med Sci Sports Exerc. 2012;44:917–25.

Chmielewski TL, Myer GD, Kauffman D, et al. Plyometric exercise in the rehabilitation of athletes: physiological responses and clinical application. J Orthop Sports Phys Ther. 2006;36:308–19.

Davids K, Glazier P, Araujo D, et al. Movement systems as dynamic systems: the functional role of variability and its implications for sports medicine. Sports Med. 2003;33:245–60.

Dejong AF, Koldenhoven RM, Hertel J. Proximal adaptations in chronic ankle instability: Systematic review and meta-analysis. Med Sci Sports Exerc. 2020;52:1563–75.

De Ridder R, Witvrouw E, Dolphens M, et al. Hip strength as an intrinsic risk factor for lateral ankle sprains in youth soccer players: a 3 season prospective study. Am J Sports Med. 2017;45:410–16

Doherty C, Bleakley C, Hertel J, et al. Lower extremity function during gait in participants with first-time acute lateral ankle sprain compared to controls. J Electromyogr Kinesiol. 2015;25:182–92.

Doherty C, Bleakley C, Hertel J, et al. Gait biomechanics in participants, six months after first-time lateral ankle sprain. Int J Sports Med. 2016a;37:577–83.

Doherty C, Bleakley C, Hertel J, et al. Recovery from a first-time lateral ankle sprain and the predictors of chronic ankle instability: a prospective cohort analysis. Am J Sports Med. 2016b;44:995–1003.

Dorn TW, Schache AG, Pandy MG. Muscle strategy shift in human running: dependence of running speed on hip and ankle muscle performance. J Exp Biol. 2012;215:1944-56.

Dragert K, Zehr E. Bilateral neuromuscular plasticity from unilateral training of the ankle dorsiflexors. Exp Brain Res. 2011;208:217–27.

Dundas MA, Gutierrez GM, Pozzi F. Neuromuscular control during stepping down in continuous gait in individuals with and without ankle instability. J Sports Science. 2014;32:926-33.

Farris DJ, Kelly LA, Cresswell AG, et al. The functional importance of human foot muscles for bipedal locomotion. PNAS. 2019;116:1645-50.

Feger MA, Donovan L, Hart JM, et al. Lower extremity muscle activation during functional exercises in patients with and without chronic ankle instability. PMR. 2014;6:602–11.

Filipa A, Byrnes R, Paterno MV, et al. Neuromuscular training improves performance on the star excursion balance test in young female athletes. J Orthop Sports Phys Ther. 2010;40:551–8.

Fong CM, Blackburn JT, Norcross MF, et al. Ankle-dorsiflexion range of motion and landing biomechanics. J Athl Train. 2011;46:5–10.

Fourchet F, McKeon PO. Foot core strengthening: an update about the intrinsic foot muscles recruitment. Br J Sports Med. 2015;49:A6.

Fraser JJ, Hertel J. Effects of a 4-week intrinsic foot muscle exercise program on a motor function: a preliminary randomized control trial. J Sports Rehab. 2019;28:339–49.

Franz JR, Kram R. Advanced age and the mechanics of uphill walking: a joint level inversive dynamic analysis. Gait Posture. 2014;39:135–40.

Friel K, McLean N, Myers C, Caceres M. Ipsilateral hip abductor weakness after inversion ankle sprain. J Athl Train. 2006;41(1):74.

Garmin database. Available at: https://support. garmin.com/en-GB/faq

Goldmann JP, Sanno M, Willwacher S, et al. The potential of toe flexor muscles to enhance performance. J Sports Sci. 2013;31:424–33.

Goo YM, Kim TH, Lim JY. The effects of gluteus maximus and abductor hallucis strengthening exercises for four weeks on the navicular drop and lower extremity muscle activity during gait with flatfoot. J Phys Ther Sci. 2016;28:911–15.

Gribble PA, Hertel J, Plisky P. Using the Star Excursion Balance Test to assess dynamic postural-control deficits and outcomes in lower extremity injury: a literature and systematic review. J Athl Train. 2012;47:339–57.

Grimmer M. Elshamanhory AA, Beckerle P. Human lower limb joint biomechanics in daily life activities: a literature-based requirement analysis for anthropomorphic robot design. Frontiers Robotics AI. 2020;7:1–17.

Grimmer M, Seyfarth A. Mimicking human-like leg function in prosthetic limbs. In: Neuro-robotics: from brain machine interfaces to rehabilitation robotics. Spring; 2014:105–55.

Hashimoto T, Sakuraba K. Strength training for the intrinsic flexor muscles of the foot: effects on muscle strength, the foot arch and dynamic parameters before and after. J Phys Ther Sci. 2014;26:373–6.

Headlee DL, Leonard JL, Hart JM, et al. Fatigue of the plantar intrinsic foot muscles increases navicular drop. J Electromyogr Kinesiol. 2008;18:420–5.

Herb CC, Hertel J. Shank-rearfoot joint coupling in young adults with chronic ankle instability: across-correlation analysis. J Sports Med Phys Fitness. 2015;55:639–46.

Hicks H. The mechanics of the foot. II. The plantar aponeurosis and the arch. J Anatomy. 1954;88:25–30.

Hogan KK, Prince JA, Hoch MC. The evaluation of the foot core system in individuals with plantar heel pain. Phys Ther Sport. 2020;42:75-81.

Honert EC, Zelik KE. Foot and shoe are responsible for the majority of soft tissue work in the early stance of walking. Hum Mov Sci. 2019;64:191–202.

Huang PY, Chen WL, Lin CF, et al. Lower extremity biomechanics in athletes with ankle instability after a 6-week integrated training program. J Athl Train. 2014;49:163–72.

Hubbard TJ, Kramer LC, Deneger CR, et al. contributing factors to chronic ankle instability. Foot Ankle Int. 2007;28:343–54.

Kelly LA, Cresswell AG, Racinais S, et al. Intrinsic foot muscles have the capacity to control deformation of the longitudinal arch. J R Soc Interface. 2014;11:20131188.

Koldenhoven RM, Hart J, Saliba S, et al. Gait kinematics at three walking speeds in individuals with chronic ankle instability and ankle sprain copers. Gait Posture. 2019;74:169–75.

Koldenhoven RM, Jaffri AH, DeJong AF, et al. Gait biofeedback and impairment-based rehabilitation for chronic ankle instability. Scand J Med Sci Sport. 2021;31:193–204.

Konor MM, Morton S, Eckerson JM, et al. Reliability of three measures of ankle dorsiflexion range of motion. Int J Sports Phys Ther. 2012;7:279–87.

Kotsifaki A, Korakakis V, Graham-Smith P, et al. Vertical and horizontal hop performance: Contributions of the hip, knee, and ankle. Sports Health. 2021;13:128–35.

Kumagai K, Abe T, Brechue WF et al. Sprint performance is related to muscle fascicle length in male 100m sprinters. J Appl Physiol. 2000;88:811–16.

Kuo AD. Energetics of actively powered locomotion using the simplest walking model. J Biomech Engineering. 2002;124:113–20.

Kuo AD, Donelan JM, Ruina A. Energetic consequences of walking like an inverted pendulum: step to step transition. Exerc Sports Sci Rev. 2005;33:88–97.

Lee DR, Choi YE. Effects of a 6-week intrinsic foot muscle exercise program on the functions of intrinsic foot muscle and dynamic balance in patients with chronic ankle instability. J Exerc Rehab. 2019;15:709–14.

Leetun DT, Ireland ML, Wilson JD, et al. core stability measures as risk factors for lower extremity injury in athletes. Med Sci Sports Exerc. 2004;36:926–34.

Leetun DT, Ireland ML, Willson, D, et al. Core stability measures as risk factors for lower extremity injury in athletes. Med Sci Sports Exerc. 2015;36:926–34.

Lewis CL, Ferris DP. Walking with increased ankle pushoff decreases hip muscle moments. J Biomech. 2008;41(10):2082–9.

Lilley T, Herb CC, Hart, et al. Lower extremity joint coupling variability during gait in young adults with and without chronic ankle instability. Sports Biomech. 2018;17:261–72.

Mackinnon CD, Winter D. Control of whole-body balance in the frontal plane during human walking. J Biomech. 1993;26:633–44.

Malliaras P, Cook JL, Kent P. Reduced ankle dorsiflexion range may increase the risk of patellar tendon injury among volleyball players. J Sci Med Sport. 2006;9:304–9.

Mason-Mackay AR, Whatman C, Reid D. The effect of reduced ankle dorsiflexion on lower extremity mechanics during landing: A systematic review. J Sci Med Sport. 2017;20:451-8.

McCann RS, Crossett ID, Terada M, et al. Hip strength and star excursion balance test deficits of patients with chronic ankle instability. J Sci Med Sport. 2017;20:992–6.

McKeon PO, Fourchet F. Freeing the foot: integrating the foot core system into rehabilitation for lower extremity injuries. Clin Sports Med. 2015;34:347–61.

McKeon PO, Ingersoll CD, Kerrigan C et al. Balance training improves function and postural control in those with chronic ankle instability. Med Sci Sports Exerc. 2008;40:1810–19.

McKeon PO, Hertel J, Bramble D, et al. The foot core system: a new paradigm for understanding intrinsic foot muscle function. Br J Sports Med. 2015;49:290.

Miller RH, Chang R, Baird Je, et al. Variability in kinematic coupling assessed by vector coding and continuous relative phase. J Biomech. 2010;43:2554–60.

Minoonejad H, Ardakani MK, Rajabi R, et al. Hop Stabilization training improves neuromuscular control in college basketball players with chronic ankle instability: a randomized control trial. J Sports Rehab. 2019;28:576–83.

Monaghan K, Delahunt E, Caulfield B. Ankle function during gait in patients with chronic ankle instability compared to controls. Clin Biomech. 2006;21:168–74.

Mooses M, Haile DW, Ojiambo R, et al. Shorter ground contact time and better running economy: evidence from female Kenyan runners. J Strength Condition Res. 2021;35:481–6.

Mulligan EP, Cook PG. Effect of plantar intrinsic muscle training on medial longitudinal arch morphology and dynamic function. Man Ther. 2013;18:425–30.

Murphy D, Connolly D, Beynnon B. Risk factors for lower extremity injury: a review of the literature. Br J Sports Med. 2003;37:13–29.

Neptune RR, McGowan CP. Muscle contributions to frontal plane angular momentum during walking. J Biomech. 2016;49:2975–81.

Ness BM, Taylor AL, Haberl MD, et al. Clinical observation and analysis of movement quality during performance on the Star Excursion Balance Test. Int J Sports Phys Ther. 2015;10:168-77.

Neumann DA. Kinesiology of the hip: a focus on muscular actions. J Orthop Sports Phys Ther. 2010;40:82–94.

Özdemir H, Söyüncü Y, Özgörgen M, et al. Effects of changes in heel fat pad thickness and elasticity on heel pain. J Am Podiatr Med Assoc. 2004;94(1):47–52.

Park H. Gait optimization with a real-time closed-loop artificial sensory feedback. Dissertation submitted – Georgia Institute of Technology, August 2017.

Peter A, Hegyi A, Finni T, et al. In vivo fascicle behavior of the flexor hallucis longus muscle at different walking speeds. Scand J Med Sci Sport. 2017;27:1716–23.

Plisky PJ, Rauh MJ, Kaminski TW, Underwood FB. Star Excursion Balance Test as a predictor of lower extremity injury in high school basketball players. J Orthop Sports Phys Ther. 2006;36:911-9.

Rabin A, Kozol Z. Measures of range of motion and strength among healthy women with differing quality of lower extremity movement during the lateral step-down test. J Orthop Sports Phys Ther. 2010;40:792–800.

Santana da Silva L, Fukuchi KR, Duarte M, et al. Effects of age and speed on the ankle-foot system's power during walking. Scientific Reports. 2020;10:14903.

Son SJ, Kim H, Seeley MK, et al. Movement strategies among groups of chronic ankle instability, coper and control. Med Sci Sports Exerc. 2017;49:1649–61.

Son SJ, Kim H, Seeley MK, et al. altered walking neurodynamics in patients with chronic ankle instability. J Athl Train. 2019;56:684–97.

Steinberg N, Dar G, Dunlop M et al. The relationship of hip muscle performance to leg, ankle, and foot injuries: a systematic review. Phys Sports Med. 2017;45:49–63.

Tang A, Bordoni B. Anatomy, bony pelvis and lower limb foot nerves. Treasure Island, FL: StatPearls Publishing; 2021.

Tudor-Locke CE, Myers AM. Methodological considerations for research and practitioners using pedometers to measure physical (ambulatory) activity. Res Q Exer Sport. 2001;72:1–12.

Tweed JL, Campbell JA, Avil SJ. Biomechanical risk factors in the development of medial tibial stress syndrome in distance runners. J Am Podiatr Med Assoc. 2008;98:436–44.

Venturini C, Ituassú NT, Teixeira LM, Deus CVO. Intra- and inter-examiner reliability of two methods of measuring active range of ankle dorsiflexion in healthy individuals. Braz J Phys Ther. 2006;10:407–11.

Verrelst R, Willems TM, De Clercq D, et al. The role of hip abductor and external rotator muscle strength in the development of exertional medial tibial pain: a prospective study. Br J Sports Med. 2014;48:1564–69.

Wahlstedt C, Rasmussen-Barr E. Anterior cruciate ligament injury and ankle dorsiflexion. Knee Surg Sports Traumatol Arthrosc. 2015;23:3202–7.

Wikstrom EA, Fournier KA, McKeon PO. Postural control differs between those with and without chronic ankle instability. Gait Posture. 2010;32:82–6.

Yamauchi J, Koyama K. Importance of toe flexor strength in vertical jump performance. J Biomech. 2020;104:109719.

Multidisciplinary management of hip and knee pain disorders

3

Effectiveness of manual therapy approaches for hip and knee pain disorders: an evidence-based approach

15

Nils Runge, Josiah Sault, Alexandra Anderson, Thomas Mitchell

Mechanisms of Manual Therapy

The adoption of manual therapy in physical therapy is well recorded through the work of esteemed innovators, including from the Mennells, who pioneered the use of pain-free therapeutic passive movements, Cyriax, Maitland and Kaltenborn, who described passive joint mobilizations and thrust manipulations, to New Zealand clinicians McKenzie and Mulligan, who combined passive and active interventions and promoted self-treatment (Pettman, 2007; MacDonald et al., 2019). For generations the concept of repositioning joints into a biomechanically "correct" position has been thought to be crucial in the easing of pain and disability in musculoskeletal conditions (Pettman, 2007; Vicenzino et al., 2007). Whilst manual therapy's roots in a purely biomechanical model have been discarded (Gyer et al., 2019; Lascurain-Aguirrebena et al., 2016), it remains a widely used treatment, with a plethora of proposed mechanisms of action. The IFO-MPT defines manual therapy as "skilled hand movements intended to produce any or all of the following effects: improve tissue extensibility; increase range of motion of the joint complex; mobilize or manipulate soft tissues and joints; induce relaxation; change muscle function; modulate pain and reduce soft tissue swelling, inflammation or movement restriction" (IFOMPT, 2016). What brings about the effect from point A (application of force) to point B (patient response) is the subject of, at times, contentious debate (Mintken et al., 2018; Kolb et al., 2020; Rabey et al., 2017). Despite this, it remains a firm fixture in conservative management of a variety of conditions (MacDonald et al., 2006; Sault et al., 2020). Inclusion of manual therapy in a patient's plan of care may produce improvements in:

- Range of motion (Weerasekara et al., 2018; Stathopoulos et al., 2019)

- Pain and function (Coulter et al., 2018; Jayaseelan et al., 2018; Xu et al., 2017; Mischke et al., 2017; Steuri et al., 2017; Hidalgo et al., 2017; Paige et al., 2017; Armijo-Olivio et al., 2016, Eckenrode et al., 2018; Sampath et al., 2016)

- Motor control and strength (Courtney et al., 2010; Haavik & Murphy, 2012; Pfluegler et al., 2020)

- Sensory detection and pain thresholds (Fernández-de-las-Peñas et al., 2017; Courtney et al., 2016; Sterling et al., 2010; Paungmali et al., 2003; Vicenzino et al., 2001)

- Psychological variables such as mood and general confidence (Walker et al., 2017; Maratos et al., 2017)

It is suggested that these improvements are related to a complex interaction of the type and dosage of mechanosensory input, local and systemic histochemical changes, peripheral, central and autonomic nervous system responses. Patient beliefs and their disposition, the clinician's preference, and the interpersonal interaction and therapeutic relationship may also be primary drivers or inhibitors of the treatment response (Bialosky et al., 2009a; Testa & Rossettini, 2016).

Local and Systematic Histochemical Mechanisms

The body's natural response to injury is to produce an inflammatory cascade promoting the healing process. When this occurs, inflammatory mediators act on peripheral nociceptors, which in turn influence pain processing (Latramoliere & Woolf, 2009). There have been several studies demonstrating that manual therapy can affect inflammation via different mechanisms, including the reduction of blood and serum level cytokines, changes in endogenous cannabinoids, altered serotonin, N-palmitoylethanolamine, anandamide, β-endorphin levels, increased blood level endogenous opiates and neuropeptides (Bialosky et al., 2009a; Plaza-Manzano et al., 2014). More recent evidence supports that spinal manipulative therapy is also able to modulate substance-P, neurotensin, oxytocin or interleukin levels and may influence cortisol levels post-intervention (Sampath et al., 2017b).

The repetitive nature of joint mobilizations may specifically influence the change in the local cellular environment (Sambajon et al., 2003), e.g., concentrations of prostaglandin PGE2 (an inflammatory mediator linked to hyperalgesia in arthritic conditions) have been altered following this form of manual therapy.

For soft tissue biased manual therapy, Crane et al. (2012) demonstrated an increased expression of genes relevant for tissue repair as well as a decreased inflammatory gene expression. Acute inflammatory responses following exercise are influenced by soft tissue mobilization (Smith et al., 1994), and in those with fibromyalgia, substance P levels have also been altered (Field et al., 2002).

Further peripheral mechanisms have been described in relation to the application of force, such as those applied during a thrust manipulation. The mechanical force can act on both nociceptive and non-nociceptive afferents (Gyer et al., 2019; Potter et al., 2005). Since afferent fibers project information to the central nervous system, dysfunction in this process can lead to chronic pain conditions. Regardless of acute or chronic pain, peripheral action on these afferent fibers can alter nociceptive signaling. Studying the response from specific receptor types to biomechanical characteristics of thrust manipulative therapy (i.e., force and displacement) have advanced our understanding of mechanisms. The mechanical force of a thrust mobilization could either stimulate or inhibit mechanosensitive and nociceptive afferent fibers in somatic tissues local to the spine (Gyer et al., 2019). Pickar and Bolton (2012) explain that during the thrust phase, muscle spindles increase their firing rate and following manipulation, some of these afferents go through a silent period, while others increase their firing interval. The short- and high-frequency barrage of action potentials can modulate the central nervous system by acting on second order neurons (Pickar & Bolton, 2012). Additionally, non-nociceptive A-β fibers from muscle spindles and facet joint mechanoreceptors may inhibit nociceptive A-δ and C fibers, a theory proposed by Melzack and Wall in the 1960s, known as *gate control* theory (Potter et al., 2005). The stimulation of paraspinal sensory afferents could be, hence, responsible for the change in peripheral and central nervous system interaction (Gyer et al., 2019). This has been suggested from observing attenuation of the stretch reflex in paraspinals during thrust manipulations, as well as reduced corticospinal and spinal reflex excitability, made possible with mitigation of spinal and corticospinal excitability (Gyer et al., 2019). Additionally, it has been suggested that manipulation reduces pro-inflammatory mediators, which relieves pain by altering peripheral inflammation and sensitization of nociceptors (Gevers-Montoro et al., 2021), which would in turn reduce sensitization of second order neurons.

Central Mechanisms

Central mechanisms are typically described by the level at which they occur; being spinal or supraspinal. The supraspinal regions of the brain involved in somatosensory-discriminative, affective, and cognitive processing of pain include the primary and secondary somatosensory cortex, anterior and posterior cingulate, insula, prefrontal cortices, and the thalamus (Kregel et al., 2015). The amygdala also plays an important role in pain processing as it forms negative emotions and painful memories, communicating with the anterior cingulate cortex and hippocampus (Thompson & Neugebauer, 2017). This typically relates to fear surrounding movements and/or patterns that may pose a threat to injury. Other important areas to note include the rostral ventromedial medulla, the periaqueductal gray and the subnucleus reticularis dorsalis, which are involved in conditioned pain modulation or pain inhibition from inducing a painful stimulus (Courtney et al., 2016).

There are different approaches to assess centrally mediated mechanisms. For obvious reasons, in humans, the effects are observed secondarily via clinical testing with quantitative sensory testing (Rolke et al., 2006) or in research settings, e.g., H-reflex testing, transcranial magnetic stimulation, conditioned pain modulation (Fryer & Pearce, 2012; Courtney et al., 2016). Animal studies provide an opportunity for direct observation of spinal and supraspinal activity in response to manual therapy. However, the transferability of their outcomes to human physiology has been questioned as they do not consistently predict the human response (Greek & Kramer, 2019). Despite this, they may provide a pre-clinical understanding of the mechanisms underlying the human response to manual therapy (Espejo et al., 2018).

Spinal Mechanisms

In studies utilizing male Sprague-Dawley rats, it was found that knee mobilization of nine minutes following capsaicin-induced ankle hyperalgesia increased the stimulus force required to elicit a flexor withdrawal response back to pre-hyperalgesia levels, which is hypothesized to be associated with spinal and supraspinal mechanisms (Sluka & Wright, 2001; Skyba et al., 2003). These effects were at least partially associated with serotonergic responses in the spinal cord (Skyba et al., 2003). Utilizing male Wistar rats, Martins et al. (2011) found that ankle mobilization following sciatic nerve crush injuries not only reduced pain behavior and increased motor recovery but suppressed glial cell activity in the dorsal horn of the spinal cord, which has been linked to long-lasting neuropathic pain.

In human studies, nociceptive flexor withdrawal reflexes were reduced following knee complex mobilizations in subjects with knee osteoarthritis, which may be associated with segmental spinal modulation and/or increased descending inhibition from the brainstem (Courtney et al., 2010). Thoracic spinal manipulation can reduce temporal summation of pain, which is a clinical correlate to wind-up at the dorsal horn of the spinal cord, whereby repeated stimulus becomes more painful over time (Randoll et al., 2017). George et al. (2006) showed a change in temporal summation following lumbar thrust manipulation compared to stationary bicycling or lumbar extension. Interestingly, while the cavitation heard during manipulation has been suggested to be unnecessary to patient clinical response (Cleland et al., 2007), the audible cavitation has been seen to correlate with a reduction in the spinal muscle stretch reflex response, which may break a hypothesized pain–spasm–pain cycle (Clark et al., 2011).

Supraspinal Mechanisms

When looking at the supraspinal effects of manual therapy, in humans, nine minutes of joint oscillatory mobilization at the knee significantly improved pressure pain thresholds at both the knee and the foot in patients with knee osteoarthritis, which is hypothesized to be related to supraspinal mechanisms (Moss et al., 2007). Additionally, changes in pressure pain thresholds at local and distal pain-free sites that have been seen following joint mobilizations likely indicate symptom mediation via the central nervous system (Lascurain-Aguirrebena et al., 2016). These changes following manual therapy may be associated with activation of the periaqueductal gray substance promoting descending noradrenergic inhibition of nociceptive transmission via sympatho-excitation (Savva et al., 2014).

Non-opioid descending pain modulation circuits utilize serotonin and noradrenaline pathways from the periaqueductal gray and rostral ventromedial medulla in the brain (Pickar, 2002). This hypoalgesic system is thought to be affected by spinal manipulation, which is supported by findings in both animal and human studies (Skyba et al., 2003;

Reed et al., 2014). Mobilization, or non-thrust techniques, produces hypoalgesia through the same mechanism and has been studied in peripheral joints as well (Courtney et al., 2016; Savva et al., 2014).

An additional supraspinal response to manual therapy occurs via alterations in neuromotor control. Researchers have noted improved reaction times in motor tasks and neural plastic changes in the cerebellum, basal ganglia, prefrontal cortex, and primary motor cortex following cervical manipulation in subjects with a history of neck pain (Daligadu et al., 2013; Haavik et al., 2010; Lelic et al., 2016). The central mechanisms cannot be fully separated; however, as studies have shown, both spinal and supraspinal effects happen in tandem. Functional magnetic resonance imaging studies in rats have shown reduced activation in the areas of the brain associated with pain processing (bilateral anterior cingulate and frontal cortex) in response to capsaicin injections following ankle joint mobilizations and at the spinal cord in response to capsaicin injections in the hind paw following knee joint mobilizations (Malisza et al., 2003). In a study of healthy human volunteers, lumbar manipulation significantly reduced central motor and alpha-motor neuron excitability via H-reflex testing compared to controls, further indicating neuromotor modulation at both the spinal cord and cortical levels (Fryer & Pearce, 2012).

Autonomic Nervous System Mechanisms

The autonomic nervous system (ANS) unconsciously regulates heart rate, respiratory rate, blood pressure, and more, whilst also innervating organs with smooth muscle. It is controlled by the hypothalamus, influences our fight-or-flight (adrenal) response, and interacts with nociceptive processing at several levels (Gyer et al., 2019). Spinal manipulation in the thoracic spine and its relation to the autonomic nervous system has been widely studied. It is believed to influence opioid independent analgesia through interactions with the ANS, including the sympathetic and parasympathetic nervous systems (Gyer et al., 2019; Sampath et al., 2015). ANS communication extending to the CNS, immune, and neuroendocrine systems strengthen the case for various mechanisms occurring simultaneously at multiple systems.

Manipulation appears to modulate hypothalamic–pituitary–adrenal (HPA) axis activity, changing salivary cortisol levels and testosterone–cortisol ratio, and has been suggested to immediately reduce oxygenated haemoglobin levels (Sampath et al., 2017a). The implications of these findings are unclear and deserve further investigation, as it may be important for the regulation of blood flow to skeletal muscle and tissue repair processing, which is a complex process, influenced by many systems (Sampath et al., 2017a).

Heart rate variability can be used to assess autonomic function by measuring low- and high-frequency bands, which are ultimately an efferent action of the parasympathetic nervous system (PNS) or both sympathetic nervous system (SNS) and PNS activity. Results of spinal manipulation on heart rate variability are not conclusive (Sampath et al., 2017a; Budgell & Polus, 2006; Ward et al., 2013), and the accuracy is questionable. However, Sampath et al. (2017a) suggested that thoracic spinal manipulation could be used to improve physiological processing in acute stages of injury (regardless of location) due to the quick response of the SNS and the longer-lasting slow response from the neuroendocrine system. The effects on blood pressure, skin blood flow and pupillary reflex has also been studied as a measure of ANS activity. Although further investigation is needed to determine the exact effects of these influences, it is suggested that manipulation might lead to opioid independent analgesia, altering reflex neural outputs through the influence of the hypothalamus and periaqueductal gray (Sampath et al., 2015; Gyer et al., 2019). Areas of the brain responsible for autonomic function, such as insular cortex, cerebellar vermis, middle temporal gyrus, visual association cortex, inferior prefrontal cortex, and anterior cingulate cortex, also appear to be affected by manipulation (Ogura et al., 2011; Sparks et al., 2013; Kenney & Ganta, 2014).

Massage therapy has also been shown to influence ANS activity with an increased response from the parasympathetic nervous system, leading to vasodilation. Implications include alterations in blood flow and disbursement of inflammatory mediators, such as prostaglandins, that may act on peripheral nociceptors leading to a more sensitized state (Holey et al., 2011). This area of research deserves further attention as there may be therapeutic benefits from spinal manipulation offered to those in chronic pain, accompanied by dysregulation of the ANS and HPA axis.

Psychological Mechanisms

Placebo effects are a collection of psycho-neurobiological responses within a patient that can be activated through the expectation of nearly any person involved in the intervention (Colloca, 2019). Similarly, a nocebo effect would be related to any negative perceived placebo response, e.g., increased pain (Barsky et al., 2002). Each of these has neurobiological effects which should not be dismissed as unimportant or invalid to an individual patient's response to intervention (Bialosky et al., 2017). Testa and Rossettini (2016) lay out the effects through changes in chemicals, areas of the brain that are activated/deactivated (associated with pain), changes in neural activity, corticospinal system excitability, reduced fatigue, and contextual factors such as therapist and patient alliance, treatment characteristics and healthcare setting. This may also extend to the physiotherapist's appearance, qualifications, and reputation, along with their personality and communication methods.

The means by which clinicians interact and communicate with their patients around and about the selection of manual therapy can contribute to the placebo or nocebo effects of therapy. One challenge in the study of manual therapy is a lack of clinician equipoise noted in many trials. Equipoise is simply the clinician in the interaction giving no indication, positive or negative, of their expectation of the effects of an intervention. This concept puts the clinician in the interaction as a neutral party. While this may be important to clinical studies, face-to-face provider interactions in a clinic are never a neutral interaction. The extent to which a clinician believes or does not believe the intervention they are providing will work may affect their patient's outcome (Cook & Sheets, 2011).

It may be that the mechanisms of, and/or responses to, manual therapy are enhanced through a lack of equipoise on the clinician's part. This may come across in the way the clinician educates their patient about the intervention, the explanation of its anticipated effects, and even their non-verbal demeanour (Bialosky et al., 2017).

On the other side of the interaction, a patient's own expectation may affect treatment outcome. Patients receiving cervical manipulation when they expect it to provide relief are more likely to experience that relief than those who do not (Bishop et al., 2013). In a study on subjects with experimentally induced low back pain, subject expectation, provider preference or equipoise, and the type of manual intervention were all found to affect the subjects' outcomes (Bishop et al., 2017). This does not relate only to manual therapy interventions but to other treatments as well. To outline this aspect further, in the clinical maze that encompasses the entirety of a patient's experience in therapy, a patient's expectation that they will improve with therapy has been shown to more strongly predict their outcome than many physical findings on examination in subjects with shoulder pain (Chester et al., 2018).

Effects of Dosage

Manual therapy techniques are wide-ranging and may be intended to focus on a specific tissue such as joint, muscle, nerve, skin, etc. Regardless of the application type, they all involve physical contact with the patient at a determined intensity for a period of time. The intensity and duration combined are considered in the dosage of manual therapy. Considerations of desired mechanism of action, patient and provider preference, and the patient's baseline level of sensitization all inform decisions made regarding dosage.

With oscillatory joint mobilizations, the frequency of oscillations may contribute to the effect of the mobilization. Piekarz and Perry (2016) examined skin conductivity, a measure of sympatho-excitation and ANS response, following three bouts of lumbar spinal mobilization of 1 minute at 3 Hz, 2 Hz, placebo, and control conditions. They found a statistically significant increase in sympatho-excitation in the 3 Hz group compared to placebo and control conditions (Piekarz & Perry, 2016). Likewise, Jowsey and Perry (2010) demonstrated that mobilizations at 0.5 Hz could also result in statistically significant sympatho-excitation compared to placebo. Interestingly, a systematic review concluded that high-velocity, low-amplitude manipulation of the spine may have no effect on autonomic function (Picchiottino et al., 2019) which may indicate that a longer duration than a single thrust is needed for ANS response with manual therapy. Indeed, the oscillatory nature of mobilization appears to be an essential component to affect a variety of outcomes. Moss et al. (2007) found that oscillatory mobilization resulted in a statistically significant improvement in both distal pressure pain thresholds and improved timed up-and-go test in subjects with knee pain compared to either manual contact or no-contact.

Conversely, different velocities of manual therapy appear to similarly attenuate temporal summation of heat pain (Penza et al., 2017). When measuring the attenuation of temporal summation of heat pain at the foot, there were no differences found with 3 bouts of lumbar non-thrust mobilizations performed at 1 Hz for 1-minute intervals and 4 lumbar thrust mobilizations in a 5-minute period. Penza et al. (2017) also measured temporal summation of heat pain at the hand, finding no changes. This suggests a localized modulatory effect at the spinal cord. The attenuation of temporal summation has also been observed following neurodynamic techniques of the upper extremity (Beneciuk et al., 2009; Bialosky et al., 2009b). These findings differ, however, from a meta-analysis by Arribas-Romano et al. (2020). Here, changes were identified in mechanical temporal summation following spinal manipulation and neural mobilizations but not found with a combination of education and low-velocity mobilizations. Although both methods of measuring temporal summation are aimed at evaluating the sensitivity of neurons at the dorsal horn of the spinal cord, it should be considered that sensitivity to thermal versus mechanical stimuli varies mechanistically, due to the receptors involved. It is probable that manual therapy has a greater effect on mechanical sensitivity rather than on thermal sensitivity.

The effects of massage and light touch also appear dependent on dosage. For example, Rapaport et al. (2012) measured cytokines, lymphocytes, and endocrine measures to better understand the effects on neuroendocrine and immune systems. They found unique responses from both touch and massage that were enhanced with repeated treatments, and also a contradistinction when increasing dosage to twice weekly. One massage per week affected circulating lymphocyte markers and cytokine expression and when repeated over 5 weeks, potentiated immune changes but had no effect on neuroendocrine function. Although single session and repeated weekly massages increased lymphocyte subsets, this decreased for touch. Neuroendocrine function was progressively enhanced when increasing massage dosage to twice weekly, with increases in cytokines and decreases in many phenotypic lymphocyte markers. Twice weekly massage also differed with increases found in pre-treatment levels of CD56+ and, in contrast to touch, increases in oxytocin, arginine–vasopressin, adrenal corticotropin hormone, and cortisol (Rapaport et al., 2012).

Depth, that is the intensity of the manual therapy intervention, should also be considered, as Testa and Rossettini (2016) describe moderate pressure massage can increase vagal activity, modify heart rate, decrease cortisol levels, improve serotonin and dopamine levels, alter cortical and spinal excitability, and inhibit nociception at subcortical and cortical levels (Field et al., 2005; Field, 2014; Sefton et al., 2011; Mancini et al., 2015).

All this to say, the dosage of intervention has unique biologic effects, therefore outcomes of massage and touch will likely vary depending on intervention technique, frequency, and length of application. Ultimately, the decision on how deeply or intensely we apply manual therapy and for how long should be guided by clinical reasoning considering the patient's condition, their baseline pain sensitization, and their preferences to achieve the greatest response. The proposed mechanisms, application and dosage of manual therapy is a developing field, and this is not unique in physical therapy given that the debates around the mechanism of effect, application and dosage of core treatments such as exercise also remain elusive. Accepting this, we shall now consider the evidence which investigates the use of manual therapy specifically with regard to hip and knee conditions.

Effectiveness of Manual Therapy for Hip Pain

Hip Osteoarthritis

Beumer et al. (2016) investigated the effectiveness of manual therapy on pain. The manual therapy techniques in the primary studies mainly included joint manipulations and/or mobilization as well as passive stretching. These authors did not find statistically significant differences between the combination of manual therapy and exercise versus minimal care at short- (3 studies) and mid- (2 studies) terms. No studies were identified for long-term follow-up in the context of this comparison. Likewise, they did not find significant differences between the combination of exercise and manual therapy versus exercise alone at the short-term (2 studies). No studies investigated mid-term or long-term follow-ups. Interestingly, they also reported no statistically significant difference between exercise alone and manual therapy alone (2 studies). The authors described that considerable heterogeneity (e.g., control interventions) decreased their confidence in the results. Consequently, they argue that it would be necessary to conduct further high-quality studies to gain greater confidence in their findings.

Sampath et al. (2016) investigated pain and function in their review. Joint manipulations and mobilizations were the main manual therapy techniques used in the primary studies, while one study also added soft tissue techniques. The authors reported low quality of evidence for a statistically significant superiority of manual therapy over "control" for pain and function post-treatment (2 studies), with medium effect sizes (Cohen, 1988). They further found low-quality evidence for a statistically significant benefit of manual therapy over control (2 studies). The effect sizes were less pronounced compared to post-treatment and were considered small. Furthermore, the authors pooled two studies for combined exercise and manual therapy versus control. They found low-quality evidence for a statistically significant benefit for pain and function post-treatment with small effect sizes. However, just one study reported on follow-up and did not find a statistically significant difference for pain and function. This was graded as low-quality evidence. The findings of this review must be considered in the context of different aspects. First, the authors combined studies with different control interventions, including exercises and minimal care, and compared those to manual therapy. Second, they evaluated only response directly after the intervention period and combined all later follow-up durations. Finally, the reported confidence intervals (CIs) for all outcomes were wide including trivial to large effect sizes.

Wang et al. (2016) focused on the effect of manual therapy versus control, reporting on pain and function as outcomes. The included studies used a variety of manual therapy techniques including manipulation, mobilization, massage, manual stretching, and traction. The authors found no statistically significant differences between manual therapy and control for pain in the immediate (6 studies), short-term (2 studies), mid-term (1 study) and long-term follow-up periods (3 studies). The quality of evidence was low to moderate. For physical function, the results were similar reporting moderate quality evidence for no significant differences between manual therapy and control at any follow-up. However, in the intermediate follow-up (1 study), significant differences were found but the clinical relevance of these effects was questionable, and CIs were wide. In contextualizing the outcomes of this review, one should note that authors combined various control interventions, including detuned ultrasound, exercise, other manual therapy, and education. Furthermore, they included studies that had a number of co-interventions in the experimental group such as education and additional exercises, making it hard to make a judgment about specific manual therapy effects.

Ceballos-Laita et al. (2019) concluded that there is high-quality evidence for manual therapy for the outcomes of pain and function. In the primary studies, mainly joint mobilizations and manipulations, as well as soft tissue techniques, were used. Caution should be applied with interpreting those results as the overall number of included studies was very low, and the authors seemed to judge the quality of evidence by using the Oxford Centre of Evidence-Based Medicine scale in an unusual fashion. It remains unclear how authors synthesized the studies, and they did not comment on effect sizes or clinical relevance of their findings. Additionally, the authors did not distinguish between follow-up durations, control interventions, and adjunct interventions in the experimental groups.

Finally, Westad et al. (2019) investigated the effects of mobilization with movement (MWM) on peripheral joint conditions. The authors found two studies investigating hip OA, which both used placebo or sham as a control intervention. Both studies showed statistically significant differences in the immediate follow-up compared to control

for pain and functional outcomes. Only one of the studies also investigated the difference at 3 months follow-up and found that there was a statistically significant difference in favoring of MWMs for pain and function. The authors concluded that there is moderate-quality evidence for an effect of MWMs in hip OA. Notably, the authors did not comment on the effect sizes and clinical relevance of their findings. Furthermore, as just one study investigated medium-term outcomes, the quality of evidence for this follow-up duration is most likely to be low to very low.

Analyzing the available research, it becomes clear that there is conflicting evidence for the benefits of manual therapy in the management of symptomatic hip OA (Table 15.1). In fact, heterogeneity between inclusion and exclusion criteria and clinical aspects of primary studies could explain the differences in results. The latter relates to the variable combinations of control interventions and the amorphous nature of manual therapy interventions (including which techniques are appropriate, how it was used and the levels of dosage or intensity). It can be concluded that the existing evidence is mostly of low to moderate quality and more high-quality studies are needed to make clear

TABLE 15.1 Results of Systematic Reviews on Manual Therapy for Hip Osteoarthritis

Study	MT combinations	Comparison	Outcome	Post-treatment	Short-term	Medium-term	Long-term
Beumer et al. (2016)	MT + EX	Minimal care	Pain	X	NS	NS	X
		EX alone	Pain	X	NS	X	X
	MT	EX	Pain	X	NS	X	X
Sampath et al. (2016)	MT	Mixed control	Pain	SE (M)	SE(S)		
			Function	SE (M)	SE(S)		
	MT+ EX	Mixed control	Pain	SE (S)	NS		
			Function	SE (S)	NS		

(Continued)

TABLE 15.1 *(Continued)*

Study	MT combinations	Comparison	Outcome	Post-treatment	Short-term	Medium-term	Long-term
Wang et al. (2016)	MT	Mixed control	Pain	NS	NS	NS	NS
			Function	NS	NS	SE (S)	NS
Ceballos-Laita et al. (2019)	MT	Mixed control	Pain	No MA – concluded MT is beneficial			
			Function	No MA – concluded MT is beneficial			
Westad et al. (2019)	MWMs	Sham	Pain	SE (?)	X	SE (?)	X
			Function	SE (?)	X	SE (?)	X

EX, exercise; M, medium effect size; MA, meta-analysis; MT, manual therapy; MWM, mobilization with movement; NS, not statistically significant; S, small effect size; SE, statistically significant effect; X, no results provided.

recommendations. It remains unclear if manual therapy in combination with exercises is more effective than exercise alone, an aspect that would be highly relevant to determine.

Femoroacetabular Impingement

To our knowledge, there are no studies that specifically focused on determining the efficacy of manual therapy for the treatment of femoroacetabular impingement (FAI). However, a meta-analysis of conservative interventions for FAI found four articles assessing short-term effects of physical therapy for FAI, of which three featured manual therapy (Mallets et al., 2019). In the primary studies, manual therapy techniques included joint and soft tissue-based mobilization and manipulation, as well as manual stretching. In this meta-analysis, physical therapy interventions as a whole had a statistically significant effect on pain and function with large effect sizes. Since manual therapy was just part of the interventional packages, the authors were unable to draw conclusions about its specific effectiveness. Additionally, the large effect sizes must be viewed in light of the wide CIs ranging from negligible to large.

Two RCTs have examined joint-based manual therapy in conjunction with other interventions for FAI. Wright et al. (2016), in a randomized controlled pilot study, found that advice and exercise with or without specific physical therapy intervention, including joint-based manual therapy and exercise, improved both pain and function in patients with FAI. Notably, the addition of physical therapy intervention did not significantly alter outcomes; however, the small number of participants and resulting wide confidence intervals in this study limit concluding the superiority of either approach. In a more recent randomized controlled clinical trial, Mansell et al. (2018) compared surgical intervention to physical therapy including joint-based manual therapy and exercise, finding no statistical difference in results on pain or function between groups at 2-year follow-up. There are several weaknesses of this study. A large proportion of individuals in the conservative care group crossed over to surgical intervention leaving the conservative arm underpowered. Additionally, wide confidence intervals indicate the results are far from definitive and should be interpreted with caution. In both the above studies, manual therapy was not a specific independent variable, rather it was included in a package of care being compared to a different approach. The majority of subjects in both of these studies reported low mean satisfaction and/or perceived improvement in their final state regardless of group allocation indicating that further research is needed to improve outcomes for patients with FAI. Based on the available evidence, no conclusions can be made for or against the use of manual therapy for FAI.

Iliotibial Band Syndrome

No systematic review exists that looked specifically at manual therapy iliotibial band syndrome (ITBS). Weckström and Söderström (2016) examined three sessions of manual therapy including soft tissue mobilization, deep friction massage, and trigger point manual therapy along the lateral thigh versus extracorporeal shock-wave therapy for pain associated with running in 24 subjects with ITBS. Both groups also performed a standard exercise program. The authors found no between-groups differences at any follow-up point for pain while treadmill running. Considering the lack of research and the design of the one existing study, no conclusion can be made regarding the benefit of manual therapy in patients with ITBS.

Greater Trochanteric Pain Syndrome

Evidence for the effectiveness of manual therapy for greater trochanteric pain syndrome (GTPS) is limited to case reports and expert opinions. This is based on the conclusion of a systematic review which identified no randomized clinical trials or cohort studies relating to manual therapy interventions (Reid, 2016). The same was found in a more recent critical review (Torres et al., 2018). Therefore, no conclusion about the benefits of manual therapy in GTPS can be made at this stage.

Effectiveness of Manual Therapy for Knee Pain

Knee Osteoarthritis

Knee OA as the most common knee complaint is also the most researched condition in this chapter. Jansen et al. (2011) investigated the effectiveness of manual therapy as an adjunct to mixed exercise therapy or strength training for knee OA. These authors did not find studies that directly compared those interventions but conducted a meta-regression of two studies to identify and assimilate the given data. They found a statistically significant benefit of mixed exercise therapy with additional manual therapy versus mixed exercise alone for pain but not for function (no effect sizes given). They further evaluated the benefit of adding manual therapy to strength training versus strength training alone but did not find a statistically significant difference. Compared to control, mixed exercise and manual therapy showed statistically significant benefits with moderate (pain) and small (physical function) effect sizes. The results should be considered in the context of what authors described as very poor quality of evidence with high risk of bias in the primary studies. They further described heterogeneity between the studies and mentioned the obvious problem that no study directly compared the different interventions.

Salamh et al. (2017) undertook a meta-analysis with sub-grouping of studies in the context of their intervention combinations and comparators. The included studies used a number of different manual therapy techniques but including mainly joint and soft tissue mobilizations. They identified just two studies investigating pain outcomes. Manual therapy alone was not better than the control group, but the combination of manual therapy with another intervention was superior to the control intervention alone with moderate effect sizes. For self-reported function, the authors included three studies comparing manual therapy plus other treatment versus other treatment alone. The pooled results showed medium to large effect sizes (Cohen, 1988) in favor of manual therapy which were statistically significant. Two studies looking at manual therapy versus other treatments for function were pooled and found small to medium effect sizes favoring manual therapy. These results should be considered in light of the lack of subgrouping around follow-up durations. Furthermore, it should be mentioned that due to lack of ethical approval and concerns around the validity of their results, the authors of this review excluded five primary studies from the meta-analysis. Finally, the reported CIs of the meta-analyses were wide. This imprecision is most likely related to the small number of participants within each meta-analysis but certainly decreases confidence in the estimate of the average effect (Higgins et al., 2021).

Xu et al. (2017) compared the effects of manual therapy with or without adjunct versus a combination of different control interventions. The main manual therapy techniques used in the included studies were Maitland joint mobilization, massage techniques, manipulations, and manual stretching. For pain (11 studies) and function (11 studies) outcomes, the authors found small to medium effect sizes in favor of manual therapy, which were statistically significant. Those findings should be considered in light of a lack of subgrouping around control treatments which included acupuncture, medication, TENS, standard care alone and exercise. The number of adjunct interventions used in control and intervention groups made it difficult to isolate the effects of manual therapy. Furthermore, they did not differentiate between follow-up durations. Even though the number of cases in the meta-analyses was larger compared to Salamh et al. (2017), the found CIs were wide and included small and large effect sizes. This imprecision decreases confidence in their estimates of the average effects (Higgins et al., 2021). Finally, the authors described that the quality of primary studies was generally poor, but they did not comment on the overall quality of evidence for each outcome.

Newberry et al. (2017) conducted a review as part of a review update on the treatment of knee OA for the US Agency for Healthcare Research and Quality. This was the only systematic review for knee OA that considered different follow-up durations and conducted meta-analyses in this context. The primary studies included in this review used mainly passive joint mobilization, self-manual therapy and acupressure. The authors reported that the quality of evidence was low for all follow-up durations and outcomes. They pooled three studies for short-term follow-up on the outcome of pain and found that there was no statistically significant effect of manual therapy over other treatments. For short- and mid-term follow-up periods on function, the authors could not pool both sets of four identified studies but concluded from their qualitative synthesis that there is potentially no effect of manual therapy over the control groups. Conversely, for long-term pain, they found two studies which they synthesized qualitatively, finding statistically significant benefits of manual therapy over control. The effect sizes were small in one study but potentially clinically relevant in the other. There were no studies that investigated function at the long-term. The included studies used a number of adjunct interventions additional to manual therapy, and it is unclear how they impacted on the found effects. General heterogeneity of primary studies and other biases of study design did not allow the conduction of a meta-analysis for many outcomes and follow-up durations. This makes it more difficult to judge the potential effect sizes. Additionally, in relation to the meta-analysis for short-term pain, significant imprecision in found CI (included even large effect sizes) makes it difficult to judge the found non-significant result (Higgins et al., 2021).

Anwer et al. (2018) investigated the effects of manual therapy compared with exercise versus other controls. In the primary studies, Maitland joint mobilization, massage and MWMs were used as manual therapy techniques. They found low-quality evidence from two studies with no significant differences between manual therapy and control for pain. However, using the same outcome measure, they pooled 5 studies and found a statistically significant benefit of manual therapy as an add-on to exercise over exercise therapy alone. The effect sizes could be considered medium to large, but the quality of evidence was low. They also found moderate quality evidence for large, statistically significant effects of exercise and manual therapy versus exercise alone on the WOMAC pain and functional subscales. High-quality evidence showed no significant differences between manual therapy and exercise on the global WOMAC scale. They found only three studies with long-term follow-up and were therefore only able to draw conclusions at short-term. Importantly, they did not separate follow-up durations, which causes difficulty for clinical interpretation. All found CIs were wide and included a range of different effect sizes from small to large.

In conclusion, there are a number of systematic reviews available examining manual therapy for knee OA but their results vary considerably (Table 15.2). All identified reviews described a high risk of bias in primary studies, as well as significant heterogeneity between them in regard to the manual therapy techniques used, intensity, frequency, combination with other treatments and controls, which reduces confidence in the found results. The imprecision in the CIs of most meta-analyses indicates that the found effect sizes should be considered with caution. The factors described above make it difficult to come up with clear conclusions about the effectiveness of manual therapy for knee OA.

Meniscal Injuries

Minimal evidence is available to support manual therapy interventions in patients with meniscal tears/injuries, with

TABLE 15.2 Results of Systematic Reviews on Manual Therapy for Knee Osteoarthritis

Study	MT combinations	Control	Outcome	Post-treatment	Short-term	Medium	Long-term
Jansen et al. (2011)	MT + EX	EX alone	Pain	SE (?)			
			Function	NS			
Salamh et al. (2017)	MT	Mixed control	Pain		NS		
			Function		SE (S -M)		
	MT + other	Other alone	Pain		SE (M)		
			Function		SE (M-L)		
Xu et al. (2017)	MT	Mixed control	Pain		SE (M)		
			Function		SE (S-M)		
Newberry et al. (2017)	MT	Mixed control	Pain	X	NS	X	SE (S)
			Function	X	NS	NS	X
Anwer et al. (2018)	MT	Mixed control	Pain		NS	X	X
	MT+ EX	EX alone	Pain		SE (L)	X	X

EX, exercise; L, large effect size; M, medium effect size; MA, meta-analysis; MT, manual therapy; NS, not statistically significant; S, small effect size; SE, statistically significant effect; X, no results provided.

no systematic reviews identified and just one relevant clinical trial. Other evidence available is limited to case series and case reports. The Mulligan "squeeze" technique for the treatment of meniscal tears has been investigated in a case series and a small RCT (Hudson et al., 2018, 2016). This sham-controlled trial included both physically active and sedentary participants who were randomized into a "squeeze" technique or manual therapy sham group (Hudson et al., 2018). Significant between-groups differences were found post-treatment favouring the "squeeze" technique in the patient-specific functional scale (large effect size). However, this was not the case in the numeric pain rating scale and knee injury and OA outcome score. As this was only one small study and no long-term outcomes were assessed, evidence for manual therapy in individuals with meniscal pathology remains scarce.

Patellar Tendinopathy

Manual therapy for patellar tendinopathy is sparsely studied. No systematic reviews were found to assess the effects of manual therapy on outcomes for patients with this condition. One review on deep friction massage for tendinopathies in different body areas did not identify any study that looked specifically at knee or hip conditions (Joseph et al., 2012). More recently, in a small (n = 10) randomized, controlled, cross-over trial in athletes with patellar tendinopathy, deep friction massage to the patellar tendon was found to immediately reduce pain on palpation utilizing a pressure sensor but did not improve range of motion or quadriceps strength (Chaves et al., 2020). All subjects acted as control subjects in the first treatment session. This consisted of a rest period acting as the control condition with pre- and post-testing. The following three sessions included 10 minutes of deep friction massage at predetermined intensities with pre- and post-testing each session. Subjects all experienced statistically significant reductions in pain with palpation compared to the control session following deep friction massage regardless of intensity. As this was a small clinical trial it is difficult to generalize the results. Additionally, subjects demonstrated similar pre-intervention pain levels with palpation before each session, which may preliminarily indicate limited carryover of the effects of deep friction massage in isolation in patellar tendinopathy. The remaining evidence on manual therapy for individuals with patellar tendinopathy is limited to uncontrolled pilot studies and case series/studies.

Patellofemoral Pain

Three different systematic reviews and meta-analyses have been published in recent years analyzing outcomes of manual therapy use in patients with patellofemoral pain (PFP). Espí-López et al. (2017) included five clinical trials which assessed variable control or placebo groups as well as intervention groups. Follow-up was between immediate and four months. No meta-analysis was conducted, and the studies were individually described. The authors suggested that there is some indication of a combined effect of manual therapy and other physical therapy interventions, but they were not able to provide strong recommendations. The lack of a clear synthesis of results as well as the number and variety of co-interventions and control in the primary studies makes it impossible to reach any conclusions from this review.

Eckenrode et al. (2018) conducted a meta-analysis in which they included nine studies featuring manual therapy. The manual therapy interventions used included joint manipulations, mobilizations, deep friction transverse massage, trigger point technique and manual stretching. The authors found three studies investigating the effectiveness of manual therapy for patients with PFP versus control at short-term on self-reported function. Statistically significant benefits for manual therapy over control with medium effect sizes were found. One study investigated long-term follow-up and did not show statistically significant between-groups differences. For pain, medium effect sizes in favor of manual therapy compared to control were found at short-term (5 studies). Combinations of manual therapy and exercise versus other treatments were investigated in two studies looking at pain outcomes. No statistical difference was found between these groups. Finally, lumbopelvic manipulation was found to be used in three studies looking at PFP, but inconsistencies in study design prohibited meta-analysis, and no clear benefits were found due to mixed results. The authors classed five out of nine studies as low risk of bias; however, they did not comment on the overall quality of evidence.

Jayaseelan et al. (2018) performed a systematic review specifically looking at joint mobilization effects in people with PFP. A meta-analysis of 12 studies could not be performed due to the variability in the type of manual therapy techniques used (lumbopelvic manipulations, MWMs local to the knee and patellofemoral mobilizations) and control interventions. The authors found that only four out of ten studies reported statistically significant advantages of manual therapy over control for function. For pain, 6 out of 9 studies showed statistically significant benefits of manual therapy compared with control. No comments were made on the overall effect sizes and no overall conclusion on the quality of the evidence was described. The authors concluded that there is conflicting evidence as to whether manual therapy adds benefit for pain and functional outcomes in patients with PFP.

Willy et al. (2019) presented a clinical practice guideline based on current evidence and expert opinion.

TABLE 15.3 Results of Systematic Reviews on Manual Therapy for Patellofemoral Pain

Study	MT combinations	Control	Outcome	Immediate	Short-term	Medium	Long-term
Espi-Lopez et al. (2017)	MT+ PT	Mixed control	Pain	No MA – concluded MT is beneficial			
			Function	No MA – concluded MT is beneficial			
Eckenrode et al. (2018)	MT	Mixed control	Pain	X	SE(M)	X	X
			Function	X	SE(M)	X	NS
	MT+ EX	Mixed control	Pain	X	NS	X	X
Jayaseelan et al. (2018)	MT	Mixed control	Pain	No MA – concluded MT is beneficial			
			Function	No MA – concluded MT is beneficial (conflicting)			

EX, exercise; M, medium effect size; MA, meta-analysis; MT, manual therapy; PT, physical therapy; NS, not statistically significant; SE, statistically significant effect; X, no results provided.

They concluded that previous reviews were of poor quality and that manual therapy as an alone intervention may not improve outcomes in patients with PFP. As a result, they recommended not using manual therapy if this detracted from the time given to exercise prescription in clinical sessions. This is in line with a recent network meta-analysis that found that adding mobilization or taping to exercises and education can potentially add some benefit, but quality of evidence was low and effects were not consistently present for all outcomes and follow-ups (Winters et al., 2021). Overall, manual therapy may be beneficial for individuals with PFP, though we can conclude it should not be used as a stand-alone treatment, but either complementary to exercise and educational interventions. Table 15.3 provides an overview of the results of the systematic reviews on PFP.

Conclusion

While evidence for the mechanisms of manual therapy is diverse, emerging, and suggests a wide array of potential mechanisms, evidence surrounding manual therapy for specific hip and knee conditions can, at best, be summarized as weak. Unfortunately, just three conditions (PFP, knee OA, hip OA) exhibit a number of systematic reviews and meta-analyses while for other conditions, research is mostly lacking. Even in these conditions, the evidence is mostly classed as low quality and the results are far from consistent, making it impossible to make strong recommendations for the use of manual therapy in any specific hip or knee condition.

Reaching a conclusion on the effectiveness of manual therapy in specific conditions of the hip and knee is difficult based on the current literature. Some individual studies show effectiveness; however, when the literature is synthesized the overall effect becomes negligible. There are several reasons for this to be the case. The type, dosage, duration and application of manual therapy in the management of hip and knee conditions is ambiguous. Current reviews did not (and potentially could not) account in their synthesis for differences regarding those parameters within the primary studies. This could have led to potential effects being masked due to the inclusion of underpowered studies, or studies with insufficient manual therapy dosage, intensity or techniques. The latter is highly relevant as many primary studies used standardized manual therapy programs that did not allow adjustments of treatment based on the individual patients. Additionally, current systematic reviews did not (and possibly could not) account for the complexity of the therapeutic interaction which includes factors like therapeutic alliance and patients' expectations, which have been shown to be relevant on clinical outcomes in musculoskeletal care (Cormier et al., 2016; Kinney et al., 2020; Parsons et al., 2007). This is especially significant as many primary studies used manual therapy as an additional adjunct (A + B versus A alone design) and did not use attention-control measures like sham interventions to account for those aspects.

Based on this, we appreciate that for clinicians, the appropriate choice and application of manual therapy techniques can be difficult. Considering the limits of the outlined evidence, there does not appear to exist a clear superiority of one type of manual therapy and the optimal dosage is also unknown. The current knowledge around the underlying mechanisms of manual therapy, as outlined earlier in this chapter, could offer an explanation for why this could be the case. One could argue that this provides greater freedom for the practitioner to individualize the treatment to a patient in front of them considering neurophysiological mechanisms of action of manual therapy, dominant pain mechanisms and treatment aims, but also allow recognition of the clinician's and patient's expectations as well as their preferences. What this means is that not only the choice of manual therapy technique but also the decision to use manual therapy overall must be based within a bio-psychosocial framework. For this, it appears invaluable for clinicians to have a good knowledge of pain mechanisms and the mechanisms of action of manual therapy. However, one could argue that it is even more important to have very good understanding of the patient in front of them including their beliefs, values, and expectations.

References

Anwer S, Alghadir A, Zafar H, Brismée J-M. Effects of orthopaedic manual therapy in knee osteoarthritis: a systematic review and meta-analysis. Physiother. 2018;104:264–76.

Armijo-Olivo S, Pitance L, Singh V, et al. Effectiveness of manual therapy and therapeutic exercise for temporomandibular disorders: Systematic review and meta-analysis. Phys Ther. 2016;96:9–25.

Arribas-Romano A, Fernández-Carnero J, Molina-Rueda F, et al. Efficacy of physical therapy on nociceptive pain processing alterations in patients with chronic musculoskeletal pain: A systematic review and meta-analysis. Pain Med. 2020;21:2502–17.

Barsky AJ, Saintfort R, Rogers MP, Borus JF. Nonspecific medication side effects and the nocebo phenomenon. JAMA. 2002;287:6227.

Beneciuk JM, Bishop MD, George SZ. Effects of upper extremity neural mobilization on thermal pain sensitivity: a sham-controlled study in asymptomatic participants. J Orthop Sports Phys Ther. 2009;39:428–38.

Beumer L, Wong J, Warden SJ, et al. Effects of exercise and manual therapy on pain associated with hip osteoarthritis: a systematic review and meta-analysis. Br J Sports Med. 2016;50:458–63.

Bialosky JE, Bishop MD, Price DD, et al. The mechanisms of manual therapy in the treatment of musculoskeletal pain: a comprehensive model. Man Ther. 2009a;14:531–8.

Bialosky JE, Bishop MD, Price DD, et al. A randomized sham-controlled trial of a neurodynamic technique in the treatment of carpal tunnel syndrome. J Orthop Sports Phys Ther. 2009b;39:709–23.

Bialosky JE, Bishop MD, Penza CW. Placebo mechanisms of manual therapy: A Sheep in Wolf's Clothing? J Orthop Sports Phys Ther. 2017;47:301–4.

Bishop MD, Mintken PE, Bialosky JE, Cleland JA. Patient expectations of benefit from interventions for neck pain and resulting influence on outcomes. J Orthop Sports Phys Ther. 2013;43:457–65.

Bishop MD, Bialosky JE, Penza CW, et al. The influence of clinical equipoise and patient preferences on outcomes of conservative manual interventions for spinal pain: an experimental study. J Pain Res. 2017;10:965–72.

Budgell B, Polus B. The effects of thoracic manipulation on heart rate variability: a controlled crossover trial. J Manipulative Physiol Ther. 2006;29:603–10.

Ceballos-Laita L, Estébanez-de-Miguel E, Martín-Nieto G, et al. Effects of non-pharmacological conservative treatment on pain, range of motion and physical function in patients with mild to moderate hip osteoarthritis. A systematic review. Complement Ther Med. 2019;42:214–22.

Chaves P, Simões D, Paço M, et al. Deep friction massage in the management of patellar tendinopathy in athletes: Short-term clinical outcomes. J. Sport Rehabil. 2020;29:860–5.

Chester R, Jerosch-Herold C, Lewis J, Shepstone L. Psychological factors are associated with the outcome of physiotherapy for people with shoulder pain: a multicentre longitudinal cohort study. Br J Sports Med. 2018;52:269–75.

Clark BC, Goss DA Jr, Walkowski S, et al. Neurophysiologic effects of spinal manipulation in patients with chronic low back pain. BMC Musculoskelet Disord. 2011;12:170.

Cleland JA, Flynn TW, Childs JD, Eberhart S. The audible pop from thoracic spine thrust manipulation and its relation to short-term outcomes in patients with neck pain. J Man Manip Ther. 2007;15:143–54.

Cohen J. Statistical power analysis for the behavioral sciences. 2nd ed. Hillsdale, NJ: L. Erlbaum Associates; 1988.

Colloca L. The placebo effect in pain therapies. Annu Rev Pharmacol Toxicol. 2019; 59:191–211.

Cook C, Sheets C. Clinical equipoise and personal equipoise: two necessary ingredients for reducing bias in manual therapy trials. J Man Manip Ther. 2011;19:55–7.

Cormier S, Lavigne GL, Choinière M, Rainville P. Expectations predict chronic pain treatment outcomes. Pain. 2016;157:329–38.

Coulter ID, Crawford C, Hurwitz EL et al. Manipulation and mobilization for treating chronic low back pain: a systematic review and meta-analysis. Spine J. 2018;18:866–79.

Courtney CA, Lewek MD, Witte PO, et al. Heightened flexor withdrawal responses in subjects with knee osteoarthritis. J Pain. 2009;10:1242–9.

Courtney CA, Witte PO, Chmell SJ, Hornby TG. Heightened flexor withdrawal response in individuals with knee osteoarthritis is modulated by joint compression and joint mobilization. J Pain. 2010;11:179–85.

Courtney CA, Steffen AD, Fernández-de-las-Peñas C, et al. Joint mobilization enhances mechanisms of conditioned pain modulation in individuals with osteoarthritis of the knee. J Orthop Sports Phys Ther. 2016;46:168–76.

Crane JD, Ogborn DI, Cupido C, et al. Massage therapy attenuates inflammatory signaling after exercise-induced muscle damage. Sci Transl Med. 2012;4:119ra13.

Daligadu J, Haavik H, Yielder PC, et al. Alterations in cortical and cerebellar motor processing in subclinical neck pain patients following spinal manipulation. J Manipulative Physiol Ther. 2013;36:527–37.

Eckenrode BJ, Kietrys DM, Parrott JS. Effectiveness of manual therapy for pain and self-reported function in individuals with patellofemoral pain: Systematic review and meta-analysis. J Orthop Sports Phys Ther. 2018;48:358–71.

Espejo JA, García-Escudero M, Oltra E. Unraveling the molecular determinants of manual therapy: an approach to integrative therapeutics for the treatment of fibromyalgia and chronic fatigue syndrome/myalgic encephalomyelitis. Int J Mol Sci. 2018;19:2673.

Espí-López GV, Arnal-Gómez A, Balasch-Bernat M, Inglés M. Effectiveness of manual therapy combined with physical therapy in treatment of patellofemoral pain syndrome: Systematic review. J Chiropr Med. 2017;16:139–46.

Fernández-de-las-Peñas C, Cleland J, Palacios-Ceña M, et al. Effectiveness of manual therapy versus surgery in pain processing due to carpal tunnel syndrome: A randomized clinical trial. Eur J Pain. 2017;21:1266–76.

Field T. Massage therapy research review. Complement Ther Clin Pract. 2014;20:224–9.

Field T, Diego M, Cullen C, et al. Fibromyalgia pain and substance P decrease and sleep improves after massage therapy. J Clin Rheumatol. 2002;8:72–6.

Field T, Hernandez-Reif M, Diego M, et al. Cortisol decreases and serotonin and dopamine increase following massage therapy. Int J Neurosci. 2005;115:1397–413.

Fryer G, Pearce AJ. The effect of lumbosacral manipulation on corticospinal and spinal reflex excitability on asymptomatic participants. J Manipulative Physiol Ther. 2012;35:86–93.

George SZ, Bishop MD, Bialosky JE, et al. Immediate effects of spinal manipulation on thermal pain sensitivity: an experimental study. BMC Musculoskelet Disord. 2006;7:68.

Gevers-Montoro C, Provencher B, Descarreaux M, et al. Neurophysiological mechanisms of chiropractic spinal manipulation for spine pain. Eur J Pain. 2021;25(7):1429–48.

Greek R, Kramer LA. How to evaluate the science of non-human animal use in biomedical research and testing: a proposed format for debate. In: Herrmann K & Jayne K (eds). Animal experimentation: working towards a paradigm change. Leiden, The Netherlands: Brill; 2019:65–87.

Gyer G, Michael J, Inklebarger J, Tedla JS. Spinal manipulation therapy: Is it all about the brain? A current review of the neurophysiological effects of manipulation. J Integr Med. 2019;17:328–37.

Haavik H, Murphy B. The role of spinal manipulation in addressing disordered sensorimotor integration and altered motor control. J Electromyogr Kinesiol. 2012;22:768–76.

Haavik Taylor H, Murphy B. The effects of spinal manipulation on central integration of dual somatosensory input observed after motor training: a crossover study. J Manipulative Physiol Ther. 2010;33:261–72.

Hidalgo B, Hall T, Bossert J, et al. The efficacy of manual therapy and exercise for treating non-specific neck pain: A systematic review. J Back Musculoskelet Rehabil. 2017;30:1149–69.

Higgins JPT, Thomas J, Chandler J, et al (eds). Cochrane Handbook for Systematic Reviews of Interventions, 6th ed. Cochrane; 2021. Available from www.training.cochrane.org/handbook

Hoeksma HL, Dekker J, Ronday HK, et al. Comparison of manual therapy and exercise therapy in osteoarthritis of the hip: A randomized clinical trial. Arthritis Rheum. 2004;51:722–9.

Holey LA, Dixon J, Selfe J. An exploratory thermographic investigation of the effects of connective tissue massage on autonomic function. J Manipulative Physiol Ther. 2011;34:457–62.

Hudson R, Richmond A, Sanchez B, et al. An alternative approach to the treatment of meniscal pathologies: A case series analysis of the Mulligan concept "squeeze" technique. Int J Sports Phys Ther. 2016;11:11.

Hudson R, Richmond A, Sanchez B, et al. Innovative treatment of clinically diagnosed meniscal tears: a randomized sham-controlled trial of the Mulligan concept 'squeeze' technique. J Man Manip Ther. 2018;26:254–63.

International Federation of Orthopaedic Manipulative Physical Therapists (IFOMPT). Educational Standards in Orthopaedic Manipulative Therapy [Internet]. Auckland: IFOMPT; 2016. Available from: https://www.ifompt.org/site/ifompt/IFOMPT%20Standards%20Document%20definitive%202016.pdf

Jansen MJ, Viechtbauer W, Lenssen AF, et al. Strength training alone, exercise therapy alone, and exercise therapy with passive manual mobilisation each reduce pain and disability in people with knee osteoarthritis: a systematic review. J Physiother. 2011;57:11–20.

Jayaseelan DJ, Scalzitti DA, Palmer G, et al. The effects of joint mobilization on individuals with patellofemoral pain: a systematic review. Clin Rehabil. 2018;32:722–33.

Joseph MF, Taft K, Moskwa M, Denegar CR. Deep friction massage to treat tendinopathy: a systematic review of a classic treatment in the face of a new paradigm of understanding. J Sport Rehabil. 2012;21:343–53.

Jowsey P, Perry J. Sympathetic nervous system effects in the hands following a grade III postero-anterior rotatory mobilisation technique applied to T4: a randomised, placebo-controlled trial. Man Ther. 2010;15:248–53.

Kenney M, Ganta C. Autonomic nervous system and immune system interactions. Compr Physiol. 2014;4:1177–200.

Kinney M, Seider J, Beaty AF, et al. The impact of therapeutic alliance in physical therapy for chronic musculoskeletal pain: A systematic review of the literature. Physiother Theory Pract. 2020;36:886–98.

Kolb WH, McDevitt AW, Young J, Shamus E. The evolution of manual therapy education: what are we waiting for? J Man Manip Ther. 2020;28:1–3.

Kregel J, Meeus M, Malfliet A et al. Structural and functional brain abnormalities in chronic low back pain: A systematic review. Semin Arthritis Rheum. 2015;45:229–37.

Lascurain-Aguirrebeña I, Newham D, Critchley DJ. Mechanism of action of spinal mobilizations: A systematic review. Spine. 2016;41:159–72.

Latremoliere A, Woolf CJ. Central sensitization: a generator of pain hypersensitivity by central neural plasticity. J Pain. 2009;10:895–926.

Lelic D, Niazi IK, Holt K et al. Manipulation of dysfunctional spinal joints affects sensorimotor integration in the prefrontal cortex: A brain source localization study. Neural Plast. 2016;2016:3704964.

MacDonald CW, Whitman JM, Cleland JA, et al. Clinical outcomes following manual physical therapy and exercise for hip osteoarthritis: A case series. J Orthop Sports Phys Ther. 2006;36:588–99.

MacDonald CW, Osmotherly PG, Parkes R, Rivett DA. The current manipulation debate: historical context to address a broken narrative. J Man Manip Ther. 2019;2:1–4.

Malisza KL, Gregorash L, Turner A, et al. Functional MRI involving painful stimulation of the ankle and the effect of physiotherapy joint mobilization. MRI. 2003;21:489–96.

Mallets E, Turner A, Durbin J, et al. Short-term outcomes of conservative treatment for femoroacetabular impingement: A systematic review and meta-analysis. Int J Sports Phys Ther. 2019;14:514–24.

Mancini F, Beaumont A-L, Hu L, et al. Touch inhibits subcortical and cortical nociceptive responses. Pain. 2015;156:1936–44.

Mansell NS, Rhon DI, Meyer J, et al. Arthroscopic surgery or physical therapy for patients with femoroacetabular impingement syndrome: A Randomized Controlled Trial with 2-year follow-up. Am J Sports Med. 2018;46:1306–14.

Maratos FA, Duarte J, Barnes C, et al. The physiological and emotional effects of touch: Assessing a hand-massage intervention with high self-critics. Psychiatry Res. 2017;250:221–7.

Martins DF, Mazzardo-Martins L, Gadotti VM, et al. Ankle joint mobilization reduces axonotmesis-induced neuropathic pain and glial activation in the spinal cord and enhances nerve regeneration in rats. Pain. 2011;152:2653–61.

Mintken PE, Rodeghero J, Cleland JA. Manual therapists - Have you lost that loving feeling?!. J Man Manip Ther. 2018;26:53–4.

Mischke JJ, Jayaseelan DJ, Sault JD, Emerson Kavchak AJ. The symptomatic and functional effects of manual physical therapy on plantar heel pain: a systematic review. J Man Manip Ther. 2017;25:3–10.

Moss P, Sluka K, Wright A. The initial effects of knee joint mobilization on osteoarthritic hyperalgesia. Man Ther. 2007;12:109–18.

Newberry SJ, FitzGerald J, SooHoo NF, et al. Treatment of Osteoarthritis of the Knee: An Update Review [Internet]. Rockville: US Agency for Healthcare Research and Quality; 2017. Report No.: 190. Available from: http://www.effectivehealthcare.ahrq.gov/index.cfm/search-for-guides-reviews-and-reports/?pageaction=displayproduct&productid=2441

Ogura T, Tashiro M, Masud M, et al. Cerebral metabolic changes in men after chiropractic spinal manipulation for neck pain. Altern Ther Health Med. 2011;17:12–7.

Paige NM, Miake-Lye IM, Booth MS P, et al. Association of spinal manipulative therapy with clinical benefit and harm for acute low back pain: Systematic review and meta-analysis. JAMA. 2017;317:1451–60.

Parsons S, Harding G, Breen A S, et al. The influence of patients' and primary care practitioners' beliefs and expectations about chronic musculoskeletal pain on the process of care: a systematic review of qualitative studies. Clin J Pain. 2007;23:91–8.

Paungmali A, O'Leary S, Souvlis T, Vicenzino B. Hypoalgesic and sympathoexcitatory effects of mobilization with movement for lateral epicondylalgia. Phys Ther. 2003;83:374–83.

Penza CW, Horn ME, George SZ, Bishop MD. Comparison of two lumbar manual therapies on temporal summation of pain in healthy volunteers. J Pain. 2017;18:1397–408.

Pettman E. A history of manipulative therapy. J Man Manip Ther. 2007;15:165–74.

Pfluegler G, Kasper J, Luedtke K. The immediate effects of passive joint mobilisation on local muscle function. A systematic review of the literature. Musculoskelet Sci Pract. 2020;45:102106.

Picchiottino M, Leboeuf-Yde C, Gagey O, Hallman DM. The acute effects of joint manipulative techniques on markers of autonomic nervous system activity: a systematic review and meta-analysis of randomized sham-controlled trials. Chiropr Man Therap. 2019;27:17.

Pickar JG. Neurophysiological effects of spinal manipulation. Spine J. 2002;2:357–71.

Pickar JG, Bolton PS. Spinal manipulative therapy and somatosensory activation. J Electromyogr Kinesiol. 2012;22:785–94.

Piekarz V, Perry J. An investigation into the effects of applying a lumbar Maitland mobilisation at different frequencies on sympathetic nervous system activity levels in the lower limb. Man Ther. 2016;23:83–9.

Plaza-Manzano G, Molina-Ortega F, Lomas-Vega R, et al. Changes in biochemical markers of pain perception and stress response after spinal manipulation. J Orthop Sports Phys Ther. 2014;44:231–9.

Potter L, McCarthy C, Oldham J. Physiological effects of spinal manipulation: a review of proposed theories. Phys Ther Rev. 2005;10:163-70.

Rabey M, Hall T, Hebron C, et al. Reconceptualising manual therapy skills in contemporary practice. Musculoskelet Sci Pract. 2017;29:28–32.

Randoll C, Gagnon-Normandin V, Tessier J, et al. The mechanism of back pain relief by spinal manipulation relies on decreased temporal summation of pain. Neuroscience. 2017;349:220–8.

Rapaport MH, Schettler P, Bresee C. A preliminary study of the effects of repeated massage on hypothalamic-pituitary-adrenal and immune function in healthy individuals: a study of mechanisms of action and dosage. J Altern Complement Med. 2012;18:789–97.

Reed WR, Sozio R, Pickar JG, Onifer SM. Effect of spinal manipulation thrust duration on trunk mechanical activation thresholds of nociceptive-specific lateral thalamic neurons. J Manipulative Physiol Ther. 2014;37:552–60.

Reid D. The management of greater trochanteric pain syndrome: A systematic literature review. J Orthop. 2016;13:15–28.

Rolke R, Baron R, Maier C, et al. Quantitative sensory testing in the German Research Network on Neuropathic Pain (DFNS): standardized protocol and reference values. Pain. 2006;123:231–43.

Salamh P, Cook C, Reiman MP, Sheets C. Treatment effectiveness and fidelity of manual therapy to the knee: A systematic review and meta-analysis. Musculoskeletal Care. 2017;15:238–48.

Sambajon VV, Cillo JE, Gassner RJ, Buckley MJ. The effects of mechanical strain on synovial fibroblasts. J Oral Maxillofac Surg. 2003;61:707-12.

Sampath KK, Mani R, Cotter JD, Tumilty S. Measureable changes in the neuro-endocrinal mechanism following spinal manipulation. Med Hypoth. 2015;85:819–24.

Sampath KK, Mani R, Miyamori T, Tumilty S. The effects of manual therapy or exercise therapy or both in people with hip osteoarthritis: a systematic review and meta-analysis. Clin Rehabil. 2016;30:1141–55.

Sampath KK, Botnmark E, Mani R, et al. Neuroendocrine response following a thoracic spinal manipulation in healthy men. J Orthop Sports Phys Ther. 2017a;47:617–27.

Sampath KK, Mani R, Cotter J, Gisselman AS, Tumilty S. Changes in biochemical markers following spinal manipulation-a systematic review and meta-analysis. Musculosk Sci Pract. 2017b;29:120–31.

Sault JD, Jayaseelan DJ, Mischke JJ, Post AA. The utilization of joint mobilization as part of a comprehensive program to manage carpal tunnel syndrome: A Systematic Review. J Manipulative Physiol Ther. 2020;43:356–70.

Savva C, Giakas G, Efstathiou M. The role of the descending inhibitory pain mechanism in musculoskeletal pain following high-velocity, low amplitude thrust manipulation: a review of the literature. J Back Musculoskelet Rehabil. 2014;27:377–82.

Schiotz EH, Cyriax JH. Manipulation: Past and Present. London: Heinemann Educational Books; 1975.

Sefton JM, Yarar C, Carpenter DM, Berry JW. Physiological and clinical changes after therapeutic massage of the neck and shoulders. Man Ther. 2011;16:487–94.

Skyba DA, Radhakrishnan R, Rohlwing JJ, et al. Joint manipulation reduces hyperalgesia by activation of monoamine receptors but not opioid or GABA receptors in the spinal cord. Pain. 2003;106:159–68.

Sluka KA, Wright A. Knee joint mobilization reduces secondary mechanical hyperalgesia induced by capsaicin injection into the ankle joint. Eur J Pain. 2001;5:81–7.

Smith LL, Keating MN, Holbert D, et al. The effects of athletic massage on delayed onset muscle soreness, creatine kinase, and neutrophil count: a preliminary report. J Orthop Sports Phys Ther. 1994;19:93–9.

Sparks C, Cleland JA, Elliott JM, et al. Using functional magnetic resonance imaging to determine if cerebral hemodynamic responses to pain change following thoracic spine thrust manipulation in healthy individuals. J Orthop Sports Phys Ther. 2013;43:340–8.

Stathopoulos N, Dimitriadis Z, Koumantakis GA. Effectiveness of Mulligan's mobilization with movement techniques on range of motion in peripheral joint pathologies: A systematic review with meta-analysis between 2008 and 2018. J Manipulative Physiol Ther. 2019;42:439–49.

Sterling M, Pedler A, Chan C, et al. Cervical lateral glide increases nociceptive flexion reflex threshold but not pressure or thermal pain thresholds in chronic whiplash associated disorders: A pilot randomised controlled trial. Man Ther. 2010;15:149–53.

Steuri R, Sattelmayer M, Elsig S, et al. Effectiveness of conservative interventions including exercise, manual therapy and medical management in adults with shoulder impingement: a systematic review and meta-analysis of RCTs. Br J Sports Med. 2017;51:1340-7.

Testa M, Rossettini G. Enhance placebo, avoid nocebo: How contextual factors affect physiotherapy outcomes. Man Ther. 2016;24:65-74.

Thompson JM, Neugebauer V. Amygdala plasticity and pain. Pain Res Manag. 2017;2017:8296501

Torres A, Fernández-Fairen M, Sueiro-Fernández J. Greater trochanteric pain syndrome and gluteus medius and minimus tendinosis: nonsurgical treatment. Pain Manag. 2018;8:45-55.

Vicenzino B, Paungmali A, Buratowski S, Wright A. Specific manipulative therapy treatment for chronic lateral epicondylalgia produces uniquely characteristic hypoalgesia. Man Ther. 2001;6:205–12.

Vicenzino B, Paungmali A, Teys P. Mulligan's mobilization-with-movement, positional faults and pain relief: current concepts from a critical review of literature. Man Ther. 2007;12:98–108.

Walker SC, Trotter PD, Swaney WT, et al. C-tactile afferents: Cutaneous mediators of oxytocin release during affiliative tactile interactions? Neuropeptides. 2017;64:27–38.

Wang Q, Wang T, Qi X, et al. Manual therapy for hip osteoarthritis: A systematic review and meta-analysis. Pain Physician. 2016;18:E1005–20.

Ward J, Coats J, Tyer K, et al. Immediate effects of anterior upper thoracic spine manipulation on cardiovascular response. J Manipulative Physiol Ther. 2013;36:101–10.

Weckström K, Söderström J. Radial extracorporeal shockwave therapy compared with manual therapy in runners with iliotibial band syndrome. J Back Musculoskelet Rehabil. 2016;29:161–70.

Weerasekara I, Osmotherly P, Snodgrass S, et al. Clinical benefits of joint mobilization on ankle sprains: A systematic review and meta-analysis. arch Phys Med Rehabil. 2018;99:1395–412.

Westad K, Tjoestolvsen F, Hebron C. The effectiveness of Mulligan's mobilisation with movement (MWM) on peripheral joints in musculoskeletal (MSK) conditions: A systematic review. Musculoskelet Sci Pract. 2019;39:157–63.

Willy RW, Hoglund LT, Barton CJ, et al. Patellofemoral pain. J Orthop Sports Phys Ther. 2019;49:CPG1–95.

Winters M, Holden S, Lura CB, et al. Comparative effectiveness of treatments for patellofemoral pain: a living systematic review with network meta-analysis. Br J Sports Med. 2021;55:369–77.

Wright AA, Hegedus EJ, Taylor JB, et al. Non-operative management of femoroacetabular impingement: A prospective, randomized controlled clinical trial pilot study. J Sci Med Sport. 2016;19:716–21.

Xu Q, Pang J, Zheng Y, et al. The effectiveness of manual therapy for relieving pain, stiffness and dysfunction in knee osteoarthritis: A systematic review and meta-analysis. Pain Physician. 2017;23:A387.

Joint-biased interventions for hip and knee pain disorders

Thomas Mitchell, Alexandra Anderson, Josiah Sault, Paul Glynn

Joint-biased Techniques in Patient-centered Care

Some practitioners debate whether manual therapy should remain a cornerstone of current musculoskeletal (MSK) practice, particularly through social media and blogs (Meakins, 2017), albeit a substantial base of research supports its positive effects on nociceptive mechanisms.

Others argue that modernization in its rationale for usage is needed and that manual therapy should be applied equilibrated with other interventions targeting the central nervous system (Mintken et al., 2018; Lluch Girbés et al., 2015). The argument against the use of manual therapy has been framed around the discrepancy between traditional teaching philosophies when matched against the evolution in the understanding of the complexity of the therapist/patient interaction and of neurophysiological responses to hands-on therapies. The classic premise of justifying the use of manual therapy through biomechanical reasoning where the correction of adverse joint mechanics or "positional faults" between articulations is, in part, informed by skill-based motion palpation assessment, has been the main area of contention and debate (Zusman, 2004; Rabey et al., 2017; Oostendorp, 2018). The ability of a clinician to perform accurate and reproducible motion assessment may be unreliable, and sham treatments have been found to be comparable in effect to specifically reasoned application of techniques (Stolz et al., 2020), although evidence to the contrary exists (Hall et al., 2010; Fritz et al., 2005).

The above accounts for a shift in clinical reasoning where manual therapy techniques are now used as a method for pain modulation as a part of a multi-modal plan of care that typically includes exercise and patient neuroscience education. Guidelines for the management of the most common knee and hip pain conditions recommend multi-modal management of the patients, which should be based on patient preference, and individualized care. Recent recommendations from Lewis et al. (2021) provide the following evidence-informed suggestions as to what clinicians can offer when encountering MSK conditions:

- ensure patients are aware of and understand all reasonable diagnosis and management options, and the harms, benefits, and expected outcomes of each

- avoid emotive language and outdated explanations when explaining symptoms and making recommendations for management

- establish what matters most to the patient and discuss this as part of the decision-making

- understand the natural course of the condition

- know the investigations that should and should not be considered, and age-related norms for investigation findings

- discuss the impact an intervention may have on the individual

An example of a pathway for osteoarthritis comes from the UK's National Institute for Health and Care Excellence (NICE, 2020) which defines core first-line management as patient education, exercise and weight loss, with reference made to the possibility of adjuncts with some evidence to support them (including manual therapy). The guidelines are set to encourage the standardization of care and reduce engagement with low-value interventions in order to improve the global quality of care and general population health. Noting the limitations of guideline-based care, recent evidence has found that individuals with knee osteoarthritis who underwent physical therapy, of which manual therapy was a major component, had less pain and functional disability at one year than patients who received an intra-articular glucocorticoid injection (Deyle et al., 2020).

Considering Resistance During Joint-biased Manual Therapy

Several manual therapy educators sought to quantify their approaches through grading systems based on tissue resistance and pain markers to give a clinical framework for the application of manual therapy (Maitland, 2001; Kaltenborn et al., 2014), and this remains a useful tool, particularly when trying to educate physical therapists on patient handling (IFOMPT Standards, Dimension 8).

Tissue resistance is akin to load deformation (i.e., tissue strain) in the stress/strain curve. This concept takes into account the properties of human tissue, both pathological and non-pathological. A significant number of physical therapist assessments utilize tissue resistance as a means to measure characteristics of musculoskeletal and other somatic tissues. In fact, resistance is characterized as any force that works opposite, or against, another applied force, and clinicians often use their perception of tissue resistance in their decision-making (Maitland, 2001). For example, when assessing a patient's physiological knee flexion range of motion in supine, the moment the clinician perceives that the weight of the leg is no longer sufficient to continue a steady rate of flexion at the knee without some facilitation from the clinician is considered to be the onset of resistance. Once onset is defined, the clinician assesses the resistance with further facilitated movement, noting how quickly the resistance builds to the point of maximal resistance. This may vary between the sudden onset of maximal resistance, or a near-linear increase in resistance to the endpoint.

For a patient with minimal to no pain, the quality of resistance may be sufficient to determine the intensity of a therapeutic intervention. With a patient with minimal resistance, but with some restriction in range, a mobilization with a small amplitude but deep into the range working near or up to end-range may be the most appropriate. For a patient with an onset of resistance early in range of motion and a more linear increase to maximal resistance, using a larger amplitude mobilization that works through the range of resistance may be the most appropriate to facilitate improving a patient's mobility (Maitland et al., 2005). Selecting the duration of a treatment may be more directly tied to a perceived reduction in tissue resistance during the mobilization and a retest of onset and maximal resistance to observe changes.

Considering Pain during Joint-biased Manual Therapy

The presence of pain is the primary reason for a patient to seek physiotherapy input (McRae & Hancock, 2017). Physical therapists should focus on the effect of nociception as pain, rather than other centrally driven processes which are less likely to respond to physical modalities (Schäfer et al., 2009). With this in mind, any passive assessment of mobility must incorporate an assessment of pain. Incorporating the concepts of onset of pain and reproduction of symptoms can help the clinician understand how the patient's

pain relates to their movement dysfunction (Beneck et al., 2005; Owens et al., 2007). The onset of pain is defined as the instant where a patient reports pain during testing. For individuals whose pain is of high severity or irritability, assessment to maximal pain may be inappropriate, meaning the assessment is modified to allow partial reproduction of symptoms over symptom reproduction at all. Conversely, if reproduction is not provoked during testing, the clinician may reach maximal tissue resistance. It follows that if a patient has a more highly irritable issue, the clinician selects a gentler technique for manual therapy, whilst if a patient does not experience discomfort or pain until very close to maximum resistance, they may be more amenable to a more aggressive technique toward end range.

The target of manual therapy can be either pain or movement limitation (hypomobility). If the patient presents with pain prior to tissue resistance, reducing pain may be the focus with the purpose of eventually addressing the tissue limitation. If there is a restriction at an adjacent joint, it may be the clinician's preference to treat the hypomobility to address both joint restriction and to achieve a modulatory effect on the patient's pain experience. Often both pain and resistance are addressed in obtaining an improved patient outcome.

Do Clinicians Treat into Pain or Avoid It?

Deciding to treat into pain greatly depends on the Severity, Irritability, Nature and Stage of healing (SINSs) (Maitland et al., 2005). An additional consideration may be the type of pain experienced by the patient (i.e., neuropathic, nociceptive, or nociplastic). Avoiding pain provocation may be the best option for a highly irritable or acute injury/condition, whereas if nociplastic pain is the predominant presentation, staying out of pain will lower the risk of an adverse reaction, such as temporal summation (Meeus & Nijs, 2007). Defining the nature of a patient's pain is collected on subjective assessment and confirmed with physical examination, where a patient may present with hyperalgesia and/or allodynia. Using small or large amplitude oscillations that are not into tissue resistance are likely most appropriate for this patient scenario. If a patient's ability to inhibit pain is intact, commonly measured via conditioned pain modulation, treating into pain may be ideal for achieving pain inhibition. Treating into pain can allow increased pain thresholds and may be progressed by moving further into restriction and pain. This process may be indicated in all types of pain and can be used to activate conditioned pain modulation, which is often impaired (Petersen et al., 2019).

Dosage of Joint-biased Manual Therapy

In selecting the parameters of manual therapy, the patient's irritability will be influenced by both central and peripheral mechanisms. The clinical reasoning as to which mechanism(s) dominate the patient presentation is important to consider in determining the application of manual therapy. A patient whose complaint is highly irritable (e.g., presentations dominated by central sensitization or a severe neuropathic pain) will likely not tolerate a large dosage of manual therapy which would be likely to exacerbate the patient's complaint. It follows that a low grade (barely into resistance, or perhaps shy of resistance), short duration, slow oscillatory technique may help reduce their symptoms. A patient with minimal pain, or whose pain is primarily dominated by peripheral nociception rather than central sensitization, may respond to greater intensity of dosage of manual therapy.

Symptom and Functional Modification During Joint-biased Manual Therapy

An alternative process in the application of manual therapy uses symptom and functional modification. This is a process where the therapist works in partnership with the patient in attempting to alter their functional limitation in real time (Lehman, 2018). If the application of a joint-biased intervention improves the patient's symptoms, this intervention gives insight into the nature of the problem, and to whether the symptoms can be immediately modified. The technique used to assess and change the patient's functional limitation then becomes the treatment artifact. The goal of symptom and functional modification is to encourage "painless" mobility to the offensive movement and allow the patient to manage their own condition through the use of self-treatment, or other adjuncts such as taping. The most common techniques used for symptom and functional modification are mobilization with movement (MWM), the brainchild of Brian Mulligan, who defines them thus: "The joint mobilizations are passive, sustained at the pain-free limit, followed by pain-free active movement" (Mulligan, 2010).

The application of the symptom and function modification principle does not involve grading the level of manual tissue resistance applied by the therapist, or working up to, or into discomfort. Instead, the minimum amount of glide applied to a joint to elicit an improvement in function is recommended. It is for the clinician to decide whether full pain elimination or reduction is sufficient (Lewis et al., 2016). These interventions are applied with different adjustments until the movement becomes most functional through attempting different glides, pressures, and refinements. Working together, the patient and clinician identify the technique which allows most symptom modification. Mulligan considered that MWMs are thus the combination of hands-on manual therapy and exercise. Although historically their effects were suggested to be related to joint positional faults (Mulligan, 2010), current reasoning guided by understanding neurophysiological mechanisms is the predominant understanding of the mechanisms of effect (Vicenzino et al., 2011). These are: (1) aim to decrease symptoms (threat) with a movement or activity; (2) evoke endogenous hypoalgesia; (3) be able to disrupt pain memories/exposure with control. It is also postulated that this approach could lead to reduction in movement avoidance behaviors and improved self-efficacy (Vicenzino et al., 2011). If a movement can be modified using a specific mobilization, it is recommended that the newly pain-free movement be repeated several times to relearn the memory of the previously pain-free action (Zusman, 2004). In terms of dosage, the minimal number of repetitions is advised to restore the movement.

Although there is no formal grading of force with the application of MWM, a cornerstone of its use is the assumption of functional positions and the progressive increase of load with movement as the condition allows. With a highly irritable patient, the most tolerable position may be first non-weight-bearing, but over time the irritability may reduce, allowing the MWM to be performed in partial or full weight-bearing, as indicated in Figure 16.1. As a patient may experience pain with different functional positions, the clinician can apply MWM in these postures. If symptoms worsen with treatment, the clinician changes the position to a lower load and more tolerable one. If there is no immediate benefit to the patient's symptom and functional modification, this approach should be discarded.

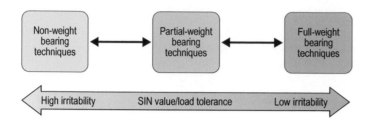

FIGURE 16.1
Progression from non-weight-bearing to full weight-bearing interventions using Mobilization with Movement (MWM) interventions.

(Redrawn and modified from McDowell et al. (2021).)

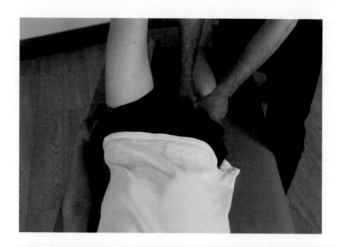

FIGURE 16.2
Supine anterior–posterior mobilization of the hip in neutral position.

Passive Joint-biased Manual Therapy Interventions for the Hip

Hip Anterior–Posterior Joint Mobilization

The least loaded position is the patient supine with the knee straight. The clinician delivers an anterior to posterior pressure through the upper femur with the hip in a neutral position (Fig. 16.2). To progress, the knee is flexed and the foot placed flat on the table. The clinician places their hands on the anterior knee and imparts an anterior to posterior (AP) force through the axis of the femur (Fig. 16.3). If a stretch is not felt in the posterior hip, the patient's foot can be placed on the lateral side of the opposite knee. If additional stretch is required, the hip can be brought up into varying degrees of flexion (Fig. 16.4).

Hip Posterior–Anterior Joint Mobilization

With the patient in the prone position, the clinician grasps and supports the patient's lower extremity with the knee flexed. The clinician's proximal hand is placed just inferior and medial to the patient's greater trochanter and a posterior to anterior (PA) pressure is applied at the posterior hip (Fig. 16.5). If a stretch is not felt anteriorly, the clinician can raise the hip into varying degrees of extension (Fig. 16.6).

Hip Posterior–Anterior Joint Mobilization with External Rotation

The patient lies prone with the knee flexed. The clinician grasps the patient's ankle with their distal hand and places

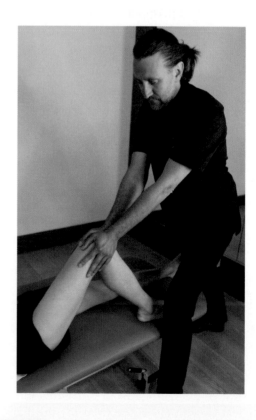

FIGURE 16.3
Supine anterior–posterior mobilization of the hip with 45 degrees of flexion.

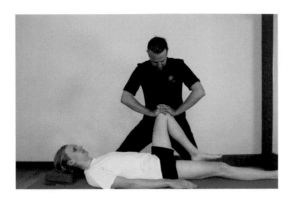

FIGURE 16.4
Supine anterior–posterior mobilization of the hip with 90 degrees of flexion.

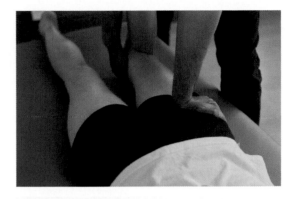

FIGURE 16.6
Prone posterior–anterior mobilization of the hip in extension.

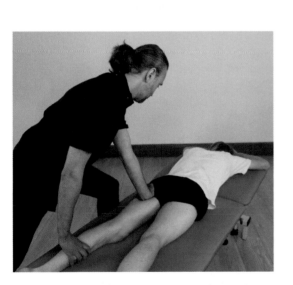

FIGURE 16.5
Prone posterior–anterior mobilization of the hip in neutral position.

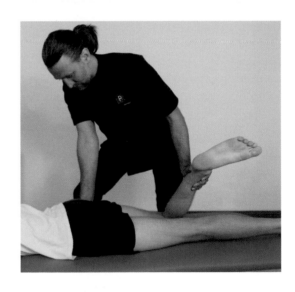

FIGURE 16.7
Prone posterior–anterior mobilization of the hip in external rotation.

the first webspace or hypothenar eminence of their proximal hand just below and medial to the patient's greater trochanter. The clinician then externally rotates the hip until they feel tissue tension begin. The lower leg is held in this position as a PA pressure is applied through their proximal hand (Fig. 16.7). This can be advanced to the "figure-of-4" position. The clinician uses their lower leg to apply downward counterforce pressure on the patient's lower leg. The clinician then places the first web space of the hand or the hypothenar eminence just below and medial to the patient's

greater trochanter and a PA downward mobilizing pressure is applied (Fig. 16.8).

Hip Anterior–Posterior Mobilization (Long Axis) with Lower Extremity Crossed

The patient is positioned in supine with the involved lower extremity placed in a figure-of-4 position. The clinician stands on the contralateral side of the patient, placing bilateral

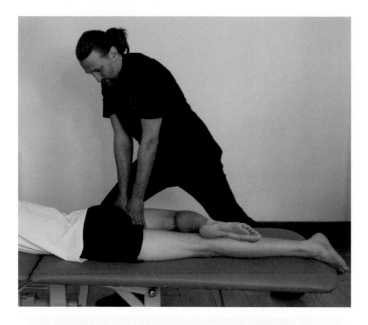

FIGURE 16.8
Prone posterior–anterior mobilization of the hip in "figure of 4" position.

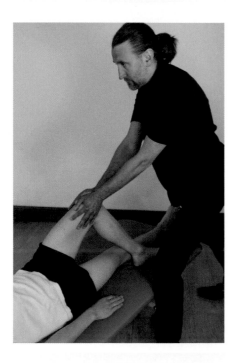

FIGURE 16.9
Supine anterior–posterior mobilization (long axis) of the hip with the lower extremity crossed.

hands at the patient's knee. Force is applied on the same axis as the femur, acting as a long-axes AP mobilization (Fig. 16.9).

Hip Distraction Thrust (Long Axis)

The patient lies supine with the clinician at the foot of the bed. The clinician grasps the ankle just above the malleoli (Fig. 16.10). The leg is raised into the resting position of 30 degrees of flexion, slight external rotation and slight abduction. The clinician leans backward to take up the slack in the tissues and provide a high-velocity, low-amplitude thrust in the inferior direction (Fig. 16.11).

Mobilization with Movement (MWM) Interventions for the Hip

The application of hip MWMs is based on the principle of combining the problem movement with a lateral glide mobilization to the proximal femur. This can be done in non-weight-bearing (supine), partial weight-bearing (4-point kneeling or with foot on a chair), and full weight-bearing (standing) (NWB, PWB, FWB). Overpressure may be added by the patient, engaging them in their treatment. As with all MWMs, self-treatment options are key to empowering the patient with their own management, potentially allowing more autonomy in controlling their pain. It is recommended that MWMs are pain-free, and they may be sustained at the

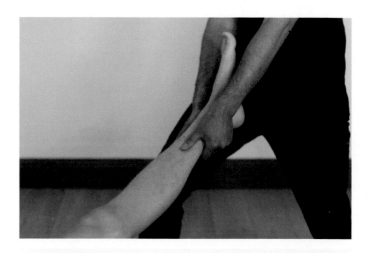

FIGURE 16.10
Hand position for a supine distraction thrust (long axis) of the hip.

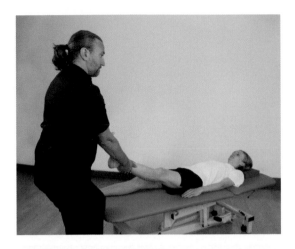

FIGURE 16.11
Supine distraction thrust (long axis) of the hip.

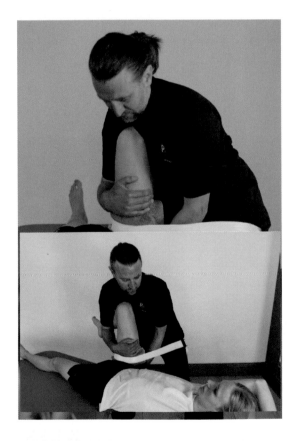

FIGURE 16.12
Belt position for lateral glide of the hip during Mobilization with Movement (MWM).

end of the range for a few seconds. Sets of 10 repetitions are commonly used, though this may be increased or decreased based on patient response.

Non-weight-bearing Position Procedures

If hip flexion is the impaired movement, the non-weight-bearing trial of MWM begins with the patient supine and the hip flexed to 90 degrees. The clinician stands at the side of the bed in a stride stance. The treatment belt is looped around the clinician's hips and around the inside of the patient's inner groin with padding as required for comfort. A lateral glide of the femur is performed through the clinician applying force through the belt through moving their pelvis away from the patient (Fig. 16.12). The patient then flexes the hip with the glide consistently held through the movement, and on return to neutral. The patient can apply overpressure with their hands, pulling the knee towards the chest to further increase range (Fig. 16.13). This treatment position can also be used for combined flexion and adduction, internal rotation (Fig. 16.14), and can be adapted for external rotation in the FABRE position (Fig. 16.15).

Partial Weight-bearing Position Procedures

Partial weight-bearing MWM for the hip requires the application of the lateral glide mobilization with the patient in a 4-point kneeling posture. Again, the lateral glide is applied

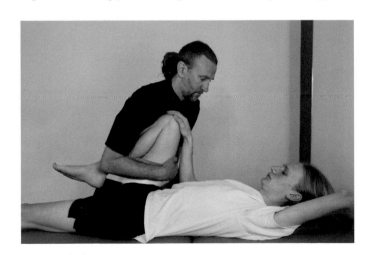

FIGURE 16.13
Supine non-weight-bearing lateral glide Mobilization with Movement (MWM) to hip flexion with overpressure.

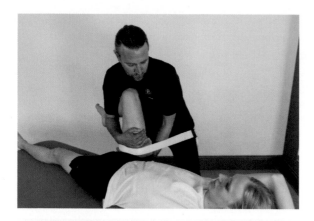

FIGURE 16.14
Supine non-weight-bearing lateral glide Mobilization with Movement (MWM) to hip internal rotation.

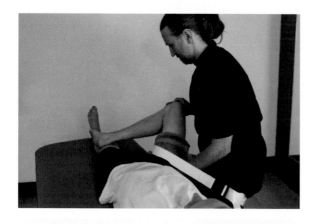

FIGURE 16.15
Supine non-weight-bearing lateral glide Mobilization with Movement (MWM) to hip external rotation.

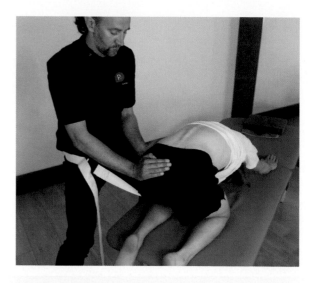

FIGURE 16.16
4-point partial weight-bearing lateral glide Mobilization with Movement (MWM) in hip flexion.

Full Weight-bearing Position Procedures

Full weight-bearing MWMs for the hip again use the lateral glide through the application of the belt, with the patient in a supported standing posture. For flexion and extension movements, the patient stands with their foot on a chair and the glide is either applied to the front leg (for flexion; Fig. 16.17) or the standing leg (for extension; Fig. 16.18). The hands of the clinician are placed on the iliac crest for lateral fixation of the pelvis, and the glide is applied through the belt prior to the impaired movement being performed by the patient. The patient can hold the treatment table for safety. With advanced sessions, the FWB technique can also be applied in the squatting position for the more active patient or those with pain in this position (Fig. 16.19).

For FWB internal or external rotation, the same position is used; however, the patient movement is either turning the body toward or away from the standing leg (Fig. 16.20).

Finally, self-MWM for the hip is an important aspect of the management of a patient's condition (McDowell et al., 2021), and can be applied successfully with the use of a track band in whichever weight-bearing position is suitable for the patient to modify their painful movement (Fig. 16.21). In conclusion, it is important to note that joint-biased interventions are not dogmatic. Using knowledge of both basic

through the clinician moving their pelvis away from the patient, with the clinician standing at the side of a bed in a stride stance (Fig. 16.16). The movement of hip flexion is performed by the patient initiating a "rocking back" movement, taking the pelvis toward the ankles. Overpressure is controlled by the patient moving further back into movement. This technique can also be combined with elements of internal and external rotation and abduction or adduction though the placement of the knee on the bed, dependent on the patient-identified functional requirement.

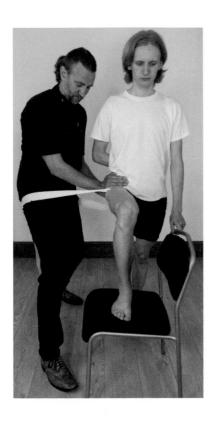

FIGURE 16.17
Semi-standing partial weight-bearing lateral glide
Mobilization with Movement (MWM) to hip flexion.

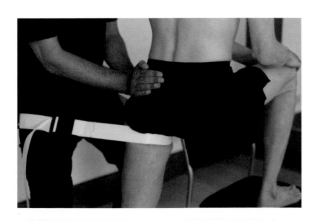

FIGURE 16.18
Semi-standing partial weight-bearing lateral glide
Mobilization with Movement (MWM) to hip extension.

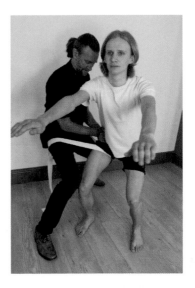

FIGURE 16.19
Squat position full weight-bearing lateral glide
Mobilization with Movement (MWM).

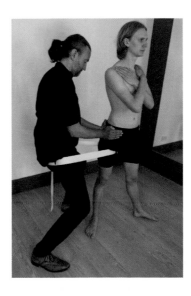

FIGURE 16.20
Standing full weight-bearing lateral glide Mobilization with
Movement (MWM) to hip rotation.

and clinical sciences, clinical reasoning and the patient's
presentation, the clinician should be creative in how they
choose and apply manual techniques.

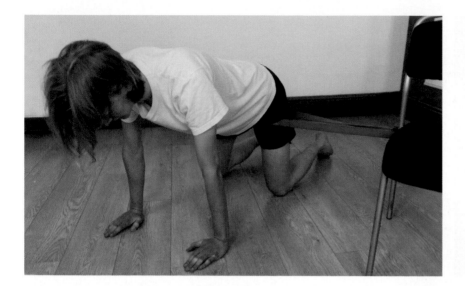

FIGURE 16.21
4-point self-lat glide MWM to hip flexion with resistance band.

Joint-biased Manual Therapy Interventions for the Knee

Proximal Tibiofibular Joint Mobilizations

Proximal Tibiofibular Joint Posterior–Medial Mobilization

With the patient in supine in hook-lying position, the clinician rests the patient's foot to their knee to assure position. The thenar eminence is placed over the anterior, proximal fibular head and fingers 2–5 are wrapped around into the popliteal fossa. Pressure is applied in a posteromedial direction and graded accordingly (Fig. 16.22).

Proximal Tibiofibular Joint Posterior–Anterior Mobilization

The patient is in prone, with the feet hanging over the edge of the table placing the ankle in a neutral position. The clinician gently grasps the proximal fibula and places their thenar eminence over the posterior fibular head. Pressure is applied in an anterolateral direction and graded accordingly (Fig. 16.23). The knee of the patient can be placed in varying degrees of flexion and extension depending on the patient presentation and goal of the intervention.

Proximal Tibiofibular Joint Caudal Glide

The patient is positioned in side-lying with the involved side up and the knees in slight flexion. The clinician places

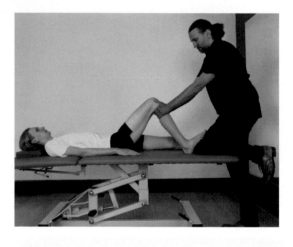

FIGURE 16.22
Supine proximal tibiofibular posterior–medial mobilization.

both thumbs on the superior fibular head. A graded mobilization is performed by applying a force in a caudal direction (Fig. 16.24).

Proximal Tibiofibular Joint Posterior-Anterior Manipulation Thrust

The clinician places their hand in the patient's popliteal fossa on the lateral aspect of the knee and pulls the soft tissue laterally until the metacarpophalangeal (MCP) joint of their hand is firmly stabilized behind the patient's fibular head. The opposite hand grasps their foot and ankle

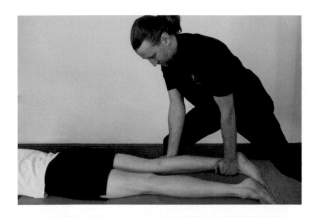

FIGURE 16.23
Prone proximal tibiofibular posterior–anterior mobilization.

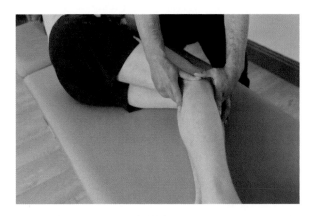

FIGURE 16.24
Side-lying proximal tibiofibular caudal glide.

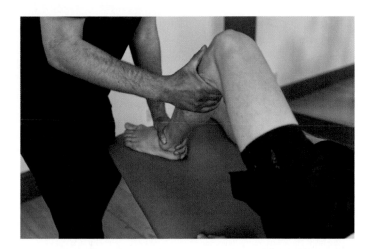

FIGURE 16.25
Hand position supine proximal tibiofibular posterior–anterior manipulation thrust.

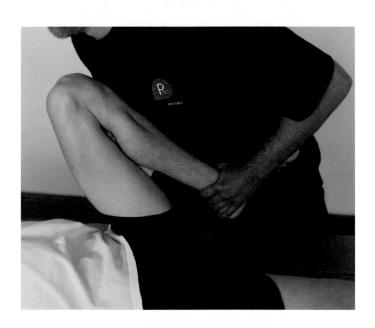

FIGURE 16.26
Supine proximal tibiofibular posterior–anterior manipulation thrust.

(Fig. 16.25). The knee is flexed, and the lower leg is externally rotated approximately 75% into tissue resistance. The clinician applies a high-velocity, low-amplitude thrust through the tibia, pushing the patient's heel towards the ipsilateral hip (Fig. 16.26).

Tibiofemoral Joint Mobilizations

Tibiofemoral Joint Anterior–Posterior Mobilization in Flexion

Mobilizing the tibia posteriorly on the femur can be performed in various degrees of knee flexion. If mobilizing the joint in a more extended position the clinician may use a towel or bolster as support under the femur. Otherwise, the knee is flexed with the foot resting on the treatment table. The clinician should place the thenar eminence on medial and lateral tibial plateaus with thumbs facing superiorly and the remaining fingers wrapping around the joint line (Fig. 16.27). The application force is applied in an AP direction.

351

CHAPTER SIXTEEN

Tibiofemoral Joint Posterior–Anterior Mobilization with Knee Extended

A PA tibiofemoral joint mobilization with the knee extended can be done with two different hand positions in the prone position. The first technique involves the supporting hand at the distal anterior tibia while the mobilizing hand is placed at the proximal posterior tibia with the heel of the hand at the joint line with fingers directed distally (Fig. 16.28). The alternate technique involves bilateral hands mobilizing at the proximal tibia with thumbs facing distally and fingers wrapping around the calf anteriorly (Fig. 16.29). For both techniques, the application force is applied in a PA direction.

Tibiofemoral Joint Posterior–Anterior Mobilization in Flexion

Similar to the AP technique, the knee can be flexed to varying degrees, using a bolster/towel. This technique can be done with the patient in supine or prone. In the supine position, the patient is positioned with the knee flexed with the clinician hand placement similar to the AP mobilization. The clinician applies a PA force, pulling the tibia anteriorly on the femur.

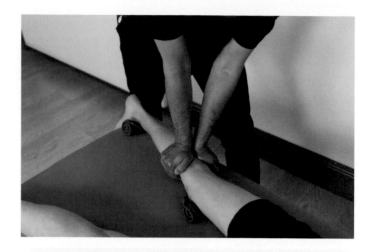

FIGURE 16.28
Prone tibiofemoral joint posterior–anterior mobilization with knee extended.

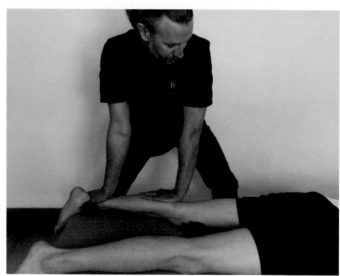

FIGURE 16.29
Prone tibiofemoral joint posterior–anterior mobilization with knee extended (alternative position of the hands).

In prone lying, the patient's knee is flexed, and the clinician can choose to rest the patient's distal tibia on their shoulder to offer stability while placing both mobilizing hands at the proximal tibia, posteriorly (Fig. 16.30). The clinician would then apply a force in the AP direction.

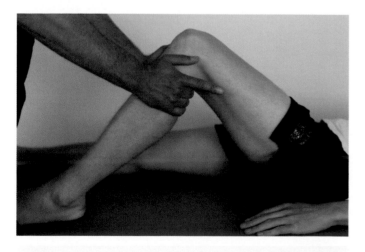

FIGURE 16.27
Supine tibiofemoral joint anterior–posterior mobilization in flexion.

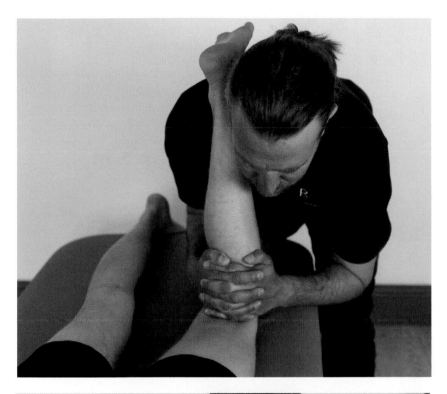

FIGURE 16.30
Prone tibiofemoral joint posterior–anterior mobilization in flexion.

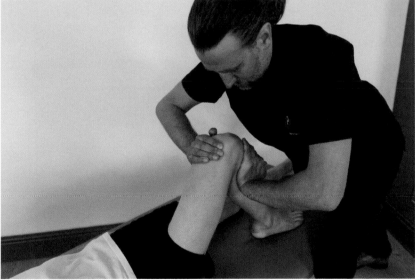

FIGURE 16.31
Supine tibiofemoral medial–lateral glide mobilization.

Tibiofemoral Joint Medial and Lateral Glide Mobilization

Either medial or lateral tibiofemoral joint mobilization can be applied in various degrees of knee flexion, using a towel/bolster as necessary. This is performed in supine with the clinician's mobilizing hand on the proximal tibia or fibula, while the femur is stabilized through contact with the bed (Fig. 16.31).

An alternative is to perform this technique in side-lying with the lower extremity flexed, the femur and distal tibia supported by a towel where the clinician places both hands at the proximal tibia or fibula based on the glide used. Force is applied towards the table to provide a medial (Fig. 16.32) or lateral (Fig. 16.33) tibiofemoral joint mobilization.

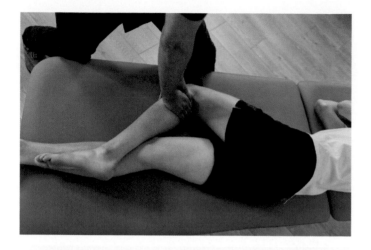

FIGURE 16.32
Side-lying tibiofemoral medial glide mobilization.

Tibiofemoral Joint Internal and External Rotation Mobilization

The patient is prone with the involved knee flexed so the distal tibia is resting on the clinician's shoulder. The clinician should stand in a staggered stance with the table at the appropriate height, with both hands surrounding the proximal tibia, using a circumferential grip. The application force is PA with a combined medial (Fig. 16.34) or lateral (Fig. 16.35) rotatory force.

Tibiofemoral Joint Posterior Mobilization

The patient is in supine with the involved lower extremity resting in extension. The clinician stands laterally to the patient's involved side, placing their thenar eminence at the proximal tibia, fingers directed distally and medially on the tibia. The other mobilizing hand grasps the distal tibia,

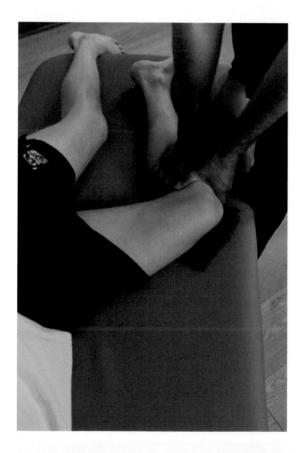

FIGURE 16.33
Side-lying tibiofemoral lateral glide mobilization.

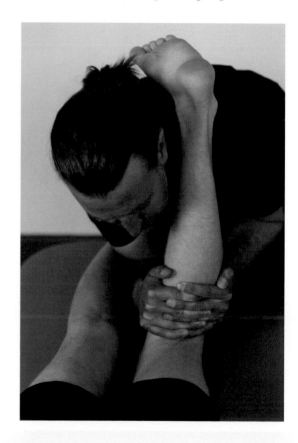

FIGURE 16.34
Prone tibiofemoral joint mobilization in internal rotation.

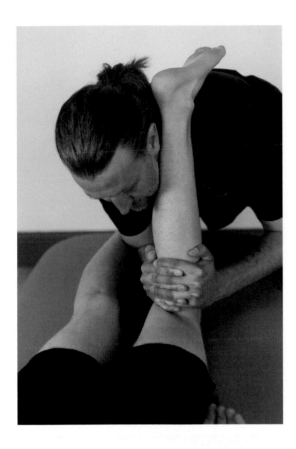

FIGURE 16.35
Prone tibiofemoral joint mobilization in external rotation.

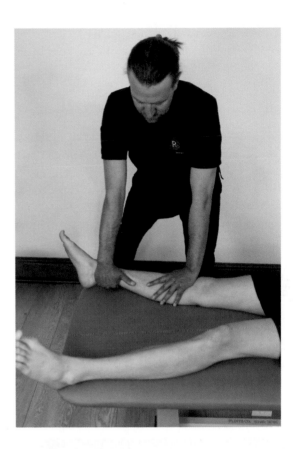

FIGURE 16.36
Supine tibiofemoral physiological posterior mobilization.

wrapping fingers medially (Fig. 16.36). A long-levered force is applied by pulling the distal tibia upwards while stabilizing the proximal tibia, providing a posterior tilt.

Tibiofemoral Joint Anterior Mobilization

The patient is positioned supine. The clinician places their proximal forearm in the popliteal space of the patient's knee. Force is applied by flexing the knee over the clinician's forearm, which acts as a wedge, providing a PA force on the tibia (Fig. 16.37).

Physiological Knee Mobilization in Flexion

The patient is supine with hip and knee flexed to 90 degrees. The clinician's mobilizing hand is the caudal hand and grasps the ankle using a lumbrical grip. The supporting hand is cephalic, resting on the knee with the fingers

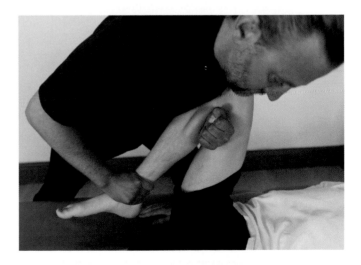

FIGURE 16.37
Supine tibiofemoral joint anterior mobilization.

on the joint line and forearm parallel against the femur (Fig. 16.38). The clinician gently flexes the knee by bringing the heel towards the buttocks.

Physiological Knee Mobilization in Extension

The patient is in supine while the clinician is standing laterally to the involved knee. The clinician places their proximal upper extremity on the medial side of the patient's involved lower leg so that the distal tibia is secured between the clinician's upper arm and trunk. This cradle hold allows for bilateral mobilizing hands to support the knee at the joint line. The clinician gently extends the knee by supporting the ankle between the elbow and trunk, while guiding the knee posteriorly (Fig. 16.39).

Patellofemoral Joint Mobilizations

Patellofemoral mobilizations can be applied in many ways, including: inferior and superior, medial and lateral, distraction and rotation glides. Patient comfort is paramount,

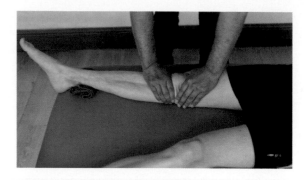

FIGURE 16.39
Supine knee physiological mobilization in extension.

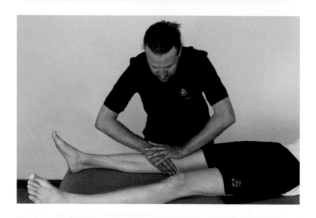

FIGURE 16.40
Supine patellofemoral joint inferior mobilization.

and typically the patient will be in supine with the knee extended, or if needed, slightly flexed with a towel behind the knee for comfort.

Inferior and Superior Mobilization

The clinician's distal hand cups the patella through their first web space and may apply distraction of the patella away from the trochlear groove. Using the palm of their proximal hand the clinician applies graded mobilizations in a caudal (Fig. 16.40) or cephalad direction (Fig. 16.41).

Medial and Lateral Glide Mobilization

For the medial glide, the clinician places their mobilizing thumbs pointing towards each other on the lateral border of the patella with the supporting fingers resting on the femur

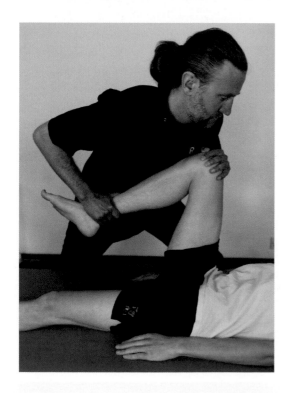

FIGURE 16.38
Supine knee physiological mobilization in flexion.

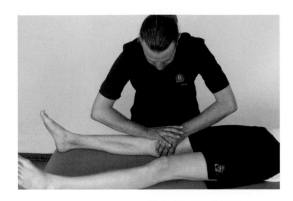

FIGURE 16.41
Supine patellofemoral joint mobilization superior.

and tibia, facing medially (Fig. 16.42). The clinician's arms are extended in a parallel line with the patella, so as not to add a compressive force. Medial force is applied with use of the thumbs in a butterfly motion. The lateral glide is performed by reaching across the patient to apply pressure to the medial border of the patella with the same method on the contralateral limb (Fig. 16.43).

Distraction

The patient is supine or long sitting with the knee extended. The clinician places their hands surrounding the patella

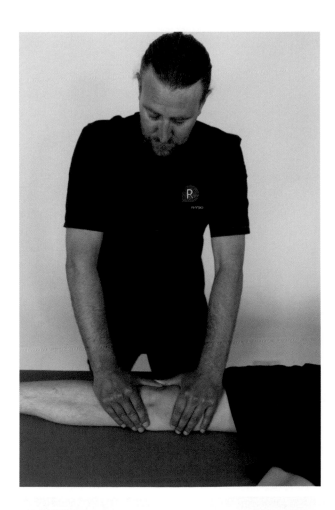

FIGURE 16.42
Supine patellofemoral joint medial glide mobilization.

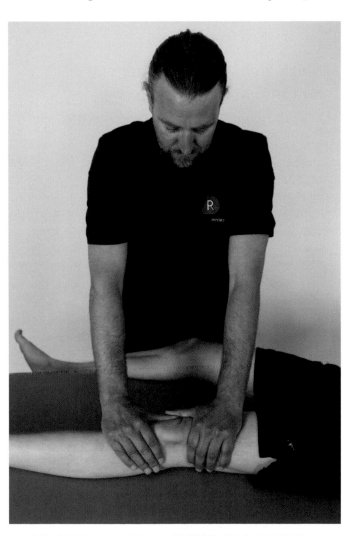

FIGURE 16.43
Supine patellofemoral joint lateral glide mobilization.

so that thumbs meet on the lateral border of the patella, while the index fingers cup the patella, meeting medially. To apply a distraction force, the fingers and thumbs squeeze together, gently lifting the patella (Fig. 16.44).

Mobilization Rotation

The patient is in supine or long sitting with the knee extended. The clinician places the mobilizing thumbs in the space between the patella and femur (medially or laterally), with the supporting index fingers on the opposite side. Application of force is applied in a clockwise or counter-clockwise moment, using a bi-manual technique (Fig. 16.45).

Mobilization with Movement (MWM) Interventions for the Knee

Non-weight-bearing Position Procedures

As the knee is the largest hinge joint in the body, medial, lateral, anterior, posterior, and medial and lateral rotation glides could all be applied using MWM, based on the patient response. If knee flexion is the painful movement and the patient has a high SINSs value, an NWB posture would likely probably be chosen first. In such a situation, the patient is supine and performs the painful movement and the clinician applies tests/various glides during active range of motion to determine which glide decreases symptoms. For a lateral glide, the clinician stabilizes the proximal tibia medially, places the mobilizing hand on the

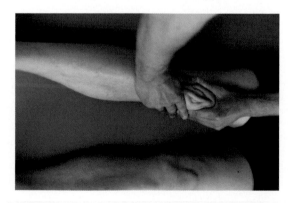

FIGURE 16.44
Supine patellofemoral joint distraction mobilization.

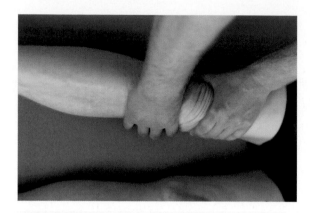

FIGURE 16.45
Supine patellofemoral joint rotation mobilization.

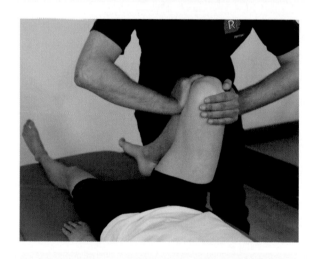

FIGURE 16.46
Non-weight-bearing lateral glide Mobilization with Movement (MWM) in knee flexion.

lateral femur and applies a sustained force medially while the patient performs active knee flexion (Fig. 16.46) and/or extension (Fig. 16.47) motions. For a medial glide, the clinician stabilizes the proximal tibia laterally, places the mobilizing hand on the medial femur and applies a sustained force medially. For internal and external rotational glide, the hands are placed on the medial and lateral aspect of the proximal tibia and the fingers linked. To create an internal rotation glide, a posterior (AP) force is applied medially and an anterior (PA) force is applied laterally. To create an external rotation lateral glide, an anterior (PA) force is applied medially and a posterior (AP) force is applied laterally. The

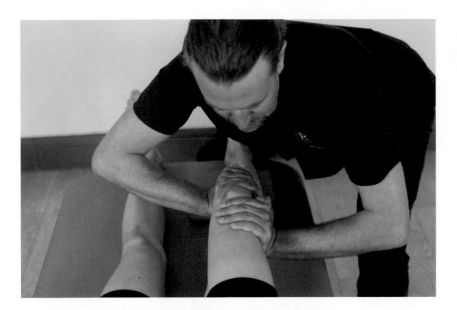

FIGURE 16.47
Non-weight-bearing lateral glide
Mobilization with Movement (MWM) to knee
extension.

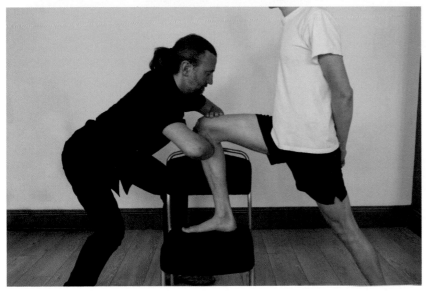

FIGURE 16.48
Full weight-bearing lateral glide Mobilization
with Movement (MWM) to knee flexion.

direction that creates the greatest symptom modification is repeated based on treatment response. The patient can apply an overpressure with a treatment belt to assist with the technique. If no pain is felt in the NWB position, then the same procedure is followed with the patient in FWB.

Full Weight-bearing Position Procedures

In FWB, the same medial or lateral glides can be applied in a foot-on-chair posture to increase the loading and functional aspect to the movement as the patient's presentation allows.

For flexion and extension movements, the patient stands with their foot on a chair and the glide is either applied to the front leg (for flexion; Fig. 16.48) or the standing leg (for extension; Fig. 16.49). The patient then actively performs a physiological mobilization by oscillating into the functional movement.

Self-MWM for the knee can be simply applied and provides an important part of self-management. If flexion is painful, the patient can be shown how to perform a knee glide using their hands to apply, and combine it with the movement (Fig. 16.50). An additional adjunct to allow

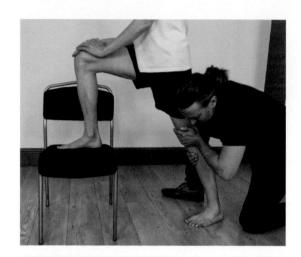

FIGURE 16.49
Full weight-bearing lateral glide Mobilization with Movement (MWM) to knee extension.

long-lasting management could be taping for medial or lateral rotation of the tibiofemoral joint.

Conclusions

The use of joint-based therapies has strong historical and cultural precedent with evidence for its benefit for pain and stiffness found in the literature. The techniques demonstrated in this chapter may provide benefit to clinicians and patients alike as part of a wider treatment package, especially where manual therapy is the patient's preference and allows individualized care.

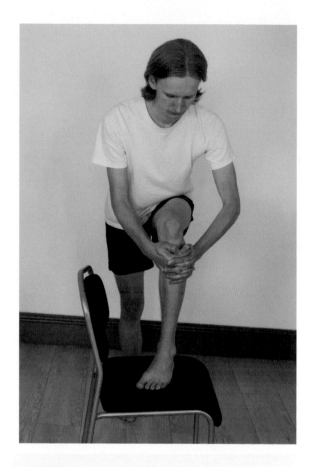

FIGURE 16.50
Full weight-bearing self-Mobilization with Movement (MWM) with lateral glide to knee flexion (patient in a semi-standing position).

References

Beneck GJ, Kulig K, Landel RF, Powers CM. The relationship between lumbar segmental motion and pain response produced by a posterior-to-anterior force in persons with nonspecific low back pain. J Orthop Sports Phys Ther. 2005;35:203–9.

Courtney CA. Mechanisms underlying the effects of manual therapy: a new look at an old concept. Manuelletherapie. 2013;17:68–72.

Deyle GD, Allen CS, Allison SC, et al. Physical therapy versus glucocorticoid injection for osteoarthritis of the knee. N Engl J Med. 2020;382:1420–9.

Fritz JM, Whitman JM, Childs JD. Lumbar spine segmental mobility assessment: an examination of validity for determining intervention strategies in patients with low back pain. Arch Phys Med Rehabil. 2005;86:1745–52.

Hall T, Briffa K, Hopper D, Robinson K. Reliability of manual examination and frequency of symptomatic cervical motion segment dysfunction in cervicogenic headache. Man Ther. 2010;15:542–6.

Kaltenborn FM, Evjenth O, Kaltenborn T, et al. Manual Mobilization of the Joints – Vol. 1: The Extremities, 8th Edition; 2014.

Lehman GJ. The role and value of symptom-modification approaches in musculoskeletal

practice. J Orthop Sports Phys Ther. 2018;48:430–5.

Lewis JS, McCreesh K, Barratt E, et al. Inter-rater reliability of the Shoulder Symptom Modification Procedure in people with shoulder pain. BMJ Open. 2016;2:e000181.

Lewis JS, Stokes EK, Gojanovic B, et al. Reframing how we care for people with persistent non-traumatic musculoskeletal pain. Suggestions for the rehabilitation community. Physiotherapy. 2021;112:143–9.

Lluch Girbés E, Meeus M, Baert I, Nijs J. Balancing "hands-on" with "hands-off" physical therapy interventions for the treatment of central sensitization pain in osteoarthritis. Man Ther. 2015;20:349–52.

Maitland G. Vertebral Manipulation. 6th ed. Oxford, UK: Butterworth-Heinemann; 2001.

Maitland GD, Banks K, Hengeveld E. Maitland's peripheral manipulation. Edinburgh; New York: Elsevier/Butterworth Heinemann; 2005.

McDowell J, Mitchell T, Mulligan B. Self-Mobilisation with Movement, a patient guide Self-Mobilisation with Movement, a patient guide. Vol. 1. Invercargill: Plane View Publishing; 2021.

McRae M, Hancock MJ. Adults attending private physiotherapy practices seek diagnosis, pain relief, improved function, education and prevention: a survey. J Physiother. 2017;63:250–6.

Meakins A. The Sports Physio [Internet]. Manual Therapy Sucks. 2017. Available from: https://www.thesports.physio/manual-therapy-sucks/

Meeus M, Nijs J. Central sensitization: a biopsychosocial explanation for chronic widespread pain in patients with fibromyalgia and chronic fatigue syndrome. Clin Rheumatol. 2007;26:465–73.

Mintken PE, Rodeghero J, Cleland JA. Manual therapists - Have you lost that loving feeling?! J Man Manip Ther. 2018;26:53–4.

Mulligan B. 'NAGs', 'SNAGSs', 'MWMs' etc. 6th ed. Wellington, NZ: Orthopaedic Physical Therapy Products; 2010.

NICE: National Institute of Health and Care Excellence Guidelines: Osteoarthritis: Care and Management [Internet]. National Institute of Health and Care Excellence; 2020. https://www.nice.org.uk/guidance/cg177/chapter/1-Recommendations#non-pharmacological-management-2

Oostendorp RAB. Credibility of manual therapy is at stake 'Where do we go from here?' J Man Manip Ther. 2018;26:189–92.

Owens EF Jr, DeVocht JW, Gudavalli MR, et al. Comparison of posteroanterior spinal stiffness measures to clinical and demographic findings at baseline in patients enrolled in a clinical study of spinal manipulation for low back pain. J Manipulat Physiol Ther. 2007;30:493–500.

Petersen KK, McPhee ME, Hoegh MS, Graven-Nielsen T. Assessment of conditioned pain modulation in healthy participants and patients with chronic pain: manifestations and implications for pain progression. Curr Opin Support Palliat Care. 2019;13:99–106.

Rabey M, Hall T, Hebron C, et al. Reconceptualising manual therapy skills in contemporary practice. Musculoskel Sci Pract. 2017;29:28–32.

Schäfer A, Hall T, Briffa K. Classification of low back-related leg pain: A proposed patho-mechanism-based approach. Man Ther. 2009;14:222–30.

Stolz M, von Piekartz H, Hall T, Schindler A, Ballenberger N. Evidence and recommendations for the use of segmental motion testing for patients with LBP: A systematic review. Musculoskel Sci Pract. 2020;45:102076.

Vicenzino B HW, Hall T RD. Mobilization with Movement: The Art and the Science. Sydney, Australia: Churchill Livingstone; 2011.

Willy RW, Hoglund LT, Barton CJ, et al. Patellofemoral pain. J Orthop Sports Phys Ther. 2019;49:CPG1–95.

Zusman M. Mechanisms of Musculoskeletal Physiotherapy. Phys Ther Rev. 2004;9:39–49.

Muscle-biased interventions for hip and knee pain disorders

César Fernández-de-las-Peñas, Gustavo Plaza-Manzano, Joseph Donnelly, Michelle Finnegan

17

Myofascial Trigger Points

Definition

Trigger points (TrPs) have varying definitions depending on the healthcare practitioner's discipline. Simons et al. (1999) defined a TrP as a "hyperirritable spot in a taut band of a skeletal muscle that is painful on compression, stretch, overload or contraction which causes localized or referred pain that is perceived distant from the TrP". The updated and current version of the *Trigger Point Manual* utilized the same definition, with new caveats (Donnelly, 2019). The key sign of a TrP is a palpable taut band with an exquisitely painful spot within the taut band producing local or referred pain (pain felt in a region remote from the source of pain). The term "referred pain" encompasses any abnormal sensation, including traditional descriptions of pain, paresthesias, dysesthesias or any other phenomena. This is consistent with the updated definition of pain by the International Association for Study of Pain (Treede et al., 2019). Additionally, a Delphi study proposed the term "referred sensation" to describe any phenomenon associated with TrPs (Fernández-de-las-Peñas & Dommertholt 2018). It is clear that TrPs may be responsible for producing numerous unpleasant sensory phenomena in patients seeking resolution to their pain interfering with activities and participation abilities.

Active and Latent Trigger Points

There are two different types of TrPs, active and latent. Active TrPs are those which reproduce local and/or referred sensory or motor symptoms that are familiar to the patient (Fernández-de-las-Peñas & Dommertholt, 2018; Donnelly, 2019). These findings are consistent with the current literature regarding active TrPs. Latent TrPs are those which produce local and/or referred pain that is not familiar to the patient. The patient commonly reports that the symptoms produced from latent TrPs are different from the symptoms they are currently experiencing (Fernández-de-las-Peñas & Dommertholt, 2018; Donnelly, 2019).

Active and latent TrPs have similar physical findings on clinical examination, e.g., taut band, painful spot, local twitch response and referred pain. The local twitch response is the most elusive in many muscles and most difficult to reproduce by clinicians in inter-rater reliability studies (Bron et al., 2007; Al-Shenqiti & Oldham, 2005; Gerwin et al., 1997). The main difference is that active TrPs reproduce familiar symptoms experienced by a patient whereas latent TrPs produce an unfamiliar report of symptoms. Nevertheless, an important, and commonly ignored topic is that both active and latent TrPs provoke motor impairments in the affected muscles, e.g., muscle weakness (Kim et al., 2017; Celik & Yeldan 2011), greater fatigability (Ge et al., 2012), muscle inhibition, increased motor irritability (Ge et al., 2014), muscle stiffness (Grabowski et al., 2018; Kisilewicz et al., 2018), muscle antagonist co-activation (Ibarra et al., 2011), and altered muscle activation patterns (Lucas et al., 2010). In fact, several studies demonstrated that treatment of latent TrPs improves range of motion (Grieve et al., 2011, 2013b; Oliveira-Campelo et al., 2013), decreases resting muscle stiffness (Albin et al., 2020; Sánchez-Infante et al., 2021; Kisilewicz et al., 2018; De Meulemeester et al., 2017; Maher et al., 2013), changes muscle flexibility (Pérez-Bellmunt et al., 2021; Basu et al., 2020), or increase in lower extremity jump performance (Devereux et al., 2019).

Manual Identification of Trigger Points

Several signs and symptoms have been proposed for a TrP diagnosis: (1) presence of a palpable taut band in a skeletal muscle (when accessible to palpation); (2) presence of a hyperirritable spot within the taut band; (3) local twitch response on snapping palpation (or needling) of the TrP; (4) presence of local and/or referred pain elicited by stimulation or palpation of the TrP; (5) jump sign; (6) restricted range of motion; and (7) pain on contraction in a shortened or lengthening position (Simons et al., 1999; Donnelly, 2019). A recent review conducted by Li et al. (2020) observed high variability in the use of TrP diagnostic criteria in clinical trials investigating physical therapy interventions for the management of myofascial pain. These investigators reported that tender painful spot, referred pain, and the local twitch response were the most popular criteria and the most frequently used combination (Li et al., 2020). These findings partially agree with a recent Delphi study concluding that taut band, spot tenderness, and referred pain are the most recommended cluster criteria for TrP diagnosis (Fernández-de-las-Peñas & Dommerholt, 2018). When these criteria are utilized by an experienced clinician, good inter-rater reliability (kappa) ranging from 0.84 to 0.88 is obtained (Gerwin et al., 1997).

Over the years, manual TrP diagnosis has been a topic of debate because previous reviews have reported poor reliability (Tough et al., 2007; Myburgh et al., 2008; Lucas et al., 2009). Several factors that may contribute to the varying results of reliability from these studies include lack of identification of taut bands, inexperienced examiners, incorrect positioning of the patient or the assessor, incorrect palpation techniques, variation in the manual force applied on the palpated point and the duration of force applied and use of superficial or deep muscles. In fact, a more recent review estimated an inter-rater agreement of κ: 0.452 for manual palpation of TrPs (Rathbone et al., 2017). These authors also found that localized tenderness (κ: 0.676) and pain recognition (κ: 0.575) were the most reliable criteria.

Sensory Mechanisms Associated with Trigger Points

Referred pain elicited by TrPs is a clinical manifestation of spinal cord sensitization, which is mediated by peripheral nociceptive activity and is facilitated by sympathetic overactivity or altered descending inhibition (Fernández-de-las-Peñas & Dommerholt, 2014).

There is evidence to support TrPs are a source of peripheral nociception. Pressure pain threshold testing is lower at TrPs than at control points, suggesting increased nociceptive sensitivity and peripheral sensitization (Stieven et al., 2021; de Cássia Correia Kälberer Pires et al., 2017; Sacramento et al., 2017; Fernández-Pérez et al., 2012). Shah et al. (2005, 2008) found significantly higher concentrations of pro-inflammatory chemical mediators (i.e., bradykinin, substance P, serotonin, and norepinephrine) in active TrPs compared to latent TrPs or muscle without TrPs. The presence of chemical mediators contributes to the presence of nociceptive (hyperalgesia) and non-nociceptive (allodynia) hyperalgesia at TrPs (Li et al., 2009; Wang et al., 2010). The application of dry needling reduces the presence of the pro-inflammatory mediators (Hsieh et al., 2012). Sympathetic facilitation and modulation are also involved in this process (Ge et al., 2006).

Despite a clear association between peripheral and central mechanisms for TrPs (Ge & Arendt-Nielsen, 2011), the role of either mechanism continues to be under debate (Fernández- de-las-Peñas & Dommerholt, 2014). Scientific evidence supports the hypothesis that TrPs are able to sensitize the spinal cord (Kuan et al., 2007) and the brain (Niddam, 2009). Clinically, the presence of multiple TrPs (spatial summation) or the presence of TrPs over prolonged periods of time (temporal summation) would first sensitize primary afferent nociceptors and second-order dorsal horn spinal cord neurons and, subsequently, supra-spinal structures by promoting long-lasting nociceptive afferent barrage into the central nervous system (Fernández-de-las-Peñas & Dommerholt, 2014).

Theoretical Construct for Trigger Points: The Integrated Hypothesis

There are several different proposed hypotheses for the pathogenesis of TrPs; however, their summary is beyond the scope of this chapter. Only a brief summary of the most common hypothesis will be reviewed. Although TrPs can result from different factors including repetitive muscle overuse, sustained overload, psychological stress, or unaccustomed eccentric exercise or loading, particular attention has been paid to injured or overloaded muscle fibers as the pathogenesis of TrPs (Gerwin et al., 2004).

The *integrated hypothesis* is the proposed model for explaining the pathogenesis of TrPs. This hypothesis suggests that an abnormal depolarization at the post-junctional membrane of motor endplates enhances sustained muscular contraction, giving rise to a localized hypoxic energy crisis that is associated with sensory and autonomic reflex arcs, which are perpetuated by sensitization mechanisms (Gerwin et al., 2004). The presence of endplate noise and endplate spikes (EMG signals from dysfunctional motor endplate region) in TrPs supports the belief that TrPs are associated with dysfunctional motor endplates (Simons et al., 2002). There is also growing evidence to support that muscle spindles are involved in TrP formation (Ge et al., 2009). Furthermore, Hong (1996) hypothesized that each TrP contains one sensitive (sensory component) and one active (motor component) locus where the abovementioned sensitization mechanisms and motor disturbances can be present. To date, the presence of these loci has not been confirmed.

Trigger Points in Hip and Knee Pain Conditions

Clinical examination of TrPs in patients with lower quadrant syndromes can be highly complex. There is a considerable overlap of pain referral patterns between different somatic structures in the lower quarter. Many of the muscles in the lower quarter are deep, and their palpation is difficult. Clinicians should be cautious of preconceived expectations of the location of TrPs and their referred pain patterns. Several textbooks use specifically designated regions of the muscle for didactic purposes; however, the clinician must palpate the entire muscle from origin to insertion to accurately identify for the presence of TrPs. The presence of TrPs in the lower quarter is highly prevalent. Latent TrPs in the lower extremity muscles have been found in 70% of asymptomatic subjects (Zuil-Escobar et al., 2016). In this chapter, the muscles most commonly involved in lower quadrant pain syndromes will be covered.

Psoas Major and Iliacus Muscles

The psoas major muscle is one of the main dynamic stabilizers of the lumbar spine and hip. Changes in the cross-sectional area of the hip flexors have been found to be associated with hip pain (Peiris et al., 2020). Because the lumbar plexus crosses the psoas muscle fibres, it can have an influence on the iliohypogastric, ilioinguinal, genitofemoral, femoral, lateral femoral cutaneous, and obturator nerves as well as the lumbosacral trunk when exiting on their respective sides of the muscle (Petchprapa et al., 2010). A similar situation occurs with the iliacus muscle. Therefore, taut bands in the psoas major or iliacus muscle can contribute to possible entrapments of the lumbar plexus with potential impact on the hip and knee regions. Entrapment of the femoral nerve can induce paresis of the quadriceps muscle (Lefevre et al., 2015). The pain referral pattern elicited by TrPs in the psoas major muscle may be into the groin area, superior part of the thigh and to the ipsilateral lumbar spine (Figure 17.1). Trigger points in the psoas major can also be related to movement impairment and coordination changes commonly observed in patients with hip pain. For example, Jasani et al. (2002) described nine patients with residual pain following total hip arthroplasty due to involvement of the psoas major muscle. The referred pain from the iliacus spreads to the lower abdomen, groin area and the iliac crest. One of the primary challenges of these muscles clinically is being able to identify TrPs. They are not easily accessible with palpation, especially in individuals who are overweight, contributing to low reliability of TrP identification (Hsieh et al., 2000).

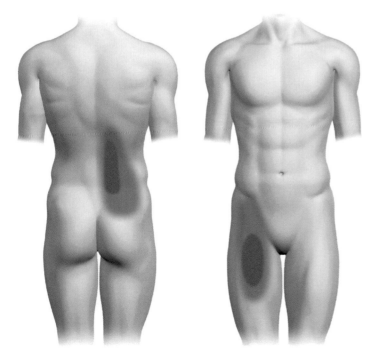

FIGURE 17.1
Referred pain elicited by trigger points in the psoas muscle.

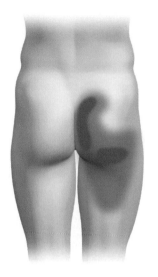
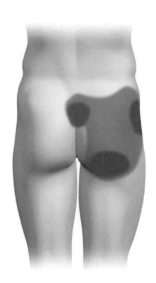
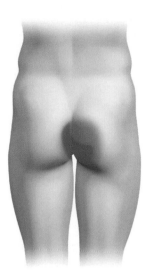

FIGURE 17.2
Referred pain elicited by trigger points in the gluteus maximus muscle.

Gluteus Maximus

The gluteus maximus is a primary extensor of the hip being assisted by the hamstring musculature. It also participates in posterior stabilization of the hip and sacroiliac joints. It has been demonstrated that the gluteus maximus exhibits atrophy in people with low back pain (Pourahmadi et al., 2020) or hip pathology (Lawrenson et al., 2019). The referred pain from this muscle typically remains in the buttock area, sacrum, sacrococcygeal region, and laterally, to the area inferior to the iliac crest (Figure 17.2). Recent studies have reported the presence of TrPs in the gluteus maximus in people with patellofemoral pain (Samani et al., 2020) and chronic pelvic pain (Fuentes-Márquez et al., 2019). Further, gluteus maximus TrPs can also contribute to complex symptoms of piriformis syndrome, also called "deep gluteal syndrome" (Fusco et al., 2018).

Gluteus Medius and Minimus Muscles

The gluteus medius muscle is a primary hip abductor and one of the main muscles responsible for lateral stabilization of the pelvis. The gluteus minimus assists the gluteus medius with hip abduction and is also a main lateral stabilizer of the hip. A meta-analysis found a decreased cross-sectional area in both muscles in individuals with hip pathology (Lawrenson et al, 2019) or low back pain (Pourahmadi et al., 2020). Additionally, deficits in the strength of these muscles are associated with the presence of patellofemoral pain syndrome (Payne et al., 2020) and low back pain (Sadler et al., 2019). It is also reported that patients with patellofemoral pain syndrome exhibit TrPs in both the affected and unaffected gluteus medius muscles (Roach et al., 2013). The inclusion of dry needling for TrPs in the gluteus medius muscle, along with an exercise program, for patients with patellofemoral pain, exhibits superior benefits compared to exercise alone (Zarei et al., 2020).

It is essential for the clinician to differentiate TrP referred pain patterns of the gluteus medius and minimus muscles. Assessment with dry needling assists the clinician in identifying TrPs in the gluteus minimus muscle as it lies deep to the gluteus medius muscle in the area where the two muscles overlap closer to the greater trochanter. Trigger points in the gluteus medius mainly refer pain to the sacroiliac joint, gluteal and lumbo-sacral regions (Figure 17.3), whereas TrPs in the gluteus minimus muscle refer pain to the iliotibial tract, gluteal region, posterior thigh, and posterior one-third of the lower leg (Figure 17.4). Samuel et al. (2007) found that active TrPs in the gluteus medius muscle were related to an L5–S1 disc prolapse. The presence of TrPs in the gluteal muscles are specific indicators for lumbar

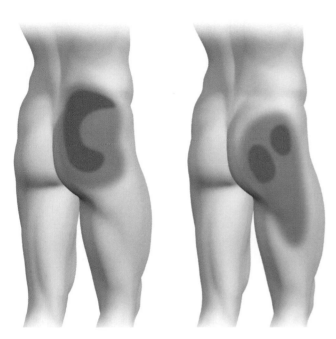

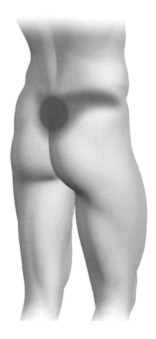

FIGURE 17.3
Referred pain elicited by trigger points in the gluteus medius muscle.

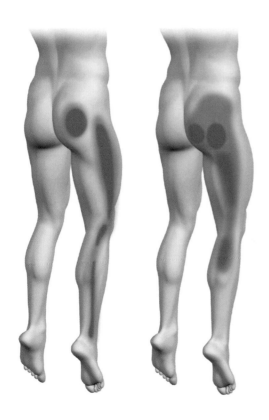

FIGURE 17.4
Referred pain elicited by trigger points in the gluteus minimus muscle.

radicular pain (Adelmanesh et al., 2016). It is possible that TrPs in this muscle group are intrinsically related to disc prolapses and the neurogenic inflammation of associated lumbar nerve rootlets or nerve roots at the related segments.

Piriformis Muscle

The piriformis muscle is a stabilizer of the sacrum and the femur. The sciatic nerve anatomically runs deep to the muscle; however, this relationship is heterogeneous (Natsis et al., 2014). Due to the variable anatomical relationship of the piriformis muscle and the sciatic nerve, TrPs and the associated taut band in this muscle may contribute to entrapment of the sciatic nerve, causing piriformis syndrome. Piriformis syndrome continues to be a controversial diagnosis for sciatic pain (Jankovic et al., 2013); however, dry needling of the piriformis muscle has been shown to be effective in individuals with this diagnosis (Tabatabaiee et al., 2019). The referred pain pattern of this muscle spreads along the proximal two-thirds of the posterior thigh and may include the sacroiliac region (Figure 17.5).

Quadriceps Musculature

The quadriceps muscle is formed by the rectus femoris, vastus medialis, vastus lateralis and vastus intermedius muscles. Its primary function is knee extension and stabilization of the patella, particularly the vastus medialis and lateralis muscles. The rectus femoris muscle also functions as a hip flexor. Active TrPs in any of these muscles may induce motor disturbances commonly observed in patients with knee pain. Active TrPs in the vastus medialis and lateralis muscles have been frequently observed in patients with knee osteoarthritis (Sánchez Romero et al., 2020), anterior knee pain (Rozenfeld et al., 2020), and following meniscectomy (Torres-Chica et al., 2015). The inclusion of dry needling of the vastus medialis muscle into a rehabilitation protocol was effective for improving range of motion and function in individuals after post-surgical reconstruction of a complete anterior cruciate ligament rupture (Velázquez-Saornil et al., 2017).

The pain referral pattern elicited by TrPs in the quadriceps muscle group includes the anterior thigh and knee area (*vastus intermedius*; Figure 17.6A), the lateral side of the thigh from the iliac crest to midportion of the lower leg (*vastus lateralis*; Figure 17.6B), and to the anterior–medial aspect of the thigh down to the medial aspect of the knee (*vastus medialis*; Figure 17.6C).

Hamstring Muscles

The hamstring muscle group is formed by the semitendinosus, semimembranosus, and biceps femoris muscles. Their primary function is knee flexion and hip extension. The sciatic nerve anatomically runs to the biceps femoris in the midportion of the thigh; therefore, taut bands on these muscles could contribute to its entrapment.

The referred pain pattern elicited by TrPs in the hamstrings is perceived as widespread posterior thigh pain (including their attachment area) and the posterior area of the knee (Figure 17.7). Patients with painful knee osteoarthritis exhibit active TrPs in the hamstring muscles

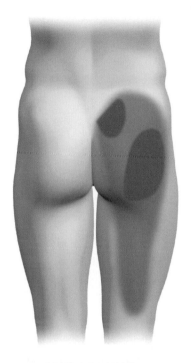

FIGURE 17.5
Referred pain elicited by trigger points in the piriformis muscle.

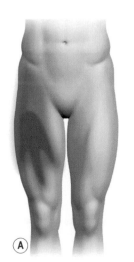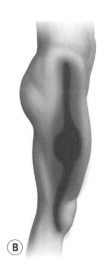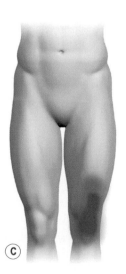

(A)   (B)   (C)

FIGURE 17.6
Referred pain elicited by trigger points in the quadriceps musculature: (A) vastus intermedius; (B) vastus lateralis; (C) vastus medialis.

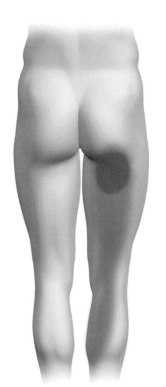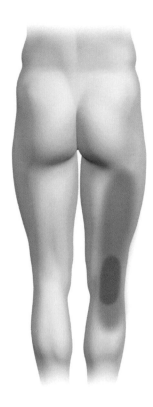

FIGURE 17.7
Referred pain elicited by trigger points in the hamstring muscles.

(Sánchez Romero et al., 2020). Additionally, manual treatment of the hamstring muscles increases muscle activity in patients with knee replacement (E Silva et al., 2018).

Adductor Muscles

The adductor musculature includes the adductor longus, adductor brevis, and adductor magnus muscles. Their main function is adduction and medial rotation of the thigh as well as hip flexion when the hip is extended. There is moderate evidence suggesting the presence of adductor musculature deficits in patients with groin pain (Kloskowska et al., 2016). The pain referral from adductor muscle TrPs extends from the femoral triangle to the knee (adductor longus and brevis; Figure 17.8A), from the pelvic floor and genitals to the internal side of the leg (adductor magnus; Figure 17.8B), and along a line within the medial aspect of the thigh (gracilis muscle; Figure 17.8C). Sánchez Romero et al. (2020) reported that TrPs in the adductor muscles were highly prevalent in individuals with painful knee osteoarthritis. Finally, since the obturator nerve merges motor and sensory branches to the adductor group muscles, this nerve

can be entrapped as it enters the thigh in the adductor canal (Craig, 2013).

Gastrocnemius and Soleus Muscles

The dynamic function of the gastrocnemius and soleus muscles is plantarflexion but it is also a stabilizer of the knee and the ankle via insertion into the Achilles tendon. The pain referral pattern from TrPs in the gastrocnemius muscle is felt deep in the lower leg, travelling along the posterior aspect of the lower leg and ankle and into the medial longitudinal arch of the foot (Figure 17.9). The soleus muscle refers pain to the distal part of the Achilles tendon and the posterior and plantar surfaces of the heel (Figure 17.10). Trigger points in the proximal part of the gastrocnemius muscles are reportedly responsible for posterior knee pain in patients after total knee replacement (Henry et al., 2012). Patients with painful knee osteoarthritis exhibit active TrPs in the gastrocnemius muscles (Sánchez Romero et al., 2020). Additionally, TrPs in these muscles can also contribute to calf pain (Grieve et al., 2013a) and can also contribute to restricted range of motion of the ankle (Grieve et al., 2011, 2013b).

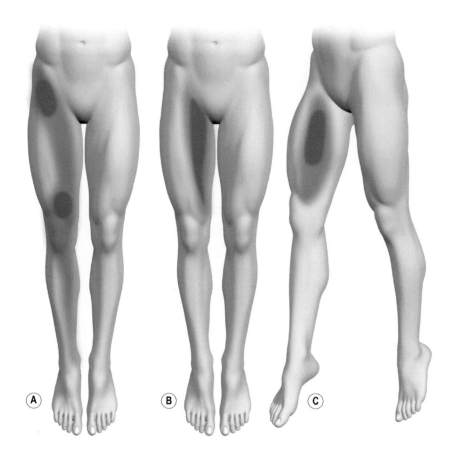

FIGURE 17.8
Referred pain elicited by trigger points in the adductor longus and brevis (A), adductor magnus (B), and gracilis (C) muscles.

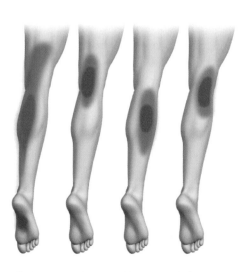

FIGURE 17.9
Referred pain elicited by trigger points in the gastrocnemius muscles.

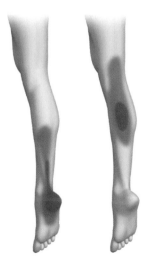

FIGURE 17.10
Referred pain elicited by trigger points in the soleus muscle.

Manual Therapy in Trigger Points: Evidence-based Approach

Clinicians can utilize several interventions for the management of TrPs, with manual therapy techniques and dry needling being the most commonly implemented (Donnelly, 2019). It is important to clarify that there is no specific "TrP manual therapy," only different manual therapy techniques for the treatment of TrPs, including TrP pressure release, soft-tissue mobilization, and stretching (Donnelly, 2019). Clinicians should select the appropriate technique based on the clinical presentation and the preference of the patient.

Current evidence supports the effectiveness of manual therapy techniques targeting TrPs for the treatment of myofascial pain in general (Wang et al., 2017), and for specific pain conditions such as primary headaches (Falsiroli Maistrello et al., 2018). In addition, Gay et al. (2013) found that muscle-biased manual therapies have a hypoalgesic effect (positive effect on pressure pain sensitivity) compared with no treatment/sham and these findings are comparable with other treatments. This hypoalgesic effect, however, does not exhibit tolerance to repetitive applications (Moraska et al., 2017). The clinical effects of manual compression are similar to the clinical effects of dry needling, at least in the cervical spine (Cagnie et al., 2015; Lew et al., 2021). Similar findings have been reported when comparing manual compression to dry needling for the management of patients with patellofemoral pain (Behrangrad et al., 2020).

Even with research supporting manual TrP techniques, it is difficult to draw firm conclusions regarding these studies since most have investigated single interventions, whereas multimodal approaches are mostly used in clinical practice. Clinical evidence supports including manual TrP release techniques into multimodal protocols for the management of several different persistent/chronic pain conditions (Jayaseelan et al., 2014; Dembowski et al., 2013; González-Iglesias et al., 2011; Segura-Pérez et al., 2017; Arias-Buría et al., 2015). This assumption is supported by a meta-analysis concluding that exercise has positive effects on pain intensity in patients with myofascial pain and that the combination of different types of exercises seems to achieve greater benefits (Mata Díz et al., 2017).

Compression Interventions

Within the literature for manual compression interventions, there are variations in the amount of pressure, duration of application, position of the muscle, and the presence or absence of pain during the intervention, with no consensus on which method is best. Hou et al. (2002) did not observe clear differences between applying a high level of pressure for shorter periods of time versus a low level of pressure for a longer period of time; both showed improvements. On the other hand, the meta-analysis by Gay et al. (2013) reported that the intensity of pressure perceived by the patient may be an important parameter for a positive effect of muscle-biased techniques.

The "ischemic compression" technique previously used for the management of TrPs has been replaced by the "pressure release" (Donnelly, 2019). This intervention was featured by a gradual increase of pressure applied to the TrP until the patient reported a moderate level of pain. The pressure is maintained until the pain is reduced. The hypothesis for that change is that no reason exists for applying an "ischemic" intervention into a TrP area which features ischemia and hypoxia. Therefore, because the TrP is already hypoxic, a pain-free technique, the "TrP pressure release technique," is currently proposed since this technique is based on pressure to tissue resistance (barrier), not on the presence of pain (Donnelly, 2019). Implementing compression manual interventions will depend on the clinical presentation of the patient. In high pain-sensitive patients (e.g., fibromyalgia), less pressure applied for a longer period of time would be more appropriate, whereas in less pain-sensitive patients (e.g., sports players), higher pressure would likely be more appropriate.

Massage/Myofascial Release/Neuromuscular Interventions

Massage, myofascial release, or neuromuscular interventions can be also applied over TrPs and surrounding tissues and fascia. Simons (2002) suggested that massage may exert a lengthening effect over a TrP. For instance, transverse strokes (Figure 17.11) provide a lengthening effect by going perpendicular to the taut band and TrP, whereas longitudinal strokes (Figure 17.12) offer a lengthening effect by following along the length of the taut band and TrP.

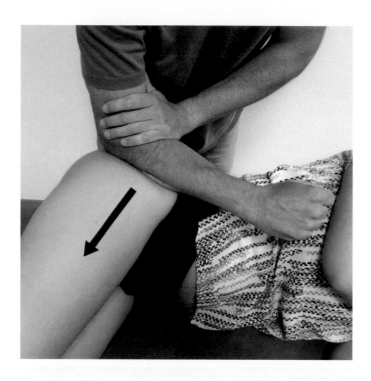

FIGURE 17.11
Transverse stroke with the elbow over the gluteus medius and minimus muscles (black arrow shows the direction of the stroke).

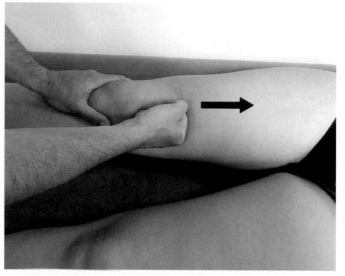

FIGURE 17.12
Longitudinal stroke with the knuckles over the vastus medialis muscle (black arrow shows the direction of the stroke).

In muscles where a pincer palpation can be applied, e.g., gastrocnemius, the therapist's fingers grasp the taut band and TrP, stroking centrifugally and elongating away from the TrP (Figure 17.13).

With any of the approaches, the most important factors to consider are the pressure and the speed of the strokes. Clinically, it is suggested that the pressure be adapted to the texture, stiffness, and character of the underlying tissue.

Stretching/Muscle Energy Interventions

There are several different methods of applying a stretching to a TrP including passive stretching (where the clinician passively stretches the muscle without the participation of the patient; Figure 17.14), active stretching (where the patient actively stretches the muscle without participation of the clinician; Figure 17.15), spray and stretch and muscle energy techniques, i.e., post-isometric relaxation (Donnelly,

2019). Despite the variety of stretching techniques, there is little evidence supporting this mode of TrP treatment. If anything, they should be used as part of a multimodal therapeutic approach, not an isolated treatment. Additionally, caution should be taken when stretching muscle tissue in individuals with hypermobility.

Dynamic Manual Therapy Interventions

Since TrPs are located within muscles responsible for contraction and movement, it may be helpful to implement dynamic interventions, which involve contraction or stretching of the affected muscle at the same time the manual technique is applied by the clinicians. Simons (2002) proposed that applying vertical or perpendicular compression over a TrP, combined with active contraction of the affected muscle, may equalize the length of the sarcomeres and consequently decrease the pain. For instance, during manual compression or a longitudinal stroke of the hamstring muscles (Figure 17.16), the patient is asked to actively contract the affected muscle. The same procedure can be applied with a muscle like the rectus femoris in a stretching position (Figure 17.17).

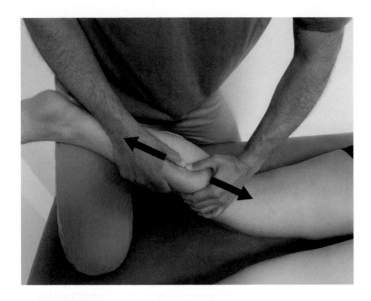

FIGURE 17.13
Longitudinal stroke with pincer palpation over the gastrocnemius muscle (black arrow shows the direction of the stroke).

Trigger Point Dry Needling: An Evidence-based Approach

Definition

The American Physical Therapy Association (APTA) defines dry needling as a "skilled intervention using a thin filiform needle to penetrate the skin that stimulates TrPs, muscles, and surrounding connective tissue for the management of musculoskeletal disorders" (APTA, 2013). Although acupuncture practitioners may refer to dry needling as "TrP acupuncture," this does not imply that dry needling would be in the exclusive domain of any healthcare discipline, and several differences, mostly in the theoretical aspects, can be found (Dommerholt & Fernández-de-las-Peñas, 2019).

Among the different needling approaches available for the management of TrPs, the technique most commonly applied consists of inserting the needle into the TrP area until local twitch responses (i.e., brief and sudden involuntary contraction of the taut band) are obtained (Dommerholt & Fernández-de-las-Peñas, 2019). Once a local twitch response is obtained, the needle is moved up and down, with no rotations, to get more local twitch responses. Clinicians should be aware of a current discussion about eliciting local twitch responses during the application of dry needling; however, this topic will be not covered in this chapter.

Clinical Reasoning for Application of Dry Needling

Clinical application of dry needling requires a thorough knowledge of the anatomy of muscles and their surrounding environment. The first step is the proper location of the TrP. In the lower extremity, most muscles are easily palpated; however, some like the psoas and piriformis are less readily palpated. Once a TrP is identified, the clinician must visualize it in a three-dimensional perspective and appreciate the depth and presence of surrounding structures, particularly those sensitive to the needle, e.g., arteries, veins, nerves, and internal organs. In the hip and knee region, the tissues at a potential risk of injury from a needle are nerves, arteries, and veins.

Before considering the application of dry needling interventions, clinicians should be aware of potential medical comorbidities and risk factors that will influence the clinical decision for dry needling appropriateness, technique, and potential adverse responses to treatment (Kearns et al., 2019). The most common adverse events usually observed after application of dry needling are pain during or after, bleeding and bruising (Brady et al., 2014). Of particular interest is post-needling soreness, a common response frequently seen in almost 60% of the patients, which is thought to be the potential consequence of the neuromuscular damage generated by the repetitive needling insertions into the muscle (Baraja-Vegas et al., 2019). In fact, intramuscular edema is observed after the application of a single session of dry needling (Baraja-Vegas et al., 2019). This minor adverse event is clinically relevant since the presence of post-needling soreness can be associated with a reluctance to receive further needling sessions by the patient, generating patient dissatisfaction, and reduction in adherence. Nevertheless, current evidence supports that this post-needling soreness disappears 48–72 hours after needling, without any intervention, suggesting that post-needling soreness may be considered as a physiological secondary effect of dry needling. Given that dry needling can induce post-needling soreness, clinicians should inform the patient of that potential event, particularly if this intervention is applied on athletes.

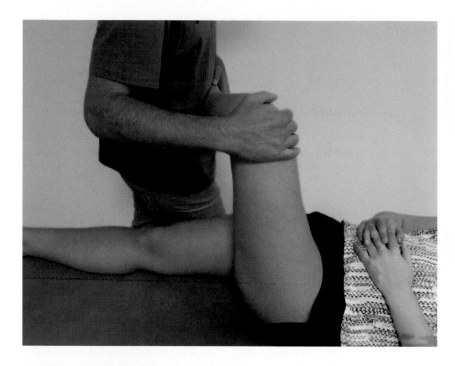

FIGURE 17.14
Passive stretching of piriformis muscle trigger point taut bands.

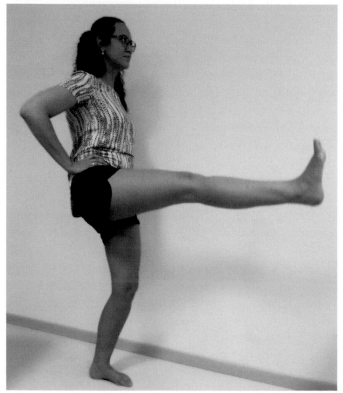

FIGURE 17.15
Active (ballistic) stretching of hamstring musculature.

Effectiveness of Dry Needling in the Hip and Knee

A review of the current literature suggests that dry needling is effective in reducing pain, but not improving function, quality of life, depression, range of motion, or strength, associated with lower quarter TrPs at short-term (Morihisa et al., 2016). These findings are also supported by a recent meta-analysis concluding that trials investigating dry needling on force production in the lower extremity did not find any significant effect (Mansfield et al., 2019). A recent meta-analysis found low to moderate evidence suggesting a positive effect of TrP dry needling on pain and related disability in patients with patellofemoral pain, but not in those with painful knee osteoarthritis or post-surgery knee pain, in the short term (Rahou-El-Bachiri et al., 2020).

The results of single clinical trials are more positive. For instance, Alaei et al. (2020) recently found that one session of dry needling is effective for decreasing hamstring tightness and increasing hamstring flexibility. Similarly, Haser et al. (2017) also reported a significant effect on muscular endurance and hip flexion range of motion in elite soccer players after the application of dry needling. These effects lasted up to 4 weeks after the intervention. Other recent clinical trials have observed positive effects of dry needling on pain and function (Ceballos-Laita

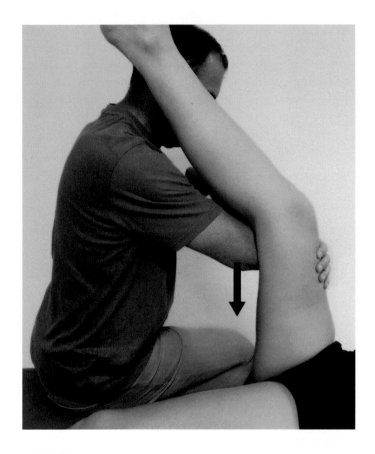

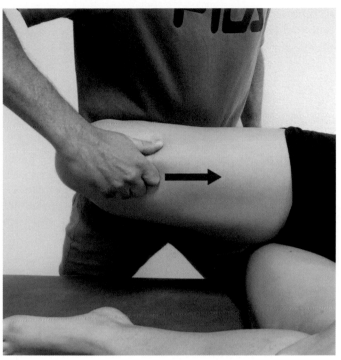

FIGURE 17.17
Dynamic longitudinal stroke of rectus femoris muscle in stretching (black arrow shows the direction of the stroke).

FIGURE 17.16
Dynamic longitudinal stroke of hamstring musculature (black arrow shows the direction of the stroke).

et al., 2019) and range of motion and muscle strength (Ceballos-Laita et al., 2021) in hip osteoarthritis patients. Interestingly, dry needling is comparable to corticoid steroid injections for improving pain and related function in patients with greater trochanteric pain syndrome (Brennan et al., 2017).

Although there is much evidence in support of dry needling, there is some evidence that its application is not always effective. For instance, the inclusion of dry needling into an exercise program for patients with painful knee osteoarthritis was not more effective than exercise alone (Sánchez-Romero et al., 2018). As a result, it is important to choose to implement dry needling not only on evidence, or lack thereof, but also the patient's symptoms, impairments, and needs.

Examples of Needling Procedures for Hip and Knee Musculature

Although the needles used are sterile, single-use and disposable, dry needling is not considered a sterile technique; therefore, the area to be needled should be visibly clean, or possibly cleaned with alcohol or soap and water. Depending on the country, there is an ongoing debate whether disinfection of the skin or the use of gloves is necessary or not (ASAP, 2007; Bachmann et al., 2014).

The length of the needle will depend on the depth of the targeted muscle. The tip of the needle is considered an extension of the clinician's hand. In fact, the clinician must have a mental representation of the area where the needle will be inserted and which structures may be encountered. Well-developed kinesthetic perception and clinical skills will permit to the clinician to appreciate change in structures (Dommerholt & Fernández-de-las-Peñas, 2019). Once removing the needling, hemostasis is usually recommended to prevent or minimize local bleeding and potential bruising. This chapter will describe the application of dry needling in some muscles.

Gluteus Medius and Minimus Muscles

The patient is positioned in side-lying position with the affected side up. The clinician will use a flat palpation/needling technique for both muscles. The needle direction is towards the pelvic bone (Figure 17.18). The most superficial muscle is the gluteus medius (15–20 mm), whereas the gluteus minimus is deeper. Strong depression of the subcutaneous tissue is essential, particularly to reach the gluteus minimus muscle. Needle contact at the periosteum is common when needling the gluteus minimus since it is deep, and also when needling the proximal portion of the gluteus medius muscle. Although needling the sciatic nerve is highly unlikely, there are deep branches of the superior gluteal vessels and superior gluteal nerve between both muscles to be aware of.

Quadriceps Muscles

The patient is positioned in supine. Each part of the quadriceps musculature can be easily needled. The vastus lateralis (Figure 17.19) and medialis (Figure 17.20) muscles are needled towards the femur. For the vastus medialis muscle, the vicinity of the saphenous nerve and popliteal artery should be considered but for the vastus lateralis muscle needling is performed without any relevant precautions.

Hamstring Muscles

The patient lies in prone with the knee slightly flexed. The biceps femoris is needled with a flat palpation technique (Figure 17.21) whereas the semimembranosus and the semitendinosus are needed with the pincer palpation technique (Figure 17.22). Clinicians should avoid the sciatic nerve by needling centrifugally from the center of the posterior part of the thigh.

Gastrocnemius Muscles

The patient lies in prone with the knee slightly flexed. The medial gastrocnemius is needled with a pincer palpation technique (Figure 17.23) and the lateral gastrocnemius is needled with a flat palpation technique (Figure 17.24). It should be noted that needling of the gastrocnemius muscles usually elicits visible and intense local twitch responses.

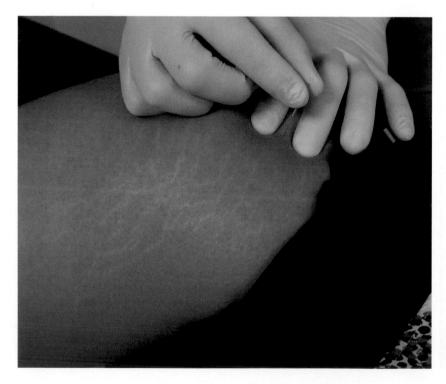

FIGURE 17.18
Dry needling of trigger points in the gluteus medius and minimus muscles.

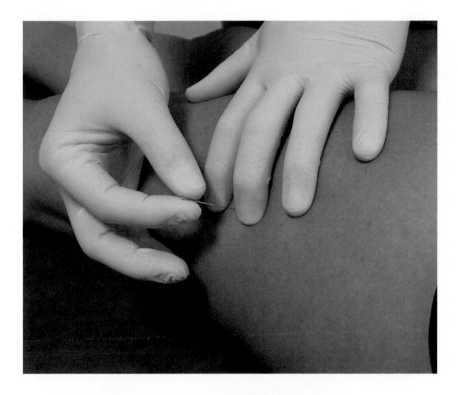

FIGURE 17.19
Dry needling of trigger points in the vastus lateralis muscle.

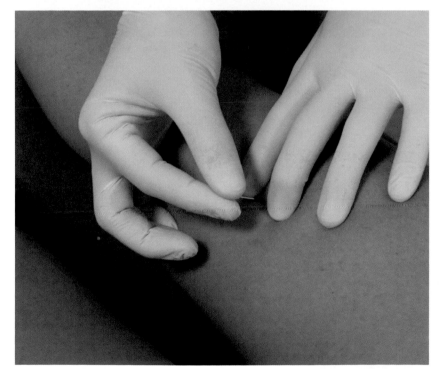

FIGURE 17.20
Dry needling of trigger points in the vastus medialis muscle.

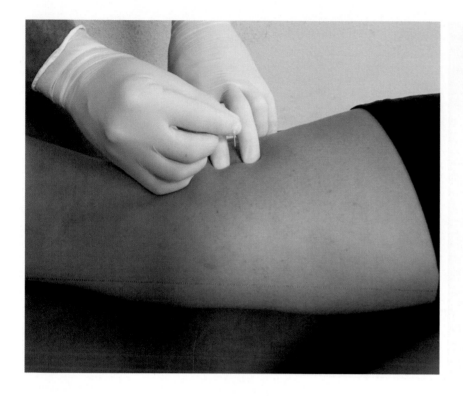

FIGURE 17.21
Dry needling (flat technique) of trigger points in the biceps femoris muscle.

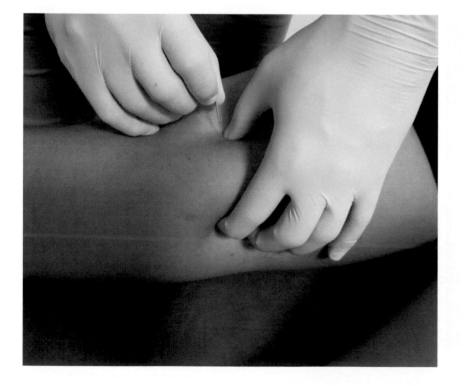

FIGURE 17.22
Dry needling (pincer technique) of trigger points in the semimembranosus and semitendinosus muscles.

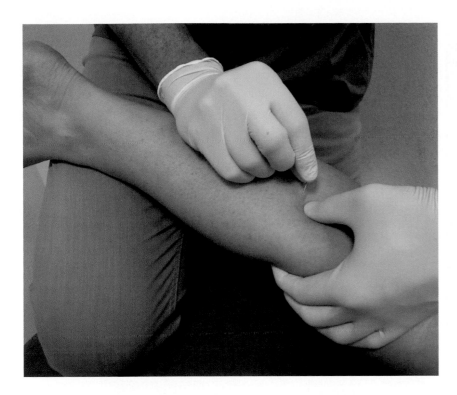

FIGURE 17.23
Dry needling (pincer technique) of trigger points in the medial gastrocnemius muscle.

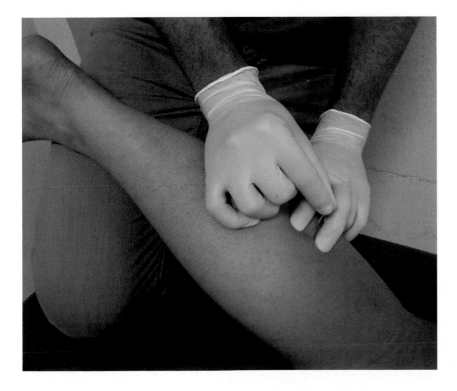

FIGURE 17.24
Dry needling (flat technique) of trigger points in the lateral gastrocnemius muscle.

A study observed that the electrical activity/intensity of subsequent local twitch responses decreases compared with the initial amplitude (Baraja-Vegas et al., 2020).

Conclusions

There are numerous muscles of the lower extremity that may present with TrPs and specific referred pain patterns that can contribute to the initiation and maintenance of symptoms in several hip and knee pain syndromes. Clinicians should examine these relevant muscles and TrPs to better characterize and manage hip and knee pain. Although much progress has been made, further studies are required to elucidate further the role of muscle TrPs in the clinical evolution of these syndromes.

References

Adelmanesh F, Jalali A, Shirvani A, et al. The diagnostic accuracy of gluteal trigger points to differentiate radicular from non- radicular low back pain. Clin J Pain. 2016;32:666–72.

Alaei P, Nakhostin Ansari N, Naghdi S, et al. Dry needling for hamstring flexibility: A single-blind randomized controlled trial. J Sport Rehabil. 2020;30(3):452–7.

Albin SR, Koppenhaver SL, MacDonald CW, et al. The effect of dry needling on gastrocnemius muscle stiffness and strength in participants with latent trigger points. J Electromyogr Kinesiol. 2020;55:102479.

Al-Shenqiti AM, Oldham JA. Test-retest reliability of myofascial trigger point detection in patients with rotator cuff tendonitis. Clin Rehabil. 2005;19:482–7.

American Physical Therapy Association (APTA). Description of dry needling in clinical practice: an educational resource paper. Alexandria, VA, USA: APTA Public Policy, Practice, and Professional Affairs Unit; 2013.

Arias-Buría JL, Valero-Alcaide R, Cleland JA, et al. Inclusion of trigger point dry needling in a multimodal physical therapy program for postoperative shoulder pain: a randomized clinical trial. J Manipulative Physiol Ther. 2015;38:179–87.

Australian Society of Acupuncture Physiotherapists (ASAP). Guidelines for safe acupuncture and dry needling practice. Australian Society of Acupuncture Physiotherapists Inc; 2007.

Bachmann S, Colla F, Gröbli C, et al. Swiss Guidelines for safe Dry Needling, Association Swiss Dry Needling Inc; 2014.

Baraja-Vegas L, Martín-Rodríguez S, Piqueras-Sanchiz F, et al. Localization of muscle edema and changes on muscle contractility after dry needling of latent trigger points in the gastrocnemius muscle. Pain Med. 2019;20:1387–94.

Baraja-Vegas L, Martín-Rodríguez S, Piqueras-Sanchiz F, et al. Electromyographic activity evolution of local twitch responses during dry needling of latent trigger points in the gastrocnemius muscle: A cross-sectional study. Pain Med. 2020;21:1224–9.

Basu S, Edgaonkar R, Baxi G, et al. Comparative study of instrument assisted soft tissue mobilisation vs ischemic compression in myofascial trigger points on upper trapezius muscle in professional badminton players. Indian J Physiother Occup Ther. 2020;14:253–8.

Behrangrad S, Abbaszadeh-Amirdehi M, Kordi Yoosefinejad A, Esmaeilnejadganji SM. Comparison of dry needling and ischaemic compression techniques on pain and function in patients with patellofemoral pain syndrome: a randomised clinical trial. Acupunct Med. 2020;38:371–9.

Brady S, McEvoy J, Dommerholt J, Doody C. Adverse events following trigger point dry needling: A prospective survey of chartered physiotherapists. J Man Manip Ther. 2014;22:134–40.

Brennan KL, Allen BC, Maldonado YM. Dry needling versus cortisone injection in the treatment of greater trochanteric pain syndrome: A noninferiority randomized clinical trial. J Orthop Sports Phys Ther. 2017;47:232–9.

Bron C, Franssen J, Wensing M, Oostendorp RAB. Interrater reliability of palpation of myofascial trigger points in three muscles. J Man Manip Ther. 2007;15:203–15.

Cagnie B, Castelein B, Pollie F, et al. Evidence for the use of ischemic compression and dry needling in the management of trigger points of the upper trapezius in patients with neck pain: A systematic review. Am J Phys Med Rehabil. 2015;94:573–83.

Ceballos-Laita L, Jiménez-Del-Barrio S, Marín-Zurdo J, et al. Effects of dry needling in hip muscles in patients with hip osteoarthritis: A randomized controlled trial. Musculoskelet Sci Pract. 2019;43:76–82.

Ceballos-Laita L, Jiménez-Del-Barrio S, Marín-Zurdo J, et al. Effectiveness of dry needling therapy on pain, hip muscle strength and physical function in patients with hip osteoarthritis: a randomized controlled trial. Arch Phys Med Rehabil. 2021;102(5):959–66.

Celik D, Yeldan I. The relationship between latent trigger point and muscle strength in healthy subjects: a double-blind study. J Back Musculoskelet Rehabil. 2011;24:251–6.

de Cássia Correia Kälberer Pires R, Salles da Rocha N, Esteves JE, Rodrigues ME. Use of pressure dynamometer in the assessment of the pressure pain threshold in trigger points in the cranio-cervical muscles in women with unilateral migraine and tension-type headache: An observational study. Int J Osteopath Med. 2017;26:28–35.

Craig A. Entrapment neuropathies of the lower extremity. PM R. 2013;5:S31–S40.

Dembowski SC, Westrick RB, Zylstra E, Johnson MR. Treatment of hamstring strain in a collegiate pole-vaulter integrating dry needling with an eccentric training program: a resident's case report. Int J Sports Phys Ther. 2013;8:328–39.

De Meulemeester KE, Castelein B, Coppieters I, et al. Comparing trigger point dry needling and manual pressure technique for the management of myofascial neck/shoulder pain: a randomized clinical trial. J Manipulative Physiol Ther. 2017;40:11–20.

Devereux F, O'Rourke B, Byrne PJ, et al. Effects of myofascial trigger point release on power and force production in the lower limb kinetic chain. J Strength Cond Res. 2019;33:2453–63.

Dommerholt J, Fernandez-de-las-Peñas C, editors. Trigger point dry needling: an evidence and clinical-based approach. 2nd ed. London: Churchill Livingstone: Elsevier; 2019.

Donnelly J, editor. Travell, Simons & Simons' Myofascial Pin and Dysfunction: The Trigger Point Manual. 3rd ed. Philadelphia: Wolters Kluwer; 2019.

E Silva DCCM, de Andrade Alexandre DJ, Silva JG. Immediate effect of myofascial release on range of motion, pain and biceps and rectus femoris muscle activity after total knee replacement. J Bodyw Mov Ther. 2018;22:930–6.

Falsiroli Maistrello L, Geri T, Gianola S, et al. Effectiveness of trigger point manual treatment on the frequency, intensity, and duration of attacks in primary headaches: A systematic review and meta-analysis of randomized controlled trials. Front Neurol. 2018;9:254.

Fernández-de-las-Peñas C, Dommerholt J. Myofascial trigger points: peripheral or central phenomenon? Curr Rheumatol Rep. 2014;16:395.

Fernández-de-las-Peñas C, Dommerholt J. International consensus on diagnostic criteria and clinical considerations of myofascial trigger points: A Delphi study. Pain Med. 2018;19:142–50.

Fernández-Pérez AM, Villaverde-Gutiérrez C, Mora-Sánchez A, et al. Muscle trigger points, pressure pain threshold, and cervical range of motion in patients with high level of disability related to acute whiplash injury. J Orthop Sports Phys Ther. 2012;42:634–41.

Fuentes-Márquez P, Valenza MC, Cabrera-Martos I, et al. Trigger points, pressure pain hyperalgesia, and mechano-sensitivity of neural tissue in women with chronic pelvic pain. Pain Med. 2019;20:5–13.

Fusco P, Di Carlo S, Scimia P, et al. Ultrasound-guided dry needling treatment of myofascial trigger points for piriformis syndrome management: A case series. J Chiropr Med. 2018;17:198–200.

Gay CW, Alappattu MJ, Coronado RA, et al. Effect of a single session of muscle-biased therapy on pain sensitivity: a systematic review and meta-analysis of randomized controlled trials. J Pain Res. 2013;6:7–22.

Ge HY, Arendt-Nielsen L. Latent myofascial trigger points. Curr Pain Head Reports. 2011;15:386–92.

Ge HY, Fernández-de-las-Penas C, Arendt-Nielsen L. Sympathetic facilitation of hyperalgesia evoked from myofascial tender and trigger points in patients with unilateral shoulder pain. Clin Neurophysiol. 2006;117:1545–50.

Ge HY, Serrao M, Andersen OK, et al. Increased H-reflex response induced by intramuscular electrical stimulation of latent myofascial trigger points. Acupunct Med. 2009;27:150–4.

Ge HY, Arendt-Nielsen L, Madeleine P. Accelerated muscle fatigability of latent myofascial trigger points in humans. Pain Med. 2012;13:957–64.

Ge HY, Monterde S, Graven-Nielsen T, Arendt-Nielsen L. Latent myofascial trigger points are associated with an increased intramuscular electromyographic activity during synergistic muscle activation. J Pain. 2014;15:181–7.

Gerwin RD, Shannon S, Hong CZ, et al. Interrater reliability in myofascial trigger point examination. Pain. 1997;69:65–73.

Gerwin RD, Dommerholt D, Shah JP. An expansion of Simons' integrated hypothesis of trigger point formation. Current Pain Head Rep. 2004;8:468–75.

González-Iglesias J, Cleland JA, del Rosario Gutierrez-Vega M, Fernández-de-las-Peñas C. Multimodal management of lateral epicondylalgia in rock climbers: a prospective case series. J Manipulative Physiol Ther. 2011;34:635–42.

Grabowski PJ, Slane LC, Thelen DG, et al. Evidence of generalized muscle stiffness in the presence of latent trigger points within infraspinatus. Arch Phys Med Rehabil. 2018;99:2257–62.

Grieve R, Clark J, Pearson E, et al. The immediate effect of soleus trigger point pressure release on restricted ankle joint dorsiflexion: A pilot randomised controlled trial. J Bodywork Mov Ther. 2011;15:42–9.

Grieve R, Barnett S, Coghill N, Cramp F. Myofascial trigger point therapy for triceps surae dysfunction: A case series. Man Ther. 2013a;18:519–25.

Grieve R, Cranston A, Henderson A, et al. The immediate effect of triceps surae myofascial trigger point therapy on restricted active ankle joint dorsiflexion in recreational runners: a crossover randomised controlled trial. J Bodyw Mov Ther. 2013b;17:453–61.

Haser C, Stöggl T, Kriner M, et al. Effect of dry needling on thigh muscle strength and hip flexion in elite soccer players. Med Sci Sports Exerc. 2017;49:378–83.

Henry R, Cahill CM, Wood G, et al. Myofascial pain in patients waitlisted for total knee arthroplasty. Pain Res Manag. 2012;17:321–7.

Hong CZ. Pathophysiology of myofascial trigger point. J Formos Med Assoc. 1996;95:93–104

Hou CR, Tsai LC, Cheng KF, et al. Immediate effects of various physical therapeutic modalities on cervical myofascial pain and trigger-point sensitivity. Arch Phys Med Rehabil. 2002;83:1406–14.

Hsieh CY, Hong CZ, Adams AH, et al. Inter-examiner reliability of the palpation of trigger points in the trunk and lower limb muscles. Arch Phys Med Rehabil. 2000;81:258–64.

Hsieh YL, Yang SA, Yang CC, Chou LW. Dry needling at myofascial trigger spots of rabbit skeletal muscles modulates the biochemicals associated with pain, inflammation, and hypoxia. Evid Complement Altern Med. 2012;2012;342165.

Ibarra JM, Ge HY, Wang C, et al. Latent myofascial trigger points are associated with an increased antagonistic muscle activity during agonist muscle contraction. J Pain. 2011;12:1282–8.

Jankovic D, Peng P, van Zundert A Brief review: piriformis syndrome: etiology, diagnosis, and management. Can J Anaesth. 2013;60:1003–12.

Jasani V, Richards P, Wynn-Jones C. Pain related to the psoas muscle after total hip replacement. J Bone Joint Surg Br. 2002;84:991–3.

Jayaseelan DJ, Moats N, Ricardo CR. Rehabilitation of proximal hamstring tendinopathy utilizing eccentric training, lumbopelvic stabilization, and trigger point dry needling: 2 case reports. J Orthop Sports Phys Ther. 2014;44:198–205.

Kisilewicz A, Janusiak M, Szafraniec R, et al. Changes in muscle stiffness of the trapezius muscle after application of ischemic compression into myofascial trigger points in professional basketball players. J Hum Kinet. 2018;64:35–45.

Kearns G, Fernández-de-las-Peñas C, Brismée JM, Gan J, Doidge J. New perspectives on dry needling following a medical model: are we screening our patients sufficiently? J Man Manip Ther. 2019;27:172–9.

Kim HA, Hwang UJ, Jung SH, et al. Comparison of shoulder strength in males with and without myofascial trigger points in the upper trapezius. Clin Biomech. 2017;49:134–8.

Kloskowska P, Morrissey D, Small C, et al. Movement patterns and muscular function before and after onset of sports-related groin pain: A systematic review with meta-analysis. Sports Med. 2016;46:1847–67.

Kuan TS, Hong CZ, Chen JT, et al. The spinal cord connections of the myofascial trigger spots. Eur J Pain. 2007;11:624–34.

Lawrenson PR, Crossley KM, Vicenzino BT, et al. Muscle size and composition in people with articular hip pathology: a systematic review with meta-analysis. Osteoarthritis Cartilage. 2019;27:181–95.

Lefevre N, Bohu Y, Klouche S, et al. Complete paralysis of the quadriceps secondary to post-traumatic iliopsoas hematoma: a systematic review. Eur J Orthop Surg Traumatol. 2015;25:39–43.

Lew J, Kim J, Nair P. Comparison of dry needling and trigger point manual therapy in patients with neck and upper back myofascial pain syndrome: a systematic review and meta-analysis. J Man Manip Ther. 2021;29(3):136–46.

Li LT, Ge HY, Yue SW, Arendt-Nielsen L. Nociceptive and non-nociceptive hypersensitivity at latent myofascial trigger points. Clin J Pain. 2009;25:132–7.

Li L, Stoop R, Clijsen R, et al. Criteria used for the diagnosis of myofascial trigger points in clinical trials on physical therapy: Updated systematic review. Clin J Pain. 2020;36:955–67.

Lucas N, Macaskill P, Irwig L, et al. Reliability of physical examination for diagnosis of myofascial trigger points: a systematic review of the literature. Clin J Pain. 2009;25:80–9.

Lucas KR, Rich PA, Polus BI. Muscle activation patterns in the scapular positioning muscles during loaded scapular plane elevation: the effects of latent myofascial trigger points. Clin Biomech. 2010;25:765–70.

Maher RM, Hayes DM, Shinohara M. Quantification of dry needling and posture effects on myofascial trigger points using ultrasound shear-wave elastography. Arch Phys Med Rehabil. 2013;94:2146–50.

Mansfield CJ, Vanetten L, Willy R, et al. The effects of needling therapies on muscle force production: A systematic review and meta-analysis. J Orthop Sports Phys Ther. 2019;49:154–70.

Mata Díz JB, de Souza J, Leopoldino A, Oliveira V. Exercise, especially combined stretching and strengthening exercise, reduces myofascial pain: A systematic review. J Physiother. 2017;63:17–22.

Moraska AF, Schmiege SJ, Mann JD, et al. Responsiveness of myofascial trigger points to single and multiple trigger point release massages: A randomized, placebo-controlled trial. Am J Phys Med Rehabil. 2017;96:639–45.

Morihisa R, Eskew J, McNamara A, Young J. Dry needling in subjects with muscular trigger points in the lower quarter: a systematic review. Int J Sports Phys Ther. 2016;11:1–14.

Myburgh C, Larsen AH, Hartvigsen J. A systematic, critical review of manual palpation for identifying myofascial triggers points: evidence and clinical significance. Arch Phys Med Rehabil. 2008;89:1169–76.

Natsis K, Totlis T, Konstantinidis GA, et al. Anatomical variations between the sciatic nerve and the piriformis muscle: a contribution to surgical anatomy in piriformis syndrome. Surg Radiol Anat. 2014;36:273–80.

Niddam DM. Brain manifestation and modulation of pain from myofascial trigger points. Curr Pain Headache Rep. 2009;13:370–5.

Oliveira-Campelo NM, de Melo CA, Alburquerque-Sendín F, Machado JP. Short- and medium-term effects of manual therapy on cervical active range of motion and pressure pain sensitivity in latent myofascial pain of the upper trapezius muscle: a randomized controlled trial. J Manipulative Physiol Ther. 2013;36:300–9.

Payne K, Payne J, Larkin T. Patellofemoral pain syndrome and pain severity is associated with asymmetry of gluteus medius muscle activation measured via ultrasound. Am J Phys Med Rehabil. 2020;99:595–601.

Peiris WL, Cicuttini FM, Constantinou M, et al. Association between hip muscle cross-sectional area and hip pain and function in individuals with mild-to-moderate hip osteoarthritis: a cross-sectional study. BMC Musculoskelet Disord. 2020;21:316.

Pérez-Bellmunt A, Simon M, López-de-Celis C, et al. Effects on neuromuscular function after ischemic compression in latent trigger points in the gastrocnemius muscles: A randomized within-participant clinical trial. J Manipulative Physiol Ther. 2021:S0161-4754(20)30156-1.

Petchprapa CN, Rosenberg ZS, Sconfienza LM, et al. MR imaging of entrapment neuropathies of the lower extremity. Part 1: The pelvis and hip. Radiographics. 2010;30:983–1000.

Pourahmadi M, Asadi M, Dommerholt J, Yeganeh A. Changes in the macroscopic morphology of hip muscles in low back pain. J Anat. 2020;236:3–20.

Rahou-El-Bachiri Y, Navarro-Santana MJ, Gómez-Chiguano GF, et al. Effects of trigger point dry needling for the management of knee pain syndromes: A systematic review and meta-analysis. J Clin Med. 2020;9:2044.

Rathbone ATL, Grosman-Rimon L, Kumbhare DA. Interrater agreement of manual palpation for identification of myofascial trigger points: A systematic review and meta-analysis. Clin J Pain. 2017;33:715–29.

Roach S, Sorenson E, Headley B, San Juan JG. Prevalence of myofascial trigger points in the hip in patellofemoral pain. Arch Phys Med Rehabil. 2013;94:522–6.

Rozenfeld E, Finestone AS, Moran U, et al. The prevalence of myofascial trigger points in hip and thigh areas in anterior knee pain patients. J Bodyw Mov Ther. 2020;24:31–8.

Sacramento LS, Camargo PR, Siqueira-Júnior AL, et al. Presence of latent myofascial trigger points and determination of pressure pain thresholds of the shoulder girdle in healthy children and young adults: A cross-sectional study. J Manipulative Physiol Therap. 2017;40:31–40.

Sadler S, Cassidy S, Peterson B, et al. Gluteus medius muscle function in people with and without low back pain: a systematic review. BMC Musculoskelet Disord. 2019;20:463.

Samani M, Ghaffarinejad F, Abolahrari-Shirazi S, et al. Prevalence and sensitivity of trigger points in lumbo-pelvic-hip muscles in patients with patellofemoral pain syndrome. J Bodyw Mov Ther. 2020;24:126–30

Samuel S, Peter A, Ramanathan K. The association of active trigger points with lumbar disc lesions. J Musculoskeletal Pain. 2007;15:11–18.

Sánchez-Infante J, Bravo-Sánchez A, Jiménez F, Abián-Vicén J. Effects of dry needling on muscle stiffness in latent myofascial trigger points: A randomized controlled trial. J Pain. 2021:S1526-5900(21)00024-9.

Sánchez-Romero EA, Pecos-Martín D, Calvo-Lobo C, et al. Effects of dry needling in an exercise program for older adults with knee osteoarthritis: A pilot clinical trial. Medicine. 2018;97:e11255.

Sánchez Romero EA, Fernández Carnero J, Villafañe JH, et al. Prevalence of myofascial trigger points in patients with mild to moderate painful knee osteoarthritis: A secondary analysis. J Clin Med. 2020;9:2561.

Segura-Pérez M, Hernández-Criado MT, Calvo-Lobo C, et al. A Multimodal Approach for Myofascial Pain Syndrome: A Prospective Study. J Manipulative Physiol Ther. 2017;40:397–403.

Shah JP, Phillips TM, Danoff JV, Gerber LH. An in vitro microanalytical technique for measuring the local biochemical milieu of human skeletal muscle. J Applied Physiol. 2005;99:1977–84.

Shah JP, Danoff JV, Desai MJ, et al. Biochemicals associated with pain and inflammation are elevated in sites near to and remote from active myofascial trigger points. Arch Phys Med Rehabil. 2008;89:16–23.

Simons D, Travell J, Simons P. Travell & Simons' Myofascial Pain & Dysfunction: The Trigger Point Manual: The Upper Half of Body. Baltimore: Williams & Wilkins; 1999.

Simons DG. Understanding effective treatments of myofascial trigger points. J Bodyw Mov Ther. 2002;6:81–8.

Simons D, Hong CZ, Simons L. Endplate potentials are common to midfiber myofascial trigger points. Am J Phys Med Rehabil. 2002;81:212–22.

Stieven FF, Ferreira GE, de Araújo FX, et al. Immediate effects of dry needling and myofascial release on local and widespread pressure pain threshold in individuals with active upper trapezius trigger points: A randomized clinical trial. J Manipulative Physiol Ther. 2021;44:95–102.

Tabatabaiee A, Takamjani IE, Sarrafzadeh J, et al. Ultrasound-guided dry needling decreases pain in patients with piriformis syndrome. Muscle Nerve. 2019;60:558–65.

Torres-Chica B, Núñez-Samper-Pizarroso C, Ortega-Santiago R, et al. Trigger points and pressure pain hypersensitivity in people with post-meniscectomy pain. Clin J Pain. 2015;31:265–72.

Tough EA, Write AR, Richards SS, Campbell J. Variability of criteria used to diagnose myofascial trigger point pain syndrome: evidence from a review of the literature. Clin J Pain. 2007;23:278–86.

Treede RD, Rief W, Barke A, et al. Chronic pain as a symptom or a disease: the IASP Classification of Chronic Pain for the International Classification of Diseases (ICD-11). Pain. 2019;160:19–27.

Velázquez-Saornil J, Ruíz-Ruíz B, Rodríguez-Sanz D, et al. Efficacy of quadriceps vastus medialis dry needling in a rehabilitation protocol after surgical reconstruction of complete anterior cruciate ligament rupture. Medicine. 2017;96:e6726.

Wang YH, Ding X, Zhang Y, et al. Ischemic compression block attenuates mechanical hyperalgesia evoked from latent myofascial trigger point. Exp Brain Res. 2010;202:265–7.

Wang R, Li X, Zhou S, et al. Manual acupuncture for myofascial pain syndrome: a systematic review and meta-analysis. Acupunct Med. 2017;35:241–50.

Zarei H, Bervis S, Piroozi S, Motealleh A. Added value of gluteus medius and quadratus lumborum dry needling in improving knee pain and function in female athletes with patellofemoral pain syndrome: A randomized clinical trial. Arch Phys Med Rehabil. 2020;101:265–74.

Zuil-Escobar JC, Martínez-Cepa CB, Martín-Urrialde JA, Gómez-Conesa A. The prevalence of latent trigger points in lower limb muscles in asymptomatic subjects. PM R. 2016;8:1055–64.

Clinical neurodynamics in the lower quadrant

18

Emilio "Louie" Puentedura, Brenton Grant, Georgina Grant

Introduction to Clinical Neurodynamics

Orthopedic Manual Physical Therapy (OMPT) is defined by the International Federation of Orthopedic Manipulative Physical Therapists (IFOMPT) as a specialized area of physical therapy for the management of neuromusculoskeletal conditions, based on clinical reasoning, using highly specific treatment approaches including manual techniques and therapeutic exercises (IFOMPT, 2021). This definition was voted on at the IFOMPT General Meeting in Cape Town in March of 2004. Before then, Maitland (1986) defined it as the selective examination and evaluation of the effects of movement, position and activities on the signs and symptoms of a neuromusculoskeletal disorder. It has always been seen as a useful approach to examine, evaluate, and treat movement problems affecting the neuromusculoskeletal system. We should think of the mechanics of the body's moving parts in terms of components comprising a chassis (skeletal framework), articulations (joints and supporting ligaments), motor (muscles and tendons), and electrical wiring (nervous system). We should also appreciate that each of the components that make up the neuromusculoskeletal system plays an important and interdependent role in its overall health and function.

In the early manual therapy systems of the 1960s and 1970s, greater emphasis was placed on the health and function of the articulations (joints), and hence, "manual therapy" became synonymous with "passive joint mobilization" and "joint manipulation" (Butler, 1991). Relatively little attention was paid to the physical health and movement of the nervous system, until the advent of published works by Grieve (1991), Breig (1978), Maitland (1986), Elvey (1986, 1997), and Butler (1991). Their seminal work opened a new frontier in manual therapy – the hypothesis that the entire nervous system is a mechanical organ that could develop "adverse tension," or impaired mobility, which could then be treated with various movement therapies. However, the concept of mobilizing the nervous system was initially met with some significant skepticism by other health professions (DiFabio, 2001). We now understand this was primarily because of the focus on the mechanical "stiffness" within the nervous system, which at the time, suggested it required aggressive stretching. The use of the term "tension" had significant limitations because it failed to consider other aspects of nervous system function, such as movement, pressure, viscoelasticity, and physiology (Shacklock, 1999, 2005a). A more appropriate term, "neurodynamics" was first proposed by Shacklock (2005a).

Neurodynamics refer to the mechanics and physiology of the nervous system within the musculoskeletal system and how these systems relate to each other (Shacklock, 1995). This considers the movement-related neurophysiological changes as well as the neuronal dynamics that are postulated to occur in the central nervous system (CNS) during physical and mental activity. A key tenet of neurodynamics is that the nervous system is capable of movement and stretch, and that there is a "normal" response (as well as abnormal) of the nervous system to movement, compression and stretch. The transition from "neural tension" to "neurodynamic" placed less emphasis on "stretching" and "tension" and more emphasis on the nervous system, the "container" in which it lives, and the various physiological mechanisms that can alter the function of the nervous system. These other mechanisms include changes to intraneural blood flow (Ogata & Naito, 1986); neural inflammation (Zochodne & Ho, 1991); mechano-sensitivity (Calvin et al., 1982); and muscle responses (Hall et al., 1998; van der Heide et al., 2001).

Neurodynamic impairments should really be conceptualized as any specific physical dysfunction (whether it be neural, muscular, or skeletal) which, it is presumed, will physically challenge the normal functioning of the nervous system. These impairments can arise from mechanical, chemical or sensitivity changes in the neuromusculoskeletal system.

Operating Definitions

In order to further facilitate understanding for the rest of this chapter, some operational definitions are provided.

Clinical Neurodynamics: This can be defined as the examination, evaluation and treatment of the mechanics and physiology of the nervous system as they relate to each other and are integrated with musculoskeletal function (Shacklock, 1995).

Neurodynamic Test: The testing procedures used in clinical neurodynamics. These can be defined as a series of body movements that produces mechanical and physiological events in the nervous system according to the movements of the test. A neurodynamic test aims to physically challenge or test the mechanics and/or physiology of a part of the nervous system.

Neurogenic Pain: Pain that is initiated or caused by a primary lesion, dysfunction, or transitory perturbation in the peripheral or central nervous system (Merskey & Bogduk, 1994).

Sensitizing Movements: Movements that increase forces in the neural structures in addition to those movements employed in the standard neurodynamic test. Sensitizing movements can be useful in loading or moving the nervous system beyond the effects of the standard neurodynamic test, i.e., strengthening the test. However, they also load and move musculoskeletal structures and are therefore not as helpful in determining the existence of a neurodynamic problem as a differentiating movement.

Differentiating Movements: Movements that emphasize or isolate the nervous system by producing movement in the neural structures in the area in question rather than moving the musculoskeletal structures in the same area. Differentiating movements place emphasis on the nervous system without affecting the other structures and are therefore used to help establish the existence of a neurodynamic problem. An example of a differentiating movement for a patient with calf pain would be the addition of cervical extension.

Sliders: Neurodynamic maneuvers performed in order to produce a sliding movement of neural structures relative to their adjacent tissues (Coppieters & Butler, 2008). Sliders involve the application of movement/stress to the nervous system proximally while releasing movement/stress distally and then reversing the sequence. Sliders allow larger ranges of motion, provide a means of distraction from the painful area, and should provide multi-tissue, non-painful, and, hopefully, fear-reducing novel inputs into the CNS. Research has shown that sliders actually result in greater excursion than simply stretching the nerve (Coppieters & Butler, 2008).

Tensioners: Neurodynamic maneuvers performed in order to produce an increase in tension (not stretch) in neural structures which may improve neural viscoelastic and physiological functions, i.e., help neural tissue cope better with increased tension (Coppieters & Butler, 2008). Tensioners are the opposite of sliders in that movement/stress is applied proximally and distally to the nervous system at the same time, and then released.

Neurophysiology of Neurodynamics

As previously stated, manual therapists were initially more focused on the mechanical aspects of neurodynamics, and unfortunately it led to a rather "mechanistic" view of the nervous system. Most textbooks describe normal nerve mechanics related to various positions, postures or movements, subsequent abnormal mechanics (patho-mechanics) and, finally, movement-based treatment aimed at restoring normal nerve movement. None of this should be disputed. However, increased understanding of nerve pain related to neurophysiological changes and the processing in the brain of nerve movement (and pain) warrants investigation and discussion.

Pathologies that affect peripheral nerves usually result in dysesthetic pain and/or nerve trunk pain (Asbury & Fields, 1984). Dysesthetic pain, as an unpleasant abnormal sensation, whether spontaneous or evoked (where light touch causes pain), often manifests as burning or tingling pain due to abnormal impulses from hyperexcitable afferent nerve fibers, which, due to injury, may become abnormal impulse generating sites (AIGS) (Devor et al., 1979; Woolf & Mannion, 1999; Asbury & Fields, 1984). AIGS may spontaneously fire as the result of mechanical or chemical stimuli such that dysesthetic pain may present as very bizarre patterns. This can be from bursts of pain in response to a stimulus, to pain that presents spontaneously with no apparent stimulus.

In contrast, nerve trunk pain commonly presents as deep, achy pain arising from nociceptors within nervous tissue that is sensitized to mechanical or chemical stimuli (Asbury & Fields, 1984; Kallakuri et al., 1998). Nerve trunk pain usually has a fairly straightforward stimulus-response relationship (Asbury & Fields, 1984). These 2 types of pain can be evoked by a variety of chemical and/or mechanical stimuli and may lead to allodynia or hyperalgesia. Allodynia is a pain sensation due to a stimulus that does not normally provoke pain, while hyperalgesia is an exaggerated pain response to stimuli that would normally be painful (Asbury & Fields, 1984; Woolf & Mannion, 1999; Nee & Butler, 2006).

Nerve Sensitivity

In order to understand nerve sensitivity, knowledge of ion channels is required. Although the complexity of ion channel regulation is not yet properly understood and the research is based on animal studies, scientists and clinicians are using the information known about ion channels to improve patient care (Barry, 1991; Louw et al., 2016). Ion channels are essentially proteins clumped together with an opening – to allow ions to flow in/out of the axon membrane (axolemma) (Devor, 2006). They are synthesized within the axon's cell body (perikaryon) based on genetic coding and are distributed along an axon to allow ions to flow in/out of the nerve to polarize and/or depolarize the membrane. Ion channels are not uniformly distributed along the axolemma with certain areas known to have higher concentrations of ion channels, such as the dorsal root ganglion (DRG), axon hillock, nodes of Ranvier and areas where the axon has lost myelin (Devor et al., 1993; Devor, 1999, 2006). Furthermore, there are countless types of ion channels, including channels that seem to respond to movement, pressure, blood flow, temperature, circulating adrenaline levels, etc. From the survival perspective, it makes sense for the nervous system to change its "sensitivity" to varying stimuli. However, the amount and type of ion channels found in the axolemma are in a constant state of change (Devor et al., 1993; Devor, 2006). Research has shown that the half-life of some ion channels may be as short as two days (Barry, 1991), and ion channels that drop out of the membrane are not necessarily replaced by the same type. Ion channel deposition is thought to be directly impacted by the environment the organism finds itself in (Barry, 1991). For example, changes in temperature around an animal with experimentally removed myelin produce higher concentrations of "cold-sensing" channels in that area; animals in stressful environments produce higher concentrations of adreno-sensitive channels, and animals that have joints with restricted movement cause upregulation of movement-sensitive ion channels (Devor et al., 1993; Devor, 2006). With higher concentrations of similar ion channels in an area, the chances of the nerve depolarizing, causing an action potential, increase. In other words, the

nerve may develop an AIGS. The nervous system can then become sensitive to various types of stimuli, such as temperature, movement, pressure, anxiety, stress, the immune system modulators, and more (Louw & Puentedura, 2013; Louw et al., 2016). The nervous system can therefore be viewed as an alarm system beautifully designed to protect the organism, and the amount and type of ion channels at any given time may be a fair representation of what the brain computes is needed for survival (Louw & Puentedura, 2013; Louw et al., 2016).

Central Nervous System processing in Neurodynamic Tests

Clinicians are familiar with the term "central sensitization" or "nociplastic pain." Central sensitization is defined as a condition in which peripheral noxious input into the CNS leads to an increased excitability where the response to normal inputs is greatly enhanced (Woolf, 2007). Repeated nociceptive stimuli, such as easily excitable AIGS, may cause low-threshold neurons with large receptive fields to depolarize in response to stimuli that would normally be benign (Woolf, 2007). It has been shown that injured neural tissue may alter its chemical makeup and reorganize synaptic contacts in the CNS such that innocuous stimuli are directed to cells that normally receive only noxious inputs (Woolf, 2007). Hence, the CNS becomes "hyperexcitable" due to a combination of decreased inhibition and increased responsiveness (facilitation) (Woolf, 2007). This is analogous to turning up the volume on the system such that innocuous stimuli begin to generate painful sensations while noxious stimuli result in an exaggerated pain response. Woolf (2000) described this process as a change in both the software and the hardware of the CNS, and the argument has been made that clinicians have the tools to impact both of these.

Clinical Neurobiomechanics in the Lower Extremity

Neurobiomechanics is the study of the normal and pathological range of motion of the nervous system. What we know is based upon increasing human research, as well as animal and cadaver studies. A key issue in the understanding of neurobiomechanics is the concept of the nervous system being considered as a continuous tissue tract.

The system is continuous mechanically via its continuous connective tissue formats, electrically via conducted impulses and, chemically via its common neurotransmitters. The nervous system being a mechanical continuum is probably most relevant to the study of neurodynamics because it implies transmission of movement (sliding/gliding) and the development of tension (stretching) within and along the system. That is, ankle dorsiflexion and knee extension lengthen and move the tibial component of the sciatic nerve distally within its neural pathway, and hip flexion adds a pull in the proximal direction. This was classically demonstrated in cadaveric studies in which the nerve roots were marked with paper markers or pins (Breig, 1978).

Another key concept in neurodynamics is that of the mechanical interface. The mechanical interface is defined as the tissue or material adjacent to the nervous system that can move independently of the system. Mechanical interfaces are central to an understanding of neurodynamics because they represent the most likely sites for the development of movement/force transmission problems. Mechanical interfaces can be hard or bony (e.g., common fibular nerve at the head of the fibula); ligamentous (tibial collateral ligament at the ankle); joints (e.g., ankle); or muscular (e.g., soleus in the leg). Mechanical interfaces can be normal, where movement and function are optimal and symptom-free, or they can be pathological, where something happens to restrict movement of the nervous system at the interface or compress the nervous tissue. Examples would include osteophytes, extensive bruising, or swelling which could occupy space at the mechanical interface resulting in restricted range of motion and independence of the nervous system and the interface. Numerous studies have shown that if the interface is injured or damaged, it may have repercussions for adjacent neural tissues. Examples include the intervertebral foramen (Choi, 2019; Zhao et al., 2020), spinal canal (Fritz et al., 1998; Park et al., 2013) and piriformis (Vij et al., 2021). If this happens, the range of motion of the nervous system can be impaired, and this would then lead to an abnormal mechanical response with neurodynamic examination.

As the nervous system winds its way through its anatomical course, it will be forced to stretch, slide (longitudinal or transverse), bend, and become compressed. We can define stretch here as the elongation of the nerve relative to its starting length. However, nerves are not solid structures and stretch causes internal compression due to displacement of nerve tissue/fluid. The physiological effects of stretch and compression include changes to intraneural blood flow, conduction and axoplasmic transport. Several studies have shown that if a peripheral nerve is held on an 8% stretch for 30 minutes, it will cause a 50% decrease in blood flow; 8.8% stretch for 1 hour will cause 70% decrease in blood flow and 15% stretch for 30 minutes will cause 80%–100% blockage in blood flow (Ogata & Naito, 1986; Gilbert et al., 2015). Research by Breig (1978), Breig and Marions (1963), Breig and el-Nadi (1966), and Breig and Troup (1979) has demonstrated that flexion of the cervical spine leads to tension in the dura and spinal cord, resulting in a cephalad movement of the cauda equina. This ultimately limits the available mobility of the sciatic nerve. Obviously, there must be some mechanical and physiological adaptations within peripheral nerves to accommodate such significant changes in length and to cope with prolonged stretching or strain. The effects of compression have also been studied with as little as 20–30 mmHg causing decreased venous blood flow and 80 mmHg causing complete blockage of intraneural blood flow (Ogata & Naito, 1986; Rydevik et al., 1981). Compression is also shown to alter axonal transport (Dahlin et al., 1993) and action potential conduction (Fern & Harrison, 1994).

Nerves can be seen to move relative to their adjacent tissues, and this motion has been described as sliding or excursion (Dilley et al., 2003; Wilgis & Murphy, 1986). Excursion occurs both longitudinally and transversely. This sliding or excursion is considered an essential aspect of neural function because it serves to dissipate tension and distribute forces within the nervous system. Instead of stretching (and thereby developing tension) the nervous system can move longitudinally and/or transversely and distribute itself along the shortest course between fixed points, and hence, it can equalize tension throughout the neural tract.

As joints move, there is nerve bed elongation (increase in length of the neural container) on the convex side of the joint, and nerve bed shortening (decrease in length of the neural container) on the concave side of the joint. When there is nerve bed elongation, the nerve glides towards the joint that is moving, and this is referred to as convergence. When there is nerve bed shortening, the nerve glides away from the joint that is moving, and this is referred to as divergence. Alshami et al. (2021) used real-time ultrasound to examine the effects of ankle dorsiflexion on the magnitude of excursion of the sciatic nerve in six positions of the neck, hip, and knee. They found that distal sciatic nerve excursion was significantly greater in positions in which the knee was extended (median 0.7–1.6 mm) compared to when the knee was flexed (median 0.5–1.4 mm) (Alshami et al., 2021).

Silva et al. (2014) conducted a systematic review of the quantitative *in vivo* longitudinal nerve excursion and strain in response to joint movements. The review included 12 studies but only 3 involved lower extremity nerves: tibial nerve (n = 1), sciatic nerve (n = 1) or both tibial and sciatic nerves (n = 1). They found absolute values of 0.7–5.2 mm for tibial nerve excursion and 0.1–3.5 mm for sciatic nerve excursion (Silva et al., 2014). They also found that the starting position and the sequencing of limb movement during neurodynamic tests affect the degree of excursion along the nerve.

Coppieters et al. (2006) examined the clinical hypothesis that strain in the nerves around the ankle and foot caused by ankle dorsiflexion can be further increased with hip flexion during the straight leg raise (SLR). They inserted linear displacement transducers into the sciatic, tibial, and plantar nerves of 8 embalmed cadavers to measure strain, and a digital caliper to measure distal excursion of the nerves during this modified SLR. They found that ankle dorsiflexion resulted in a significant strain and distal excursion of the tibial nerve. Similarly, Bueno-Gracia et al. (2019b) used linear displacement transducers and digital calipers to investigate the mechanical behavior of the sciatic nerve and biceps femoris muscle in the proximal thigh with ankle dorsiflexion at different degrees of hip flexion during the SLR in 11 cadaver lower extremities. They found that ankle dorsiflexion at different degrees of hip flexion during the SLR produced changes in the strain and excursion of the sciatic nerve in the upper thigh, whereas the biceps femoris muscle at the same location was not affected by ankle movement (Bueno-Gracia et al., 2019b).

The sequence of movements has also been shown to affect the distribution of symptoms in response to neurodynamic testing (Montaner-Cuello et al., 2020; Bueno-Gracia et al., 2019a, 2021; Coppieters et al., 2015). These authors reported a greater likelihood of producing a response that is localized to the region that is moved first or more strongly during a neurodynamic maneuver.

The Base Tests for the Lower Extremity

Butler (1991) proposed a base test system for neurodynamic evaluations. It was a clinically intuitive system that evolved for ease of handling and to fulfill a perceived clinical demand. It was based on existing tests and the basic principles of neurodynamics already discussed, and in most clinical situations, the tests can be refined or adapted based upon reasoned diagnoses and the clinical presentation of the patient with back and lower extremity symptoms. A *positive* neurodynamic test is one that reproduces a familiar symptom; is changed by the movement of a body segment away from the site of symptoms; there are differences in the test response from side to side; or what is known to be normal in asymptomatic individuals (Nee & Butler, 2006; Shacklock, 2005b). While a positive test does not identify a specific area of injury, it is suggestive of increased mechano-sensitivity somewhere along the neural tissue tract (Shacklock, 2005b; Nee & Butler, 2006).

The tests for the back and lower extremity include the SLR; the seated slump test; long-sit slump test; prone knee bend and the side-lying slump. Wherever possible, it is recommended that neurodynamic tests be performed actively before passively. This allows the therapist to gauge the patient's ability and willingness to move and provides an approximate measure of the range of motion likely to be encountered during the passive test. It may also decrease the patient's fears and anxieties about the test and symptoms likely to be elicited. Finally, if the active movement is found to be extremely sensitive, a reasoned decision may be made not to perform the tests passively in order to avoid symptom exacerbation.

Some important handling issues with respect to the performance of the lower extremity neurodynamic tests include:

- Only perform them if you have a clinical rationale for doing so. Establish clinical reasoning hypotheses prior to the test regarding pathobiology, likely specific dysfunctions to be found on examination, precautions, and sources of symptoms.

- Explain to the patient exactly what you are going to do and what you want them to do. It is vital to have the patient comfortable about reporting any responses to testing, anywhere in their body.

- Perform the test on the less painful side or non-painful side first. If there is little difference between sides, perform the test on the left side first for consistency.

- Starting positions should be consistent each time, and any variations from normal practice should be noted/recorded (use of pillows, etc.).

- Note symptom responses including area and nature (type of response) with the addition of each component of the test.

- Watch for antalgic postures and other compensatory movements during the tests (e.g., cervical movements or hamstring muscle activity).

- Test for symmetry between sides.

- Explain your findings to your patient.

- Repeat the test gently a number of times before recording an actual measurement.

Straight Leg Raise Active Test

If the patient has described a symptom-provoking position or movement, have them demonstrate it for you and observe the mechanics involved. If possible, perform a quick structural differentiation. For example, the patient may report low back and posterior thigh symptoms when kicking their leg forward. Have them demonstrate the symptomatic position for their back and thigh pain, maintain that position, then ask them to move their neck to see if that alters their back and thigh symptoms.

A simple protocol for the active evaluation of the SLR test might be to have the patient walk or swing their affected leg. Alternatively, the patient could lie supine and actively elevate their leg while keeping their knee extended.

Straight Leg Raise Passive Test

Description

This test is performed with the patient in supine, with arms by the side, and the tested side close to the edge of the exam-ination table, without a pillow if possible, and with body straight. The therapist stands on the side to be tested facing the patient and then places one hand under the ankle and the other hand above the patella. Keeping the knee extended, the therapist should flex the hip in the perpendicular plane (avoiding hip abduction or adduction; Figure 18.1) The patient's leg should be taken short of, to, or into sensory or motor responses depending on clinical reasoning.

Structural Differentiation

The final component of the test (structural differentiation) may often be overlooked by clinicians. If distal symptoms have been reported (e.g., calf or heel), the patient can be asked to flex, or an assistant could passively flex the cervical spine and any change in the distal symptoms would

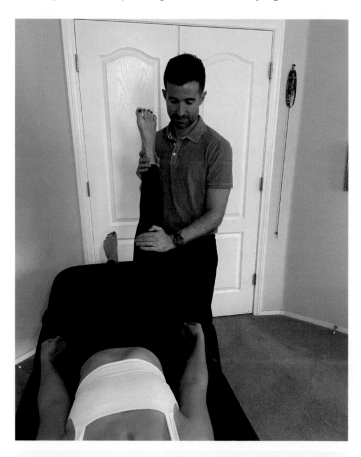

FIGURE 18.1
Straight leg raise passive test with hip flexion and knee extension.

constitute a positive structural differentiation. If proximal symptoms have been reported (e.g., buttock or posterior thigh), the ankle may be dorsiflexed and, again, any change in the proximal symptoms will constitute a positive structural differentiation.

Sensitizing Movements

Frequently used sensitizing movements include hip adduction and/or hip medial rotation (which are thought to lengthen the sciatic nerve as it exists the sciatic foramen), ankle dorsiflexion (which is thought to lengthen the tibial and plantar nerves; Figure 18.2) and ankle plantarflexion with inversion (which is thought to lengthen the superficial fibular nerve; Figure 18.3). However, there is little evidence

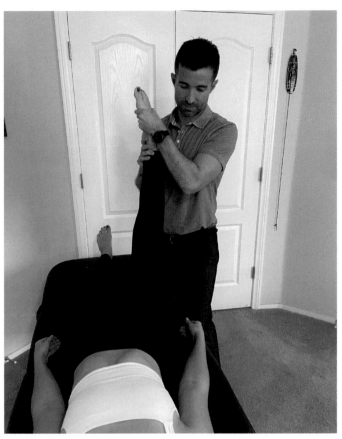

FIGURE 18.3
Straight leg raise passive test with hip flexion and knee extension including ankle plantarflexion with inversion for the superficial fibular nerve.

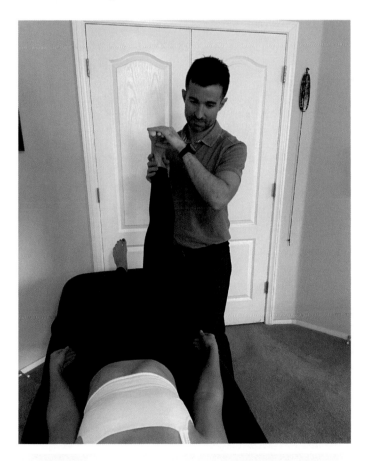

FIGURE 18.2
Straight leg raise passive test with hip flexion and knee extension including ankle dorsiflexion for the tibial and plantar nerves.

that these sensitizing movements create any greater tension or stress on the peripheral nerves that they target.

Expected Responses

A pattern of frequently reported and observed responses includes posterior thigh, posterior knee and posterior calf symptoms extending to the foot (Herrington et al., 2008). These responses may indicate neural mechano-sensitivity and result in protective muscle contraction of the hamstrings. In a recent review, Weppler and Magnusson (2010) suggested that observed changes in tissue flexibility following hamstring stretching may result, not from affecting the mechanical properties of the muscle being stretched, but from changes in the individual's perception of stretch or pain.

Indications for the SLR

A therapist would consider using the SLR test in the clinic where, after detailed subjective evaluation, objective examination and evaluation, there is a hypothesis of neurogenic pain in the lower limb, or that the source of the disorder lies in the sciatic nerve pathways and receptive fields. Alternatively, the patient may have indicated a pain-provoking movement or position that is similar to the test (e.g., kicking a football).

Seated Slump Active Test

A simple protocol for the active evaluation of the seated slump test is to have the patient sit comfortably over the edge of the treatment table with thighs well supported. Checking for symptom reproduction with each active movement component, ask them to: (1) slouch their back and round their shoulders; (2) move their chin to their chest; (3) straighten their knee on their affected side, if possible; (4) dorsiflex their ankle if they were able to achieve full knee extension; and (5) lift their head back up to neutral and see if symptoms are changed.

This can be done on the unaffected side first, if necessary; however, as this is an active movement test, the patient can decide how far to take each movement component based on the symptoms that may or may not be provoked.

Seated Slump Passive Test

Description

This test can be considered as a SLR test in a seated position, so that head, neck, and trunk movements can be added to load tissues further and increase input into the central nervous system. The test components should be performed actively with instruction from the therapist, and if necessary, some components may be performed passively. The patient should start by sitting up straight with thighs well supported and ankles uncrossed (Figure 18.4). Hands behind the back are not absolutely necessary, but this may help with the consistency of test performance. The patient is then asked to slump or "sag in the middle back" while still looking forward (Figure 18.5). This is the first component of the test and should be performed without cervical motion to assess symptom response, if any. The second

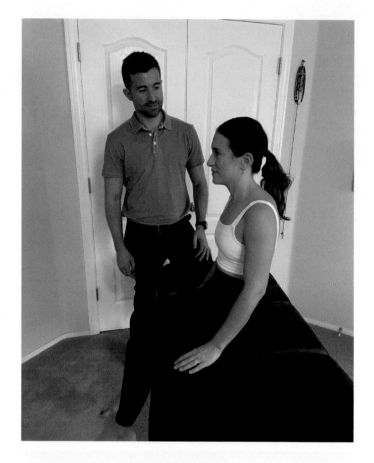

FIGURE 18.4
Seated slump passive test. Initial position with the patient sitting up straight with thighs well supported and ankles uncrossed.

component is cervical flexion, and the patient should be asked to move as far into their range as possible (Figure 18.6). The response, if any, is assessed. No overpressure needs to be applied but the therapist can place their forearm along the upper thoracic spine and hand behind the patient's head to monitor for antalgic movement out of cervical flexion and trunk flexion with further test components. Now the patient is asked to extend the knee (on the less- or non-painful side first) and again, the symptom response is assessed (Figure 18.7).

Structural Differentiation

If distal symptoms have been reported (e.g., calf or heel), the patient can be asked to lift their head back up (release

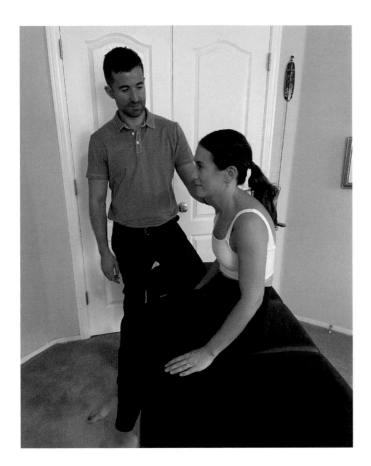

FIGURE 18.5
Seated slump passive test. The patient is asked to slump or "sag in the middle back" while still looking forward.

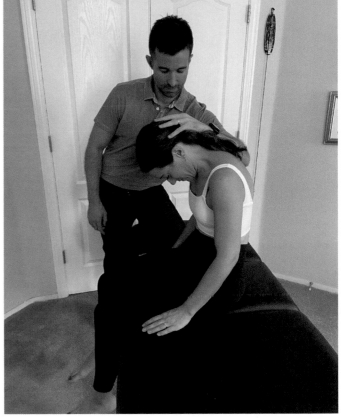

FIGURE 18.6
Seated slump passive test. The patient is asked to flex the cervical spine at her end-range of motion. The therapist can fix this position.

cervical flexion) (Figure 18.8) and any change in the distal symptoms would constitute a positive structural differentiation. If proximal symptoms have been reported (e.g., back or buttock), the test can be repeated with ankle dorsiflexion prior to the knee extension, and release of the ankle dorsiflexion causing any change in the proximal symptoms will constitute a positive structural differentiation.

Sensitizing Movements

The slump test may be sensitized by the addition of foot and ankle dorsiflexion, hip flexion and performing the test with the other leg already extended. The order of movements can also be varied to suit clinical reasoning.

Expected Responses

In most cases, patients may report central T8–T9 area symptoms when cervical flexion is added; they will be unable to fully extend their knee owing to symptoms in the posterior thigh, and knee symptoms will ease when the cervical spine is extended. Walsh et al. (2007) examined the normative sensory responses to the slump test in 84 asymptomatic subjects and recorded the prevalence, intensity, location, and nature of responses at each stage of the test – slumped sitting; knee extension; ankle dorsiflexion; and cervical extension. They found 97.6% of the subjects reported a sensory response, and prevalence of responses increased significantly from 29.8% at slump sitting to 94% at knee extension, and decreased significantly from

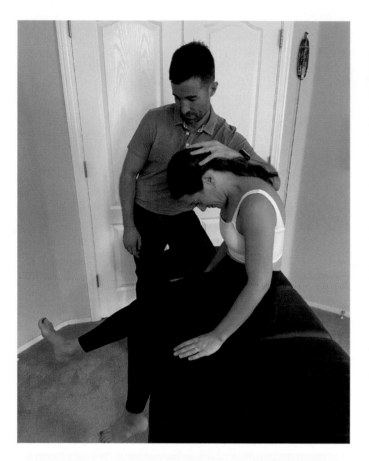

FIGURE 18.7
Seated slump passive test. The patient is asked to extend the knee.

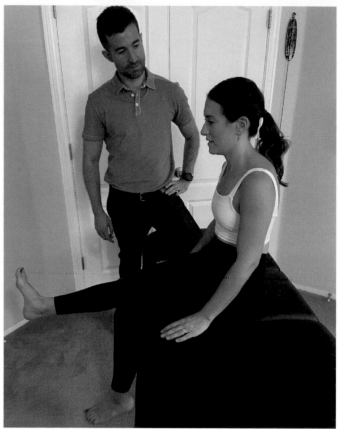

FIGURE 18.8
Seated slump passive test. The patient can be asked to lift their head back up (release cervical flexion) if distal symptoms in the lower extremity appear.

97.6% at ankle dorsiflexion to 65.5% at cervical extension (Walsh et al., 2007). Median intensity of responses increased significantly from 0/10 at slump sitting, through 4/10 at knee extension, to 6/10 at ankle dorsiflexion, and then decreased significantly to 2/10 at cervical extension (Walsh et al., 2007). Location of responses were at the back or neck during slump sitting, and then with subsequent movements, responses were located most commonly in the posterior thigh, knee, and calf (Walsh et al., 2007). The most common descriptors for the sensory responses were "stretch," "tight," and "pull" (Walsh et al., 2007).

Indications for the Seated Slump

A therapist would consider using the seated slump test in the clinic where, after detailed subjective evaluation, objective examination and evaluation, there is a hypothesis of lumbar nerve root impingement or irritation causing neurogenic pain in the lower limb. The seated slump test has been found to be more sensitive (0.84) than the SLR (0.52) in patients with lumbar disc herniations, and therefore a negative slump test can effectively rule out a lumbar disc herniation (Majlesi et al., 2008).

Side-lying Slump Test

Description

The side-lying slump test can be considered an extension of the prone knee bend (PKB) test. In the PKB test, the patient is prone close to the side of the treatment table and is asked

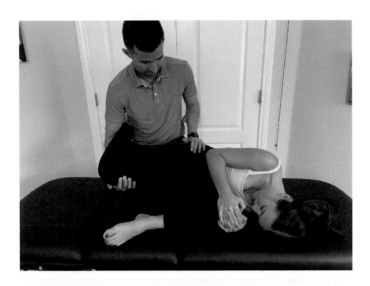

FIGURE 18.9
Side-lying slump test. The therapist stands behind the patient and flexes the superior side knee so that the patient's ankle is resting on the therapist's hip and places a hand under the knee to support the leg.

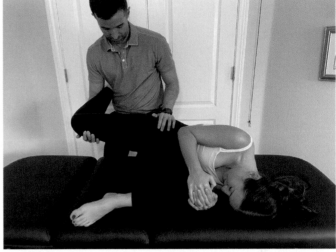

FIGURE 18.10
Side-lying slump test. The therapist stabilizing the pelvis with the other hand introduces hip extension.

to flex the knee actively without flexing the hip. Some studies have reported a positive PKB in the presence of upper lumbar disc herniation (Asquier et al., 1996; Kreitz et al., 1996); however, the test is limited by the inability to differentiate symptom responses structurally. By placing the patient in side-lying and performing the side-lying slump test (or femoral slump test), additional loading can be placed on the PKB by spinal flexion. The patient is asked to hold the knee on the side on which they are lying and is encouraged to touch it with the forehead to prompt cervical flexion. The therapist stands behind the patient and flexes the other knee so that the patient's ankle is resting on the therapist's hip and places a hand under the knee to support the leg (Figure 18.9). The therapist then stabilizes the pelvis with the other hand and introduces hip extension to the point of evoked symptoms (Figure 18.10). If that position is held, the therapist can then assess symptom response to changes in head and neck movements (cervical extension) (Figure 18.11).

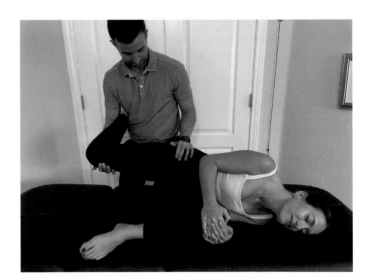

FIGURE 18.11
Side-lying slump test. Cervical extension to decrease neural tension.

Structural Differentiation

If anterior thigh symptoms have been reported, the patient can be asked to extend their cervical spine and any change in the thigh symptoms would constitute a positive structural differentiation.

Sensitizing Movements

The side-lying slump test is purported to examine the neurodynamics of the peripheral nerve pathways in the anterior, medial, and lateral thigh region, as well as the saphenous nerve which passes anteriorly below the knee. Therefore, the test may be sensitized by the addition of knee flexion and hip extension with the thigh in the sagittal plane for the femoral nerve. In an *in vivo* study using ultrasound imaging, Sierra-Silvestre et al. (2018) recorded femoral nerve excursion in the proximal thigh/groin region of 30 asymptomatic subjects. Scans were taken during knee flexion in supine and in a semi-seated position, and during cervical flexion in side-lying slump. They reported significantly greater longitudinal excursion (sliding) of the femoral nerve with knee flexion in supine (mean: 3.6 ± 2.0 mm) compared to sitting (mean: 1.1 ± 1.3 mm) (Sierra-Silvestre et al., 2018). Cervical flexion in side-lying did not result in longitudinal excursion (mean: 0.0 ± 0.3 mm), but there was medial excursion (mean: 1.1 ± 0.5 mm) (Sierra-Silvestre et al., 2018). Clinicians may introduce hip adduction to target the lateral femoral cutaneous nerve (Figure 18.12), and hip abduction to target the obturator nerve (Figure 18.13), but there does not appear to be any biomechanical or anatomical studies to confirm this.

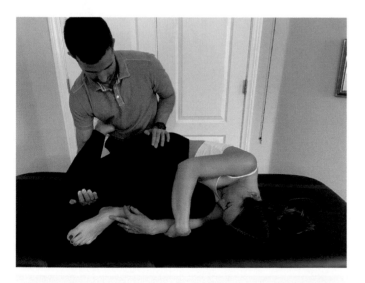

FIGURE 18.12
Side-lying slump test. The therapist can introduce hip adduction to target the lateral femoral cutaneous nerve.

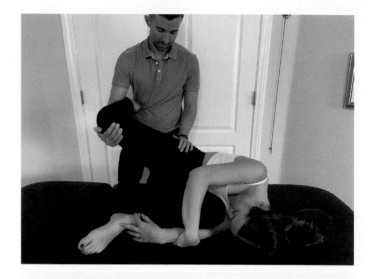

FIGURE 18.13
Side-lying slump test. The therapist can introduce hip abduction to target the obturator nerve.

Expected Responses

The side-lying slump test was performed in trunk slump and neutral positions, with cervical extension used as the structural differentiation in 32 asymptomatic subjects (16 females) (Lai et al., 2012). Hip extension angle and visual analog scale (VAS) of thigh pain was measured during the test, and results showed the decrease of nerve tension significantly increased hip extension range of motion and lowered pain intensity (Lai et al., 2012).

Indications for the Side-lying Slump

A therapist would consider using the side-lying slump test in the clinic where, after detailed subjective evaluation, objective examination and evaluation, there is a hypothesis of neurogenic pain in the anterior thigh, or upper/mid lumbar nerve root compression (Trainor & Pinnington, 2011). Good inter-tester reliability was found for the side-lying slump test (kappa coefficient: 0.71) in 4 patients with mid lumbar nerve root compression confirmed with magnetic resonance imaging (MRI) (Trainor & Pinnington, 2011). In a cross-sectional pilot study of 12 patients with unilateral patellofemoral pain syndrome (PFPS), Vegstein et al. (2019) compared the PKB test and side-lying slump test to detect increased levels of mechano-sensitivity in the leg with PFPS. They reported that both tests provoked stronger responses in the leg with PFPS compared to the asymptomatic leg (Vegstein et al., 2019). However, because of the small sample size, they could not determine the reliability of the tests.

Clinical Application of Neurodynamics in Low Back and Lower Extremity Pain

It is important to remember that healthy mechanics of the nervous system within the back and lower extremities enables pain-free posture and movement. In the presence of mechanical impairment (patho-mechanics) of neural tissues, e.g., nerve entrapment, symptoms may be provoked during activities of daily living such as bending down to reach the floor. The aim of using neurodynamic tests in assessment is to stimulate mechanically by moving neural tissues in order to gain an impression of their mobility and sensitivity to mechanical stresses. The purpose of treatment via these tests is to improve mechanical and physiological function (Shacklock, 2005a).

Mechanosensitivity is the chief mechanism that enables nerves to elicit nociception for pain to be experienced with movement. If a nerve is not mechanically sensitive, then it will not respond (provide nociception) to mechanical forces applied to it. Mechanosensitivity can be defined as the ease with which impulses can be activated from a site in the nervous system when a mechanical force is applied. Normal nerves can be mechanosensitive (given sufficient force) and therefore, respond to applied forces (Rosenblueth et al., 1953; Julian & Goldman, 1962; Lee et al., 2005; Lindquist et al., 1973). This is a key fact to keep in mind when making judgments about whether the neural tissues within the back and lower limb contribute to the problem. Responses to neurodynamic tests in the lower limb are either *normal* or *abnormal*, and then either *relevant* or *irrelevant* (Shacklock, 2005b). *Normal* neurodynamic test responses would be considered those that are in a normal location (relative to normative data), normal quality of symptoms, and normal range of movement for the lower limb. *Abnormal* neurodynamic test responses would be considered those that are in a different location than normal, different quality of symptoms and/or range of movement of the limb is less than the uninvolved side. In most cases, there may be a reproduction of the patient's symptoms. The next clinical question to

consider would be whether the test responses are *relevant* or *irrelevant*. Relevance, in this case, would mean that the test responses are causally related to the patient's current problem. In most cases, this can be clarified by asking the patient, "is that a familiar symptom to you?" The symptoms evoked on a neurodynamic test can be inferred to be neurogenic (positive test in a clinical sense):

1. if structural differentiation supports a neurogenic source

2. if there are differences left to right, and to known normal responses

3. if the test reproduces the patient's symptoms or associated symptoms

4. if there is support from other data such as history, area of symptoms, imaging tests, etc.

The greater the number of the above items present, the stronger the case for a clinically *relevant* test finding or result. Clinically, the information required from neurodynamic tests is symptom response, the resistance encountered and changes to symptom response and resistance encountered as each component of the test is added or subtracted. This information, along with the patient history, subjective and objective examination, etc., should give the clinician the ability to provisionally diagnose the site of neuropathodynamics and then re-assess after whichever treatment might be administered. It is important to realize that the treatment need not be a mobilizing technique for the nervous system, as the clinician may decide to mobilize or treat the mechanical interface, or perhaps he/she may decide the problem is not peripheral neurogenic in nature but rather a "central processing enhancement" in which patient neuroscience education/reassurance may be the treatment of choice. It is also important to remember that sensitivity to a neurodynamic test could be from a combination of primary (tissue-based) or secondary (CNS-based) processes (Butler, 2000).

Treatment

A recent meta-analysis of 13 animal and 5 human studies found evidence that joint and nerve mobilizations positively influence various neuroimmune responses (Lutke Schipholt et al., 2021). Also, Maxwell et al. (2020) conducted a systematic review of the effects of spinal manipulative therapy on lower limb neurodynamic test outcomes in adults. They found limited evidence to suggest spinal manipulative therapy improved range of motion during neurodynamic tests and was more effective than some other interventions (Maxwell et al., 2020). In a randomized controlled trial involving 60 participants with nerve-related leg pain, Ferreira et al. (2016) found that adding neurodynamic treatment to advice to remain active did not improve leg pain and disability at 2 weeks. However, Hall et al. (2017) disputed the reporting by Ferreira et al. (2016) and noted that there was indeed a significantly larger improvement for leg pain, back pain, function and global perceived effect in favor of neurodynamic treatment at 4 weeks (as well as function and global perceived effect immediately after treatment). Hall et al. (2017) believed that these were valuable outcomes that should have been reported but were not.

Kurt et al. (2020), in a prospective randomized clinical trial, randomized 41 patients with low back pain to either neurodynamic mobilization or electrotherapy. They found both groups demonstrated a significant decrease in pain and functional disability, whereas only the neurodynamic mobilization group showed a significant increase in SLR range (Kurt et al., 2020).

Plaza-Manzano et al. (2020) found that the addition of neurodynamic mobilization to a motor control exercise program led to reductions in neuropathic symptoms and mechanical sensitivity (SLR) but did not result in greater changes in pain, related disability, or pressure pain threshold over motor control exercises program alone in subjects with lumbar radiculopathy.

Finally, Rade et al. (2017) reported that displacement or excursion of the conus medullaris on the symptomatic side was significantly reduced in 15 patients with sciatic symptoms due to subacute lumbar disc herniation. In a follow-on study, Pesonen et al. (2019) reported on a controlled radiologic study to determine whether changes in spinal cord displacement with the SLR test at 1.5-year follow-up were accompanied by changes in clinical symptoms. Fourteen patients with sciatic symptoms due to a subacute single-level posterolateral lumbar disc herniation were reassessed clinically and radiologically at 1.5 years follow-up with a 1.5T MRI scanner. Displacement of the conus medullaris during the unilateral and bilateral SLR was quantified reliably with a randomized procedure and compared between SLR tests and to data from baseline. When compared to baseline

values, their data showed a significant increase in neural sliding, and particularly of 2.52 mm (p ≤0.001) with the symptomatic SLR (Pesonen et al., 2019). They noted the increase in neural sliding correlated significantly with a decrease in both radicular symptoms and LBP. Multivariate regression models confirmed the improvement of neural sliding effects as the main variable associated with the improvement of clinical symptoms (Pesonen et al., 2019).

A review of the available evidence supports the use of neurodynamic assessment and treatment in some individuals with back and lower extremity impairments. With any neurodynamic treatments, reassessment should be continual, and include clinical evaluation along with patient feedback. Patient education is paramount, and should include a brief discussion of neurodynamics, the neurobiology of pain and the continuity of the nervous system. Additionally, if there is a central sensitization component to the symptoms, this should also be addressed, along with any perceived or real fear of movement the patient may have. This can reduce the threat value associated with their pain experience.

Next, clinicians have found it useful to treat any impairment in non-neural tissues so as to reduce any mechanical forces the "container" may be placed on the nervous tissue. Interventions utilized may include joint mobilization/ manipulation, stretching, soft-tissue work and therapeutic exercise. A detailed discussion of these interventions is beyond the scope of this chapter. Any of the above interventions, if utilized, should be followed by a reassessment of the provocative neurodynamic test to determine if a change has occurred. If change occurs, treatment may be discontinued for that day, or specific neurodynamic interventions (either active or passive) may be added to the treatment.

It is clinically useful to break neurodynamic treatments down into one of two approaches, "sliders" or "tensioners," each of which has its own indications and clinical usefulness (Nee & Butler, 2006; Coppieters & Butler, 2008). With a sliding or gliding technique, combined movements of at least 2 joints are alternated in such a way that one movement elongates the nerve bed while the other movement shortens the nerve bed. This results in the nerve being mobilized through a large degree of longitudinal excursion with a minimum amount of tension. These techniques should be non-provocative and may be more tolerable to patients than tensioning techniques.

Castellote-Caballero et al. (2013) completed a pilot study on the effects of a neurodynamic sliding technique on hamstring flexibility in healthy male soccer players with decreased hamstring muscle flexibility. Compared to a no intervention control group, there was a significant improvement in hamstring flexibility for the neurodynamic sliding group (Castellote-Caballero et al., 2013). A year later, Castellote-Caballero et al. (2014) conducted a randomized double-blinded controlled trial involving 120 subjects with short hamstring syndrome randomized to 1 of 3 groups: neurodynamic sliding, hamstring stretching, and placebo control. Each subject's dominant leg was measured for SLR range of motion before and after interventions. They reported that the neurodynamic sliding technique increased hamstring flexibility to a greater degree than static hamstring stretching and no stretching (control) in healthy subjects with short hamstring syndrome (Castellote-Caballero et al., 2014).

With a tensioning technique, elongation of the nerve bed is obtained by moving one or several joints such that the "tension" within the nerve is elevated (Coppieters & Butler, 2008). These techniques are, by nature, more stressful to the neural tissue and should be used with caution as they may irritate the patient with neural mechano-sensitivity. They should not be static stretches and should always involve gentle oscillations into and out of resistance. These techniques are generally indicated for patients who experience symptoms as a result of impairments in the neural tissue's ability to elongate, hence the goal is to restore the physical capabilities of the neural tissue to tolerate movement.

The tension is increased to the point of a mild stretching sensation, or, in the case of non-irritable patients, may be taken to the onset of mild symptoms at the end of the oscillation. Any of the active or passive neurodynamic tests can be used as "tensioners." Sets and repetitions should be determined by the irritability of the patients as well as the response (positive or negative) to the interventions. Finally, techniques aimed at non-neural structures can be combined with neurodynamic interventions, such as graded lumbar rotation mobilization techniques, lower extremity distraction mobilizations or prone extensions.

Conclusion

Clinicians should keep in mind the underlying principles of neurobiomechanics; that is, the nervous system is a continuous tract that is subject to slide, glide, bend, and stretch as it travels through its mechanical interface. Symptoms can arise as a result of intrinsic or extrinsic impairments anywhere along this tortuous course. Clinicians can render meaningful interventions that have a direct impact on the space, movement, and blood supply for the nervous system in addition to producing beneficial neurophysiological effects. Neurodynamic interventions (either passive or active) should involve smooth, controlled, gentle, and large amplitude movements. Sustained stretching is rarely indicated. Finally, it is important to mention, neurodynamic interventions are but a small part of the overall patient-centered treatment approach that encompasses multiple interventions.

References

Alshami AM, Alshammari TK, Almuhaish MI, et al. Sciatic nerve excursion during neural mobilization with ankle movement using dynamic ultrasound imaging: a cross-sectional study. J Ultrasound. 2021, doi: 10.1007/s40477-021-00595-7.

Asbury AK, Fields HL. Pain due to peripheral nerve damage: an hypothesis. Neurology. 1984;34:1587–90.

Asquier C, Troussier B, Chirossel JP, et al. Femoral neuralgia due to degenerative spinal disease. A retrospective clinical and radio-anatomical study of one hundred cases. Rev Rhum Engl Ed. 1996;63:278–84.

Barry SR. Clinical implications of basic neuroscience research. I: Protein kinases, ionic channels, and genes. Arch Phys Med Rehabil. 1991;72:998–1008.

Breig A. Adverse Mechanical Tension in the Central Nervous System: An Analysis of Cause and Effect: Relief by Functional Neurosurgery. Wiley; 1978.

Breig A, Marions O. Biomechanics of the lumbosacral nerve roots. Acta Radiol Diagn. 1963;1:1141–60.

Breig A, El-Nadi AF. Biomechanics of the cervical spinal cord. Relief of contact pressure on and overstretching of the spinal cord. Acta Radiol Diagn. 1966;4:602–24.

Breig A, Troup JD. Biomechanical considerations in the straight-leg-raising test. Cadaveric and clinical studies of the effects of medial hip rotation. Spine. 1979;4:242–50.

Bueno-Gracia E, Malo-Urries M, Borrella-Andres S, et al. Neurodynamic test of the peroneal nerve: Study of the normal response in asymptomatic subjects. Musculoskelet Sci Pract. 2019a;43:117-21.

Bueno-Gracia E, Perez-Bellmunt A, Estebanez-de-Miguel E, et al. Differential movement of the sciatic nerve and hamstrings during the straight leg raise with ankle dorsiflexion: Implications for diagnosis of neural aspect to hamstring disorders. Musculoskelet Sci Pract. 2019b;43:91–5.

Bueno-Gracia E, Malo-Urries M, Montaner-Cuello A, et al. Normal response to tibial neurodynamic test in asymptomatic subjects. J Back Musculoskelet Rehabil. 2021;34:243–9.

Butler DS. Mobilisation of the Nervous System. Melbourne: Churchill Livingstone; 1991.

Butler DS. The Sensitive Nervous System. Adelaide: Noigroup; 2000.

Calvin WH, Devor M, Howe JF. Can neuralgias arise from minor demyelination? Spontaneous firing, mechanosensitivity, and afterdischarge from conducting axons. Exp Neurol. 1982;75:755–63.

Castellote-Caballero Y, Valenza MC, Martin-Martin L, et al. Effects of a neurodynamic sliding technique on hamstring flexibility in healthy male soccer players. A pilot study. Phys Ther Sport. 2013;14:156–62.

Castellote-Caballero Y, Valenza MC, Puentedura EJ, et al. Immediate effects of neurodynamic sliding versus muscle stretching on hamstring flexibility in subjects with short hamstring syndrome. J Sports Med. 2014;2014:127471.

Choi YK. Lumbar foraminal neuropathy: an update on non-surgical management. Korean J Pain. 2019;32:147–59.

Coppieters MW, Alshami AM, Babri AS, et al. Strain and excursion of the sciatic, tibial, and plantar nerves during a modified straight leg raising test. J Orthop Res. 2006;24:1883–9.

Coppieters MW, Butler DS. Do 'sliders' slide and 'tensioners' tension? An analysis of neurodynamic techniques and considerations regarding their application. Man Ther. 2008;13:213–21.

Coppieters MW, Crooke JL, Lawrenson PR, et al. A modified straight leg raise test to differentiate between sural nerve pathology and Achilles tendinopathy. A cross-sectional cadaver study. Man Ther. 2015;20:587–91.

Dahlin LB, Archer DR, Mclean WG. Axonal transport and morphological changes following nerve compression. An experimental study in the rabbit vagus nerve. J Hand Surg Br. 1993;18:106-10.

Devor M. Unexplained peculiarities of the dorsal root ganglion. Pain. 1999;S6:S27–S35.

Devor M. Sodium channels and mechanisms of neuropathic pain. J Pain. 2006;7:S3–S12.

Devor M, Schonfeld D, Seltzer Z, Wall PD. Two modes of cutaneous reinnervation following peripheral nerve injury. J Comp Neurol. 1979;185:211–20.

Devor M, Govrin-Lippmann R, Angelides K. Na+ channel immunolocalization in peripheral mammalian axons and changes following nerve injury and neuroma formation. J Neurosci. 1993;13:1976–92.

Difabio RP. Neural mobilization: the impossible. J Orthop Sports Phys Ther. 2001;31:224–5.

Dilley A, Lynn B, Greening J, Deleon N. Quantitative in vivo studies of median nerve sliding in response to wrist, elbow, shoulder and neck movements. Clin Biomech. 2003;18:899-907.

Elvey RL. Treatment of arm pain associated with abnormal brachial plexus tension. Aust J Physiother. 1986;32:225–30.

Elvey RL. Physical evaluation of the peripheral nervous system in disorders of pain and dysfunction. J Hand Ther. 1997;10:122–9.

Fern R, Harrison PJ. The contribution of ischaemia and deformation to the conduction block generated by compression of the cat sciatic nerve. Exp Physiol. 1994;79:583–92.

Ferreira G, Stieven F, Araujo F, et al. Neurodynamic treatment did not improve pain and disability at two weeks in patients with chronic nerve-related leg pain: a randomised trial. J Physiother. 2016;62:197–202.

Fritz JM, Delitto A, Welch WC, Erhard RE. Lumbar spinal stenosis: a review of current concepts in evaluation, management, and outcome measurements. Arch Phys Med Rehabil. 1998;79:700–8.

Gilbert KK, Roger James C, Apte G, et al. Effects of simulated neural mobilization on fluid movement in cadaveric peripheral nerve sections: implications for the treatment of neuropathic pain and dysfunction. J Man Manip Ther. 2015;23:219–25.

Grieve GP. Mobilisation of the Spine: A Primary Handbook of Clinical Method. University of Michigan, Churchill Livingstone; 1991.

Hall T, Zusman M, Elvey R. Adverse mechanical tension in the nervous system? Analysis of straight leg raise. Man Ther. 1998;3:140–6.

Hall T, Coppieters MW, Nee R, et al. Neurodynamic treatment improves leg pain, back pain, function and global perceived effect at 4 weeks in patients with chronic nerve-related leg pain. J Physiother. 2017;63:59.

Herrington L, Bendix K, Cornwell C, et al. What is the normal response to structural differentiation within the slump and straight leg raise tests? Man Ther. 2008;13:289–94.

IFOMT. OMPT Definition [Online access]. 2021. Available: https://www.ifompt.org/About+IFOMPT/OMPT+Definition.html

Julian FJ, Goldman DE. The effects of mechanical stimulation on some electrical properties of axons. J Gen Physiol. 1962;46:297–313.

Kallakuri S, Cavanaugh JM, Blagoev DC. An immunohistochemical study of innervation of lumbar spinal dura and longitudinal ligaments. Spine. 1998;23:403–11.

Kreitz BG, Cote P, Yong-Hing, K. Crossed femoral stretching test. A case report. Spine. 1996;21:1584–6.

Kurt V, Aras O, Buker N. Comparison of conservative treatment with and without neural mobilization for patients with low back pain: A prospective, randomized clinical trial. J Back Musculoskelet Rehabil. 2020;33:969–75.

Lai WH, Shih YF, Lin PL, et al. Normal neurodynamic responses of the femoral slump test. Man Ther. 2012;17:126–32.

Lee Y, Lee CH, Oh U. Painful channels in sensory neurons. Mol Cells. 2005;20:315–24.

Lindquist C, Nilsson BY, Skoglund CR. Obervations on the mechanical sensitivity of sympathetic and other types of small-diameter nerve fibers. Brain Res. 1973;49:432–5.

Louw A, Puentedura EJ. Therapeutic Neuroscience Education: Teaching Patients about Pain: A Guide for Clinicians. Minnesota: OPTP; 2013.

Louw A, Puentedura EJ, Zimney K, Schmidt S. Know Pain, Know Gain? A perspective on pain neuroscience education in physical therapy. J Orthop Sports Phys Ther. 2016;46:131–4.

Lutke Schipholt IJ, Coppieters MW, Meijer OG, et al. Effects of joint and nerve mobilisation on neuroimmune responses in animals and humans with neuromusculoskeletal conditions: a systematic review and meta-analysis. Pain Rep. 2021;6:e927.

Maitland GD. Vertebral Manipulation. London: Butterworths; 1986.

Majlesi J, Togay H, Unalan H, Toprak S. The sensitivity and specificity of the Slump and the Straight Leg Raising tests in patients with lumbar disc herniation. J Clin Rheumatol. 2008;14:87–91.

Maxwell CM, Lauchlan DT, Dall PM. The effects of spinal manipulative therapy on lower limb neurodynamic test outcomes in adults: a systematic review. J Man Manip Ther. 2020;28:4-14.

Merskey H, Bogduk N. Classification of Chronic Pain. Seattle: IASP Press; 1994.

Montaner-Cuello A, Bueno-Gracia E, Bueno-Aranzabal M et al. Normal response to sural neurodynamic test in asymptomatic participants. A cross-sectional study. Musculoskelet Sci Pract. 2020;50:102258.

Nee RJ, Butler DS. Management of peripheral neuropathic pain: Integrating neurobiology, neurodynamics, and clinical evidence. Phys Ther Sport. 2006;7:36–49.

Ogata K, Naito, M. Blood flow of peripheral nerve effects of dissection, stretching and compression. J Hand Surg Br. 1986;11:10–14.

Park HW, Park KS, Park MS, et al. The comparisons of surgical outcomes and clinical characteristics between the far lateral lumbar disc herniations and the paramedian lumbar disc herniations. Korean J Spine. 2013;10:155–9.

Pesonen J, Rade M, Kononen M, et al. Normalization of spinal cord displacement with the straight leg raise and resolution of sciatica in patients with lumbar intervertebral disc herniation: A 1.5-year follow-up study. Spine. 2019;44:1064–77.

Plaza-Manzano G, Cancela-Cilleruelo I, Fernandez-de-las-Peñas C, et al. Effects of adding a neurodynamic mobilization to motor control training in patients with lumbar radiculopathy due to disc herniation: A Randomized Clinical Trial. Am J Phys Med Rehabil. 2020;99:124–32.

Rade M, Pesonen J, Kononen M, et al. Reduced spinal cord movement with the straight leg raise test in patients with lumbar intervertebral disc herniation. Spine. 2017;42:1117–24.

Rosenblueth A, Buylla RA, Ramos JG. The responses of axons to mechanical stimuli. Acta Physiol Lat Am. 1953;3:204–15.

Rydevik B, Lundborg G, Bagge, U. Effects of graded compression on intraneural blood flow: An in vivo study on rabbit tibial nerve. J Hand Surg. 1981;6:3–12.

Shacklock M. Neurodynamics. Physiotherapy. 1995;81:9–16.

Shacklock MO. The clinical application of central pain mechanisms in manual therapy. Aust J Physiother. 1999;45:215–21.

Shacklock M. Improving application of neurodynamic (neural tension) testing and treatments: a message to researchers and clinicians. Man Ther. 2005a;10:175–9.

Shacklock MO. Clinical Neurodynamics: A new system of musculoskeletal treatment. Sydney, Elsevier Butterworth-Heinemann; 2005b.

Sierra-Silvestre E, Bosello F, Fernandez-Carnero J, et al. Femoral nerve excursion with knee and neck movements in supine, sitting and side-lying slump: An in vivo study using ultrasound imaging. Musculoskelet Sci Pract. 2018;37:58–63.

Silva A, Manso A, Andrade R, et al. Quantitative in vivo longitudinal nerve excursion and strain in response to joint movement: A systematic literature review. Clin Biomech. 2014;29:839–47.

Trainor K, Pinnington MA. Reliability and diagnostic validity of the slump knee bend neurodynamic test for upper/mid lumbar nerve root compression: a pilot study. Physiother. 2011;97:59–64.

Van Der Heide B, Allison GT, Zusman M. Pain and muscular responses to a neural tissue provocation test in the upper limb. Man Ther. 2001;6:154–62.

Vegstein K, Robinson HS, Jensen, R. Neurodynamic tests for patellofemoral pain syndrome: a pilot study. Chiropr Man Therap. 2019;27:26.

Vij N, Kiernan H, Bisht R, et al. Surgical and non-surgical treatment options for piriformis syndrome: A literature review. Anesth Pain Med. 2021;11:e112825.

Walsh J, Flatley M, Johnston N, Bennett K. Slump test: sensory responses in asymptomatic subjects. J Man Manip Ther. 2007;15:231–8.

Weppler CH, Magnusson SP. Increasing muscle extensibility: a matter of increasing length or modifying sensation? Phys Ther. 2010;90:438–49.

Wilgis EF, Murphy R. The significance of longitudinal excursion in peripheral nerves. Hand Clin. 1986;2:761–6.

Woolf CJ. Pain. Neurobiol Dis. 2000;7:504–10.

Woolf CJ. Central sensitization: uncovering the relation between pain and plasticity. Anesthesiology. 2007;106:864–7.

Woolf CJ, Mannion RJ. Neuropathic pain: aetiology, symptoms, mechanisms, and management. Lancet. 1999;353;1959–64.

Zhao Q, Yang Y, Wu P, et al. Biomechanical study of the C5-C8 cervical extraforaminal ligaments. J Orthop Surg Res. 2020;15:477.

Zochodne DW, Ho LT. Stimulation-induced peripheral nerve hyperemia: mediation by fibers innervating vasa nervorum? Brain Res. 1991;546:113–8.

19

Exercise programs for hip and knee pain disorders

César Fernández-de-las-Peñas, Jill Cook, Madhan K. Ramanathan, Sergio Muela-Fernández, Scot Morrison

Introduction

Exercise-based management of hip and knee injuries involves strategically applying stress to the relevant tissue to drive desired adaptations. This process has been defined as the "SAID Principle" (Specific Adaptation to Imposed Demand), and it should underpin continuous clinical reasoning throughout management. In the context of rehabilitation, exercise prescription (ExRx) is used to address any limitations identified as barriers to function, participation and performance. When the principle of SAID is applied, the ExRx emerges from the intersection of the personal patient's current presentation and their goals.

In general, rehabilitation goals will broadly cluster around range of motion (ROM), force output (strength), energy system development (ESD), and other tissue-specific adaptations. There are also other clinical objectives such as pain, health or improved performance where the causal impact of ExRx is less clear. While important, the role ExRx plays in these outcomes is poorly understood at this time. This chapter aims to provide an ExRx framework that allows the clinician to treat hip and knee disorders with a sound rationale and evidence base. Exercises can be isolated to a single joint or involve the whole kinetic chain and they can be performed non-weight-bearing or weight-bearing.

Clinical Reasoning for the Application of Exercise Programs

A Framework for Exercise Prescription

The fundamental principles of exercise prescription must drive exercise selection, dosage, and progression. The idea of progressive overload complements the SAID principle to achieve the desired goals. As structures adapt to the demands they are exposed to, future programming of the exercise program must be progressed to ensure these adaptations continue. ExRx is flawed when the stress becomes "different" instead of "progressive." Two examples where this can occur are progressing from constrained to compound exercises or adding instability to an exercise in place of overload. In the first example, the individual can "cheat" and select a movement solution that shifts force away from the target tissue and in the second, there is no actual overload (Sigward et al., 2018; Lawrence & Carlson, 2015). In both cases, the changes lead to a decrease in the load through the relevant tissue and thus failure to achieve the goal of progressive overload.

The particular exercise chosen is only a small component of the overall exercise prescription process, which requires the manipulation of multiple factors. This error is observed when resistance training and strength training, which are not synonymous, are conflated. Strength training involves the deliberate process of increasing the force that can be produced against some external resistance (Schoenfeld et al., 2021). In contrast, resistance training is merely the process of adding resistance to a movement. This may not hit the minimum effective dosage necessary to see adaptations in strength but can still lead to improved function and decreased pain through processes such as graded exposure or learning of the task (Table 19.1).

A review of exercise adaptations exceeds the scope of this chapter, but the general goals of strength, hypertrophy, and connective tissue adaptation deserve attention. Resistance training has traditionally been prescribed based on repetition "zones" that were proposed to align with specific adaptations; however, this model may be overly simplistic. A recent review by Schoenfeld et al. (2021) suggested that strength adaptations seem to favor heavier loads largely independent of volume. And hypertrophy appears to be more independent of load once a minimum threshold (~30% 1 repetition maximum (RM)) is met, with adaptations tending to reflect the effort and total volume load. Despite this, Schoenfeld et al. (2021) still suggest moderate intensities as generally the most practical approach for hypertrophy (Table 19.2). Connective tissue adaptations require an understanding of prescription based on the SAID principle. In tendons, a systematic review and meta-analysis demonstrated that external loads exceeding 70% of 1RM were necessary to cause adaptation (Bohm et al., 2015). Further work done by Arampatsis et al. (2020) shows this threshold may be even higher, with loads of over 90% MVC necessary to achieve optimal strain in the Achilles tendon. Aside from muscle, bone and tendon adaptations there are also neural changes in the central nervous system

CHAPTER NINTEEN

TABLE 19.1 Training Variables

Training Variable	Measure	Prescription	Impact
Intensity	External load added or torque at joint	% of rep max (85% RM) or reps at load (e.g., 5RM)	See Table 19.2
Effort	Proximity to failure	Reps in reserve or rating of perceived exertion	Fatigue, motor unit recruitment, hypertrophy
Tempo/Velocity	Speed of movement	Metronome or descriptive term (e.g., maximal, controlled, etc.)	Stress and strain on tissue, accumulation of fatigue
Volume	Total repetitions per workout Volume load = reps × load Volume = reps per set × sets	Assigned by total exercises sets and reps	Muscular, energetic, and connective tissue adaptations
Rest	Time	Complete rest - time between efforts Active rest - time of alternative activity between efforts	Fatigue and force capabilities on subsequent sets, motor unit recruitment
Frequency	Sessions per time period	Per desired time interval (generally weekly)	Total dosage and recovery abilities

(Modified from Lorenz & Morrison, 2015.)

TABLE 19.2 Training Intensity

Intensity Training Zones	Goal	Intensity as % 1RM (Rep Range)
Zone 1	Hypertrophy, skill, work capacity, rate of force with high rate	<50% (>15 reps)
Zone 2	Hypertrophy default	50%–75% (10–15 RM)
Zone 3	General strength, connective tissue, hypertrophy, rate of force with intent	75%–86% (5–10 RM)
Zone 4	Max strength, connective tissue, hypertrophy	90%+ (1–4 RM)

(Modified from Lorenz & Morrison, 2015; Schoenfeld et al., 2021; Haff & Triplett, 2016.)

that affect the response to overload. Specific adaptations to exercise, such as adding visual or auditory cues and timing to repetition execution can improve neural responses (Rio et al., 2016). In summary, it is important to determine what the desired adaptations are through a thorough evaluation and assessment and ensure programming reflects these goals by honoring the SAID principle.

Exercise Prescription

Exercise selection requires a few fundamental principles to guide the process. First, the external load imposed by the programming is only part of what determines the internal loads experienced by the tissues. Torque at the joint is the product of the moment arm (distance from resistance to joint), the total force applied, and the angle it is applied at. Because of this, all of these factors must be considered when selecting an exercise. This chapter uses a continuum model to give the sports medicine professional a loose framework for identifying and selecting movements.

Exercise prescription tends to be full of vaguely defined concepts with terms like "functional" used in a manner so broad as to lose any real meaning. Biomechanically unsound concepts like open kinetic chain and closed kinetic chain also fall into this category as they do not accurately represent the forces experienced by the system (Knudson, 2007). Because of these clarity issues, this chapter will approach exercise selection based on general movement biases and the concept of constraints. A movement bias is operationally defined as the predominant joint(s) around which the movement is organized. Figure 19.1 shows the "Hip Hinge Continuum" as a method for categorizing exercises (John, 2013). This model is a way to understand and organize compound exercises based on the relative contribution of the hip and knee. The clinician can orientate the specific exercise to the continuum, in order to have a reasonable approximation of its demands. This allows the clinician to determine whether the exercise selected is likely to address the stated goals. As a general heuristic "hinge" movements shift demands to the hip while "squat" movements have a greater knee demand. Using this continuum allows the clinician to initially categorize an exercise as well as come up with progressions and regressions for it. This can then be compared to the literature on muscle demands during exercise in order to predict actual demands. It must be stressed that these data frequently contain confounders and do not necessarily represent actual mechanical

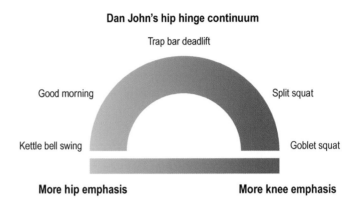

Dan John's hip hinge continuum

FIGURE 19.1
The "Hip Hinge Continuum" as a method for categorizing exercises.
(Modified from John, 2013.)

tension on the muscle or tendon for each exercise. Reports on muscular demands and progression of exercise (often based exclusively on EMG data) should be interpreted with caution since examined loads are not normalized and EMG can be problematic. As a result, these studies may give a general idea of muscles recruited with the lift, but shouldn't be the main driver of decision-making as they are unlikely to predict actual internal loads or eventual adaptations. A clear example of this can be seen in the study by Delmore et al. (2014), where loaded side-lying adduction exercise was compared to body-weight sumo squats. There was a significant difference in relative intensity for the adductor muscles in these exercises and the sumo squat showed a low level of activity. This is contrasted by biomechanical modeling showing over 50% of the net hip extension moment comes from the adductor magnus during a loaded squat, which agrees with findings from a 10-week intervention study that found the adductors were the most hypertrophied muscle group after a squat-based training program (Vigotsky & Bryanton, 2016; Kubo et al., 2019).

Evidence supports the application of localized exercises for the injured or painful area, i.e., quadriceps exercises for patellofemoral pain, hamstring exercises for biceps femoris strain/tear, or gastrocnemius and soleus exercises for Achilles tendinopathy. Less constrained exercises are commonly used to improve function and performance further and integrate the tissue/motion segment back into a compound movement. The hip displacement continuum allows

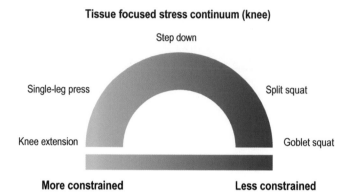

Tissue focused stress continuum (knee)

Step down

Single-leg press   Split squat

Knee extension   Goblet squat

More constrained   **Less constrained**

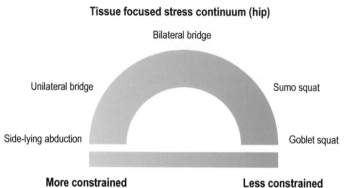

Tissue focused stress continuum (hip)

Bilateral bridge

Unilateral bridge   Sumo squat

Side-lying abduction   Goblet squat

More constrained   **Less constrained**

FIGURE 19.2
Examples of the tissue focused stress continuum principle.

for the global categorization of compound lower body exercises. This categorization can be further refined by introducing the idea of constraints that determine the degrees of freedom available for that movement (Figure 19.2). An exercise can be considered highly constrained when the performance of the movement can only be accomplished by limited options such as during single-joint movements. This reduction in movement options ensures that any loads placed on the system are constrained to the selected tissue. For instance, during a constrained Nordic hamstring exercise, the hamstring is significantly loaded while there is very little hamstring load during a more unconstrained squat (van Dyk et al., 2019; Vigotsky & Bryanton, 2016; Kubo et al., 2019). The use of constraints allows the clinician to prescribe movements that have a higher probability of loading relevant tissue in order to ensure SAID is occurring at the desired system and level. In contrast, a less constrained exercise can be used to load the kinetic chain in order to ensure integration of local adaptions back into larger movement patterns.

Which Type of Contraction Should be Applied During Exercise Programs?

There is extensive literature trying to determine which type of contraction, i.e., eccentric, concentric, isometric, is more effective for improving pain and related function in lower limb pain, particularly in tendinopathies. To date, it seems that eccentric, concentric or isometric contractions exhibit

similar effects in individuals with tendinopathies, probably because of these tissues' non-contractile properties (Bohm et al., 2015; Clifford et al., 2020). It also appears that when the maximal load or effort is matched, morphologic changes in the muscle are equivalent albeit through slightly different pathways (Franchi et al., 2017). Therefore, ExRx should generally use combined movements with isolated contractions being implemented under specific circumstances, e.g., isolated isometrics to avoid painful ROM, accentuated eccentrics as part of a progressive loading exercise program according to patient presentation and established goals.

Progression of Exercise Loading

Tissue stress is probably the key factor for properly designed exercise programs. Knowledge of muscle and connective tissue properties, force applications, tissue injury (bone, ligament, tendon, muscle, nerve) and tissue healing principles and timelines (e.g., inflammation, proliferation, maturation) is an important precursor for developing a suitable and safe exercise program. The main difference faced by the clinician in ExRx is the presence of pathology which results in a more volatile presentation. Because of this, symptom response and exercise intensity as a percentage of maximal voluntary contraction (%MVC) must be considered.

A variety of exercise programs have been investigated for treating hip and knee problems. A unique problem that clinicians face in ExRx is how to dose exercise in the presence of pain. For instance, eccentric strength training, while potentially effective in the management of hip-knee problems, can also be associated with higher rates of delayed onset muscle soreness (DOMS) (Morawetz et al., 2020). There have been a number of models for how to solve this problem. Alfredson et al. (1998) recommended an increase in load when pain or discomfort during the exercise for Achilles tendinopathy decreased. Stanish et al. (1986) proposed that the appropriate load for tendinopathy is that one when pain or discomfort is experienced in the last set of repetitions of the exercise. Based on the current body of literature the appropriate clinical question is "what level of pain or discomfort should be permitted?" While Silbernagel et al. (2001) allowed activity-based pain when treating tendinopathy to reach 5 (moderate intensity) on a numerical pain rate scale, clinicians should consider that pain intensity is a subjective outcome and so a fixed acceptable number may not be realistic. A meta-analysis by Smith et al. (2017) concluded that painful exercises offer better, although small, benefits at short-term (moderate quality of evidence) and equal long-term outcomes over pain-free exercises in the management of chronic musculoskeletal pain. So, while pain during exercise is not a barrier for successful clinical outcomes, it must be properly monitored (Smith et al., 2017). This is consistent with postoperative exercise programs being progressive and graded according to the stage of tissue healing while avoiding any aggravation of pain, swelling, or a deterioration of other clinical signs such as ROM, strength and function of the patient.

Exercise intensity in ExRx can be based on objective measures such as using a repetition maximum or maximal isometric test, or even velocity-based estimates of the patient's 1RM. However, this is often complicated by tissue healing status which makes subjective estimates of effort like repetitions in reserve (RIR) an appealing alternative. This is an approach where the clinician asks the individual to make an estimate of how many more repetitions, they believe they could have completed if they hadn't stopped the set. This can be estimated at any time but is typically done immediately following the end of the set. A numerical estimate is given based on the patient's perception of their ability and recorded as "estimated reps in reserve." This approach has been proposed as an acceptable alternative to the use of more traditional methods with acceptable reliability in several studies (Helms et al., 2016; Lovegrove et al., 2021). It should be noted, however, that this approach almost always results in a lower intensity than intended since most subjects underestimate their abilities and seem to frequently anchor the perception of effort on discomfort (Steele et al., 2017; Armes et al., 2020). To mitigate these downsides, it is recommended that those using this approach take the following steps. Only use estimates of 2–3 RIR or less to make decisions and regularly use a set performed to momentary muscular failure (MMF) (inability to perform a subsequent rep without loss of form) to anchor the patient's perception of maximal effort (0 RIR) to what it actually feels like (MMF). All patients should be instructed clearly to separate effort from discomfort or pain, and RIR use should be limited to moderate or lower rep ranges.

Periodization of Exercise

Periodization is the sequential planning of training to achieve desired adaptions at specific time points (Plisk & Stone, 2003). This is done by adjusting training parameters to expose the trainee to the stressors that will result in the desired adaptation at the appropriate time points (Plisk & Stone, 2003; Evans, 2019; Lorenz & Morrison, 2015). In spite of its popularity it is surrounded by mystique and is poorly understood. For a detailed discussion of this subject and its application to rehabilitations see Lorenz & Morrison (2015), but fundamentally it is about manipulation of intensity and volume. Three broad categories of periodization have emerged: linear, block, and undulating. While there are differences, the foundational aspects are the same. The most traditional method is linear, which starts with higher volumes and lower intensities and then progresses to higher intensities and lower volumes in a progressive and sequential manner (Evans, 2019; Lorenz & Morrison, 2015). Block periodization uses discrete time periods to focus on addressing a specific aspect while secondary capacities are stimulated just enough to maintain a training effect. Finally, undulating approaches alternate between a higher volume or a higher intensity emphasis on a more frequent basis than the other two (typically progressed daily or weekly) (Evans, 2019; Lorenz & Morrison, 2015). While there are many significant concerns with periodization dogma, the principles of progressive overload and SAID appear to be "eminently sensible" (Kiely, 2012). For rehabilitation it is very hard to beat the model laid out by Al Vermeil in his training hierarchy (Figure 19.3). This model typically starts with building general physical capacity to prepare the individual

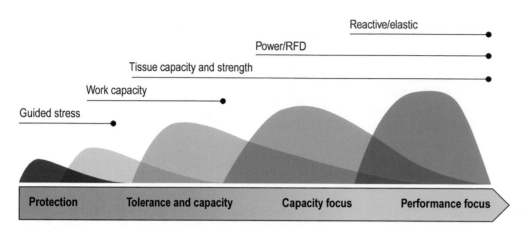

FIGURE 19.3
Vermeil's hierarchy adapted for rehabilitation.
(From Morrison, 2020.)

to tolerate the future training. In rehabilitation it often becomes necessary to add a tissue protection phase before work capacity when there are contraindications based on tissue healing timeframes. It then continues to progress through a classic linear approach building from strength to the rate at which the force is expressed to the realization of this training by working on reactive ability. This process has each phase preparing the individual for the next one in a logical and sequential manner with return to performance at the end (Panariello et al., 2017). While this model will not always suit, it is also recommended that the rehabilitation professional have a general plan for progression of exercise that honors the principles of progressive overload and SAID. This allows continued progress towards the overall goal without being distracted by necessary regressions and lateralizations that may occur along the way.

Adherence to Exercise Programs

Since exercise adaptations proceed in a dose response manner, adherence to the exercise program plays a major role in outcomes. Many factors modify adherence, including the patient's self-efficacy, personal beliefs, accessibility or fear-avoidance behaviors. The healthcare professional may enhance adherence to exercise programs by adapting their program to these limitations. Self-efficacy has been defined as "the belief and conviction that one can successfully perform a given activity" and should play a substantial role in the way the clinician approaches ExRx for the individual (Fletcher & Banasik, 2001). One potential efficacy modifier is the number of exercises prescribed, with emerging data showing a single exercise elicited similar outcomes to multiple exercises (Littlewood et al., 2016). Emerging data

support these ideas, such as a meta-analysis by Nicolson et al. (2017), who found behavioral graded exercises, which gradually increase intensity and exercise integration into ADLs, were better at increasing patient motivation than other strategies such as counseling, action coping plans or audio/video exercise cues. Clinicians should identify and consider patients' preferences and appropriate progressions to improve exercise adherence.

Evidence for Exercise for Hip and Knee Disorders

Moderate to strong evidence supports the use of exercise programs for addressing pain and improving function in conditions of the hip and knee such as patellofemoral pain (Clijsen et al., 2014), knee osteoarthritis (Bartholdy et al., 2017), and meniscus tear (Swart et al., 2016), as well as potentially reducing the risk of overuse injuries (Lauersen et al., 2014, 2018). Most clinical practice guidelines recommend exercise programs as a first-line intervention for the management of patellofemoral pain (Wallis et al., 2021), knee osteoarthritis (Arden et al., 2021), or hip osteoarthritis (Cibulka et al., 2017). Similarly, strengthening exercises are also strongly recommended in clinical practice guidelines after anterior cruciate ligament (ACL) reconstruction (Andrade et al., 2020), and pain with meniscal injury and other associated cartilage lesions (Logerstedt et al., 2018).

Various types of exercises including stretching, stabilization, strengthening, motor control, proprioceptive, graded activity and aerobic are described in the literature for hip and knee conditions. Saltychev et al. (2018) found that all these exercise types exhibit similar effects for decreasing pain symptoms in individuals with patellofemoral pain: strengthening (decrease pain on a 100-point scale –65.0, 95%CI –87.7 to –48.3), weight-bearing (–40.0, 95%CI –49.4 to –30.6), neuromuscular facilitation combined with aerobic exercise and stretching (–60.1, 95%CI –66.9 to –54.5), or postural stabilization (–24.4, 95%CI –33.5 to –15.3) exercises. The type of exercise should be adapted to patient characteristics and based on clinical reasoning.

Are There Subgroups of Patients Who Will Benefit from Exercise?

Classification systems have been proposed throughout the literature, by developing clinical prediction rules, suggesting that subgroups of patients may respond differently to exercise programs; however, it is unknown which individuals with hip or knee problems would benefit most from which type of exercise. In fact, clinical prediction rules have not been validated with high-quality randomized clinical trials and currently cannot be recommended (Walsh et al., 2021).

Potential Effects of Exercise

Exercise may be effective for reducing pain and improving function through two mechanisms. The first hypothesis is that exercise leads to positive effects by changing connective tissue, neural tissue and even bone properties. For example, Gérard et al. (2020) observed that an eccentric strength-training exercise program induced architectural adaptations on the long head of the biceps femoris muscle and an increase in eccentric hamstring strength. However, while muscular changes could be able to explain improvements in function, any extrapolation to changes in pain are tenuous at best.

Exercise has been shown to exhibit an analgesic effect which is not fully understood but is thought to be due to multiple factors including graded exposure, local changes, descending pathways, and central nociceptive changes (Vaegter et al., 2014). The effects of exercise in individuals with chronic pain exhibiting central sensitization might be slightly different and, therefore, opposite clinical outcomes may occur. For instance, inappropriate exercise may induce hyperalgesia instead of hypoalgesia in a patient with chronic pain (Daenen et al., 2015), and hyperalgesia

may also cause ExRx that is innocuous from a traditional perspective to be detrimental as well. An ongoing consideration of the patient's pain experience is a necessary component of proper exercise progression.

Types of Exercises

Stretching Exercises

Flexibility and the role of stretching exercises have a conflicting body of evidence, an exploration of which is also beyond the scope of this chapter. Stretching includes multiple approaches such as static, ballistic, proprioceptive neuromuscular facilitation, post-isometric relaxation, and activated isolated stretching. In general, current data do not support the idea of tissue changes during stretching with an alteration in tolerance to stretch explaining most ROM changes seen (Weppler & Magnusson, 2010). In contrast to this, the body of evidence points to eccentric training through full range leading to similar ROM changes as stretching with associated performance adaptations (O'Sullivan et al., 2012). As a result, it is suggested, when time is limited, resistance training with a ROM emphasis should be used as the primary approach to increasing ROM. If stretching is included, dosage recommendations for duration and frequency are heterogeneous, but a general target of 5 times a week accumulating at least 5 minutes of stretch seems indicated (Thomas et al., 2018).

Independent of the form of stretching applied, the common assumptions that stretching prevents injury, increases muscle strength and/or reduces delayed muscle onset soreness after exercise do not appear to be supported by the literature. Two previous Cochrane reviews concluded that evidence did not support that stretching exercises reduce the risk of lower extremity limb soft-tissue injuries (Yeung et al., 2011) or prevent or reduce muscle soreness after exercise (Herbert et al., 2011). Similarly, the effect of stretching exercises on muscle strength has been found to be trivial (Konrad et al., 2021).

Strength and Hypertrophy Training

Strengthening exercises for the management of lower extremity conditions have been investigated, although evidence of effectiveness is generally inconclusive in many of these (Geneen et al., 2017). The progression of load is critical for any strengthening exercise program where strength changes are the goal. This is an issue since many times progressive overload is failed such as the report by Minshull and Gleeson (2017) that principles of training were inconsistently applied and inadequately reported in clinical trials investigating exercise programs in people with knee osteoarthritis.

In strength training the consideration of intensity, duration, and frequency of the exercise is important for appropriate ExRx. The energy demands and volume load of the exercise and session can be modulated by varying intensity (%RM), sets, repetitions, rest intervals, velocity and intent. In line with the more traditional zones discussed previously, Kraemer & Ratamess (2004) recommended 1–6 repetitions for strength, 6–12 repetitions for hypertrophy, and 12–15 repetitions for endurance, based on fatigue towards the end of the stated number of repetitions (Kraemer & Ratamess, 2004). More recently, Schoenfeld et al. (2014) observed that a hypertrophy (3 sets of 10 repetitions with a 90-sec rest) and a strength (7 sets of 3 repetitions with a 3-min rest) program were equally effective for muscle size (hypertrophy) but the latter was superior for enhancing maximal strength. The weekly frequency and volume of training is also important for appropriate progression. Current evidence indicates that training twice a week promotes superior strength outcomes than training once a week but there may be limited benefits associated with higher frequencies (Schoenfeld et al., 2019). For hypertrophy a goal of 10 sets per week per muscle group with a weekly frequency that makes this volume easily achieved seems consistent with current evidence (Schoenfeld et al., 2017, 2019).

Exercises for the Lower Extremity

The exercises chosen must be based on the adaptations desired. As these neuromusculoskeletal adaptations occur, the practice of the daily tasks and movements specific to the population must also be considered as these are two distinct goals. When treating subjects with a more volatile presentation, such as higher levels of pain or post-surgery, a starting point substantially less than what can be tolerated may reduce the probability of overshooting their capacity. This allows the clinician to build up to a level of tolerance instead of overdoing it from the start. It also offers the opportunity to take advantage of the repeated bout effect where initial exercise conveys a protective aspect to exercise-related

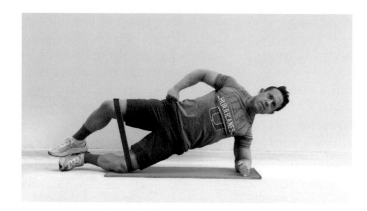

FIGURE 19.4
"Clam shell position" with a band in a "side-bridge" position.

soreness in subsequent bouts. The following section reviews some of the more common exercises along with EMG data and their place in the continuum.

Gluteal Musculature

Globally, most movements on the "hinge" side of the continuum will involve the gluteals, although they also play a significant role in squatting. Several exercises for the gluteal musculature (i.e., gluteus maximus, gluteus medius, and gluteus minimus) will be discussed, although gluteal muscles are used during most compound lower body exercises.

The gluteus medius and minimus musculature can be strengthened in both non-weight-bearing (i.e., side-lying hip abduction) or weight-bearing (i.e., lateral lunge, dip test, standing hip abduction) positions. Macadam et al. (2015) reported that side-bridge with hip abduction exercise, also called "side plank" provokes the highest activity of gluteus medius; however, this exercise also needs a proper control of the trunk. For instance, mixed exercises could be also applied by using a band in a "side-bridge" position (Figure 19.4). A more recent review revealed that variations of the "hip hitch-pelvic drop" exercise are able to generate higher activity in both gluteus medius and minimus segments (Moore et al., 2020). If clinicians aim to focus on the gluteus minimus muscle, from a basic hip hitch–pelvic drop exercise, the patient can progress to a "lateral step-up" (Figure 19.5).

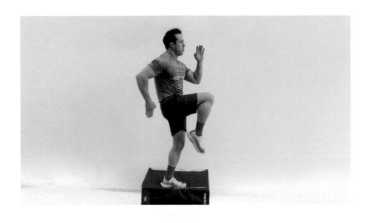

FIGURE 19.5
"Lateral step-up" on a box.

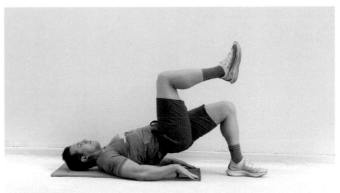

FIGURE 19.7
Single-leg bridge with knees flexed exercise.

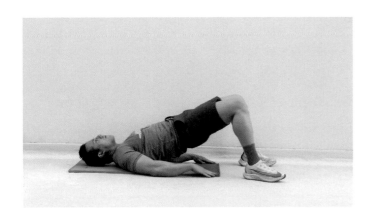

FIGURE 19.6
Bilateral hip extension exercise (bridge) combined with hip abduction. A band can be used for resisting abduction.

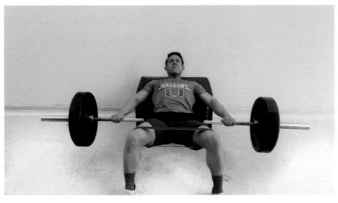

FIGURE 19.8
The "barbell hip thrust" exercise.

The gluteus maximus muscle is targeted with hip extension (knees flexed for decreasing hamstring activity). Again, non-weight-bearing (e.g., double-leg bridge, frontal plank with bent leg hip extension) and weight-bearing (e.g., single-leg wall squat with other leg knee extended, front squat) exercises can be applied. First, clinicians must consider that at a fixed load, unilateral exercises, e.g., single-leg bridge-knees flexed (Figure 19.6), impose a higher relative intensity on the limb than the bilateral version of that exercise, e.g., double-leg bridge. Exercises provoking high-level activation of gluteus maximus include "step-up," "lateral step-up," "belt squat," "split squat," or "traditional lunge"

(Neto et al., 2020). The review by Macadam and Feser (2019) concluded that hip extension combined with hip abduction (Figure 19.7) or external rotation resulted in higher activity of the gluteus maximus. It is also relevant to consider the synergestic role gluteus maximus plays with hamstring or erector spinae musculature; therefore, clinicians can constrain the exercise to target a specific muscle, e.g., during a bridge the gluteus maximus may be better addressed with a flexed knee, whereas hamstring demands go up as the knees are extended. The "barbell hip thrust" exercise (Figure 19.8) is a good option for increasing the load during bridge variations (Neto et al., 2019).

Hamstring Musculature

Exercise programs, including the Nordic hamstring exercise (NHE) (van Dyk et al., 2019) or other types of exercise (Vatovec et al., 2020), have been shown to improve architecture and strength in the hamstring musculature and may reduce the risk of hamstring injuries.

Towards the hinge side of the continuum for strengthening the posterior musculature of the lower quadrant (i.e., gluteus maximus, hamstrings, and erector spinae) is the "deadlift." Several variations of this exercise are proposed: regular deadlift (lifted from the floor with arms outside the thighs), Romanian deadlift (more hip dominant with a more limited ROM), or sumo deadlift (wide stance regular deadlift where the hands are between the thighs while lifting). The deadlift does a great job of developing the posterior chain; however, an interesting literature review found that activation of erector spinae and quadriceps muscles was higher than activation of the gluteus maximus and biceps femoris during deadlift exercises, but they urge caution in interpretation based on methodology issues (Martín-Fuentes et al., 2020).

For individuals looking to challenge the posterior chain in a more constrained exercise a "single-leg bridge" with knee flexed (see Figure 19.7) is a good starting point. Progression occurs by increasing the moment arm by extending the knee, adding load or adding a variation such as the "heel strike against ball exercise" (Figure 19.9).

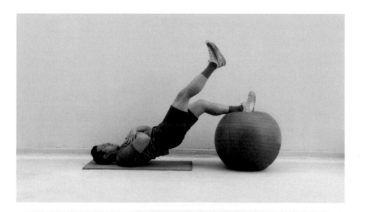

FIGURE 19.9
The "heel strike against ball exercise." The subject can increase the speed and amplitude for increasing the difficulty of the exercise.

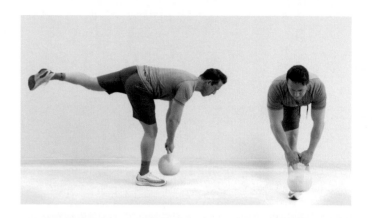

FIGURE 19.10
"The Arabesque". The patient can use a kettlebell for increasing the load.

Alternatively, a less constrained standing unilateral exercise such as the "Arabesque" can be progressively loaded as well (Figure 19.10).

Quadriceps Musculature

Progressive exercise training of the quadriceps muscle is frequently recommended for those with patellofemoral pain (Chapter 3), knee osteoarthritis (Chapter 4), patellar tendinopathy (Chapter 2), and after ACL reconstruction.

The "squat" falls on the right side of the hip hinge continuum by adding in the knee to the movement execution. The squat has a large number of variations which can increase or decrease the load on the knee extensor mechanism without change in the external load. For instance, performing a bilateral squat on a slight declination by placing a step under the heel increases the moment arm at the knee, which leads to more load on the knee extension complex (Figure 19.11). A "single-leg decline squat" constrains this movement by removing the ability to weight shift and also increases load assuming external load cannot be added. The load on the tissue can be decreased or increased by using the other lower extremity muscles and joints (Figure 19.12). Another squat variant is the "Spanish squat" (Figure 19.13), which constrains the motion to being almost predominantly at the knee (similar to a leg extension) (Basas et al., 2018). This is a great option for achieving high loads at the knee without the need for any external loads. Finally, squats can be performed in a "split" stance leading to significant control

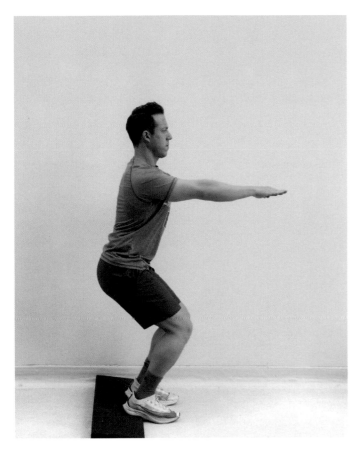

FIGURE 19.11
Bilateral "squat" with a slight declination by placing a step under the heel for increasing the load on the patellar tendon.

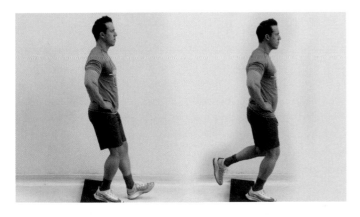

FIGURE 19.12
"Single-leg decline squat" with declination. The first figure is more towards the right of the hip hinge (knee) and the second more to the left (hip).

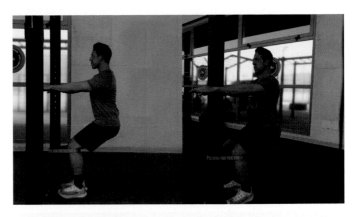

FIGURE 19.13
"Spanish" squat with a muscle belt.

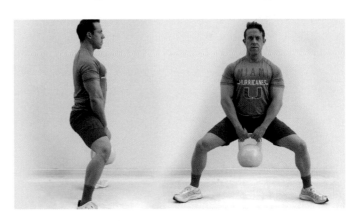

FIGURE 19.14
The "sumo squat." A kettlebell, dumbbell, or barbell can be used to increase the load.

over the forces at the knee. Changes in the shin angle and trunk lean of the lead and trail limb will control whether the loads are focused or distributed between the front and rear knee. Contrary to popular belief, advice to keep the "knee behind the toes" is not at all supported and positive shin angles should be used during squats and its variants to focus torque at the knee (Hofmann et al., 2017; Schütz et al., 2014).

Adductor Musculature

Diminished strength on the adductor squeeze test is a feature of athletes with groin pain (Mosler et al., 2015). For the adductor muscles the "sumo squat" (Figure 19.14)

413

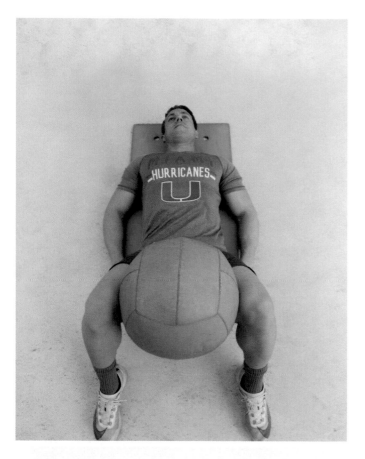

FIGURE 19.15
"Isometric ball squeeze." The subject performs an isometric contraction by squeezing their knees against the ball.

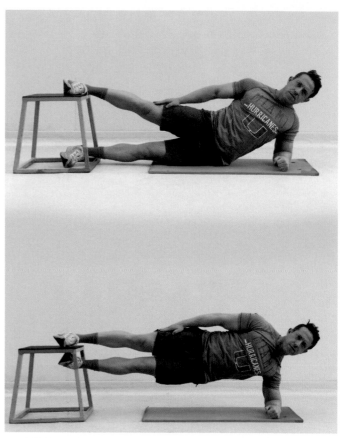

FIGURE 19.16
"Copenhagen adduction exercise." A box or chair supports the ankle/knee and the individual supports himself on his elbow in a side plank position.

and other squat variations are a minimally constrained method that significantly targets the adductor magnus. In contrast, a constrained exercise such as the "isometric ball squeeze" (Figure 19.15) allows the clinician to ensure that any overload is occurring in the adductor complex. The "Copenhagen adduction exercise" (Figure 19.16) is a way to achieve high intensity for the adductor musculature using only body weight and it has been shown to be effective for improving the adduction strength; however, due to its higher loads, a progressive approach should be used to avoid DOMS (Serner et al., 2014).

Conclusion

Exercise plays an important role in the management of hip and knee problems. This chapter has outlined some basic principles of exercise prescription that should be considered in the clinical setting. A comprehensive assessment is required to ensure safe and suitable prescription and progression. The exercise program demands must be matched to the clinical presentation based on the concepts of SAID and progressive overload. Clinicians may use the basic principles outlined in this chapter as a guide for exercise prescription to meet the needs of each individual with hip and knee pain problems.

References

Alfredson H, Pietilä T, Jonsson P, et al. Heavy-load eccentric calf muscle training for the treatment of chronic Achilles tendinosis. Am J Sports Med. 1998;26:360–6.

Andrade R, Pereira R, van Cingel R, et al. How should clinicians rehabilitate patients after ACL reconstruction? A systematic review of clinical practice guidelines (CPGs) with a focus on quality appraisal (AGREE II). Br J Sports Med. 2020;54:512–51.

Arampatzis A, Mersmann F, Bohm S. Individualized muscle-tendon assessment and training. Front Physiol. 2020;11:723.

Arden NK, Perry TA, Bannuru RR, et al. Non-surgical management of knee osteoarthritis: comparison of ESCEO and OARSI 2019 guidelines. Nat Rev Rheumatol. 2021;17:59–66.

Armes C, Standish-Hunt H, Androulakis-Korakakis P, et al. "Just One More Rep!" – Ability to predict proximity to task failure in resistance trained persons. Front Psychol. 2020;11:565416.

Bartholdy C, Juhl C, Christensen R, et al. The role of muscle strengthening in exercise therapy for knee osteoarthritis: A systematic review and meta-regression analysis of randomized trials. Semin Arthritis Rheum. 2017;47:9–21.

Basas A, Cook J, Gómez MA, et al. Effects of a strength protocol combined with electrical stimulation on patellar tendinopathy: 42 months retrospective follow-up on 6 high-level jumping athletes. Phys Ther Sport. 2018;34:105–12.

Bohm S, Mersmann F, Arampatzis A. Human tendon adaptation in response to mechanical loading: a systematic review and meta-analysis of exercise intervention studies on healthy adults. Sports Med Open. 2015;1:7.

Cibulka MT, Bloom NJ, Enseki KR, et al. Hip pain and mobility deficits-hip osteoarthritis: Revision 2017. J Orthop Sports Phys Ther. 2017;47:A1–A37.

Clifford C, Challoumas D, Paul L, et al. Effectiveness of isometric exercise in the management of tendinopathy: a systematic review and meta-analysis of randomised trials. BMJ Open Sport Exerc Med. 2020;6:e000760.

Clijsen R, Fuchs J, Taeymans J. Effectiveness of exercise therapy in treatment of patients with patellofemoral pain syndrome: systematic review and meta-analysis. Phys Ther. 2014;94:1697–708.

Daenen L, Varkey E, Kellmann M, Nijs J. Exercise, not to exercise, or how to exercise in patients with chronic pain? Applying science to practice. Clin J Pain. 2015;31:108–14.

Delmore RJ, Laudner KG, Torry MR. Adductor longus activation during common hip exercises. J Sport Rehabil. 2014;23:79–87.

Evans JW. Periodized resistance training for enhancing skeletal muscle hypertrophy and strength: A mini-review. *Front Physiol.* 2019;10:13.

Fletcher JS, Banasik JL. Exercise self-efficacy. Clin Excell Nurse Pract. 2001;5:134–43.

Franchi MV, Reeves ND, Narici MV. Skeletal muscle remodeling in response to eccentric vs. concentric loading: Morphological, molecular, and metabolic adaptations. Front Physiol. 2017;8:447.

Geneen LJ, Moore RA, Clarke C, et al. Physical activity and exercise for chronic pain in adults: an overview of Cochrane Reviews. Cochrane Database Syst Rev. 2017;4:CD011279.

Gérard R, Gojon L, Decleve P, Van Cant J. The effects of eccentric training on biceps femoris architecture and strength: A systematic review with meta-analysis. J Athl Train. 2020;55:501-14.

Haff G, Triplett NT. Essentials of Strength Training and Conditioning. NSCA; 2016.

Helms ER, Cronin J, Storey A, Zourdos MC. Application of the repetitions in reserve-based rating of perceived exertion scale for resistance training. Strength Cond J. 2016;38:42–9.

Herbert RD, de Noronha M, Kamper SJ. Stretching to prevent or reduce muscle soreness after exercise. Cochrane Database Syst Rev. 2011;7:CD004577.

Hofmann CL, Holyoak DT, Juris PM. Trunk and shank position influences patellofemoral joint stress in the lead and trail limbs during the forward lunge exercise. J Orthop Sports Phys Ther. 2017;47:31–40.

Houglum P. Therapeutic exercise for musculoskeletal injuries. Champaign, IL: Human Kinetics; 2005.

John D. Intervention. On Target Publications; 2013

Kiely J. Periodization paradigms in the 21st century: evidence-led or tradition-driven? Int J Sports Physiol Perform. 2012;7:242–50.

Knudson D. Fundamentals of Biomechanics. 2nd ed. Switzerland AG: Springer; 2007.

Konrad A, Močnik R, Titze S, et al. The influence of stretching the hip flexor muscles on performance parameters: A systematic review with meta-analysis. Int J Environ Res Public Health. 2021;18:1936.

Kraemer WJ, Ratamess NA. Fundamentals of resistance training: progression and exercise prescription. Med Sci Sports Exerc. 2004;36:674-88.

Kubo K, Ikebukuro T, Yata H. Effects of squat training with different depths on lower limb muscle volumes. Eur J Appl Physiol. 2019;119:1933–42.

Lauersen JB, Bertelsen DM, Andersen LB. The effectiveness of exercise interventions to prevent sports injuries: a systematic review and meta-analysis of randomised controlled trials. Br J Sports Med. 2014;48:871–7.

Lauersen JB, Andersen TE, Andersen LB. Strength training as superior, dose-dependent and safe prevention of acute and overuse sports injuries: a systematic review, qualitative analysis and meta-analysis. Br J Sports Med. 2018;52:1557–63.

Lawrence MA, Carlson LA. Effects of an unstable load on force and muscle activation during a parallel back squat. J Strength Cond Res. 2015;29:2949–53.

Littlewood C, Bateman M, Brown K, et al. A self-managed single exercise programme versus usual physiotherapy treatment for rotator cuff tendinopathy: a randomised controlled trial (the SELF study). Clin Rehabil. 2016;30:686–96.

Logerstedt DS, Scalzitti DA, Bennell KL, et al. Knee pain and mobility impairments: Meniscal and articular cartilage lesions Revision 2018. J Orthop Sports Phys Ther. 2018;48:A1–A50.

Lorenz D, Morrison S. Current concepts in periodization of strength and conditioning for the sports physical therapist. Int J Sports Phys Ther. 2015;10:734–47.

Lovegrove S, Hughes LJ, Mansfield SK, et al. Repetitions in reserve is a reliable tool for prescribing resistance training load. J Strength Cond Res. 2021 Epub Ahead of Print.

Macadam P, Feser EH. Examination of gluteus maximus electromyographic excitation associated with dynamic hip extension during body weight exercise: A systematic review. Int J Sports Phys Ther. 2019;14:14–31.

Macadam P, Cronin J, Contreras B. An examination of the gluteal muscle activity associated with dynamic hip abduction and hip external rotation exercise: A systematic review. Int J Sports Phys Ther. 2015;10:573–91.

Martín-Fuentes I, Oliva-Lozano JM, Muyor JM. Electromyographic activity in deadlift exercise and its variants. A systematic review. PLoS One. 2020;15:e0229507.

Minshull C, Gleeson N. Considerations of the principles of resistance training in exercise studies for the management of knee osteoarthritis: A systematic review. Arch Phys Med Rehabil. 2017;98:1842–51.

Moore D, Semciw AI, Pizzari T. Systematic review and meta-analysis of common therapeutic exercises that generate highest muscle activity in the gluteus medius and gluteus minimus segments. Int J Sports Phys Ther. 2020;15:856–81.

Morawetz D, Blank C, Koller A, et al. Sex-related differences after a single bout of maximal eccentric exercise in response to acute effects: a systematic review and meta-analysis. J Strength Cond Res. 2020;34:2697–707.

Morrison S. Optimal Loading: ExRx for Rehabilitation Professionals. Professional Course; 2020.

Morrison S, Ward P, duManoir G. Energy system development and load management through the rehabilitation and return to play process. Int J Sports Phys Ther. 2017;12:697–710.

Mosler AB, Agricola R, Weir A, et al. Which factors differentiate athletes with hip/groin pain from those without? A systematic review with meta-analysis. Br J Sports Med. 2015;49:810.

Neto WK, Vieira TL, Gama EF. Barbell hip thrust, muscular activation and performance: A systematic review. J Sports Sci Med. 2019;18:198–206.

Neto WK, Soares EG, Vieira TL, et al. Gluteus maximus activation during common strength and hypertrophy exercises: A systematic review. J Sports Sci Med. 2020;19:195–203.

Nicolson PJA, Bennell KL, Dobson FL, et al. Interventions to increase adherence to therapeutic exercise in older adults with low back pain and/or hip/knee osteoarthritis: a systematic review and meta-analysis. Br J Sports Med. 2017;51:791–99.

O'Sullivan K, McAuliffe S, Deburca N. The effects of eccentric training on lower limb flexibility: a systematic review. Br J Sports Med. 2012;46:838–45.

Panariello RA, Stump TJ, Allen AA. Rehabilitation and return to play following anterior cruciate ligament reconstruction. Oper Techn Sport Med. 2017;25:181–93.

Plisk SS, Stone M H. Periodization strategies. Strength Cond J .2003;25:19–37.

Rio E, Kidgell D, Moseley GL, et al. Tendon neuroplastic training: changing the way we think about tendon rehabilitation: a narrative review. Br J Sports Med. 2016;50:209–15.

Saltychev M, Dutton RA, Laimi K, et al. Effectiveness of conservative treatment for patellofemoral pain syndrome: A systematic review and meta-analysis. J Rehabil Med. 2018;50:393–401.

Schoenfeld BJ, Ratamess NA, Peterson MD, et al. Effects of different volume-equated resistance training loading strategies on muscular adaptations in well-trained men. J Strength Cond Res. 2014;28:2909–18.

Schoenfeld BJ, Ogborn D, Krieger J. Dose-response relationship between weekly resistance training volume and increases in muscle mass: A systematic review and meta-analysis. J Sports Sci. 2017;35:1073–82.

Schoenfeld BJ, Grgic J, Krieger J. How many times per week should a muscle be trained to maximize muscle hypertrophy? A systematic review and meta-analysis of studies examining the effects of resistance training frequency. J Sports Sci. 2019;37:1286–95.

Schoenfeld BJ, Grgic J, Every DWV, Plotkin DL. Loading recommendations for muscle strength, hypertrophy, and local endurance: A re-examination of the repetition continuum. Sports. 2021;9:32.

Schütz P, List R, Zemp R, et al. Joint angles of the ankle, knee, and hip and loading conditions during split squats. J Appl Biomech. 2014;30:373-80.

Serner A, Jakobsen MD, Andersen LL, et al. EMG evaluation of hip adduction exercises for soccer players: implications for exercise selection in prevention and treatment of groin injuries. Br J Sports Med. 2014;48:1108–14.

Sigward SM, Chan MS, Lin P, et al. Compensatory strategies that reduce knee extensor demands during a bilateral squat change from 3 to 5 months following anterior cruciate ligament reconstruction. J Orthop Sports Phys Ther. 2018;48:713–18.

Silbernagel KG, Thomeé R, Thomeé P, et al. Eccentric overload training for patients with chronic Achilles tendon pain: a randomised controlled study with reliability testing of the evaluation methods. Scand J Med Sci Sports. 2001;11:197–206.

Smith BE, Hendrick P, Smith TO, et al. Should exercises be painful in the management of chronic musculoskeletal pain? A systematic review and meta-analysis. Br J Sports Med. 2017;51:1679–87.

Stanish WD, Rubinovich RM, Curwin S. Eccentric exercise in chronic tendinitis. Clin Orthop Relat Res. 1986:65–8.

Steele J, Endres A, Fisher J, et al. Ability to predict repetitions to momentary failure is not perfectly accurate, though improves with resistance training experience. Peer J. 2017;5:e4105.

Swart NM, van Oudenaarde K, Reijnierse M, et al. Effectiveness of exercise therapy for meniscal lesions in adults: A systematic review and meta-analysis. J Sci Med Sport. 2016;19:990-8.

Thomas E, Bianco A, Paoli A, Palma A. The relation between stretching typology and stretching duration: The effects on range of motion. Int J Sports Med. 2018;39:243–54.

Vaegter HB, Handberg G, Graven-Nielsen T. Similarities between exercise-induced hypoalgesia and conditioned pain modulation in humans. Pain. 2014;155:158–67.

van Dyk N, Behan FP, Whiteley R. Including the Nordic hamstring exercise in injury prevention programmes halves the rate of hamstring injuries: a systematic review and meta-analysis of 8459 athletes. Br J Sports Med. 2019;53:1362–70.

Vatovec R, Kozinc Ž, Šarabon N. Exercise interventions to prevent hamstring injuries in athletes: A systematic review and meta-analysis. Eur J Sport Sci. 2020;20:992–1004.

Vigotsky A, Bryanton M. Relative muscle contributions to net joint moments in the barbell back squat. American Society of Biomechanics 40th Annual Meeting. North Carolina State University, Raleigh, NC; 2016.

Wallis JA, Roddy L, Bottrell J, et al. A systematic review of Clinical Practice Guidelines for physical therapist management of patellofemoral pain. Phys Ther. 2021;101(3):pzab021.

Walsh ME, French HP, Wallace E, et al. Existing validated clinical prediction rules for predicting response to physio-therapy interventions for musculoskeletal conditions have limited clinical value: A systematic review. J Clin Epidemiol. 2021;135:90–102.

Weppler CH, Magnusson SP. Increasing muscle extensibility: A matter of increasing length or modifying sensation? Phys Ther. 2010;90:438–49.

Winters M, Holden S, Lura CB, et al. Comparative effectiveness of treatments for patellofemoral pain: a living systematic review with network meta-analysis. Br J Sports Med. 2020;55(7):369–77.

Yeung SS, Yeung EW, Gillespie LD. Interventions for preventing lower limb soft-tissue running injuries. Cochrane Database Syst Rev. 2011;7:CD001256.

Pain neuroscience education: treating the brain in hip and knee pain syndromes

Emilio "Louie" Puentedura, Thomas Longbottom

Introduction

Whenever a person has pain in their lower extremity, their experience of that pain is complex, individualized and 100% produced by their brain (Moseley 2003a; Moseley 2007). We now know that pain is a decision by the brain, based on subjective perception (Moseley 2007; Louw & Puentedura, 2013; Louw et al., 2018), and it is quite distinct from nociception. Nociception is merely the signaling of noxious stimulation and is a subcategory of somatosensation (Dubin & Patapoutian, 2010). It is the neural processing of that nociception by the brain that may or may not result in a pain experience. While a person will always be aware of their experience of pain, nociception can be present without any awareness. Take, for instance, the activation of nociceptors when stepping barefoot on a Lego block, causing the reflexive withdrawal of the foot to avoid tissue damage before that information ever reaches the conscious perception of pain. For a more complex example, consider the case of victims of severe trauma who do not register the subjective experience of pain despite their injuries. It is the false assumption that pain and nociception are synonymous that forms the basis of the Cartesian model of pain (1664) which assumes that tissue injury or disease states are directly correlated with pain (Haldeman, 1990; Goldberg, 2008; Louw & Puentedura, 2013; Louw et al., 2018). We know the concept of the greater the severity of injury or disease state causing the greater pain experience to be untrue. And yet, it is this outdated Cartesian thinking that continues to be the prevailing model we use for treating pain (Goldberg, 2008). More and more pain researchers believe that this outdated model of seeking "which tissues are to blame" (i.e., which tissues are providing nociception) and then focusing solely on those tissues may in fact be a significant contributor to the increased epidemic of chronic pain worldwide (Haldeman, 1990; Goldberg, 2008; Louw & Puentedura, 2013; Louw et al., 2018).

For any clinician interested in treating people with hip and knee pain, especially chronic hip or knee pain, the brain should be the primary target for directing treatment (Melzack, 2001). It has now been well established that the central nervous system (CNS) undergoes several significant changes in people with chronic pain, and it is these changes that contribute to the development and maintenance of chronic pain states (Flor et al., 1997; Flor, 2000; Schmidt-Wilcke et al., 2006; Apkarian et al., 2009; Tracey & Bushnell, 2009). Understanding these changes within the CNS is important, as treatment should aim to restore these changes as a means to ease the pain and suffering of the patient with chronic pain. This chapter will focus on four observed changes within the brain and spinal cord (CNS) related to pain and then discuss treatment options to restore these changes.

The Neuromatrix

Contrary to the historical view of pain being experienced and controlled in a single or discrete area within the brain (Melzack, 2001), we can now appreciate that multiple areas of the brain are activated during a pain experience (Flor, 2000, 2003; Melzack, 2001; Moseley 2003a; Puentedura & Louw, 2012; Louw et al., 2015a). This widespread brain activation during a pain experience has become known as the pain neuromatrix (Figure 20.1) (Melzack, 2001). It is defined as a pattern of nerve impulses generated by a distributed neural network within the brain (Melzack, 2001). Pain is therefore experienced (produced) by the output of this widely distributed neural network in the brain rather than directly by sensory input evoked by injury, inflammation, or other pathology (Melzack, 2001; Moseley 2003a; Puentedura & Louw, 2012). Although care should be taken with generalization, it is now understood that certain areas are commonly activated during any pain experience and these areas have become synonymous with the "pain neuromatrix" (Melzack, 2001; Flor, 2003; Moseley, 2003a; Puentedura & Louw, 2012). Functional MRI (fMRI) and positron emission tomography (PET) scans have shown that the most common areas associated with the pain neuromatrix are the anterior cingulate cortex, primary sensory cortex, amygdala, thalamus, anterior insula, and prefrontal and posterior parietal cortices (Flor, 2000, 2003; Moseley, 2003a). When a person is asked to perform a painful task or is administered experimental pain whilst undergoing brain scans, these increasingly active brain areas communicate with each other, developing a pain map or a pain neurotag (Puentedura & Louw, 2012; Louw & Puentedura, 2013).

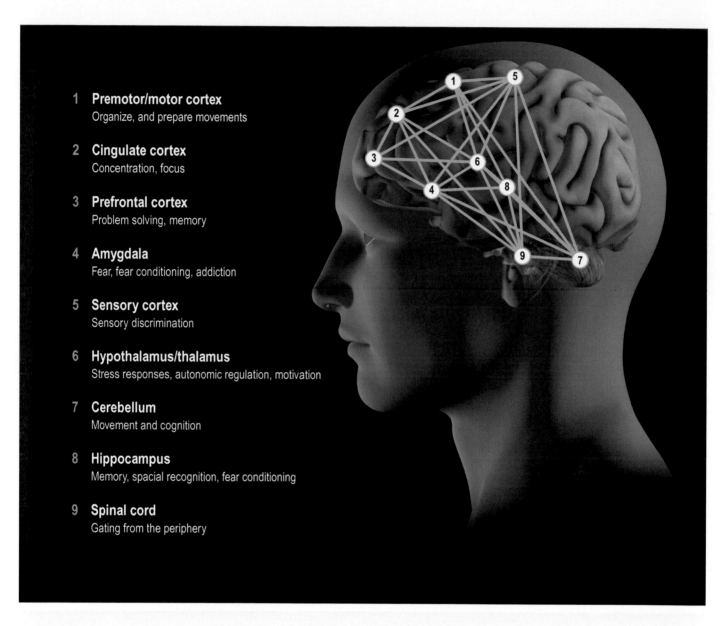

1 **Premotor/motor cortex**
Organize, and prepare movements

2 **Cingulate cortex**
Concentration, focus

3 **Prefrontal cortex**
Problem solving, memory

4 **Amygdala**
Fear, fear conditioning, addiction

5 **Sensory cortex**
Sensory discrimination

6 **Hypothalamus/thalamus**
Stress responses, autonomic regulation, motivation

7 **Cerebellum**
Movement and cognition

8 **Hippocampus**
Memory, spacial recognition, fear conditioning

9 **Spinal cord**
Gating from the periphery

FIGURE 20.1
Widespread brain activation during a pain experience seen as a pain neurotag, which involves several common brain areas.
(Redrawn from Puentedura EJ, Louw A. A neuroscience approach to managing athletes with low back pain. Phys Ther Sport. 2012;13:123–33.)

An important and relevant concept is related to the Hebbian theory commonly described as proposing that neurons that fire together, wire together (Shatz, 1992; Keysers & Gazzola, 2014). More precisely, Hebb proposed that "When an axon of cell A is near enough to excite a Cell B and repeatedly or persistently takes part in firing it, some growth process or metabolic change takes place in one or both cells such that A's efficiency, as one of the cells firing B, is increased" (Hebb, 1949, p. 62). This describes a basic mechanism for synaptic plasticity wherein an increase in synaptic efficacy arises from the presynaptic cell's repeated and persistent stimulation of the postsynaptic cell. The brain of a person with chronic pain, then, may become more proficient in running its pain map. This CNS synaptic plasticity occurs both at spinal and supraspinal levels. Clinically, less stimulation may be needed to activate the pain map, which is the hallmark of central sensitization (Woolf, 2007; Nijs et al., 2010). Furthermore, the activation of the pain neuromatrix can be influenced by neighboring neural circuits, likely influencing the individual pain experience (Figure 20.2) (Puentedura & Louw, 2012). The fact that a person's pain map can be tuned up or down by the adjacent maps in regard to the individual's knowledge, experiences, beliefs, etc., makes each person's pain experience more individualized and complicated. A skilled clinician should recognize that a pain experience can be associated with multiple and various issues that may all need to be addressed in treatment.

The clinician should also be cognizant that neuroplastic changes involving activation of the pain neuromatrix can be targeted to down-regulate or dissociate normal somatosensation, movement, and other functions also associated with the multimodal neuromatrix that, to be clear, is not isolated to pain signals alone (Iannetti & Mouraux,

2010). Rather than being a rigid pathway dedicated to pain information, the neuromatrix includes neuronal regions involved in a variety of roles, including such functions as cognition, emotion, sensation, motion, and motivation (Ossipov et al., 2010). When motor cortex activation for motor control exercises is associated with the pain neuromatrix, for example, a person may justifiably exhibit difficulty executing the desired precise motor control activities (Moseley & Hodges, 2002). The multimodal nature of the neurons in the pain neuromatrix can explain other issues commonly seen in persons with chronic pain such as problems with focus and concentration, regulating body temperature, sleep disturbance, short term memory issues and more (Sapolsky, 1994; Luerding et al., 2008). Understanding this multimodal nature of the pain neuromatrix and its potential neuroplasticity may be key in helping a person manage chronic pain, and explanation of these concepts is a cornerstone of Pain Neuroscience Education (PNE) (Louw et al., 2011a; Louw & Puentedura, 2013).

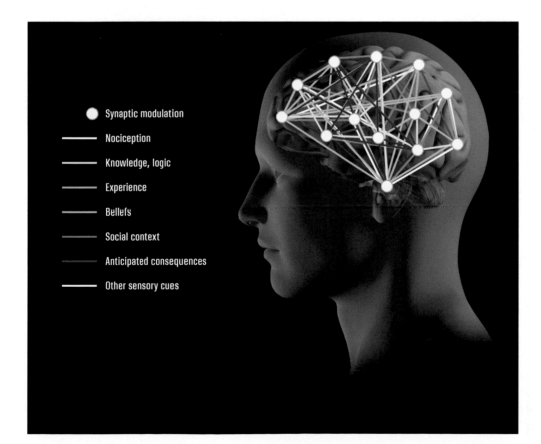

Synaptic modulation

Nociception

Knowledge, logic

Experience

Beliefs

Social context

Anticipated consequences

Other sensory cues

FIGURE 20.2
The activation of the pain neuromatrix (shown in red) can be influenced by neighboring neural circuits involved with knowledge and logic (yellow), past experience (green), beliefs about pain (blue), etc. and these neighboring circuits can modulate the pain experience.
(Redrawn from Puentedura EJ, Louw A. A neuroscience approach to managing athletes with low back pain. Phys Ther Sport. 2012;13:123–33.)

CHAPTER TWENTY

Structural Changes in the Brain

Studies comparing brain structure between healthy individuals and those suffering from chronic pain have looked at changes in gray and white matter volume (Apkarian et al., 2004; Schmidt-Wilcke, 2008; Schmidt-Wilcke et al., 2008). It is now well established that in people with chronic pain, various areas of the brain undergo volume changes including the dorsolateral prefrontal cortex, right anterior thalamus, brainstem, and somatosensory, posterior parietal, insular and cingulate cortices (Apkarian et al., 2004; Schmidt-Wilcke et al., 2008). The extent of changes in brain density has been correlated to pain intensity (Schmidt-Wilcke et al., 2006). Indeed, there is a growing body of evidence that acute pain and particularly pain intensity may be a consequential predictor in the development of chronic pain (Woolf & Salter, 2005; Jull et al., 2007; Woolf, 2007). Of particular interest to clinicians is the potential to restore gray matter following decreases associated with chronic pain (Rodriguez-Raecke et al., 2009). Interventions aimed at altering information to the brain with modalities like cognitive behavioral therapy, mobility training, and others aimed at affecting nociception have the ability to restore gray matter, resulting also in positive effects on pain, pain catastrophization and disability (de Lange et al., 2008, Rodriguez-Raecke et al., 2009; Gwilym et al., 2010; Seminowicz et al., 2011, 2013). The take-away message from a growing body of evidence is the suggestion that strategies aimed at structural reorganization in the brain may be useful as a means of treating chronic pain (Apkarian et al., 2004; de Lange et al., 2008; Schmidt-Wilcke, 2008; Schmidt-Wilcke et al., 2008; Rodriguez-Raecke et al., 2009; Gwilym et al., 2010; Seminowicz et al., 2011; Wand et al., 2011; Seminowicz et al., 2013).

Functional Changes in the Brain

Cortical areas of the brain can be mapped by observing neuron activity during sensory stimulation or motor activity. Modification of these cortical maps is possible via varied or altered sensory or motor input, with use-dependent and experience-dependent remodeling of the cortical map having implications for rehabilitation (Liepert et al., 2000; Barnes & Finnerty, 2010; Xerri, 2012). The relative quickness with which these changes in the cortical map can occur can be astounding. For example, one study has demonstrated

that change in the cortical map associated with the fingers can occur when the four fingers are webbed together for a period of only 30 minutes (Stavrinou et al., 2007). This has implications for the importance of strategies to maintain normal sensory and motor cortical representation early in a pain experience that has the potential to change this functional organization (Moseley, 2004a, 2005).

Descending Pathways

A notable factor in a person's pain experience is the brain's descending anti-nociceptive system (Fields et al., 2005; Giesecke et al., 2006). It is well established that various neurophysiological mechanisms in the CNS, particularly the midbrain, regulate information that the brain receives from the periphery. This bidirectional system allows information to be enhanced (facilitation) or down-regulated (inhibition). The midbrain periaqueductal gray (PAG) is noted to integrate inputs from the limbic forebrain and diencephalon with the nociceptive input received by the dorsal horn (Bandler & Keay, 1996). Further, functional neuroimaging studies in humans indicate that PAG activation by nociceptive inputs is modulated by attention, emotion, expectation of pain, and expectation-related placebo analgesia (Tracey et al., 2002; Parry et al., 2008; Wiech & Tracey, 2009). Considering that patients with chronic pain display a decreased ability to engage the endogenous mechanisms of the brain it is commonly believed that the PAG is negatively affected in patients with chronic pain (Peyron et al., 2000, Sterling et al., 2001; Nijs et al., 2012). For example, it has been shown that in patients with chronic low back pain there are lesser increases in blood flow in the PAG than controls when exposed to equally painful stimuli (Giesecke et al., 2006). The decreased ability of the PAG to alter sensory information, such as touch, is likely a part of the clinical manifestation of central sensitization (Woolf, 2007; Nijs et al., 2011).

Management

Many changes occur to the CNS and brain in people with chronic hip and knee pain, and this chapter has only discussed four specific changes. Obviously, addressing and making corrections to these changes will be vital if clinicians are to help these people with their chronic pain. This statement is supported by the emerging evidence for the use of treatments aimed at restoring these changes in the CNS and brain, such as restoring laterality (Gormley & Brydges, 2016; Phillips et al., 2020), graded motor imagery (Moseley, 2004b, 2006; Daly & Bialocerkowski, 2009; Bowering et al., 2013), sensory discrimination (Moseley & Wiech, 2009), and PNE (Moseley, 2002; Moseley et al., 2004; Louw et al., 2011a). Understanding that pain is an output produced by the brain, based on perception of threat, is the cornerstone of PNE.

Traditionally, clinicians have either followed a top-down (cognitive) approach or a bottom-up (nociceptive modulation) approach, such as manual therapy and exercise to treat hip and knee pain. We would argue that these two approaches need not be mutually exclusive. Looking at a patient with chronic hip and knee pain as having *either* a cognitive or a nociceptive tissue problem can be seen as contrary to the modern neuroscience view of pain. It would merely perpetuate Cartesian thinking about pain and lead the clinician to determine if pain is *either* physical or psychological. Pain is *both* and therefore treatment must address both. For example, PNE has shown compelling evidence for treating people with chronic pain (Louw et al., 2011, 2016), but it has been shown to be best if combined with movement-based therapies such as manual therapy and exercise (Ryan et al., 2010; Louw et al., 2011a, 2016).

In a case series involving 12 patients scheduled for total knee arthroplasty (TKA), Louw et al. (2019a) provided preoperative PNE and looked for immediate effects. They reported statistically lower scores for the Tampa Scale of Kinesiophobia (TSK), increased Pain Pressure Thresholds (PPT), and improved beliefs about their upcoming surgery. But there were no significant changes for knee pain, function, or knee flexion range of motion, suggesting that education by itself seemed to have no immediate effects on physical outcome measures. In a second study of 120 patients scheduled for TKA, Louw et al. (2019b) compared patients who received traditional group hospital preoperative education on its own versus those who received an additional 30-minute group PNE session. They tracked pain, function, fear of movement, and pain catastrophization at baseline, 1, 3, and 6 months post-surgery. There were no significant differences in any outcome measures between the two groups over time, and both groups demonstrated similar improvements over time suggesting that the 30-minute group PNE session was not sufficient to change key outcome measures. In both of the studies by Louw et al., the designs were limited by patient access and hospital administration parameters. Both studies found improved patient satisfaction scores and improved beliefs about pain post-TKA but no changes or differences in pain, function, and physical outcome measures.

A recent study protocol by Larsen et al. (2020) might well provide further insight into the value of PNE for chronic pain in patients after TKA. The researchers have proposed a randomized controlled superiority trial involving 120 patients with moderate-to-severe chronic pain after TKA. Patients will be randomly assigned to one of two interventions – a 12-week neuromuscular exercise training program combined with PNE or 2 sessions of PNE given over 6 weeks. Assessment will be performed at baseline before intervention and at 3, 6, and 12 months after start of intervention. Primary outcome measures proposed are changes in the Knee Injury and Osteoarthritis Outcome Score[4] (KOOS[4]) as well as pain, function, Fear-Avoidance Beliefs Questionnaire (FABQ), Global Perceived Effect, and the Pain Catastrophization Scale. They will also assess physical performance measures of walking, stair climbing, and chair standing tests as well as tests of muscle strength and power.

Briones-Cantero et al. (2020) investigated the effects of including motor imagery (MI) (a component of PNE) into early physical therapy on pain, disability, pressure pain thresholds (PPTs), and range of motion in the early postsurgical phase after TKA. They reported that the application of MI to early physiotherapy was effective for improving pain and disability, but not range of motion or pressure pain sensitivity, in the early postsurgical phase after TKA in people with knee osteoarthritis.

The studies discussed so far can be seen as primary top-down approaches in an attempt to alter the way the CNS and brain *perceives* pain. Bottom-up approaches can be seen as attempts to alter the information (input) the CNS and brain *receives* to determine if pain is an appropriate output. Most of the current research on PNE alone (education only) suggests that it is not very effective for outcomes such as pain and disability, however it does appear to be effective for patient satisfaction and altering their beliefs about pain. Research has shown that transcutaneous electrical neuromuscular stimulation (TENS) and electrical stimulation, via the pain gate, can have an effect on the information received by the dorsal horn of the spinal cord and ultimately the brain, pain neuromatrix and change a person's pain experience in the short term (Wall, 1996; Melzack, 1999). Manual therapy, e.g., joint mobilization and manipulation, exercise, needling techniques, etc., have been shown to exert endogenous effects and positively affect a person's pain state in the short term (Vicenzino et al., 1996; Sterling et al., 2001; George et al., 2006; Fernandez-Carnero et al., 2008). Today's evidence-informed clinician utilizing sound clinical reasoning and an updated knowledge of pain neuroscience and pain mechanisms should approach treatment from the perspective of altering "danger information" to the CNS and brain as a means to minimize threat and ultimately the patient's pain experience. To do this effectively requires restructuring the meaning of information received by the CNS and brain, and restructuring (rewiring) the CNS and brain so that alternatives to pain as an output can be instigated in patients with chronic hip and knee pain.

Pain Neuroscience Education – Restructuring the Meaning

Research into educational strategies for patients with chronic pain shows an increased use of PNE (Moseley, 2003b, 2004c, 2005; Moseley et al., 2004), which aims to reduce pain and disability by helping patients gain an increased understanding of neurobiological and neurophysiological processes involved in their pain experience (Ryan et al., 2010; Louw et al., 2011a). PNE differs from traditional education strategies in that it does not focus on anatomical or biomechanical explanations for pain, but rather on neurophysiology, neurobiology, processing and representation and meaning of pain (Moseley, 2005; Meeus et al., 2010; Ryan et al., 2010). It has been demonstrated that patients are quite capable of understanding the neurophysiology of pain, while healthcare professionals tend to underestimate their patients' ability to understand the complex issues related to pain (Moseley, 2003a). Different systematic reviews suggest strong evidence for PNE addressing pain, disability and physical performance in musculoskeletal pain, particularly spinal disorders (Louw et al., 2011a, 2016; Watson et al., 2019). Studies which utilized PNE have been shown to decrease fear and change a patient's perception of their pain (Moseley, 2003c), have an immediate effect on improvements in patients' attitudes about pain (Moseley, 2003c), improvements in pain, cognition and physical performance (Moseley, 2004c), increased pain thresholds during physical tasks (Moseley et al., 2004), improved outcomes of therapeutic exercises (Moseley, 2002), and significantly reduced widespread brain activity characteristic of a pain experience (Moseley, 2005).

Despite the explosive growth in research on PNE and the improved understanding of pain by many healthcare providers, there are still many who continue to hold to Cartesian thinking and will persist in dichotomizing their patients' pain as either mostly physical or mostly psychological. If they believe it is mostly psychological, they might argue that PNE is the approach that is needed. This thinking has led PNE to be viewed as the provision of lengthy one-on-one psycho-educational sessions around a table, trying to get a patient to change their beliefs about pain – in other words, restructuring the meaning of the patient's pain experience. However, as noted earlier in this chapter and evidenced in the research, PNE should be provided *in conjunction with* movement-based treatments. We should acknowledge that we cannot simply "talk our patients out of pain" (Shala et al., 2021). Movement, when applied and utilized in conjunction with PNE is better understood, less feared and has different meaning. It is understood that pain felt during movement is not necessarily due to injury but from an extra-sensitive nervous system (Louw et al., 2013).

In regards to structural changes within the CNS and brain, no studies specific to PNE have been reported; however, some studies have shown an increase in gray matter in the brain following cognitive behavioral therapy (CBT) (de Lange et al., 2008; Seminowicz et al., 2013). PNE is similar in many ways to CBT in that PNE is cognitive therapy and in its ability to restructure the meaning of pain. PNE can be seen as the "C" in CBT in that it aims to restructure threat and meaning of pain, which is a cornerstone of CBT (Bennett & Nelson, 2006; Ang et al., 2010). Future studies should investigate if these increases in gray matter can be correlated to the cognitive restructuring and more directly specific to PNE.

To date no studies have been reported on whether or not PNE is associated with functional changes in body maps within the brain. PNE may have an effect on the PAG and anti-nociceptive system. Indirectly, PNE is associated

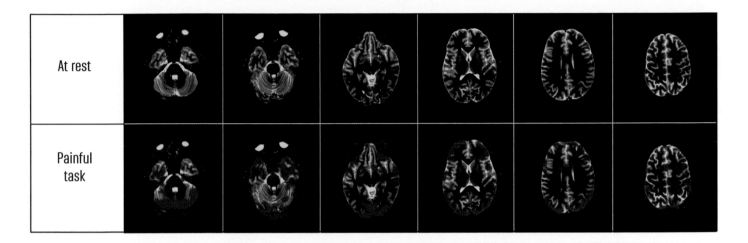

FIGURE 20.3
Functional magnetic resonance images (fMRI) of a subject at rest (top) and while performing a painful task (bottom) showing widespread brain activation via blood oxygen level dependent (BOLD) technique.

(From Louw A, Puentedura EJ, Diener I, Peoples RR. Pre-operative therapeutic neuroscience education for lumbar radiculopathy: a single-case fMRI report. Physiother Theory Pract. 2015;31:496–508.)

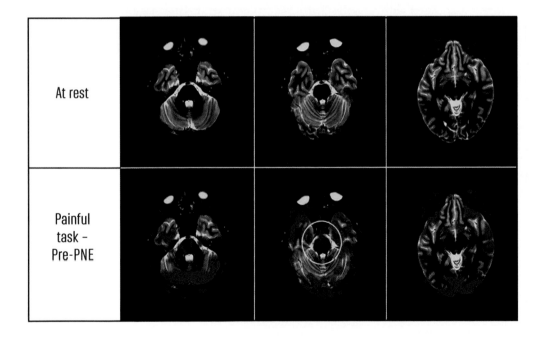

FIGURE 20.4
In the pre-PNE imaging, the widespread brain activation seen via blood oxygen level dependent (BOLD) technique when the subject performs a painful task (bottom image) shows activation of the periaqueductal gray region of the brain (circled).

(From Louw A, Puentedura EJ, Diener I, Peoples RR. Pre-operative therapeutic neuroscience education for lumbar radiculopathy: a single-case fMRI report. Physiother Theory Pract. 2015;31:496–508.)

with decreased levels of pain experience, increase in PPT and ability to exercise and move better despite pain (Louw et al., 2011a). In a functional magnetic resonance imaging (fMRI) case study utilizing PNE preoperatively for lumbar radiculopathy, pre- and post-PNE changes to the PAG were observed (Louw et al., 2015a). During a painful task, the patient displayed widespread brain activity (Figure 20.3). Closer analysis revealed significant activation of the PAG (Figure 20.4). Although cause and effect cannot be determined from a case study, it is plausible that the PAG was activated in response to a threatening movement this patient associated with a painful task. However, following PNE the same painful task did not result in a similar activation of the PAG (Figure 20.5). As the aim of the PNE was to

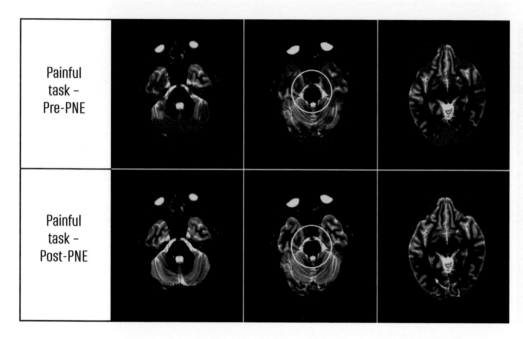

Painful task – Pre-PNE
Painful task – Post-PNE

FIGURE 20.5
In the post-PNE imaging, the widespread brain activation seen via blood oxygen level dependent (BOLD) technique when the subject performs a painful task (bottom image) shows decreased brain activation and almost no increase in activation of the periaqueductal gray region of the brain (circled).

(From Louw A, Puentedura EJ, Diener I, Peoples RR. Pre-operative therapeutic neuroscience education for lumbar radiculopathy: a single-case fMRI report. Physiother Theory Pract. 2015;31:496–508.)

reconceptualize the pain and decrease fear associated with movement, we could argue that, in this case, after the PNE the PAG did not need activation, since the incoming nociception was understood and determined not a threat. Further research should investigate the specific effect of PNE on the anti-nociceptive systems, such as the PAG.

Graded Motor Imagery – Restructuring Brain/Body Maps

Therapeutic interventions targeted towards correcting the observed functional changes within the brain have gained increased attention, especially in advanced pain states such as complex regional pain syndrome (CRPS) (Daly & Bialocerkowski, 2009; Wand et al., 2011). Graded motor imagery (GMI) is a structured, sequential series of cortical exercises aimed at reestablishing the cortical deficits described previously (Moseley, 2004b, 2006; Daly & Bialocerkowski, 2009; Bowering et al., 2013). GMI includes strategies such as normalizing a person's ability to recognize left or right body parts or movements (laterality); motor imagery or visualization of static and dynamic use of a body part; and mirror therapy. GMI has shown increasing evidence as a means to positively influence pain states such as CRPS (McCabe et al., 2003; Moseley, 2004b, 2006; Daly & Bialocerkowski, 2009; Bowering et al., 2013) and it may have some use in patients with chronic hip and

knee pain. Additional strategies aimed at restructuring cortical maps, such as sensory discrimination, graphesthesia and two-point discrimination have been proposed and utilized alongside GMI to help facilitate these cortical changes (Moseley, 2008; Moseley et al., 2008; Moseley & Wiech, 2009; Luomajoki & Moseley, 2011). Unfortunately, there does not appear to be any research showing these altered cortical maps in patients with chronic hip and knee pain, nor any research showing that patients with chronic hip and knee pain have altered left–right discrimination (laterality) or other sensory discrimination. It has been observed in people with chronic pain (Louw et al., 2015b, 2017) and might therefore be present regardless of where pain is felt.

Traditional "hands-on" treatments such as manual therapy if being precise, specific and even vocalizing the intent and findings, such as a caudal hip distraction or posterior glide of the tibia on a stationary femur, could be seen as a form of cortical restructuring. As we gain more and more insight into the exact cortical changes that occur (i.e., two-point discrimination, smudging of body maps), treatments can become more deliberate and targeted towards creating a bottom-up feed of appropriate sensory information to the brain-senses (touch, sight, sound, etc.) used to help the brain understand more; localize a part better; develop less threat; and restore body parts.

Conclusion

There have been 25 years of understanding pain neuroscience and teaching it to patients. We have discovered and learned so much that we are well beyond Cartesian thinking, and yet we still have so much to learn. This new neuroscientific view of pain, especially chronic musculoskeletal pain, has created significant advances for patients and clinicians. For patients, understanding the true nature of pain and the realization that the brain is eminently capable of neuroplastic change provides hope and people with chronic hip and knee pain can consider non-surgical and non-pharmacological help. For the clinician, there is also excitement and hope. Instead of viewing patients with chronic pain as the most difficult or challenging to treat, they can be seen as the most rewarding when changes for the better occur. The advances described in this chapter should encourage clinicians to boldly create new paradigms and new treatments.

References

Ang DC, Chakr R, Mazzuca S, et al. Cognitive-behavioral therapy attenuates nociceptive responding in patients with fibromyalgia: a pilot study. Arthritis Care Res. 2010;62:618–23.

Apkarian AV, Sosa Y, Sonty S, et al. Chronic back pain is associated with decreased prefrontal and thalamic gray matter density. J Neurosci. 2004;24:10410–5.

Apkarian AV, Baliki MN, Geha PY. Towards a theory of chronic pain. Prog Neurobiol. 2009;87:81–97.

Bandler R, Keay KA. Columnar organization in the midbrain periaqueductal gray and the integration of emotional expression. Progr Brain Res. 1996;107:285–300.

Barnes SJ, Finnerty GT. Sensory experience and cortical rewiring. Neuroscientist. 2010;16:186–98.

Bennett R, Nelson D. Cognitive behavioral therapy for fibromyalgia. Nat Clin Pract Rheumatol. 2006;2:416–24.

Bowering KJ, O'Connell NE, Tabor A, et al. The effects of graded motor imagery and its components on chronic pain: a systematic review and meta-analysis. J Pain. 2013;14:3–13.

Briones-Cantero M, Fernandez-de-las-Peñas C, Lluch-Girbes E, et al. Effects of adding motor imagery to early physical therapy in patients with knee osteoarthritis who had received total knee arthroplasty: A Randomized Clinical Trial. Pain Med. 2020;21:3548–55.

Daly AE, Bialocerkowski AE. Does evidence support physiotherapy management of adult Complex Regional Pain Syndrome Type One? A systematic review. Eur J Pain. 2009;13:339–53.

de Lange FP, Koers A, Kalkman JS, et al. Increase in prefrontal cortical volume following cognitive behavioural therapy in patients with chronic fatigue syndrome. Brain. 2008;131:2172–80.

Dubin AE, Patapoutian A. Nociceptors: the sensors of the pain pathway. J Clin Invest. 2010;120:3760–72.

Fernandez-Carnero J, Fernandez-de-las-Peñas C, Cleland JA. Immediate hypoalgesic and motor effects after a single cervical spine manipulation in subjects with lateral epicondylalgia. J Manipulative Physiol Ther. 2008;31:675–81.

Fields HL, Basbaum AI, Heinricher MR. Central nervous system mechanisms of pain modulation. In: McMahon S, Koltzenburg M (ed). Wall and Melzack's Textbook of Pain. 5th ed. Edinburgh: Elsevier; 2005.

Flor H. The functional organization of the brain in chronic pain. Prog Brain Res. 2000; 129: 313-22.

Flor H. The image of pain. Annual scientific meeting of The Pain Society (Britain). Glasgow, Scotland; 2003.

Flor H, Braun C, Elbert T, Birbaumer N. Extensive reorganization of primary somatosensory cortex in chronic back pain patients. Neurosci Lett. 1997;224:5–8.

George SZ, Bishop MD, Bialosky JE, et al. Immediate effects of spinal manipulation on thermal pain sensitivity: an experimental study. BMC Musculoskelet Disord. 2006;7:68.

Giesecke T, Gracely RH, Clauw DJ, et al. [Central pain processing in chronic low back pain. Evidence for reduced pain inhibition]. Schmerz. 2006;20(5):411–4, 6–7.

Goldberg JS. Revisiting the Cartesian model of pain. Med Hypotheses. 2008;70:1029–33.

Gormley G, Brydges R. Difficulty with right-left discrimination: A clinical problem? CMAJ. 2016;188:98–9.

Gwilym SE, Filippini N, Douaud G, et al. Thalamic atrophy associated with painful osteoarthritis of the hip is reversible after arthroplasty: a longitudinal voxel-based morphometric study. Arthritis Rheum. 2010;62:2930–40.

Haldeman S. Presidential address, North American Spine Society: failure of the pathology model to predict back pain. Spine. 1990;15:718-24.

Hebb DO. The organization of behavior: A neruophysiological theory. New York: Wiley; 1949.

Iannetti GD, Mouraux A. From the neuromatrix to the pain matrix (and back). Exp Brain Res. 2010;205:1–12.

Jull G, Sterling M, Kenardy J, Beller E. Does the presence of sensory hypersensitivity influence outcomes of physical rehabilitation for chronic whiplash? A preliminary RCT. Pain. 2007;129:28–34.

Keysers C, Gazzola V. Hebbian learning and predictive mirror neurons for actions, sensations and emotions. Philos Trans R Soc Lond B Biol Sci. 2014;369:20130175.

Larsen JB, Skou ST, Arendt-Nielsen L, et al. Neuromuscular exercise and pain neuroscience education compared with pain neuroscience education alone in patients with chronic pain after primary total knee arthroplasty: study protocol for the NEPNEP randomized controlled trial. Trials. 2020;21:218.

Liepert J, Bauder H, Wolfgang HR, et al. Treatment-induced cortical reorganization after stroke in humans. Stroke. 2000;31:1210–6.

Louw A, Puentedura EJ. Therapeutic Neuroscience Education. Minneapolis, MN: OPTP; 2013.

Louw A, Diener I, Butler DS, Puentedura EJ. The effect of neuroscience education on pain, disability, anxiety, and stress in chronic musculoskeletal pain. Arch Phys Med Rehabil. 2011a;92:2041–56.

Louw A, Puentedura EL, Mintken P. Use of an abbreviated neuroscience education approach in the treatment of chronic low back pain: A case report. Physiother Theory Pract. 2011b;28:50–62.

Louw A, Butler DS, Diener I, Puentedura EJ. Development of a pre-operative neuroscience educational program for patients with lumbar radiculopathy. Am J Phys Med Rehabil. 2013;92:446–52.

Louw A, Puentedura EJ, Diener I, Peoples RR. Pre-operative therapeutic neuroscience education for lumbar radiculopathy: a single-case fMRI report. Physiother Theory Pract. 2015a;31:496–508.

Louw A, Schmidt SG, Louw C, Puentedura EJ. Moving without moving: immediate management following lumbar spine surgery using a graded motor imagery approach: a case report. Physiother Theory Pract. 2015b;31:509–17.

Louw A, Zimney K, Puentedura EJ, Diener I. The efficacy of pain neuroscience education on musculoskeletal pain: A systematic review of the literature. Physiother Theory Pract. 2016;32:332-55.

Louw A, Puentedura EJ, Reese D, et al. Immediate effects of mirror therapy in patients with shoulder pain and decreased range of motion. Arch Phys Med Rehabil. 2017;98:1941–7.

Louw A, Puentedura EJ, Schmidt S, Zimney K. Pain Neuroscience Education: Teaching People about Pain. 2nd ed. Minneapolis, MN: Orthopedic Physical Therapy Products (OPTP); 2018:536.

Louw A, Puentedura EJ, Reed J, et al. A controlled clinical trial of pre-operative pain neuroscience education for patients about to undergo total knee arthroplasty. Clin Rehabil. 2019a; 33:1722–31.

Louw A, Zimney K, Reed J, et al. Immediate pre-operative outcomes of pain neuroscience education for patients undergoing total knee arthroplasty: A case series. Physiother Theory Pract. 2019b;35:543–53

Luerding R, Weigand T, Bogdahn U, Schmidt-Wilcke T. Working memory performance is correlated with local brain morphology in the medial frontal and anterior cingulate cortex in fibromyalgia patients: structural correlates of pain-cognition interaction. Brain. 2008;131:3222–31.

Luomajoki H, Moseley GL. Tactile acuity and lumbopelvic motor control in patients with back pain and healthy controls. Br J Sports Med. 2011;45:437–40.

McCabe CS, Haigh RC, Ring EFR, et al. A controlled pilot study of the utility of mirror visual feedback in the treatment of complex regional pain syndrome (type 1). Rheumatology. 2003;42:97–101.

Meeus M, Nijs J, Van Oosterwijck J, et al. Pain physiology education improves pain beliefs in patients with chronic fatigue syndrome compared with pacing and self-management education: A double-blind Randomized Controlled Trial. Arch Phys Med Rehabil. 2010;91:1153–9.

Melzack R. From the gate to the neuromatrix. Pain. 1999;S6:S121–6.

Melzack R. Pain and the neuromatrix in the brain. J Dental Education. 2001;65:1378–82.

Moseley L. Combined physiotherapy and education is efficacious for chronic low back pain. Aust J Physiother. 2002;48:297–302.

Moseley GL. A pain neuromatrix approach to patients with chronic pain. Man Ther. 2003a;8:130–40.

Moseley GL. Unraveling the barriers to reconceptualization of the problem in chronic pain: the actual and perceived ability of patients and health professionals to understand the neurophysiology. J Pain. 2003b;4:184–9.

Moseley GL. Joining forces – combining cognition-targeted motor control training with group or individual pain physiology education: A successful treatment for chronic low back pain. J Man Manipul Ther. 2003c;11:88–94.

Moseley GL. Why do people with complex regional pain syndrome take longer to recognize their affected hand? Neurology. 2004a;62:2182–6.

Moseley GL. Graded motor imagery is effective for long standing complex regional pain syndrome. Pain. 2004b;108:192–8.

Moseley GL. Evidence for a direct relationship between cognitive and physical change during an education intervention in people with chronic low back pain. Eur J Pain. 2004c;8:39–45.

Moseley GL. Widespread brain activity during an abdominal task markedly reduced after pain physiology education: fMRI evaluation of a single patient with chronic low back pain. Aust J Physiother. 2005;51:49–52.

Moseley GL. Graded motor imagery for pathologic pain: a randomized controlled trial. Neurology. 2006;67:2129–34.

Moseley GL. Reconceptualising pain acording to modern pain sciences. Phys Ther Rev. 2007;12:169–78.

Moseley GL. I can't find it! Distorted body image and tactile dysfunction in patients with chronic back pain. Pain. 2008;140:239–43.

Moseley GL, Hodges PW. Chronic pain and motor control. In: Jull G, Boyling J, editors. Grieves Modern Manual Therapy of the Vertebral Column. 4 ed. Edinburgh: Churchill-Livingstone; 2002.

Moseley GL, Wiech K. The effect of tactile discrimination training is enhanced when patients watch the reflected image of their unaffected limb during training. Pain. 2009;144:314–9.

Moseley GL, Nicholas MK, Hodges PW. A randomized controlled trial of intensive neurophysiology education in chronic low back pain. Clin J Pain. 2004;20:324–30.

Moseley GL, Sim DF, Henry ML, Souvlis T. Experimental hand pain delays recognition of the contralateral hand--evidence that acute and chronic pain have opposite effects on information processing? Brain Res Cogn Brain Res. 2005;25:188–94.

Moseley GL, Zalucki NM, Wiech K. Tactile discrimination, but not tactile stimulation alone, reduces chronic limb pain. Pain. 2008;137:600–8.

Nijs J, Van Houdenhove B, Oostendorp RA. Recognition of central sensitization in patients with musculoskeletal pain: Application of pain neurophysiology in manual therapy practice. Man Ther. 2010;15:135–41.

Nijs J, Meeus M, Van Oosterwijck J, et al. Treatment of central sensitization in patients with 'unexplained' chronic pain: what options do we have? Expert Opin Pharmacother. 2011;12:1087–98.

Nijs J, Kosek E, Van Oosterwijck J, Meeus M. Dysfunctional endogenous analgesia during exercise in patients with chronic pain: to exercise or not to exercise? Pain Physician. 2012;15: ES205–13.

Ossipov MH, Dussor GO, Porreca F. Central modulation of pain. J Clin Invest. 2010;120:3779-87.

Parry DM, Macmillan FM, Koutsikou S, et al. Separation of A- versus C-nociceptive inputs into spinal-brainstem circuits. Neuroscience. 2008;152:1076–85.

Peyron R, Laurent B, Garcia-Larrea L. Functional imaging of brain responses to pain. A review and meta- analysis (2000). Neurophysiol Clin. 2000;30:263–88.

Phillips N, Hach S, Mannion J, Moran R. Effect of acute experimental hand pain on left-right discrimination response latency for hand recognition. Physiother Theory Pract. 2020;36:1232–40.

Puentedura EJ, Louw A. A neuroscience approach to managing athletes with low back pain. Phys Ther Sport. 2012;13:123–33.

Rodriguez-Raecke R, Niemeier A, Ihle K, et al. Brain gray matter decrease in chronic pain is the consequence and not the cause of pain. J Neurosci. 2009;29:13746–50.

Ryan CG, Gray HG, Newton M, Granat MH. Pain biology education and exercise classes compared to pain biology education alone for individuals with chronic low back pain: a pilot randomised controlled trial. Man Ther. 2010;15:382–7.

Sapolsky RM. Why Zebras Don't Get Ulcers. New York: Freeman; 1994.

Schmidt-Wilcke T. Variations in brain volume and regional morphology associated with chronic pain. Curr Rheumatol Rep. 2008;10: 467-74.

Schmidt-Wilcke T, Leinisch E, Ganssbauer S, et al. Affective components and intensity of pain correlate with structural differences in gray matter in chronic back pain patients. Pain. 2006;125:89–97.

Schmidt-Wilcke T, Ganssbauer S, Neuner T, et al. Subtle grey matter changes between migraine patients and healthy controls. Cephalalgia. 2008;28:1–4.

Seminowicz DA, Wideman TH, Naso L, et al. Effective treatment of chronic low back pain in humans reverses abnormal brain anatomy and function. J Neurosci. 2011;31:7540–50.

Seminowicz DA, Shpaner M, Keaser ML, et al. Cognitive-behavioral therapy increases prefrontal cortex gray matter in patients with chronic pain. J Pain. 2013;14:1573–84.

Shala R, Roussel N, Lorimer Moseley G, et al. Can we just talk our patients out of pain? Should pain neuroscience education be our only tool? J Man Manip Ther. 2021;29:1–3.

Shatz CJ. The developing brain. Sci Am. 1992;267:60–7.

Stavrinou ML, Della Penna S, Pizzella V, et al. Temporal dynamics of plastic changes in human primary somatosensory cortex after finger webbing. Cereb Cortex. 2007;17:2134–42.

Sterling M, Jull G, Wright A. Cervical mobilisation: concurrent effects on pain, sympathetic nervous system activity and motor activity. Man Ther. 2001;6:72–81.

Tracey I, Bushnell MC. How neuroimaging studies have challenged us to rethink: is chronic pain a disease? J Pain. 2009;10:1113–20.

Tracey I, Ploghaus A, Gati JS, et al. Imaging attentional modulation of pain in the periaqueductal gray in humans. J Neurosci. 2002;22:2748–52.

Vicenzino B, Collins D, Wright A. The initial effects of a cervical spine manipulative physiotherapy treatment on the pain and dysfunction of lateral epicondylalgia. Pain. 1996;68:69–74.

Wall PD. Comments after 30 years of the gate control theory. Pain Forum. 1996;5:12–22.

Wand BM, Parkitny L, O'Connell NE, et al. Cortical changes in chronic low back pain: current state of the art and implications for clinical practice. Man Ther. 2011;16:15–20.

Watson JA, Ryan CG, Cooper L, et al. Pain neuroscience education for adults with chronic musculoskeletal pain: A mixed-methods systematic review and meta-analysis. J Pain. 2019;20:1140.e1–e22.

Wiech K, Tracey I. The influence of negative emotions on pain: behavioral effects and neural mechanisms. Neuroimage. 2009;47: 987–94.

Woolf CJ. Central sensitization: uncovering the relation between pain and plasticity. Anesthesiology. 2007;106:864–7.

Woolf CJ, Salter MW. Plasticity and pain: the role of the dorsal horn. In: McMahon S, Koltzenburg M (editors). Wall and Melzack's Textbook of Pain. 5th ed. Edinburgh: Elsevier; 2005.

Xerri C. Plasticity of cortical maps: multiple triggers for adaptive reorganization following brain damage and spinal cord injury. Neuroscientist. 2012;18:133–48.

What is multimodal management? Integrating hands-on and hands-off interventions for chronic pain in the lower extremity

César Fernández-de-las-Peñas, Emilio "Louie" Puentedura

Introduction

In this concluding chapter, we propose an integrated clinical perspective for the goals of this textbook – to describe multimodal complementary treatments for patients with hip and knee pain conditions – within a broader biopsychosocial context and integrating pain neuroscience. Proper management of hip and knee pain conditions highlights the relevance of multiple risk factors, including psychosocial factors, health status, and comorbid pain disorders, associated with the transition from acute to chronic status. Therefore, a proper understanding of the pain spectrum of a particular patient, the complex mosaic of factors in which pain emerges and persists, and clinical decision-making and integration of treatment plans are the focus of this chapter. We wish to highlight that while each individual chapter in this book has focused on a particular treatment approach, e.g., joint-biased manual therapies, dry needling, soft-tissue interventions, appropriate to a particular concept of hip and knee pain conditions, e.g., anterior cruciate ligament (ACL) rupture, knee or hip osteoarthritis (OA), current treatment clinical models for chronic pain are pointing to the importance of treatments simultaneously targeting multiple levels of the person. It would be extremely rare for a patient in daily clinical practice to receive just one single intervention.

This chapter encourages clinicians to find an equilibrium between hands-on (bottom up) and hands-off (top down) interventions in individuals with chronic pain (Lluch-Girbés et al., 2015). In fact, evidence supports that the application of manual (hands-on) interventions with pain neuroscience education (hands-off) is effective for the management of complex conditions such as low back pain (Louw et al., 2017a).

Underlying the Nature of Pain: Clinical Understanding

Tissue damage is considered the proximal basis for activation of nociception, giving rise to either inflammatory, nociceptive, or neuropathic pain. It may be initiated by a medical disease or by injury, and whether tissue damage is real or not is often unclear both clinically and on imaging. If a medical disease is the cause of the reported pain symptoms, it must be identified (see Chapter 5) and, following identification, appropriate treatment should be applied. Similarly, after a knee injury, e.g., ACL or meniscus rupture (see Chapter 7), rehabilitation protocols based on tissue healing will be applied. These specific situations would seem to be easy to manage, although in real life it is not as easy as it seems and some of these patients will also develop chronic pain. In fact, tissue damage does not necessarily correlate with the extent of reported pain as it is seen in people with knee or hip OA (see Chapter 4). This situation is attributable to the fact that injury, while sufficient on its own to produce nociception, also contributes to pain onset within a matrix of multiple risk determinants. Certain persistence of pain after the initial period of tissue healing appears to be a process of this same broad matrix of factors and not solely due to a tissue injury. "Tissue healing" is an elusive (theoretical) concept. This uncertainty about whether "healing" has truly occurred within a pre-determined period of "time of usual healing" is surely a fundamental assumption behind many treatment approaches. Several factors, internal or external, will be involved in the natural process of "tissue healing," and sometimes damage can never be reversed (such as in OA). Therefore, proper clinical reasoning based on pain neuroscience must be adapted to all patients.

When no specific cause (e.g., medical condition or tissue damage) is identified, the situation becomes more complex, and the clinician should understand why a particular patient reports pain in the absence of tissue damage or any underlying medical pathology. This type of clinical situation is entirely avoidable at this stage with our current understanding of pain. Extensive evidence indicates that pain is not tied to a peripheral stimulus but may be also maintained by central neural contributions (see Chapter 20). Consequently, the evaluation of a particular patient for only physical causes will also require multimodal evaluation for a proper understanding of the role of psychosocial factors and behaviors which are inextricably part of the pain conundrum. The clinician must consider whether the pain, particularly if it is persistent, should be considered functional or dysfunctional (Woolf, 2004), in that the direction of treatment will necessarily be adapted. Pain arising from altered nociception despite there being no evidence of actual or threatened tissue damage causing the activation of peripheral nociceptors or evidence for disease or lesion of the somatosensory system causing the pain (e.g., central sensitization) is now labeled as "nociplastic pain" by the International Association for the Study of Pain (Kosek et al., 2016). Therefore, identification of the dominant pain mechanism in a particular patient would lead to different clinical reasoning.

Clinical Reasoning for Multimodal Treatment Approaches

It is clear that patients with hip and knee pain may have complex presentations. The current textbook provides many therapeutic management strategies according to different perspectives regarding sources of nociception, and how nociception is maintained. In addition, chapters detail rehabilitation protocols for specific conditions, e.g., tendinopathy, femoroacetabular impingement (FAI) or ACL rupture, whereas others describe interventions, e.g., joint-biased (see Chapter 16), soft tissue-biased (see Chapter 17), nerve-biased (see Chapter 18), that can be applied to any particular knee or hip pain condition, based on the presence of musculoskeletal dysfunctions.

Clinical and scientific evidence support that the management of individuals with hip and knee pain disorders must be multimodal since each intervention will include different components of treatment required by the biopsychosocial paradigm within the complexity of these disorders. In fact, we suggest that therapies described in this book be viewed as stepping-stones to an eventual full set of therapeutic interventions within the framework of personalized medicine: tailoring the treatments from the patient's point of view. Each component treatment will have some efficacy for some part of the complex disease process, i.e., pain, function, disability, or emotional.

The challenge facing clinicians managing hip and knee pain conditions is how to determine the treatment plan for each patient, who is likely to present differently in terms of clinical presentation and associated factors. In such a scenario, clinicians should determine (identify) if the presentation of that patient exhibits a peripheral input or central input dominance. If the clinician identifies that a patient with hip or knee pain seems to be mediated primarily by peripheral nociception, specific treatment of the affected tissue (if identified), and application of an exercise program and functional activities is encouraged. If the clinician identifies that a patient with hip or knee pain seems to be primarily mediated by altered central processing, more complex and integrative approaches, e.g., pharmacological, physical, or cognitive, should be encouraged. In these patients, clinicians need to think beyond specific tissues and integrate current knowledge on pain processes (Nijs et al., 2013). A multimodal approach is where clinical decision-making becomes more difficult, since most trials generally focus on just one or two treatments, and for a given patient population that may or may not represent the particular patient in the clinic.

An important step for managing chronic pain is the active participation of the patient in this process. Patient-centered care involves shared decision-making with an interaction between the clinician and the patient. Patient beliefs, preferences, and expectations must be considered by the clinician to understand these values from the patient's perspective since they will clearly interact with the therapeutic process. Similarly, clinician preferences and personal communication with the patient about the "positive" or "negative" effects of an intervention should be integrated with this process.

Educating the patient about their situation and the full scope of associated problems is an important part of the treatment plan. Clinicians should consider potential neurophysiologic and cognitive mechanisms underlying the effects (positive and negative) of any intervention that they will apply on a particular patient (see Chapter 20). Addressing neurophysiologic and cognitive mechanisms, putative though they may be, is particularly important in patients with chronic hip and knee pain since it is helpful to encourage patients to choose among various treatment options after the explanation of the benefits and risks of each therapeutic approach. Asking the patient to participate in the clinical and therapeutic decision processes will allow them to take responsibility for the management of their condition, which is highly relevant when the pain is chronic. This would be highly important in patients with hip and knee pain where exercise programs will represent a milestone step in the therapeutic process, and they will involve active patient participation.

Integrating Different Interventions into Contemporary Pain Science

When providing any particular intervention to patients with hip or knee pain, therapists are advised to integrate contemporary pain neuroscience reasoning when providing a treatment plan. Per evidence-based recommendations (see Chapter 15), isolated interventions such as exercise, manual therapy or education can be effective for the management of these patients. Therefore, it would be reasonable to expect that combining two evidence-based treatment approaches should lead to better clinical outcomes; however, current evidence is conflicting.

Some meta-analyses reported that the combination of exercise therapy plus manual mobilization exhibits small to moderate effect sizes on pain and function when compared to exercise therapy alone in people with knee (Jansen et al., 2011) or hip (Sampath et al., 2016) OA. Nevertheless, these benefits are mostly observed at short rather than long term (Jansen et al., 2011; Sampath et al., 2016). Similarly, low-to-moderate evidence suggests that combining dry needling with other interventions is more effective at short term, but not long term, for improving pain and disability in people with neck symptoms associated with muscle pain (Fernández-de-las-Peñas et al., 2021). In contrast, other meta-analyses did not observe the benefits of combining exercise with manual therapy in individuals with hip OA (Beumer et al., 2016) or with neck pain (Fredin & Lorås, 2017) when compared with the application of either intervention alone.

A couple of questions for the clinician may arise: (1) should all patients with hip or knee pain receive manual therapy and exercise?; (2) which interventions should be applied first, manual therapies or exercise or other? For instance, since hands-on treatments improve pain and function in the short term, clinicians may consider applying manual therapies to optimize active exercise programs in patients with knee or hip chronic pain. The pitfall when doing this relates to the message that such hands-on interventions give to (are perceived by) the patient. The message may strengthen the patient's biomedical view that (more) pain relates to (more) tissue damage, which is a typical maladaptive belief reducing long-term recovery and the patient's independence. Clearly, educating the patient on the central pain modulatory effects of both manual therapy and exercise is critical for treatment and a home exercise program will be essential for maintaining these positive treatment effects. For instance, pain education can be applied before the application of hands-on interventions, although this could be changed depending on the patient. This allows the patient to gain a broader understanding of their problem. Hands-on (bottom-up) interventions may be applied for decreasing "firing nociception" to the central nervous system and also facilitating descending inhibition (Courtney et al., 2016) before hands-off (top-down) interventions, e.g., exercise (Louw et al., 2017b). Similarly, clinicians should be aware that patients with central pain processing exhibit an abnormal pain response to exercise, and their response could be contrary to what is expected, leading to an aggravation of symptoms. Again, an integration between the hands-on and hand-off approaches would be needed here for determining exercise progression (see Chapter 19) and increasing adherence to the program.

Conclusions

Available evidence indicates that both peripheral and central factors contribute to pain in most patients with hip and knee pain conditions. Better targeted interventions and, in particular, integration of treatments forms an essential step to address multifactorial factors involved in each individual patient. This textbook describes several treatments, each with compelling evidence for clinical consideration, that when integrated into a comprehensive treatment approach tailored to such findings, we believe will improve treatment outcomes for patients with hip and knee pain problems.

References

Beumer L, Wong J, Warden SJ, et al. Effects of exercise and manual therapy on pain associated with hip osteoarthritis: a systematic review and meta-analysis. Br J Sports Med. 2016;50:458–63.

Courtney CA, Steffen AD, Fernández-de-las-Peñas C, et al. Joint mobilization enhances mechanisms of conditioned pain modulation in individuals with osteoarthritis of the knee. J Orthop Sports Phys Ther. 2016;46:168–76.

Fernández-de-las-Peñas C, Plaza-Manzano G, Sanchez-Infante J, et al. Is dry needling effective when combined with other therapies for myofascial trigger points associated with neck pain symptoms? A systematic review and meta-analysis. Pain Res Manag. 2021;2021:8836427.

Fredin K, Lorås H. Manual therapy, exercise therapy or combined treatment in the management of adult neck pain: A systematic review and meta-analysis. Musculoskelet Sci Pract. 2017;31:62–71.

Jansen MJ, Viechtbauer W, Lenssen AF, et al. Strength training alone, exercise therapy alone, and exercise therapy with passive manual mobilisation each reduce pain and disability in people with knee osteoarthritis: a systematic review. J Physiother. 2011;57:11–20.

Kosek E, Cohen M, Baron R, et al. Do we need a third mechanistic descriptor for chronic pain states? Pain. 2016;157:1382–6.

Lluch Girbés E, Meeus M, Baert I, Nijs J. Balancing "hands-on" with "hands-off" physical therapy interventions for the treatment of central sensitization pain in osteoarthritis. Man Ther. 2015;20(2):349–52.

Louw A, Farrell K, Landers M, et al. The effect of manual therapy and neuroplasticity education on chronic low back pain: a randomized clinical trial. J Man Manip Ther. 2017a;25:227–34.

Louw A, Nijs J, Puentedura EJ. A clinical perspective on a pain neuroscience education approach to manual therapy. J Man Manip Ther. 2017b;25:160–8.

Nijs J, Roussel N, Paul van Wilgen C, et al. Thinking beyond muscles and joints: therapists' and patients' attitudes and beliefs regarding chronic musculoskeletal pain are key to applying effective treatment. Man Ther. 2013;18:96–102.

Sampath KK, Mani R, Miyamori T, Tumilty S. The effects of manual therapy or exercise therapy or both in people with hip osteoarthritis: a systematic review and meta-analysis. Clin Rehabil. 2016;30:1141–55.

Woolf CJ. Pain: moving from symptom control toward mechanism-specific pharmacologic management. Annals Internal Med. 2004;140:441–51.

FIGURE 1.1 Bony hip morphology. (A) Normal shaped femur. (B) Cam morphology. (C) Pincer morphology. (D) Acetabular dysplasia. (Reproduced with permission from Mosler et al., 2018b.)

FIGURE 4.2 Assessment of (A) pressure pain thresholds, (B) temporal summation of pain, and (C) conditioned pain modulation (CPM) and a comparison between healthy subjects and patients with severe osteoarthritis (OA). (Modified from Arendt-Nielsen et al., 2015a.)

FIGURE 5.4 Key components of rehabilitation of FAI syndrome. (Adapted from Heerey et al., 2018; Short et al., 2021.)

FIGURE 6.4 (A) The Extender. The thigh is stabilized in 90 degrees of hip flexion while the knee is actively extended just prior to the point of pain. (B) The Diver. From an upright trunk position, simultaneously stretching the arms forward as the standing hip is flexed. The standing knee position is maintained at 10–20 degrees throughout. (C) The Glider. From a starting position with upright trunk, the motion is started by gliding backward with one leg and stopped prior to pain onset. (Adapted from Askling et al., 2013.)

FIGURE 14.8 Foot core system. (Adapted from McKeon et al., 2015.)

FIGURE 16.1 Progression from non-weight-bearing to full weight-bearing interventions using Mobilization with Movement (MWM) interventions. (Redrawn and modified from McDowell et al., 2021.)

FIGURE 19.1 The "Hip Hinge Continuum" as a method for categorizing exercises. (Modified from John, 2013.)

FIGURE 19.3 Vermeil's hierarchy adapted for rehabilitation. (From Morrison, 2020.)

FIGURE 20.1 Widespread brain activation during a pain experience seen as a pain neurotag, which involves several common brain areas. (Redrawn from Puentedura EJ, Louw A. A neuroscience approach to managing athletes with low back pain. Phys Ther Sport. 2012;13:123–33.)

FIGURE 20.2 The activation of the pain neuromatrix (shown in red) can be influenced by neighboring neural circuits involved with knowledge and logic (yellow), past experience (green), beliefs about pain (blue), etc. and these neighboring circuits can modulate the pain experience. (Redrawn from Puentedura EJ, Louw A. A neuroscience approach to managing athletes with low back pain. Phys Ther Sport. 2012;13:123–33.)

FIGURE 20.3 Functional magnetic resonance images (fMRI) of a subject at rest (top) and while performing a painful task (bottom) showing widespread brain activation via blood oxygen level dependent (BOLD) technique. (From Louw A, Puentedura EJ, Diener I, Peoples RR. Pre-operative therapeutic neuroscience education for lumbar radiculopathy: a single-case fMRI report. Physiother Theory Pract. 2015;31:496–508.)

FIGURE 20.4 In the pre-PNE imaging, the widespread brain activation seen via blood oxygen level dependent (BOLD) technique when the subject performs a painful task (bottom image) shows activation of the periaqueductal gray region of the brain (circled). (From Louw A, Puentedura EJ, Diener I, Peoples RR. Pre-operative therapeutic neuroscience education for lumbar radiculopathy: a single-case fMRI report. Physiother Theory Pract. 2015;31:496–508.)

FIGURE 20.5 In the post-PNE imaging, the widespread brain activation seen via blood oxygen level dependent (BOLD) technique when the subject performs a painful task (bottom image) shows decreased brain activation and almost no increase in activation of the periaqueductal gray region of the brain (circled). (From Louw A, Puentedura EJ, Diener I, Peoples RR. Pre-operative therapeutic neuroscience education for lumbar radiculopathy: a single-case fMRI report. Physiother Theory Pract. 2015;31:496–508.)

Index

Index

Index

Index

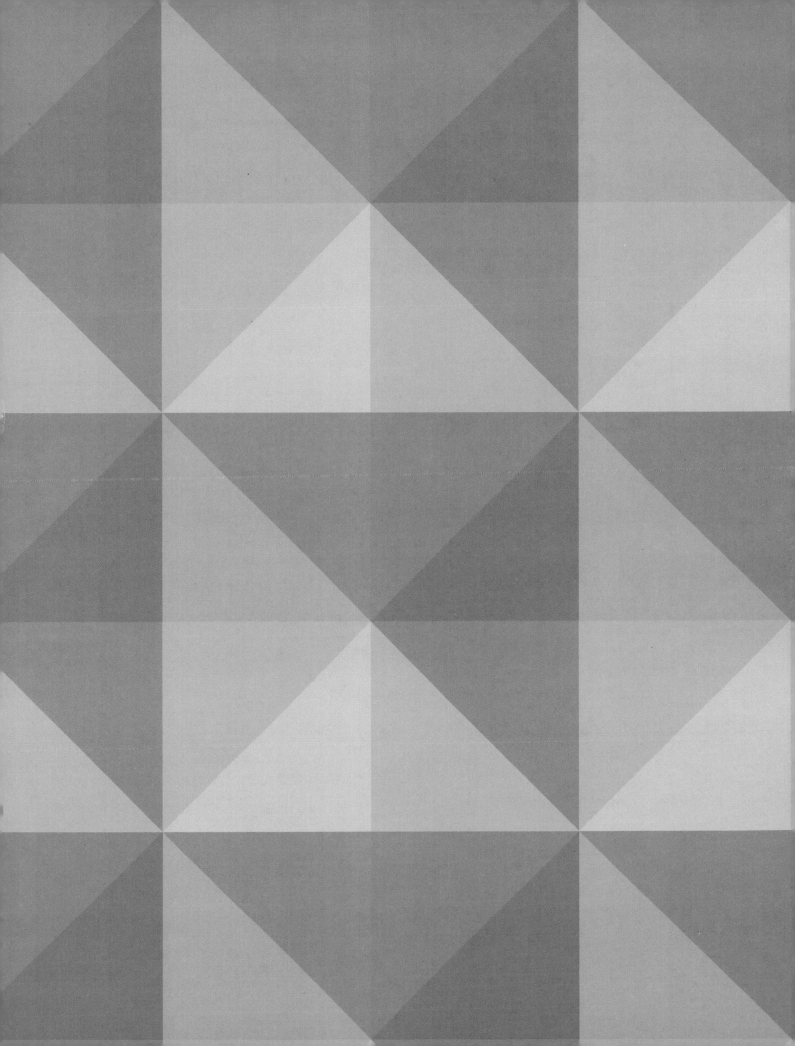